Atlas of
COSMETIC AND RECONSTRUCTIVE PERIODONTAL SURGERY

Atlas of
COSMETIC AND RECONSTRUCTIVE PERIODONTAL SURGERY

Edward S. Cohen, DMD

Assistant Clinical Professor
School of Dental Medicine
Tufts University
Boston, Massachusetts

Second Edition

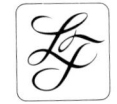

Lea & Febiger
PHILADELPHIA · BALTIMORE · HONG KONG
LONDON · MUNICH · SYDNEY · TOKYO

A WAVERLY COMPANY
1994

Lea & Febiger
Box 3024
200 Chester Field Parkway
Malvern, Pennsylvania 19355-9725
U.S.A.
(215) 251-2230

Executive Editor–Darlene Barela Cooke
Development Editor–Sharon R. Zinner
Project Editor–Denise Wilson
Production Manager–Michael DeNardo

First Edition, 1988
Reprinted, 1989

Library of Congress Cataloging-in-Publication Data

Cohen, Edward S.
    Atlas of cosmetic and reconstructive periodontal surgery / Edward S. Cohen. — 2nd ed.
      p. cm.
    Rev. ed. of: Atlas of periodontal surgery. 1988.
    Includes bibliographical references and index.
    ISBN 0-8121-1518-X
    1. Periodontium—Surgery—Atlases. I. Cohen, Edward S. Atlas of periodontal surgery. II. Title.
    [DNLM: 1. Periodontium—surgery—atlases. WU 17 C678a 1994]
RK361.C57 1994
617.6'32—dc20
DNLM/DLC
for Library of Congress   93-23929
                                                                             CIP

NOTE: Although the author(s) and the publisher have taken reasonable steps to ensure the accuracy of the drug information included in this text before publication, drug information may change without notice and readers are advised to consult the manufacturer's packaging inserts before prescribing medications.

Reprints of chapters may be purchased from Lea & Febiger in quantities of 100 or more. Contact Sally Grande in the Sales Department.

Copyright © 1994 by Lea & Febiger. Copyright under the International Copyright Union. All Rights Reserved. This book is protected by copyright. *No part of it may be reproduced in any manner or by any means without written permission from the publisher.*

Printed in the United States of America

Print number: 5 4 3 2 1

Dedicated to my wife, Judith,
and our children, Jasson, Koren,
and Aaron

PREFACE TO THE SECOND EDITION

This surgical atlas was originally published with the intent of being the most complete periodontal surgical atlas and in 1988 it was. Since that time, there have been many important advances. The emphasis in periodontics has clearly shifted toward *reconstructive periodontics*. Guided tissue regeneration, biomechanical root preparation, predictable bone regeneration procedures, and cosmetic root coverage have made reconstructive periodontics a reality.

This edition will reflect these changes with new chapters on *biomechanical root preparation, guided tissue regeneration, cosmetic gingival reconstruction, cosmetic treatment of the maxillary anterior teeth, and ridge augmentation, and expansion of the chapter on inductive osseous surgery*. A new chapter has also been added on *sutures and suturing*. All other chapters have been brought up to date, again with the intention of again making this the most complete periodontal surgical atlas.

Any book of this kind requires the help of others in order to be completed. In this regard, a special thanks must go to all those clinicians who so unselfishly contributed material for this edition (alphabetically): Burton Becker, Gerald M. Bowers, Daniel Buser, Robert Del Castillo, Stuart Froum, Bernard Gantes, Gary Golovic, Jan Gottlow, Claude G. Ibbott, L. Laurell, James T. Mellovig, Sture Nyman, Knut Selvig, Richard H. Shanaman, Athenos Spiros, Sigmond Stahl, Dennis P. Tarnow, and Theodore West.

Special acknowledgments must be extended to W.R. Gore Associates, Flagstaff, AZ and Guidor AB, Gothenburg, Sweden (Guided Tissue Regeneration, Chapter 13) and Ethicon, Inc., Somerville, NJ (Sutures and Suturing, Chapter 2) for their help and permission for parts of their clinical manuals to be incorporated into this atlas.

To my dear friends and associates Bob Ullrich (artwork) and Harry Maskell (photography), without whose talent and expertise this book most surely would not have been completed, I again say thank you.

Boston, Massachusetts Edward S. Cohen

PREFACE TO THE FIRST EDITION

Periodontology is both an art and science; as practiced daily, however, it is predominantly a surgical specialty. Although the major periodontal textbooks contain surgical sections, their general nature and scope do not allow for an in-depth analysis of any one specific area. It is for this reason that this text is devoted solely to the art of periodontics and designed for the student, general practitioner, and specialist.

Each procedure has been illustrated and laid out in a step-by-step fashion. Clinical examples have been used secondarily only to supplement illustrations. The descriptive nature of the text is meant to be both brief and simple. Each chapter presents indications, contraindications, advantages, disadvantages, and related problems for each procedure.

This atlas incorporates most of the general techniques and concepts that are outlined in the major textbooks. It can, therefore, easily be used as a supplement to any of these textbooks.

In the course of writing this text, careful attention has been paid to faithfully describing the procedures as they were outlined originally, as well as attempting to give credit to their originators. Any oversights are unintentional and would gladly be corrected in the future. In this regard credit must be given to Glickman's Clinical Periodontology for serving as the model to base the drawings of gingivectomy on and Lindhes: Clinical Periodontology for serving as a guide for the chapter on furcations.

I would like to thank my colleagues Edward Allen, Raul Caffesse, Jose Carvalho, Giovanni Castellucci, David Garber, Barry Jaye, and Edwin Rosenberg for their clinical contributions; Mark Hirsh, Mayer Liebman, and Peter Ferrigno for their helpful suggestions; and my assistants Jeanne McCormack, Rebecca Mugherini, Christine Roberts, and Judith Cohen for their patient help.

Special notes of acknowledgment must be given to Harry W. Maskell for his photographic excellence; to Robert H. Ullrich, Jr., medical illustrator, for his creative genius in the designing and drawing of the illustrations; and to the educational media department of the New England Medical Center for the pictorial overlays.

Boston, Massachusetts   Edward S. Cohen

SPECIAL TRIBUTE

A special tribute must be extended to my former teacher, Dr. Irving Glickman. Not only did he teach me the principles of periodontology, he taught me a philosophy and an academic approach that has sustained me in this difficult undertaking. Thank you.

CONTENTS

Chapter 1   BASICS 1
Basic Incisions
Classification of Surgical Procedures
General Surgical Considerations

Chapter 2   SUTURES AND SUTURING 9
Goals
Materials
Requirements
Suturing
Techniques

Chapter 3   SCALING, ROOT PLANING, AND CURETTAGE 31
Scaling and Root Planing
Curettage
Flap Debridement Surgery
Excisional New Attachment Procedure (E.N.A.P.) and Modified ENAP
Modified Widman Flap

Chapter 4   GINGIVECTOMY AND GINGIVOPLASTY 51
Gingivectomy
Gingivoplasty
Edentulous, Retromolar, and Tuberosity Areas
Common Reasons for Failure

Chapter 5   MUCOGINGIVAL SURGERY 65
Tissue Barrier Concept
General Considerations
Classification of Procedures
Periodontal Flaps—Positioned and Repositioned
Free Soft-Tissue Autograft
Laterally Positioned Pedicle Flaps
Double Papilla Laterally Positioned Flaps
Frenulectomy (Frenectomy) and Frenulotomy (Frenotomy)

| Chapter | 6 | PALATAL FLAPS | 137 |

Partial-Thickness Palatal Flap
Modified Partial-Thickness Palatal Flap
Distal Wedge
Palatal Approach to Implant Placement

| Chapter | 7 | COSMETIC TREATMENT OF MAXILLARY ANTERIOR POCKETING | 165 |

Modified Surgical Approach for Maxillary Anterior Esthetics: The Curtain Procedure
Papillary Preservation Technique

| Chapter | 8 | BIOMECHANICAL ROOT PREPARATION | 177 |

Citric Acid
Tetracycline HCL
Fibronectin
Biochemical Approach to Periodontal Regeneration
Conclusion

| Chapter | 9 | COSMETIC ROOT COVERAGE: GINGIVAL AUGMENTATION | 189 |

Cosmetic Gingival Reconstruction
Grafting for Root Coverage
Classification of Gingival Recession
Procedural Modifications
Subepithelial Connective Tissue Graft
Subpedicle Connective Tissue Graft
Semilunar Flap
Transpositional Flap
Connective Tissue Pedicle Graft
Guided Tissue Regeneration and Gingival Recession

| Chapter | 10 | RIDGE AUGMENTATION | 233 |

Classification of Ridge Defects
Full-Thickness Soft-Tissue Grafts
Pouch Procedure
Ridge Augmentation—Improved Technique
Subepithelial Connective Tissue Graft for Ridge Augmentation
Socket Preservation (Ridge Augmentation)

| Chapter | 11 | RESECTIVE OSSEOUS SURGERY | 259 |

Historical Review
Rationale and Objectives
Tissue Management
Terminology and Methods
Osteoplasty
Ostectomy
Osseous Management of Teeth with Furcations
Biologic Width
Basic Rules of Osseous Surgery
Forced Eruption

| Chapter | 12 | INDUCTIVE OSSEOUS SURGERY | 285 |

Definitions
Intrabony Defects
Selection of Graft Material
Alloplasts—Ceramics
Allografts
Treatment of Periodontal Furcations with Coronally Positioned Flaps and Citric Acid
Guided Tissue Regeneration

Chapter 13	GUIDED TISSUE REGENERATION	323

           INTRODUCTION
               Animal Studies
               Human Studies
        NONRESORBABLE MEMBRANES
        BIORESORBABLE MEMBRANES
           Nonresorbable Membranes
           Biodegradable Membranes
           RIDGE AUGMENTATION

Chapter 14	FURCATIONS	369

                 Diagnosis
              Classification
                Treatment
               Terminology
      Mandibular Molar Furcations
         Maxillary Furcations
    Periodontal–Endodontal Problems

BIBLIOGRAPHY	403
INDEX	417

1

BASICS

BASIC INCISIONS

Periodontal disease is multifaceted in the nature, scope, and types of problems created (e.g., mucogingival problems, osseous deformities, gingival enlargement); therefore, many types of treatment exist (see Fig. 1-1). *There is no one way to approach a single problem or procedure.* Training, ability, philosophy, and objectives ultimately determine final treatment selection.

1. CURETTAGE: The removal of the inner epithelial lining, epithelial attachment, and underlying inflamed connective tissue on the inner aspect of the pocket. This is a closed surgical procedure (Fig. 1-2A).
2. GINGIVECTOMY: The excisional removal of tissue for treatment of suprabony pockets. This procedure is indicated where bone loss is horizontal and there is an adequate zone of attached keratinized gingiva (Fig. 1-2B).
3. FULL-THICKNESS (MUCOPERIOSTEAL) FLAP: A flap designed to gain access and visibility for osseous surgery, relocation of frenulum, maintenance of the attached tissue, and pocket elimination. The incision can be sulcular, crestal, or inverse bevel, depending on the amount of attached tissue present (Fig. 1-2C).
4. PARTIAL OR SPLIT-THICKNESS (MUCOSAL) FLAP: A flap designed to retain and maintain the periosteal covering over the bone. A sharp dissection technique parallel to the bone is used in this procedure. It is indicated mostly in areas of thin bony plates and for mucogingival procedures (Fig. 1-2D).
5. MODIFIED FULL-THICKNESS (MUCOPERIOSTEAL) FLAP: A flap for which a first-stage gingivectomy incision is used for pocket reduction or elimination, followed by a secondary inverse bevel incision to the crest of the bone. This technique requires an adequate zone of attached keratinized gingiva and is used primarily on the palate, on enlarged tissue, or in areas where limited access may prevent a primary inverse bevel incision (Fig. 1-2E).

Tables 1-1 and 1-2 compare the various treatment procedures. These should be used only as a general guide in deciding which technique to use. Table 1-3 is a comparative analysis of the various surgical techniques.

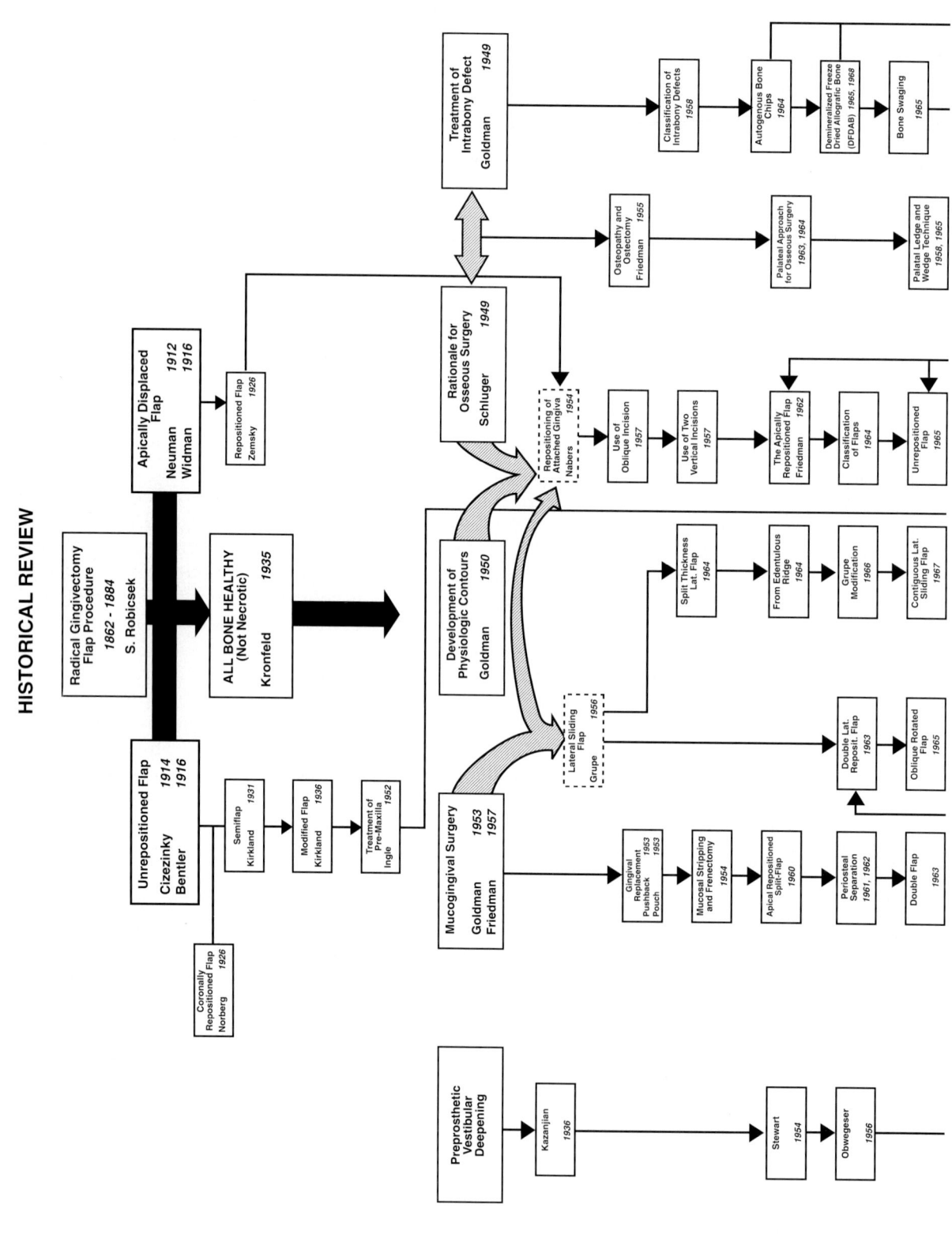

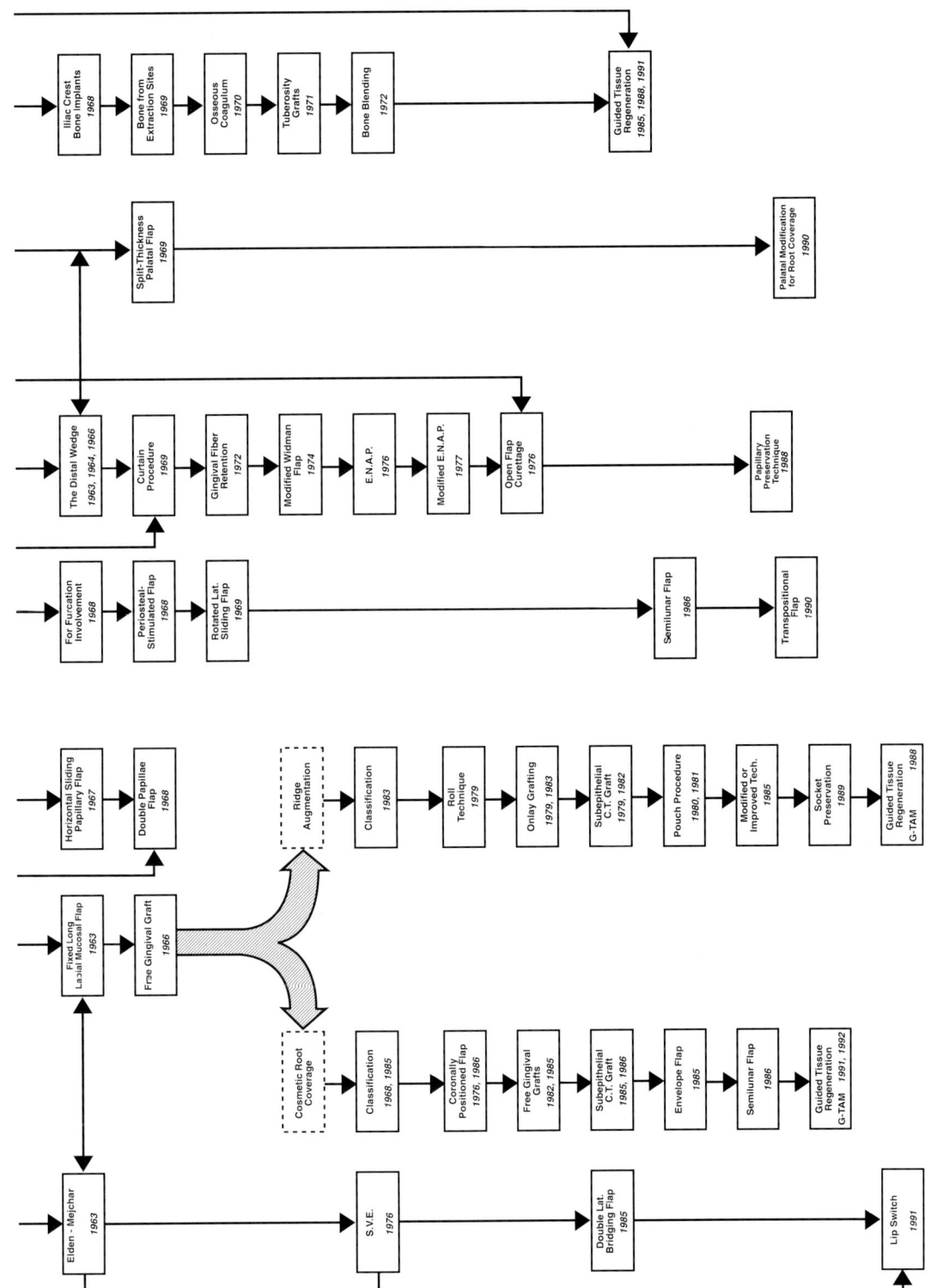

Fig. 1-1. Historical Review.

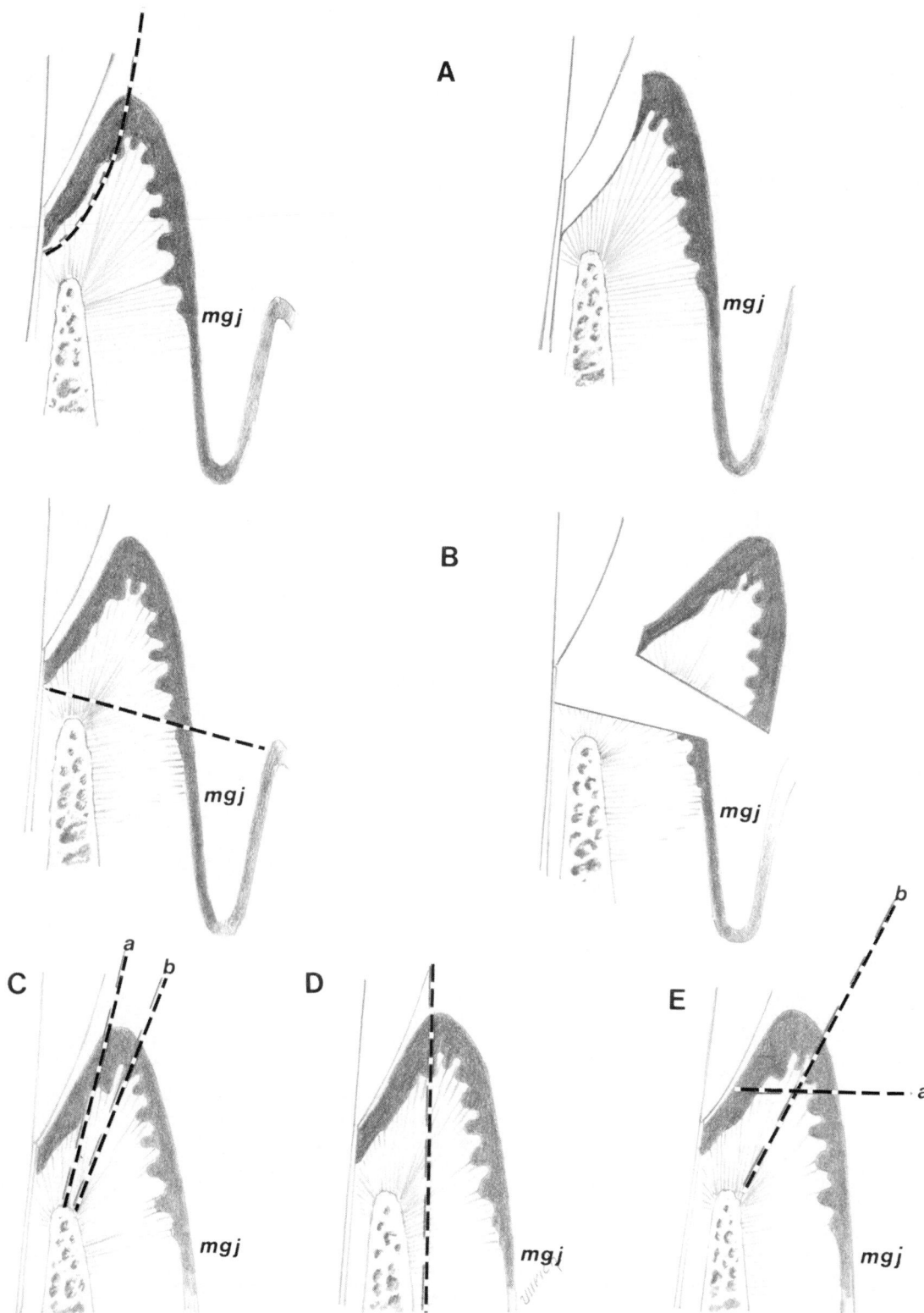

Fig. 1-2. Outline of Basic Incisions. **A,** Curettage incision and removal of inflamed inner pocket wall. **B,** Gingivectomy incision and subsequent removal of excised tissue (note incision is above mucogingival junction [mgj]). **C,** Sulcular (a) and crestal (b) incisions for full-thickness mucoperiosteal flaps. **D,** Partial-thickness incisions for partial-thickness flaps. **E,** Modified flap incisions for ledge-and-wedge techniques.

Basics

Table 1-1. Comparison of Open (Gingivectomy) vs. Closed (Flap) Procedures

	Open (Gingivectomy)	Closed (Partial- or Full-Thickness Flaps)
Healing	Secondary intention	Primary intention
Time requirement for completion of procedure	Fast	Slower
Reattachment	No	Possible
Degree of difficulty	Low	High
Bleeding postoperatively	Yes	Minimum
Visibility for osseous surgery	Inadequate	Good
Ability to treat osseous irregularities and defects	Inadequate	Good
Preservation of keratinized gingiva	No	Yes

Table 1-2. Comparison of Full-Thickness and Partial-Thickness Flaps

	Full Thickness (Mucoperiosteal)	Partial Thickness (Mucosal)
Healing	Primary intention	Secondary intention
Degree of difficulty	Moderate	High
Pocket elimination	Yes	Yes
Osseous surgery, resective or inductive	Yes	No
Periosteal retention	No	Yes
Relocation of frenum	Yes	Yes
Widen zone of keratinized gingiva	No	Yes
Increase of *attached* keratinized gingiva	Yes	Yes
Combine with other mucogingival procedures	No	Yes
Suture variability	Low	High
Presence of a thin periodontium—dehiscence or fenestration	No	Yes
Bleeding and tissue trauma	Limited	Greater

CLASSIFICATION OF SURGICAL PROCEDURES

I. CORRECTION OF SOFT-TISSUE POCKETS
  A. CLOSED PROCEDURES
    1. Curettage
    2. Excisional new attachment procedure (E.N.A.P.) and modified E.N.A.P.
    3. Modified Widman flap
    4. Apically positioned (repositioned) flap
      a. Full-thickness (partial-full-thickness)
      b. Partial-thickness
    5. Palatal flap
      a. Full-thickness
      b. Partial-thickness
    6. Distal wedge procedure
      a. Tuberosity
      b. Retromolar area
  B. OPEN PROCEDURES
    1. Gingivectomy
    2. Gingivoplasty

II. SURGERY FOR CORRECTION OF OSSEOUS DEFORMITIES AND OSSEOUS ENHANCEMENT PROCEDURES
  A. CLOSED PROCEDURES
    1. Full-thickness or partial-thickness flaps
      a. Apically positioned flap
      b. Unpositioned flap
      c. Modified flap
      d. Modified Widman flap
    2. Distal wedge procedure
    3. Palatal flap
  B. OPEN PROCEDURES
    1. Gingivectomy
      a. Rotary abrasives

Table 1-3. Comparative Analysis of Five Gingival Surgical Procedures

Procedure	I	II	III	Description
Curettage				Scaling and root planing for removal of calculus, plaque, cementum Curette inner inflamed wall of pocket
E.N.A.P.				Mark pocket with probe Scallop internal beveled incision to base of pocket Remove incised epithelium and granulation tissue Root plane Position flap and suture to presurgical level
Modified Widman flap				Primary incision ½ to 1 mm from margin to crest of bone Reflect flap 2 to 3 mm off bone 2° sulcular releasing incision Horizontal 3° incision above crest of bone Remove epithelium and granulation tissue Scale and root plane Reposition flap and suture with interrupted sutures
Apically positioned full-thickness flap				Sulcular, crestal, or labially positioned inverse beveled incision to bone Flap completed, reflected off of bone Flap is apically positioned and sutured
Apically positioned partial-thickness flap				Crestal incision with blade parallel to long axis of tooth Flap raised by sharp dissection Periosteum retained over bone Flap is apically positioned at or below alveolar crest

Modified from Kinoshita, S., and Wen, R. C.: Color Atlas of Periodontics. St. Louis, Mosby–Year Book, 1985.

      b. Interproximal denudation
      c. Intrabony pocket procedure
    2. Prichard procedures for osseous fill
  C. GUIDED TISSUE REGENERATION
III. CORRECTION OF MUCOGINGIVAL PROBLEMS
  A. PRESERVATION OF EXISTING ATTACHED GINGIVA
    1. Apically positioned (repositioned) flap
      a. Full-thickness
      b. Partial-thickness
    2. Frenectomy or frenotomy
    3. Modified Widman flap
  B. INCREASING DIMENSION OF EXISTING ATTACHED GINGIVA
    1. Mucosal stripping
    2. Periosteal separation
    3. Laterally positioned flap (pedicle)
      a. Full-thickness
      b. Partial-thickness
      c. Periosteal stimulated
      d. Partial-full-thickness
    4. Papillary flaps
      a. Double papillae
      b. Rotated papillae
      c. Horizontal papillae
    5. Edlan-Mejchar, subperiosteal vestibular extension (S.V.E.) operation, or double lateral bridging flap
    6. Free soft-tissue autografts
      a. Partial-thickness
      b. Full-thickness

7. Connective tissue autograft
8. Subepithelial connective tissue graft
IV. PROCEDURES COMMONLY USED FOR ROOT COVERAGE
   A. PEDICLE FLAPS (FULL- OR PARTIAL-THICKNESS)
      1. Laterally positioned flaps
      2. Double papillae flaps
      3. Coronally positioned flaps
      4. Periosteal stimulated flaps
      5. Semilunar flap
      6. Rotated or transpositional pedicle flap
   B. FREE SOFT-TISSUE AUTOGRAFTS
      1. Full-thickness
      2. Partial-thickness
   C. SUBEPITHELIAL CONNECTIVE TISSUE GRAFT

GENERAL SURGICAL CONSIDERATIONS

Presurgical Considerations

1. A complete medical history should be taken, and any underlying systemic disease (i.e., hypertension, diabetes, or hemorrhagic disorders) should be under adequate control. Medications should be carefully noted, and medical consultations and preoperative laboratory work should be performed where indicated. It is important to note that the medical history consists of a review of drug abuse, transfusions, and alternative life styles in attempting to determine AIDS (HIV) risk. This should be combined with a thorough oral exam (ulcers, candidiasis, hairy leukoplakia, etc.). *NOTE:* **The best protection against AIDS and hepatitis is proper barrier technique and sterilization at all times.**
2. Blood pressure should be recorded.
3. Definitive surgical therapy should be considered only after adequate plaque control, scaling, root planing, and all necessary restorative, prosthetic, endodontic, orthodontic, and occlusal stabilization and splinting procedures have been completed and the case reevaluated. *Without proper plaque control there is no need for surgery.*
4. A surgical consent form should be completed in all cases, and periodontal documentation (including tissue quality, pocket depths, radiographs, and models) is a must.

SURGICAL CONSIDERATIONS

1. Procedural selection should be based on the following:
   a. Simplicity
   b. Predictability
   c. Efficiency
   d. Mucogingival considerations
   e. Underlying osseous topography
   f. Anatomic and physical limitations (e.g., small mouth, gagging, mental foramen)
   g. Age and systemic factors (cardiac arrythmias and murmurs, diabetes, history of radiation treatment, hyparathyroidism, hyperthyroidism, etc.)
2. All incisions should be clean, smooth, and definite. Indecision usually results in an uneven, ragged incision, which requires more healing time.
3. All flaps should be designed for maximum utilization and retention of keratinized gingival tissue so as to maintain a functional zone of attached keratinized gingiva and prevent needless secondary procedures.
4. Flap design should allow for adequate access and visibility.
5. Involvement of adjacent noninvolved areas should be avoided.
6. Flap design should prevent unnecessary bone exposure with resultant possible loss and dehiscence or fenestration formation.
7. Where possible, primary intention procedures are preferred to those of secondary intention.
8. The base of a flap should be as wide as the coronal aspect to allow for adequate vascularity.
9. Tissue tags should be removed to allow for rapid healing and prevent regrowth of granulation tissue.
10. Adequate flap stabilization is necessary to prevent displacement, unnecessary bleeding, hematoma formation, bone exposure, and possible infection.

2

SUTURES AND SUTURING

GOALS

A surgical suture is one that approximates the adjacent cut surfaces or compresses blood vessels to stop bleeding. Suturing is performed to
1. Provide an adequate tension of wound closure without dead space but loose enough to obviate tissue ischemia and necrosis
2. Maintain hemostasis
3. Permit primary intention healing
4. Provide support for tissue margins until they have healed and the support is no longer needed
5. Reduce postoperative pain
6. Prevent bone exposure resulting in delayed healing and unnecessary resorption
7. Permit proper flap position

SUTURE MATERIAL

Surgical sutures have been used to close wounds since prehistoric times (50,000 to 30,000 B.C.) (Macht and Krizek, 1978). Ancient Egyptian manuscripts such as the Edwin Smith papyrus (1600 B.C.) gave us the first written description of their use dating back as early as 4000 B.C. (Macht and Krizek, 1978). Many materials have been used throughout the centuries, such as gold, silver, hemp, facia, hair, linen, bark, and many others. Yet none has provided all the desired characteristics.

Qualities of the Ideal Suture Material

The following qualities of the ideal suture material are compiled from Postlethwait (1971), Varma et al. (1974), and Ethicon (1985):
1. Pliability, for ease of handling
2. Knot security
3. Sterilizable
4. Appropriate elasticity
5. Nonreactivity
6. Adequate tensile strength for wound healing
7. Chemical biodegradability as opposed to foreign body breakdown.

With the possible exception of coated Vicryl, none of the sutures available today meets these criteria. Table 2-1 lists the various suture materials—natural, synthetic, absorbable (digested by body enzymes or hydrolyzed), and nonabsorbable—available for periodontal use.

USAGE

1. Silk and synthetic sutures are employed most often.
2. Gut sutures are used only when retrieval is difficult, if not impossible. The limited physical characteristics of gut sutures do not warrant their use any other time
3. When using gut (plain or chromic) sutures, it is often advantageous to soak the package in warm water for a half-hour prior to use and to pull gently but firmly on the suture when opened. This will remove the kinks and straighten the suture. Finally, lubricating the suture lightly with petrolatum or sterile bone wax will prevent brittleness.
4. Monofilament sutures are recommended for bone augmentation procedures to prevent "wicking" and to reduce the inflammatory response and permit longer retention (10 to 14 days).
5. Gore-tex coated Vicryl sutures are recommended for guided tissue regeneration procedures.

Table 2-1. Suture materials

Suture	Raw Material	Absorption	Suture Tensile Strength
Plain gut	Collagen from healthy mammals	Digested by body enzymes within 70 days	+ (Least)
Chromic gut	Collagen from healthy mammals treated with chromic salts	Digested by body enzymes within 90 days	+
Coated Vicryl (polyglactin 910)	Copolymer of lactide and glycolide coated with polyglactin 370 and calcium stearate	Hydrolysis 56–70 days	+++
Dexon (polyglycolic acid)	Homopolymer of glycolic acid coated with polaxamer 188	Slow hydrolysis after 60–90 days	+++
PDS (polydi-oxanone)	Polyester polymer	Slow hydrolysis 180–210 days	++++
Surgical silk	Natural protein fiber of raw silk. Treated with silicon protein or wax	Usually cannot be found after 2 years	++
Nylon Duralon Ethilon	Polyamide polymer	Degrades at a rate of 15–20% per year	+++
Nylon Nurolon Surgilon	Polyamide polymer	Degrades at a rate of 15–20% per year	+++
Polyester Mersilene Dacron Ethibond	Polyester Polyethylene Terephthalate	Nonabsorbable	+++
Prolene (polypro-pylene)	Polymer of propylene	Nonabsorbable	+++
Gor-Tex	Expanded polytetrafluoro-ethylene (ePTFE)	Nonabsorbable	+++
Monocryl	Poliglecaprone 25 Copolymer of glycolide and caprolactone	Hydrolysis 90–120 days	++++

Tissue Reaction	Knot Tensile Strength	Types	Uses	Ease of Handling
Moderate ++++	+++	Plain	Rapidly healing mucosa Avoid suture removal	+
Moderate but less than plain gut ++++	+++	Chromic	As above Slower absorption	+
Mild ++	++	Braided coated	Subepithelial Mucosal surfaces Vessel ligation All types of general closure	++++
Mild ++	++	Braided coated	Subepithelial sutures Mucosal surfaces Vessel ligation	+++ ++++
Slight +	++	Monofilament	Absorbable suture with extended wound support	++
Moderate ++++	+ (least)	Braided	Mucosal surfaces	++++
Extremely low 0–+	++	Monofilament	Skin closure	++
Extremely low 0–+	++	Braided	Skin closure Mucosal surfaces	++++
Minimal +	+++	Braided	Cardiovascular and plastic surgery General surgery	+++
Minimal + transient acute reaction	++	Monofilament	General, plastic, cardiovascular, skin, ophthalmology	++
Extremely low 0–+	++	Monofilament	All types of soft-tissue approximation and cardiovascular surgery	++++
Minimal +	+++	Monofilament	Soft-tissue closure	Most pliable Synthetic absorbable monofilament ever

KNOTS AND KNOT TYING

"Suture security is the ability of the knot and material to maintain tissue approximation during the healing process (Thacker et al., 1975). Failure is generally the result of untying due to knot slippage or breakage. *Since the knot strength is always less than the tensile strength of the material,* when a force is applied the site of disruption is always the knot (Thacker et al., 1975; Worsfield, 1961). This is because shear forces produced in the knot lead to breakage.

Knot slippage or security is a function of the coefficient of friction within the knot (Hermann, 1971; Price 1948). This is determined by the nature of the material, the suture diameter, and type of knot. Monofilament and coated sutures (teflon, silicon) have a low coefficient of friction and a high degree of slippage; braided and twisted sutures such as uncoated dacron and catgut have greater knot security because of their high coefficient of friction (Taylor, 1938).

It is interesting to note that basic suture silk, although extremely user friendly, is distinctly inferior in terms of strength and knot security compared to other materials (Hermann, 1971). It also shows a high degree of tissue reaction (Taylor, 1978; Postlethwait, 1968) and the addition of wax or silicon to reduce the tissue reaction and prevent *wicking* further diminishes knot security (Hermann, 1971).

Knot selection is the last of the variables, and the one over which surgeons have the most influence. Knot security has been found to vary greatly among clinicians, and even security of knots tied by the same clinician varies at different times (Hermann, 1971).

A sutured knot has three components (Fig. 2-1) (Thacker et al., 1975):
1. The *loop* created by the knot (Fig. 2-1A)
2. The *knot* itself, which is composed of a number of tight "throws" (Fig. 2-1B): each throw represents a weave of the two strands
3. The *ears,* which are the cut ends of the suture.

In Figure 2-2, we see the four knots most commonly used in periodontal surgery. In a study, Thacker (1975) found that the *granny* knot was the least secure, always requiring more throws or ties to achieve the same knot strength as the square or surgical knot. For materials with a high degree of slippage (monofilament or coated sutures), flat and square throws were recommended with *all additional throws being squared.* Cutting the *ears* of the suture too short is contraindicated when slippage is great because the knot will come untied if the slippage exceeds the length of the *ears.* Loosely tied knots were shown to have the highest degree of slippage, while in tight knots slippage was not a significant factor.

PRINCIPLES OF SUTURING

Ethicon (1985) recommends the following principles for knot tying:
1. The completed knot must be tight, firm, and tied so that slippage will not occur.
2. To avoid *wicking of bacteria,* knots should not be placed in incision lines.
3. Knots should be small and the ends cut short (2 to 3 mm).
4. Avoid excessive tension to finer gauge materials as breakage may occur.
5. Avoid using a jerking motion, which may break the suture.
6. Avoid crushing or crimping of suture materials by not using hemostats or needle holders on them except on the free end for tying.
7. *Do not* tie suture too tightly as tissue necrosis may occur. Knot tension should not produce tissue blanching.
8. Maintain adequate traction on one end while tying to avoid loosening the first loop.
9. The surgeons and square knot strength, although generally not needing more than two throws, will have increased strength with an additional throw.
10. Granny knots and coated and monofilament sutures do require additional throws for knot security and to prevent slippage. Coated Vicryl will hold with four throws—two full square knots.

Sutures should be removed as atraumatically and as cleanly as possible. Ethicon (1985) recommends the following principles for suture removal:
1. The area should be swabbed with hydrogen peroxide for removal of encrusted necrotic debris, blood, and serum from about the sutures.
2. A sharp suture scissors should be used to cut the loops of individual or continuous sutures about the teeth. It is often helpful to use a No. 23 explorer to help lift the sutures if they are within the sulcus or in close opposition to the tissue. This will avoid tissue damage and unnecessary pain.
3. A cotton pliers is now used to remove the sutures. The location of the knots should be noted so that they can be removed first. This will prevent unnecessary entrapment under the flap.

NOTE: Sutures should be removed in 7 to 10 days to prevent epithelialization or *wicking* about the suture.

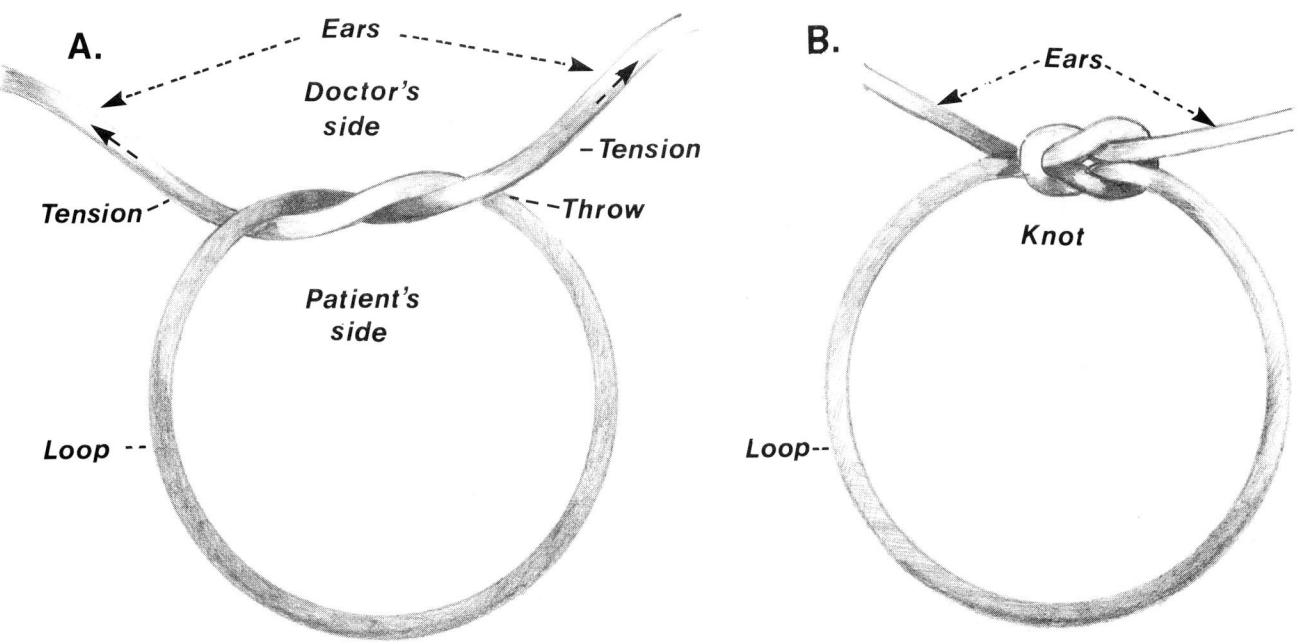

Fig. 2-1. Knot Anatomy. **A,** Various knot components prior to completion. **B,** Completed knot anatomy.

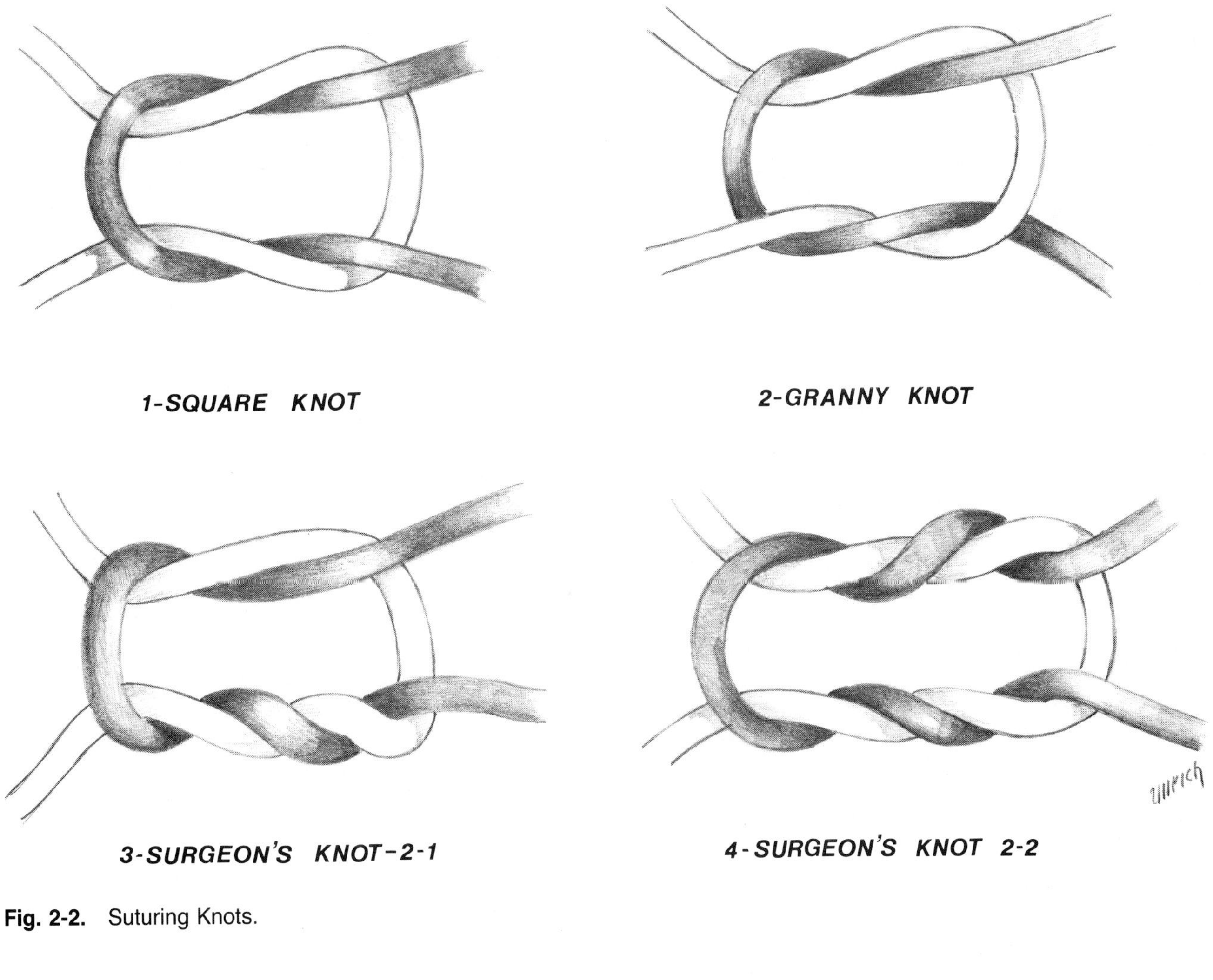

1-SQUARE KNOT

2-GRANNY KNOT

3-SURGEON'S KNOT-2-1

4-SURGEON'S KNOT 2-2

Fig. 2-2. Suturing Knots.

Surgical Needles

Most surgical needles are fabricated from heat-treated steel and possess a micro-silicon finish to diminish tissue drag and a tip that is extremely sharp and has undergone electropolishing (Ethicon, 1985). The surgical needle has a basic design composed of three parts (Fig. 2-3):

1. The *eye* which is *swaged* (eyeless) and permits the suture and needle to act as a single unit to decrease trauma.
2. The *body* which is the widest point of the needle and is also referred to as the *grasping area*. The body comes in a number of shapes (round, oval, rectangular, trapezoid, or side-flattened).
3. The *point* which runs from the tip to the maximum cross-sectional area of the body. The point also comes in a number of different shapes (conventional cutting, reverse cutting, side cutting, tapercut, taper, blunt) (Fig. 2-4).

Needle Holder Selection

Ethicon (1985) gives the following pointers for selecting a needle holder:

1. Use an approximate size for the given needle. The smaller the needle, the smaller the needle holder required.
2. Needles should be grasped one-quarter to one-half the distance from the *swaged* area to point as shown in Figure 2-5.
3. The tips of the jaws of the needleholder should meet before the remaining portions of the jaws.
4. The needle should be placed securely in the tips of the jaws and should not rock, twist, or turn.
5. Do not overclose the needle holder. It should close only to the first or second rachet. This will avoid damaging or notching the needle.
6. Pass the needle holder so it is always directed by the surgeon's thumb.
7. *Do not use digital pressure on the tissue; this may puncture a glove.*

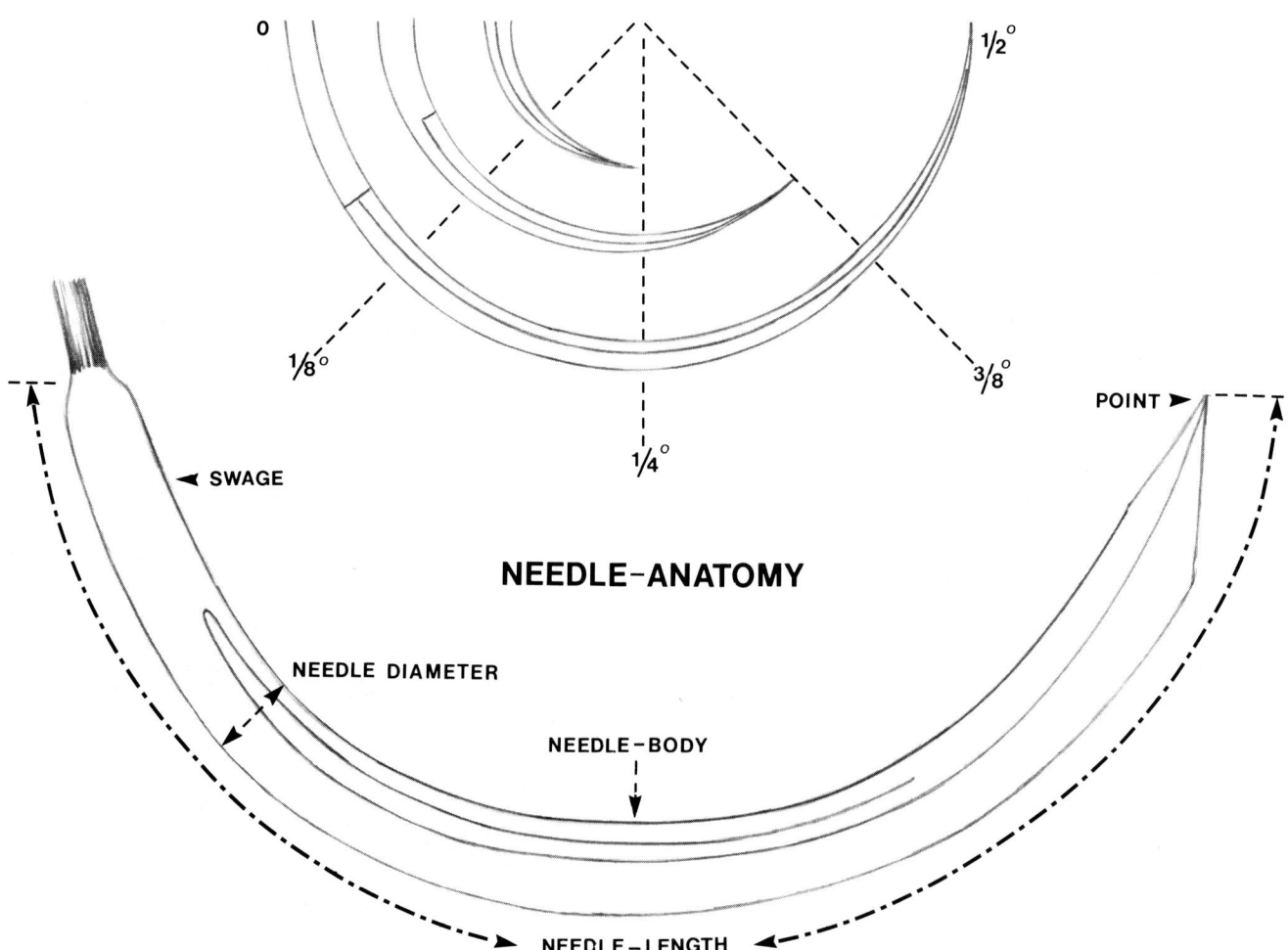

Fig. 2-3. Needle Anatomy. Needles are described by their arc. Most periodontal surgical needles are three-eighths or one-half curvature. Different components of the needle are described.

Sutures and Suturing

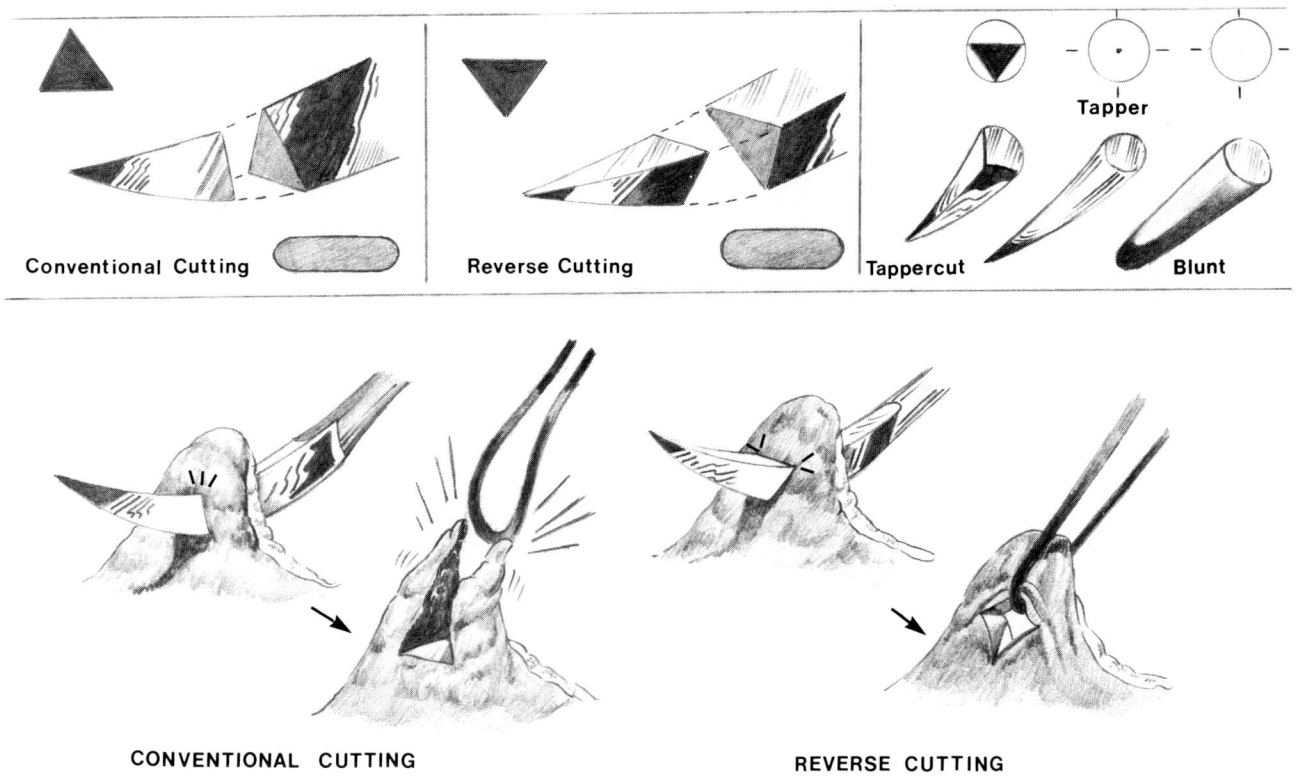

Fig. 2-4. Cutting Needles. Both outline and cross-sectional views of the various forms of cutting needle are shown. Conventional cutting and reverse cutting are also shown.

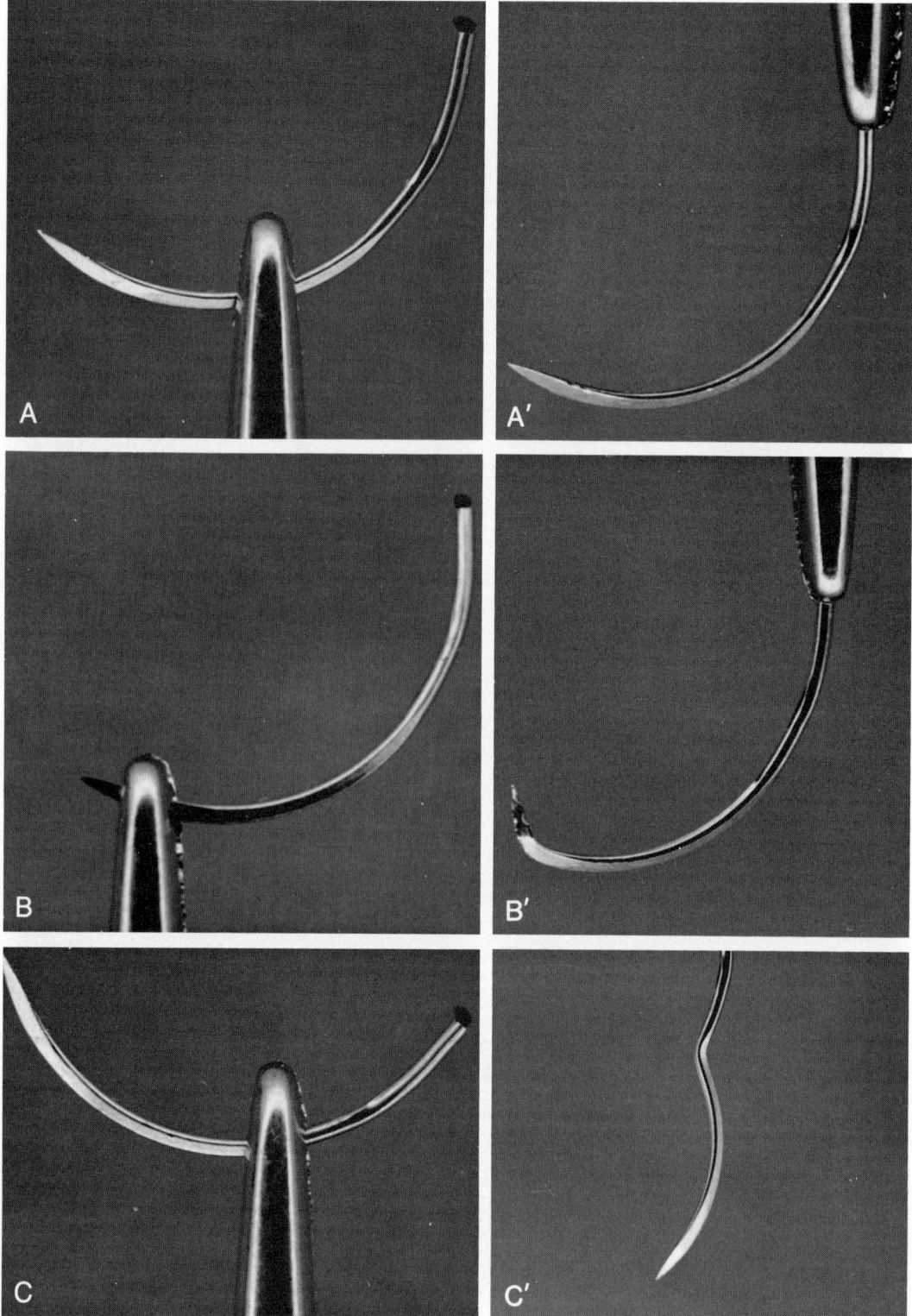

Fig. 2-5. Correct Handling of Suture Needles. **A**, Needle holder holding suture needle just anterior to curvature; correct position; **A′**, suture needle undamaged. **B**, suture needle held incorrectly at tip; **B′**, tip of suture needle damaged. **C**, Suture needle held incorrectly behind curvature; **C′**, needle bent as a result.

Placement of Needle in Tissue

Ethicon (1985) gives the following principles for placing the needle in tissue:
1. Force should always be applied in the direction that follows the curvature of the needle.
2. Suturing should always be from a movable to a nonmovable tissue.
3. Avoid excessive tissue bites with small needles as it will be difficult to retrieve them.
4. Use only sharp needles with minimal force. Replace dull needles.
5. Grasp the needle in the body one-quarter to one-half of the length from the swaged area. Do not hold the swaged area; this may bend or break the needle. Do not grasp the point area as damage or notching may result (Fig. 2-5).
6. Never force the needle through the tissue.
7. Avoid retrieving the needle from the tissue by the tip. This will damage or dull the needle. Attempt to grasp the body as far back as possible.
8. Sutures should be placed in keratinized tissue whenever possible.
9. An adequate tissue *bite* is required to prevent the flap from tearing.

SUTURING TECHNIQUES

Different suturing techniques may employ either periosteal or nonperiosteal suture placement.
1. Interrupted
   a. Figure eight
   b. Circumferential director loop
   c. Mattress—vertical or horizontal
   d. Intrapapillary
2. Continuous
   a. Papillary sling
   b. Vertical mattress
   c. Locking

The choice of technique is generally made on the basis of a combination of the individual operator's preference, educational background, and skill level, as well as surgical requirements.

PERIOSTEAL SUTURING

Periosteal suturing generally requires a high degree of dexterity in both flap management and suture placement. Small needles (P-3), fine sutures (4-0 to 6-0) and proper needle holders are a basic requirement.

Technique

The 5 steps used in periosteal suturing (Chaiken, 1977) are seen in Figure 2-6.

1. *Penetration:* The needle point is positioned perpendicular (90°) to the tissue surface and underlying bone. It is then inserted completely through the tissue until the bone is engaged. This is as opposed to the usual 30° needle insertion angle (Fig. 2-6A).
2. *Rotation:* The body of the needle is now rotated about the needle point in the direction opposite to that in which the needle is intended to travel. The needle point is held lightly against the bone so as not to damage or dull the needle point (Fig. 2-6B).
3. *Glide:* The needle point is now permitted to glide against the bone for only a short distance. Care must be taken not to lift or damage the periosteum (Fig. 2-6C).
4. *Rotation:* As the needle glides against the bone, it is rotated about the body, following its circumferenced outline. In this way, the needle will not be pushed through the tissue resulting in lifting or tearing of the periosteum (Fig. 2-6D,E).
5. *Exit:* The final stage of gliding and rotation is needle exit. The needle is made to exit the tissue through the gentle application of pressure from above, thus allowing the tip to pierce the tissue. If digital pressure is to be used, care must be used to avoid personal injury (Fig. 2-6F).

INTERRUPTED SUTURES

Indications

Interrupted sutures are most often used for the following:
1. Vertical incision
2. Tuberosity and retromolar areas
3. Bone regeneration procedures with or without guided tissue regeneration
4. Widman flaps, open flap curettage, unrepositioned flaps, or apically positioned flaps where maximum interproximal coverage is required
5. Edentulous areas
6. Partial or split-thickness flaps
7. Osseointegrated implants

Types

In Figure 2-7 we see the four most commonly used interrupted sutures:
1. Circumferential, direct, or loop (Fig. 2-7A)
2. Figure-eight (Fig. 2-7B)
3. Vertical or horizontal mattress (Fig. 2-7C)
4. Interstitial papillary placement (Fig. 2-7D)

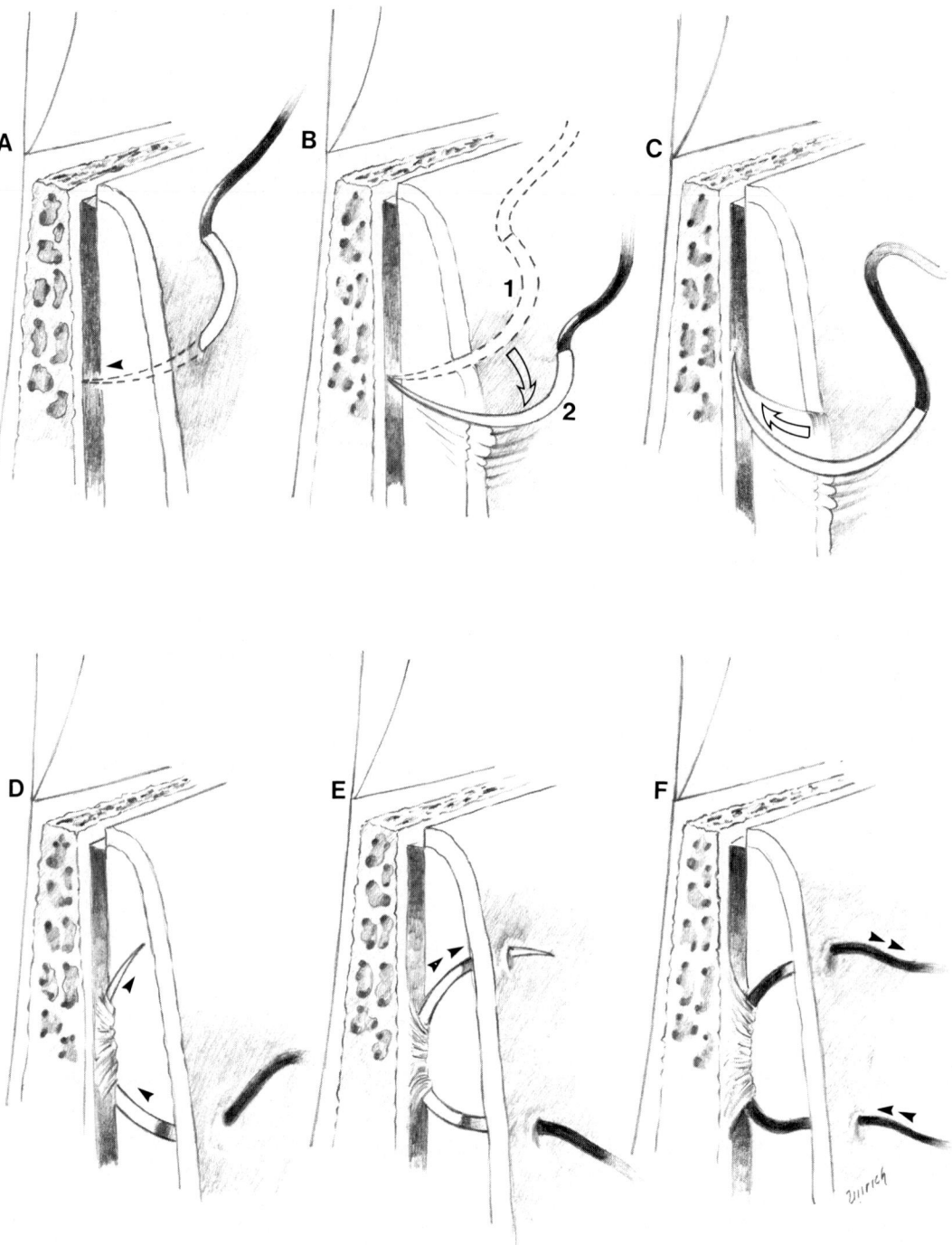

Fig. 2-6. Periosteal Suturing. **A,** Needle penetration; needle point is perpendicular to bone. **B,** Rotation of needle body about point. **C, D,** The needle is moved along the bone below the periosteum. **E,** Rotation about needle body permitting point to exit periosteum and tissue. **F,** Completed periosteal suture.

Technique

Figure-Eight and Circumferential Sutures

Suturing is begun on the buccal surface 3 to 4 mm from the tip of the papilla so as to prevent tearing of the thinned papilla. The needle is first inserted into the outer surface of the buccal flap and then either through the outer epithelialized surface *(figure-eight)* (Fig. 2-8B) or through the connective tissue under the surface *(circumferential)* (Fig. 2-8A) of the lingual flap. The needle is then returned through the embrasure and tied buccally.

When interproximal closure is critical, the circumferential suture will permit greater coaptation and **tucking-down** of the papilla because of the lack of intervening suture material between the tips of the papilla.

Mattress Sutures

Mattress sutures are used for greater flap security and control; they permit more precise flap placement, especially when combined with periosteal stabilization. They also allow for good papillary stabilization and placement. *The vertical mattress suture is recommended for use with bone regeneration procedures because it permits maximum tissue closure while avoiding suture contact with the implant material, thus preventing wicking.*

VERTICAL MATTRESS TECHNIQUE. The flap is stabilized, and a P-3 needle is inserted 7 to 10 mm apical to the tip of the papilla. It is passed through the periosteum (if periosteal sutures are being used), emerging again from the epithelialized surface of the flap 2 to 3 mm from the tip of the papilla. The needle is brought through the embrasure, where the technique is again repeated lingually or palatally. The suture is then tied buccally (Fig. 2-9B).

HORIZONTAL MATTRESS TECHNIQUE. A P-3 needle is inserted 7 to 8 mm apical and to one side of the midline of the papilla, emerging again 4 to 5 mm through the epithelialized surface on the opposing side of the midline (Fig. 2-9A). The suture may or may not be brought through the periosteum. The needle is then passed through the embrasure, and the suture, after being repeated lingually or palatally, is tied buccally. For greater papillary stability and control the double parallel strands of this suture can be made to cross over the tops of the papillae. This is the double crossed over suture.

Intrapapillary Placement

This technique is recommended for use only with modified Widman flaps and regeneration procedures in which there is adequate thickness of the papillary tissue.

A P-3 needle is inserted buccally 4 to 5 mm from the tip of the papilla and passed through the tissue, emerging from the very tip of the papilla. This is repeated lingually and tied buccally, thus permitting exact tip-to-tip placement of the flaps (Fig. 2-7D).

Sling Suture

The sling suture is primarily used for a flap that has been raised on only one side of a tooth, involving only one or two adjacent papillae. It is most often used in coronally and laterally positioned flaps. The technique involves use of one of the interrupted sutures, which is either anchored about the adjacent tooth (Fig. 2-10) or slung around the tooth to hold both papillae (Fig. 2-11).

CONTINUOUS SUTURES

When multiple teeth are involved, the continuous suture is preferred.

Advantages

1. Can include as many teeth as required
2. Minimizes the need for multiple knots
3. Simplicity
4. The teeth are used to anchor the flap
5. Permits precise flap placement
6. Avoids the need for periosteal sutures
7. Allows independent placement and tension of buccal and lingual or palatal flaps. Buccal flaps can be positioned loosely while lingual and palatal flaps are pulled more tightly about the teeth.
8. Greater distribution of forces on the flaps

Disadvantages

The main disadvantage of continuous sutures is that if the suture breaks the flap may become loose or the suture may come untied from multiple teeth.

Types

The choice of continuous suture depends on the operator's preference. These too can be periosteal or nonperiosteal:
1. Independent sling suture
2. Mattress sutures
   a. Vertical
   b. Horizontal
3. Continuous locking

Technique

Independent Sling Suture

The continuous sling suture (Fig. 2-12), although most often begun as a continuation of tuberosity or retromolar suturing (Fig. 2-12, 1), can also be started with a looped suture about the terminal papilla (buccal, lingual, or palatal). It is then continued through the next interproximal embrasure (Fig. 2-12, 2) in such a manner that the suture is made to encircle the neck of the tooth (Fig. 2-12, 3). The needle is then passed either over the papilla and through the outer epithelialized surface or underneath and through the connective tissue undersurface of the papilla. The needle is passed again through the embrasure and continued anteriorly (Fig. 2-12, 4). This procedure is repeated through each successive embrasure until all papillae have been engaged.

Note: For maximum flap control, it is best to pass the needle through the connective tissue undersurface of the papilla.

A terminal end loop (Fig. 2-12, 5) is then used if a single flap has been reflected or if the flaps are to be sutured independently. In this manner, the flaps are tied against the teeth, as opposed to each other.

TERMINAL END LOOP. Upon completion of suturing, the suture is tied off against the tooth, as opposed to the other flap. This is accomplished by leaving a loose loop of approximately 1 cm length of suture material before the last embrasure. When the last papilla is sutured and the needle is returned through the embrasure, the terminal end loop is used to tie the final knot (Fig. 2-12, 6-9).

MODIFICATION. When two flaps have been reflected and after the first flap has been sutured (Fig. 2-13, 1), it is often desirable to continue about the distal surface of the last tooth (Fig. 2-13, 2), repeating the procedure on the opposing flap (Fig. 2-13, 3) and then tying off in a terminal end loop (Fig. 2-13, 4, 5).

ALTERNATIVE PROCEDURE. This technique simultaneously slings together both the buccal and lingual or palatal flaps.

Indications

1. When flap position is not critical
2. When buccal periosteal sutures are used for buccal flap position and stabilization.
3. When maximum closure is desired (unreposition or Widman flaps or bone regeneration)

Technique

After the initial buccal and lingual tie, the suture is passed bucally about the neck of the tooth interdentally and through the lingual flap. It is then again brought interdentally through the buccal papilla and back interdentally about the lingual surface of the tooth to the buccal papilla. Then it is brought about the lingual papilla and then about the buccal surface of the tooth. This alternating buccal–lingual suturing is continued until the suture is tied off with a terminal end loop (Fig. 2-14).

Vertical and Horizontal Mattress Suture

When greater papillary control and stability and more precise placement are required, or to prevent flap movement, vertical or horizontal mattress sutures are used. This is most often the case on the palate, where additional tension is often required, or when the papillary tissue is thin and friable.

TECHNIQUE. The procedure is identical to that previously described for the independent papillary sling suture (Fig. 2-12), except that vertical or horizontal mattress sutures are substituted for the simple papillary sling. The technique is similar to that previously described for the interrupted mattress sutures.

Locking

The continuous locking suture is indicated primarily for long edentulous areas, tuberosities, or retromolar areas. It has the advantage of avoiding the multiple knots of interrupted sutures. If the suture is broken, however, it may completely untie.

TECHNIQUE. The procedure is simple and repetitive. A single interrupted suture is used to make the initial tie. The needle is next inserted through the outer surface of the buccal flap and the underlying surface of the lingual flap. The needle is then passed through the remaining loop of the suture, and the suture is pulled tightly, thus locking it. This procedure is continued until the final suture is tied off at the terminal end (Fig. 2-15).

Sutures and Suturing

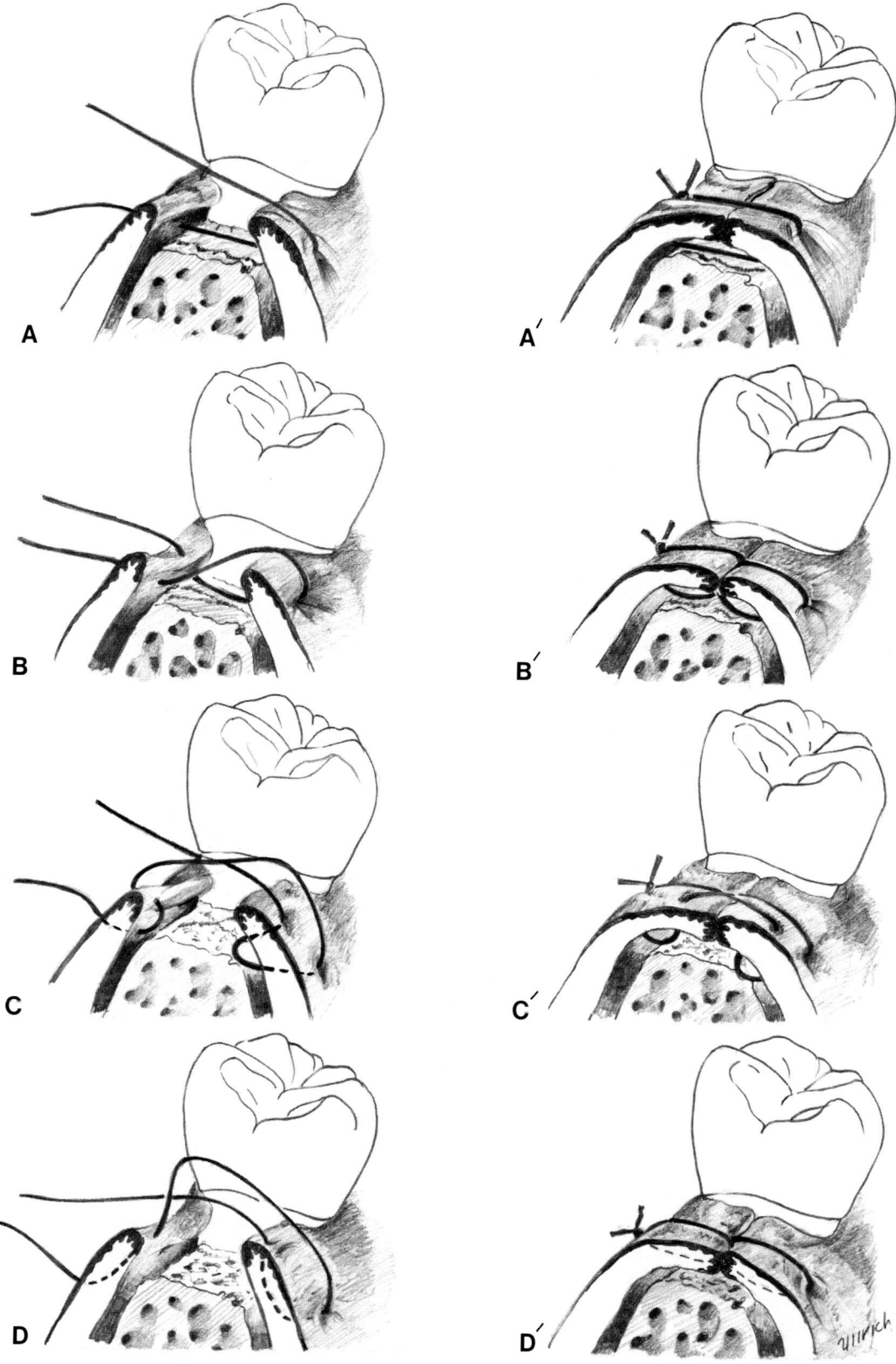

Fig. 2-7. Four Interrupted Sutures. **A,** Circumferential. **B,** Figure-eight. **C,** Vertical mattress. **D,** Intrapapillary.

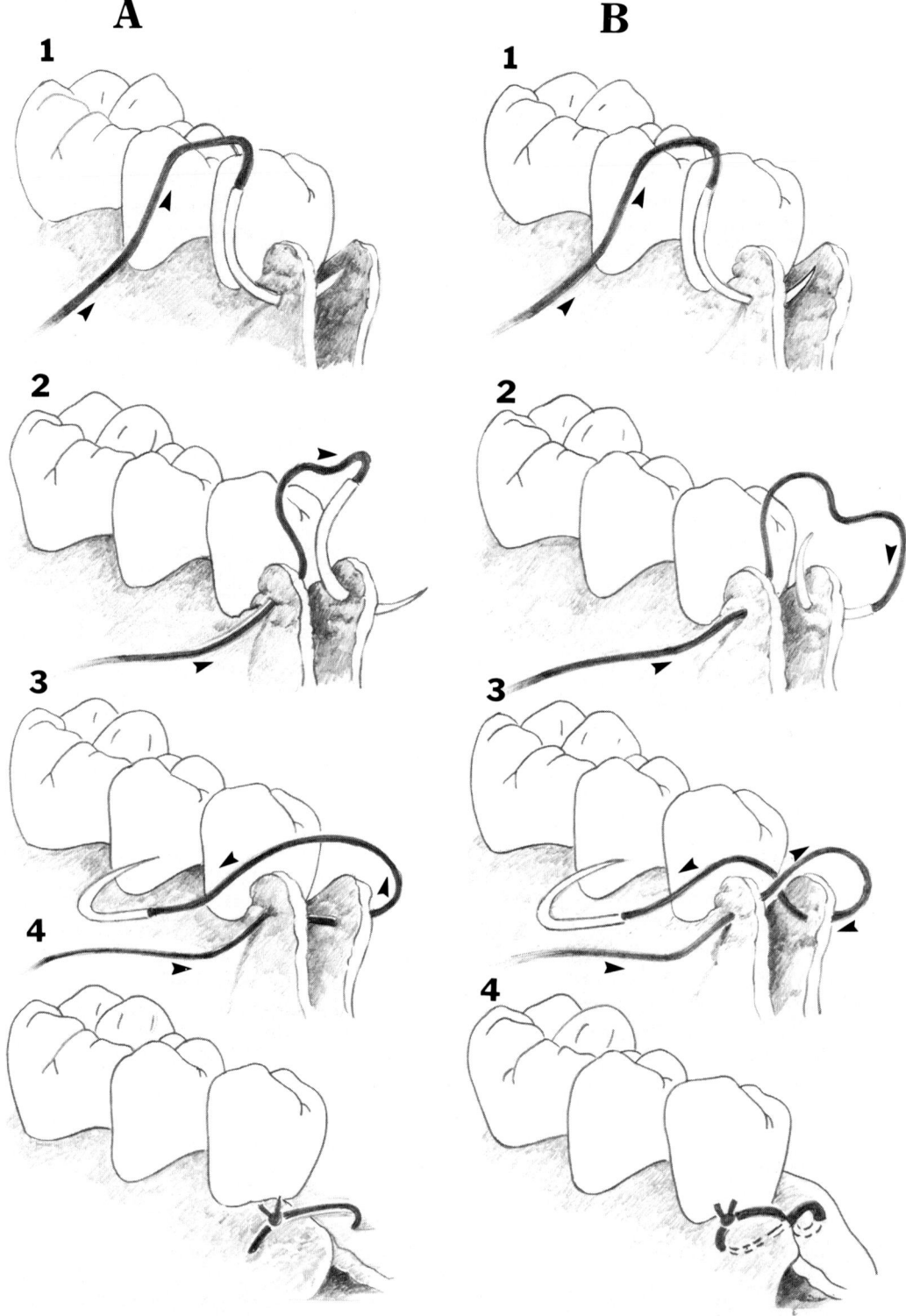

Fig. 2-8. **A,** Circumferential suture. **B,** Figure-eight suture.

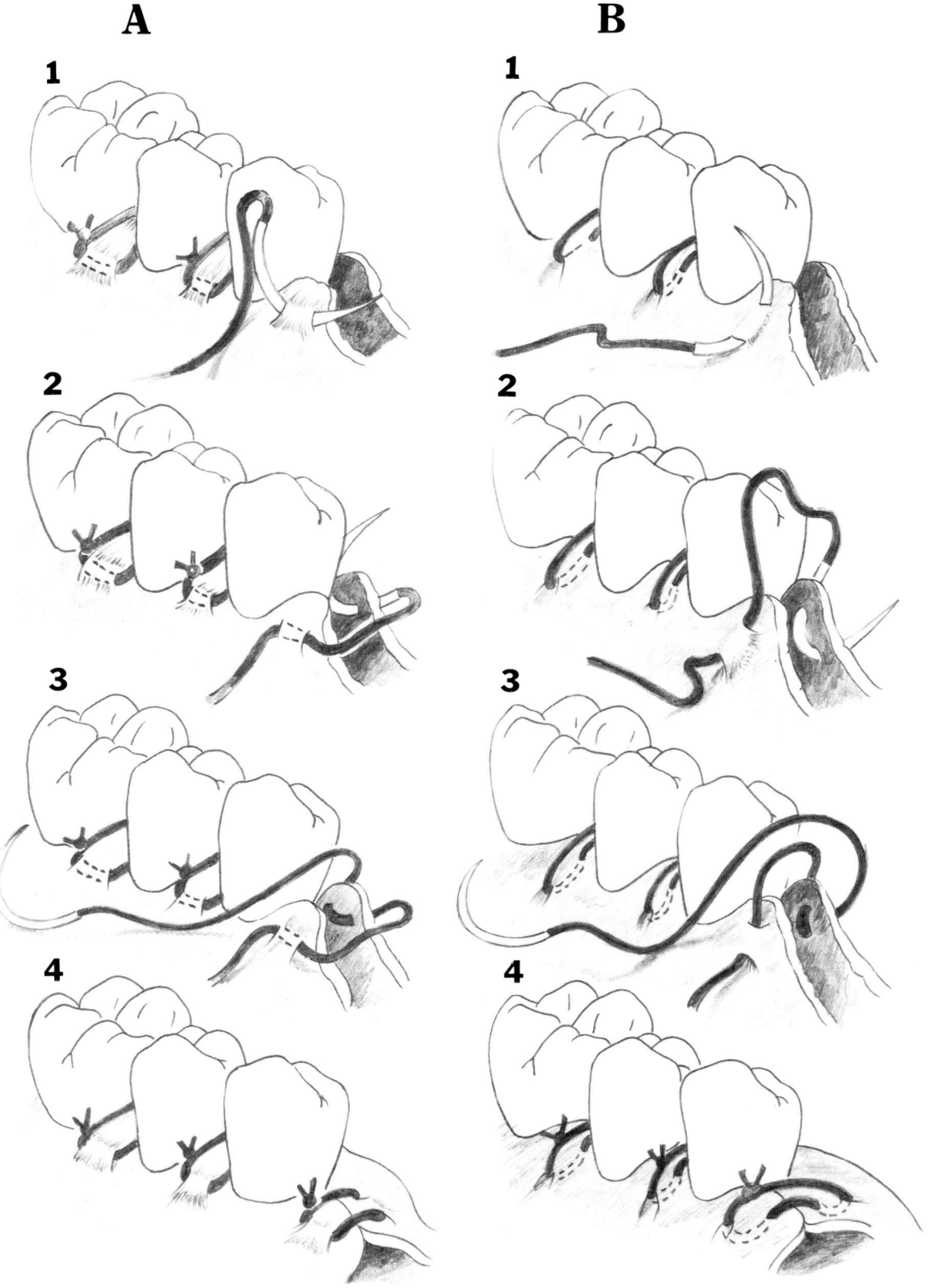

Fig. 2-9. **A,** Horizontal mattress suture. **B,** Vertical mattress suture.

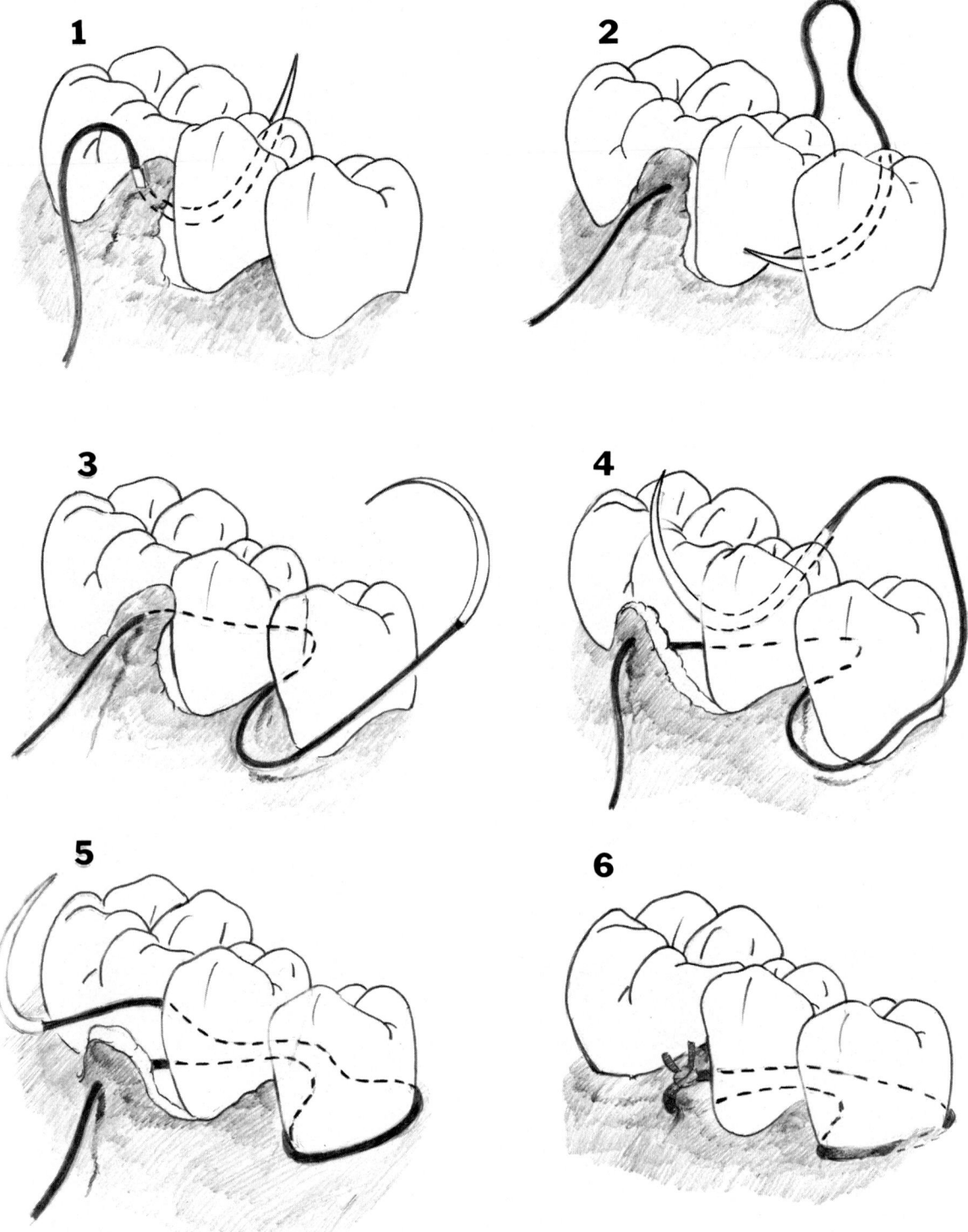

Fig. 2-10. Sling Suture About Adjacent Tooth.

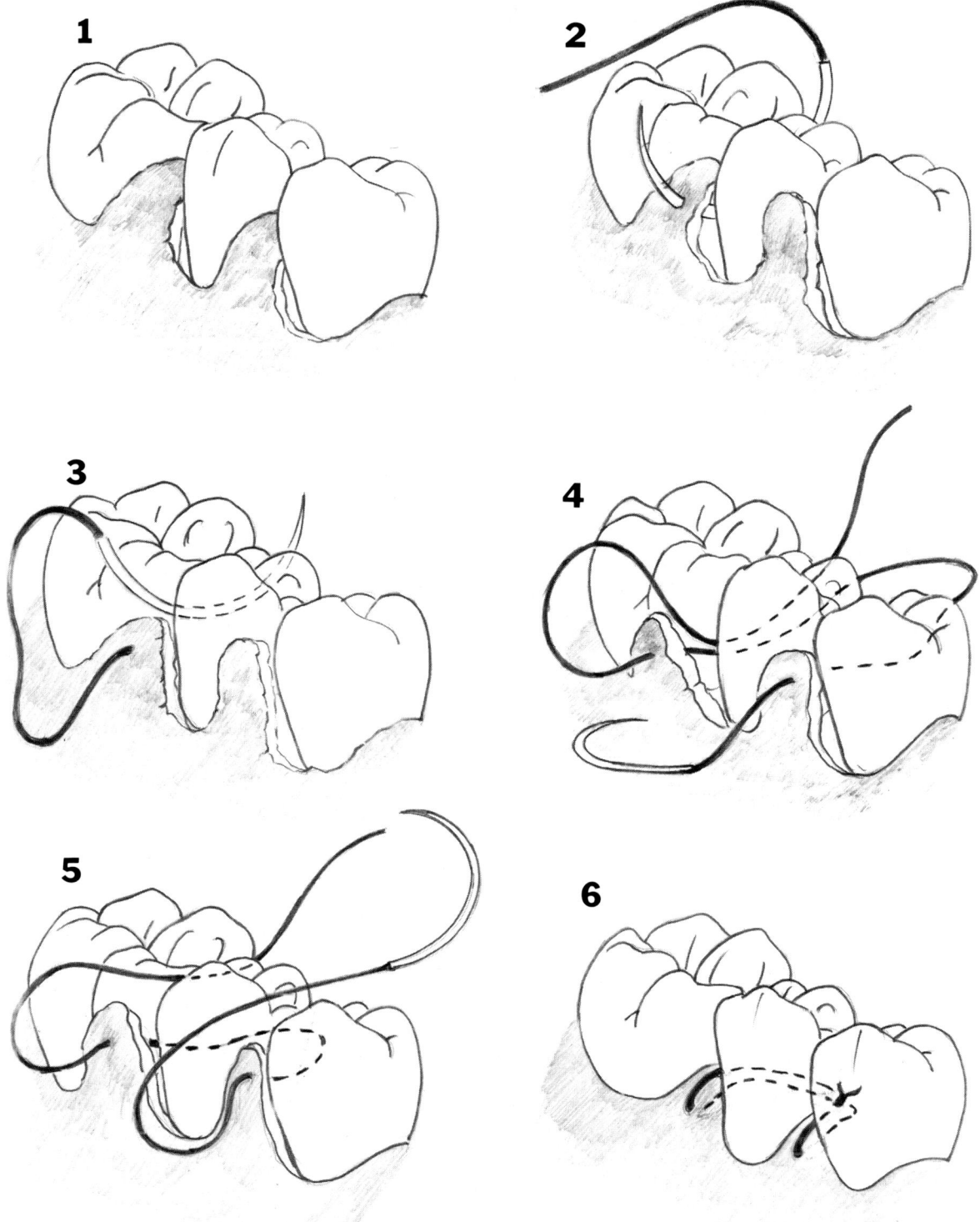

Fig. 2-11. Sling Suture About Single Tooth.

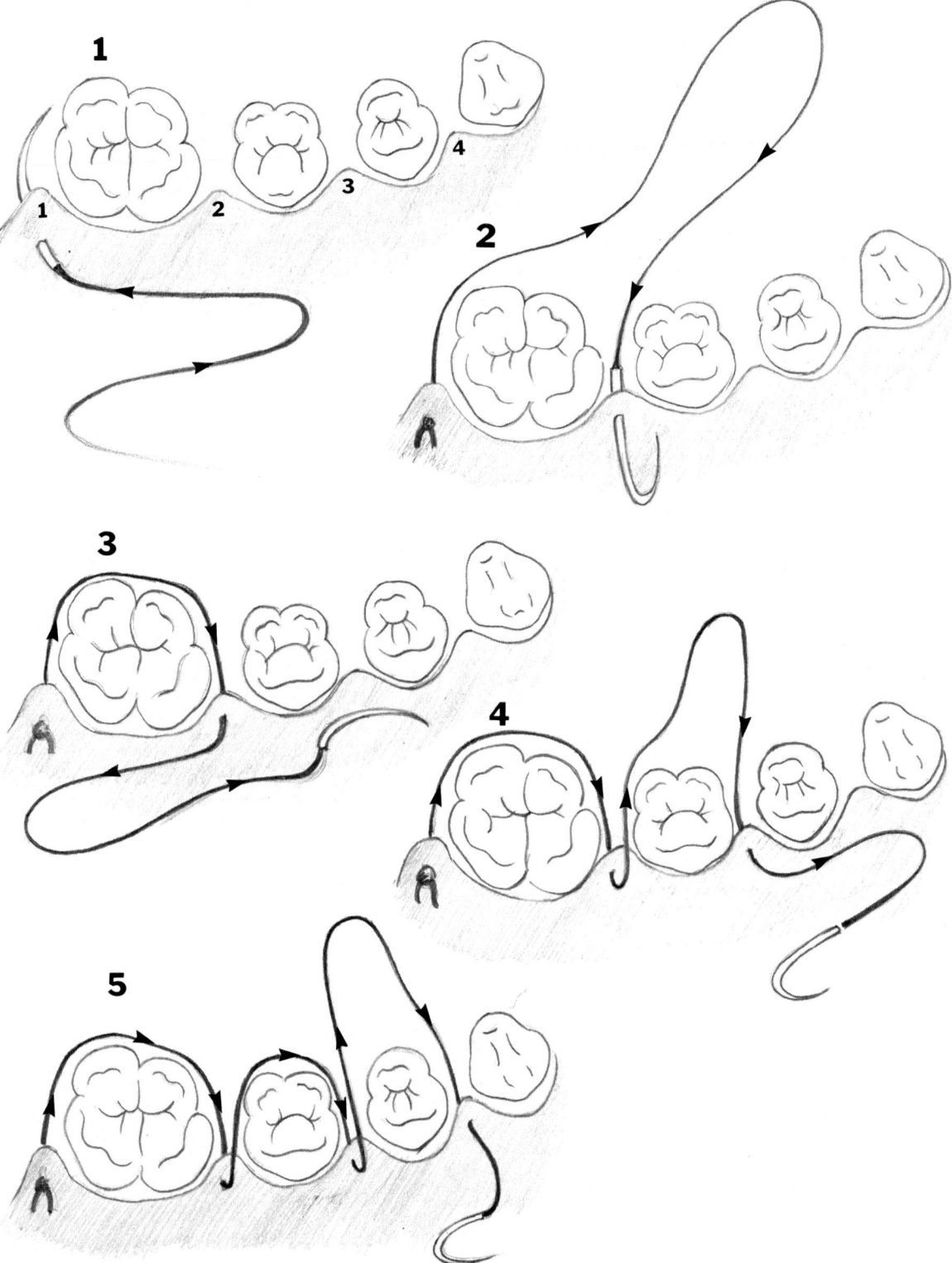

Fig. 2-12. Continuous Sling Suture with Terminal End Loop.

Sutures and Suturing

27

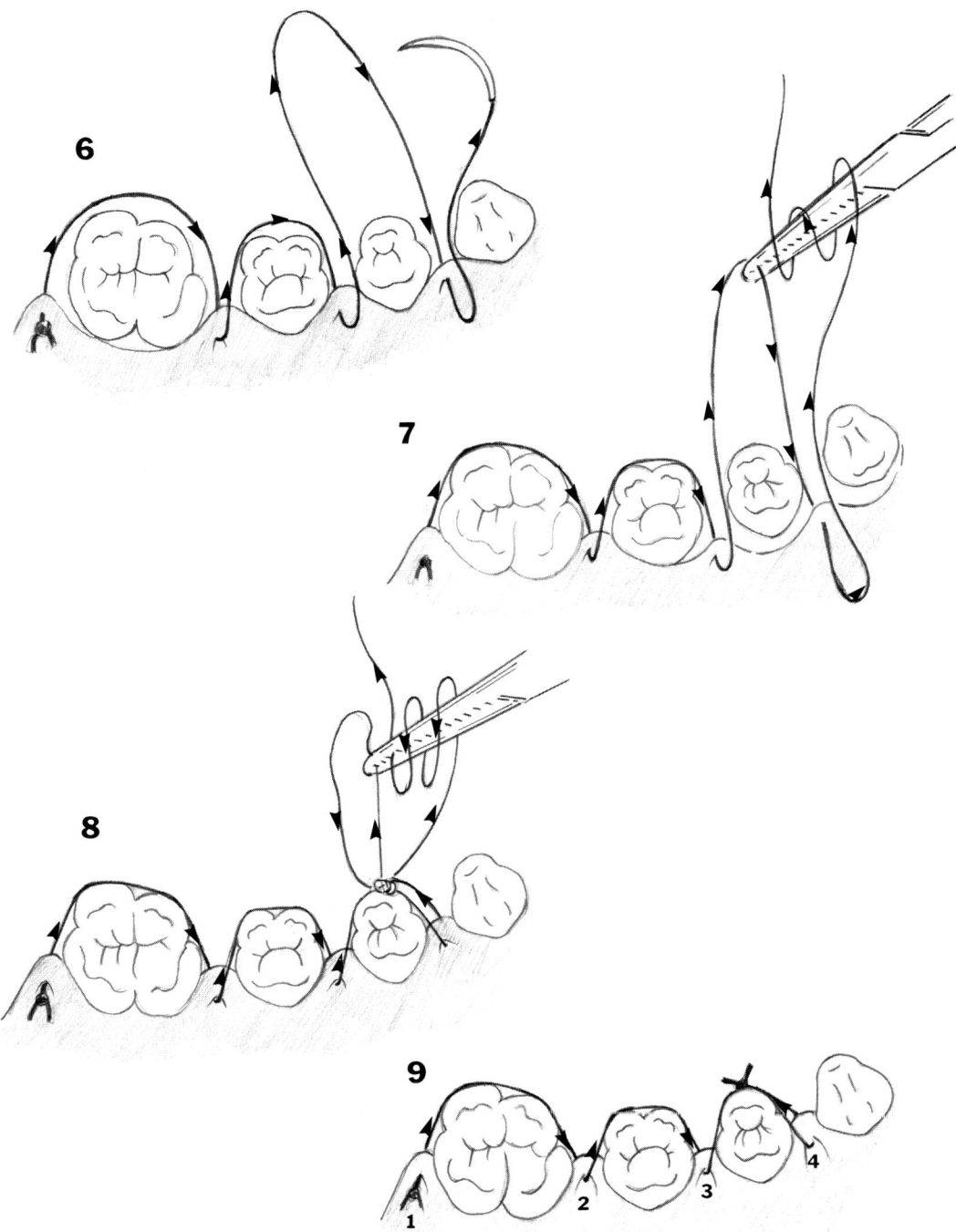

Fig. 2-12 (continued). Continuous Sling Suture with Terminal End Loop.

28 Sutures and Suturing

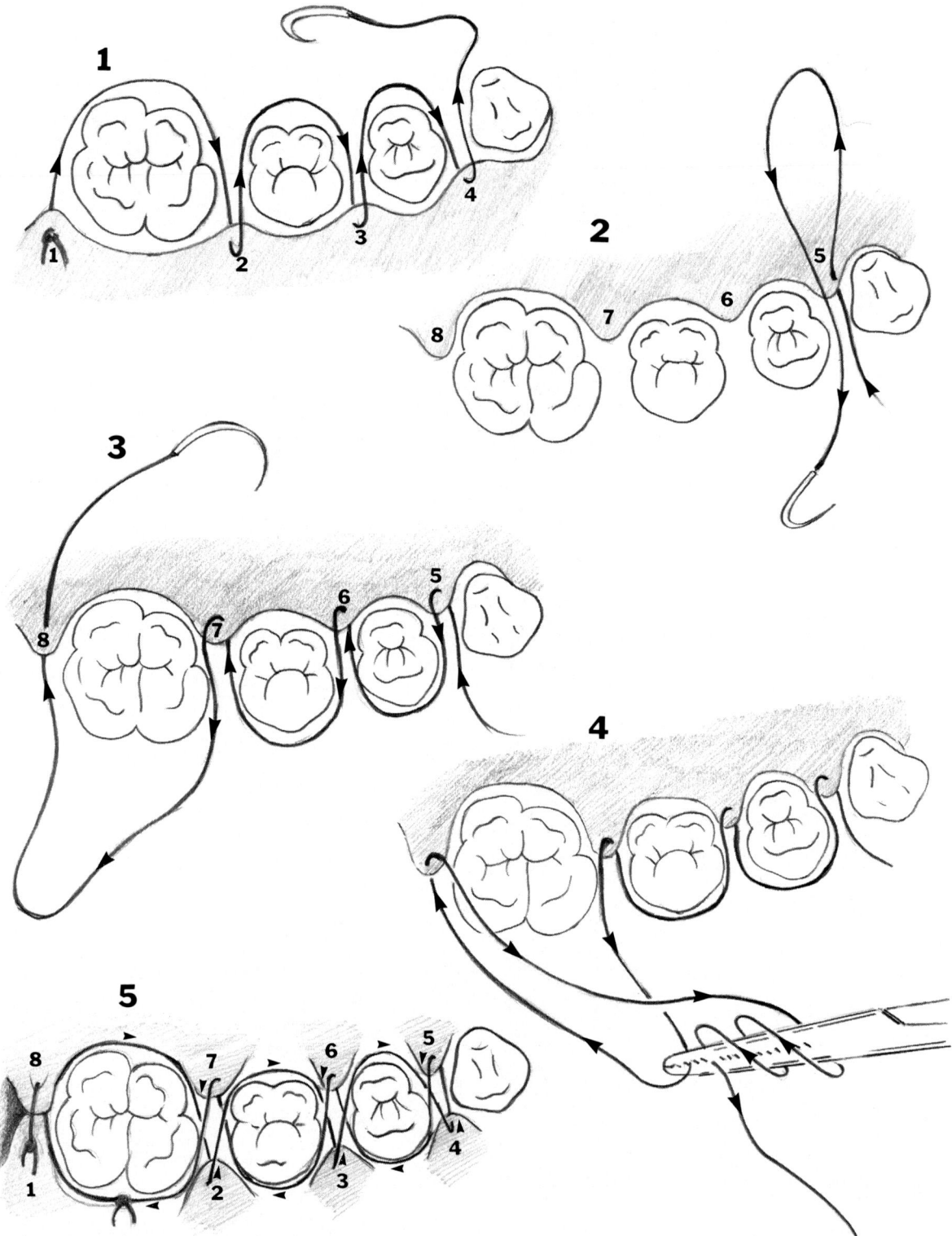

Fig. 2-13. Continuous Independent Sling Sutures of Individual Flaps.

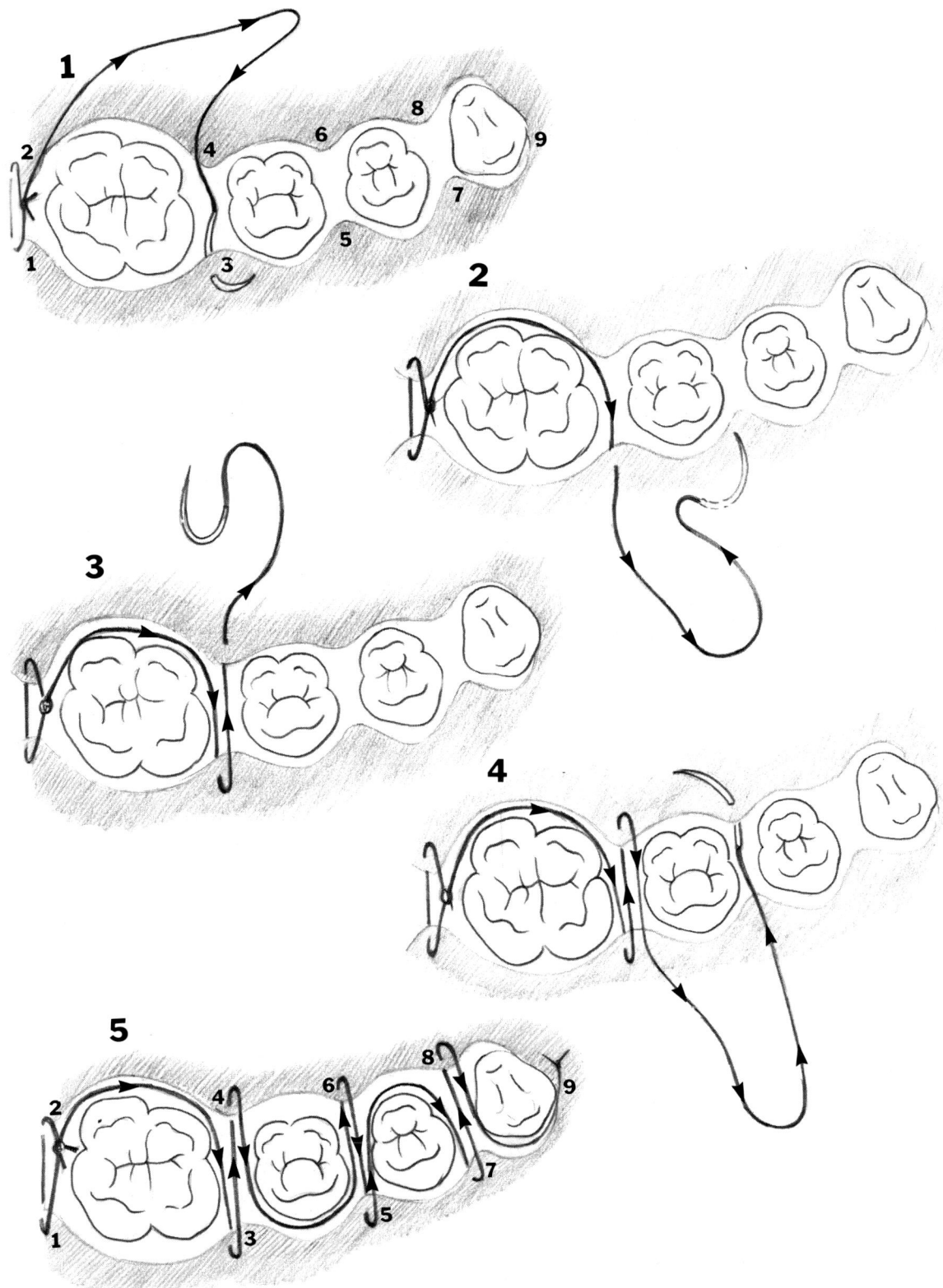

Fig. 2-14. Modification of Continuous Sling Suture. Technique permits simultaneous suturing of both flaps.

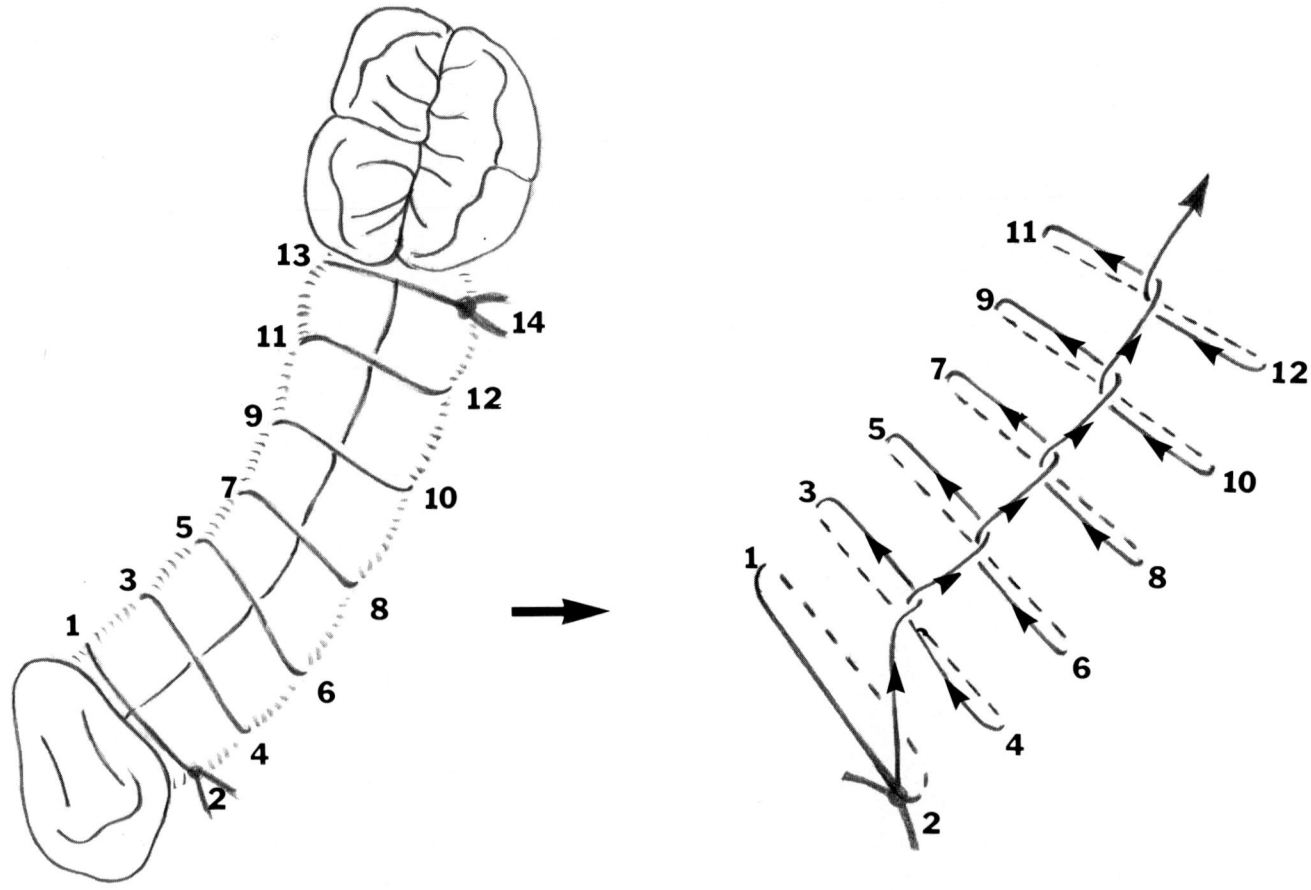

Fig. 2-15. Continuous Locking Suture Used Primarily for Edentulous Areas.

3

SCALING, ROOT PLANING, AND CURETTAGE

SCALING AND ROOT PLANING

Scaling is the removal of plaque, calculus, and stain from the crown and root surfaces. This is as opposed to *root planing*, which is the definitive removal of cementum or dentin from the root surface in an attempt to smooth rough surfaces, remove soft and/or necrotic cementum, eliminate bacteria, reduce impregnated toxins, and dislodge calculus. Without clean, smooth, hard roots the results of curettage may be limited since rough roots are foci for plaque accumulation and attachment of calculus.

Scaling and root planing are the first steps in the overall treatment of adult periodontitis. They are geared toward reducing gingival inflammation and eliminating the subgingival pathologic microorganisms that are responsible. In areas of minimal pocketing where inflammation can be controlled and disease progression stopped, no further treatment is indicated. Walker and Ash (1976), Waerhaug (1978), Caffesse et al. (1986), and Buchanan and Robertson (1987) have all shown that in pockets greater than 3 mm, the ability to remove all calculus is significantly reduced and that there is a low predictability for detection of residual calculus by instrumentation or x-ray studies. The inability to remove calculus in furcations and concavities is even greater (Maitia et al., 1986). Although less effective in these deeper pockets, scaling and root planing are still an important contributor to the reduction of inflammation and control of subgingival bacteria (Sato et al., 1993).

CURETTAGE

Curettage is a closed, definitive surgical procedure performed under local anesthesia and aimed at pocket reduction, elimination, reattachment, or new attachment. It is indicated primarily for edematous suprabony pockets, where shrinkage and a reduction of inflammation will result in a shallow sulcus, or prior to surgery for pocket elimination to reduce inflammation (Hirschfeld, 1952). It is performed with sharp curettes in an attempt to remove (1) the sulcular epithelium and the epithelial attachment, and (2) the inflamed connective tissue of the pocket wall (Fig. 3-1).

It is important to note that although scaling, root planing, and curettage are difficult, time-consuming, and often tedious procedures, they are basic to periodontal therapy and should be mastered by all clinicians.

The consensus report of the Proceedings of the World Workshop in Clinical Periodontics (1989) came to the following conclusions: "Gingival curettage as a *separate* procedure has no justifiable application during active therapy for chronic adult periodontitis. Gingival curettage is not indicated if new attachment is the goal of therapy. This conclusion was arrived at due to the difficulty of assessing what if any the beneficial effects of curettage were since they are almost always combined with root instrumentation." They further pointed out that studies have not been able to find any significant differences between scaling and root planing with and without curettage.

Indications

1. Edematous and inflamed tissues
2. Shallow pockets
3. Suprabony pockets

4. As part of initial preparation prior to open surgical procedures in an attempt to achieve tissue quality that can be handled easily
5. Progressive attachment or alveolar bone loss
6. Increased levels of pathogenic microorganisms

Contraindications

1. Fibrotic tissue
2. Deep pockets
3. Furcation involvements
4. Treatment of underlying osseous defects

Procedure

1. Scaling, root planing, and curettage require local anesthesia to control pain and hemorrhage. Figure 3-2,1 outlines the three critical areas of treatment: A, the root surface; B, the sulcular epithelium; and C, the underlying connective tissue.
2. Step one is subgingival scaling for removal of calculus, plaque, and soft cementum. The scaler is placed in the pocket with the bevel at an angle between 45° and 90° to the tooth and drawn in a vertical, oblique, or horizontal motion (Fig. 3-2,2).
3. Sharp curettes are then placed into the pocket with the cutting edge toward the tissue. Digital pressure to support the gingival tissue enhances the cutting efficiency of the curette. The curette is moved generally in a circular or horizontal motion about the tooth. The sulcular epithelium and epithelial attachment are removed first (Fig. 3-2,3).
4. Once the epithelial lining is removed (Fig. 3-2,4), the inflamed connective tissue of the inner pocket wall and that above the alveolar crest are removed (Fig. 3-2,5).
5. Upon completion of the procedure, the area is flushed and all tissue tags are removed. Digital pressure is now applied to ensure proper tissue adaptation and clot formation. Suturing is indicated if the col area has been disrupted and the papillae have been separated. A periodontal dressing may be necessary.
6. Healing will result in a shrunken, firm, well adapted, well contoured tissue (Fig. 3-2,6)

The procedure is clinically depicted in Figure 3-3, and the results that may be attained are shown in Figure 3-4.

FLAP DEBRIDEMENT SURGERY

These procedures permit the surgical debridement of root surfaces and removal of soft tissue following the reflection of a mucoperiosteal flap. They have been described as open flap curettage, modified E.N.A.P., and, most notably, the modified Widman flap. They are repositioned (unrepositioned) flaps whose primary purpose is to gain access to the roots for definitive scaling and root planing in areas where pockets are 4 mm or more. *Their purpose is for control of chronic adult periodontitis and not for gaining new attachment.*

EXCISIONAL NEW ATTACHMENT PROCEDURE (E.N.A.P.) AND MODIFIED E.N.A.P.

The excisional new attachment procedure (E.N.A.P.), as outlined by Yukna et al. (1976), was an attempt to overcome some of the limitations of closed gingival curettage and gain new attachment in areas of suprabony pockets. The E.N.A.P., unlike scaling and curettage, was developed to ensure complete removal of sulcular epithelium, epithelial attachment, granulated and inflamed connective tissue, subgingival calculus, and softened cementum. *Basically, it is curettage with a surgical blade, which increases access and visibility with minimal tissue reflection.*

When performing the E.N.A.P., the dentist uses a scalpel or sharp knife for a definitive sulcular incision, which allows greater access to and visibility of the roots for the removal of calculus and softened cementum. No vertical incisions are made, and the procedure is confined to the keratinized tissue. The sharp, clean incision of E.N.A.P. heals faster than the ragged incision of curettage. This procedure is easy to perform and within the capabilities of the general dentist.

Indications

1. Suprabony pockets
2. Adequate keratinized tissue
3. When esthetics are unimportant

Advantages

1. Improved root visualization
2. Complete removal of sulcular epithelium and epithelial attachment
3. Minimal gingival trauma
4. No loss of keratinized gingiva

Disadvantages

1. Difficult to determine apical extent of epithelial attachment
2. Does not result in new attachment

Contraindications

1. Pockets exceed mucogingival junction
2. Edematous tissue
3. Lack of keratinized tissue
4. Osseous defects have to be treated
5. Hyperplastic tissue
6. Close root proximity
7. Furcation involvement
8. Probing depths of 3 mm or less

Procedure

1. Scaling and root planing are performed at least 1 week before the E.N.A.P. procedure, which increases the healing potential.
2. Adequate anesthesia is given, after which pockets are checked to make sure the zone of keratinized tissue is adequate and the pockets do not exceed the mucogingival junction (Fig. 3-5A,B).
3. With a No. 11 or No. 15 scalpel blade, a scalloped, partial-thickness, inverse beveled incision is made (Fig. 3-5C) from the crest of the gingiva to the base of the sulcus (Fig. 3-5D).
4. The incisions are carried facially, lingually, and interproximally as far as possible (Fig. 3-5E). The papilla is thinned interproximally (Fig. 3-5F) to remove any inflamed connective tissue and the triangular wedge of interproximal tissue. This tissue is difficult to remove once the flap is free.
5. With scalers and curettes, the inflamed granulated and excised tissues are removed. All tissue tags are carefully removed. The root is scaled hard and smooth, free of calculus and softened cementum (Fig. 3-5G,H), and the area is flushed with normal saline to remove debris, blood clots, and tissue tags.
6. Interproximal sutures are used to position the tissue as closely as possible to the presurgical height and to adapt the papillae and tissue tightly about the necks of the teeth. Primary closure is desirable (Fig. 3-5I,J).
7. A periodontal dressing is now placed interproximally, without being forced.

The procedure is shown clinically in Figure 3-6.

Modified E.N.A.P. Technique Modification

In 1977, Fredi and Rosenfeld modified the technique by advocating a partial-thickness, inverse beveled incision down to the crest of the bone (Fig. 3-7,1) to completely remove tissue about the periodontal ligament (Fig. 3-7,2). The flaps were then sutured at the presurgical height (Fig. 3-7,3). The technique is basically the same in all other aspects.

MODIFIED WIDMAN FLAP

A report describing the modified Widman flap procedure was published by Ramfjord and Nissle in 1974. This procedure not only became a principal procedure of Ramfjord's long-term study on surgical techniques, but has also had a profound impact on how many clinicians treat periodontal disease. It was an extension or a progression of the Widman flap (apically displaced flap) procedure, which the authors found to have a rather "unpredictable ratio between success and failures. . . ."

The technique as outlined is technically demanding and extremely exacting. It is described as *a modification of subgingival curettage*. The flaps are raised by the use of small vertical incisions to gain access to the roots. This allows easier removal of calculus and less mechanical trauma in removal of the pocket lining than that afforded by closed gingival curettage. The aim is to get maximum healing with minimum loss of periodontal tissue.

Advantages

1. Minimal bone removal
2. Immediate close postsurgical contact of healthy collagenous tissue with the tooth surface.
3. Maximum conservation of periodontal tissue
4. Esthetic desirability
5. Facilitation of oral hygiene
6. Less root exposure with less sensitivity
7. Less mechanical trauma than closed curettage

Disadvantages

1. Technically demanding and exacting
2. Requires a high degree of technical skill
3. Interproximal flaps require exact placement
4. Immediate unfavorable interproximal contours when dressings are first removed

The original article shows no clinical examples of the procedures, and the drawings are extremely basic. This apparent lack of detail has resulted in some confusion by clinicians as to the exact technique.

Procedure

1. Sterile technique is recommended.
2. Adequate anesthesia is used to control pain and hemorrhage.
3. Figure 3-8A represents the basic outline of the incisions, showing an exaggerated scalloped palatal incision with maximum preservation of interproximal tissue. Buccally, if pockets are

greater than 2 mm, the inverse bevel is made ½ to 1 mm away from the free gingival margin.
4. The initial or primary incision is an inverse beveled, partial-thickness, thinning incision made with a No. 11 or No. 15 scalpel blade held parallel to the long axis of the tooth and directed toward the crest of bone. Palatally, the incision is more angulated, permitting thinning of the tissue (Fig. 3-8b) This is especially important interproximally, where the papillae must be thinned adequately to remove all remnants of epithelium to promote reattachment of connective tissue. *Note:* The removal of all epithelial remnants has been shown to be impossible (Bahat et al., 1984; Fisher et al., 1982).
5. Small vertical incisions are now made 2 to 3 mm apically, and the flap is raised, separating the periosteum (Fig. 3-8B,C) and exposing only a small amount of alveolar bone.
6. A secondary sulcular incision is made about the neck of the teeth from the base of the sulcus to the alveolar crest (Fig. 3-8D,E). This frees the inner or secondary flap.
7. The buccal and lingual flaps are now either pushed aside or held back to allow interproximal incisions to be made to remove the loosened collar of tissue at the alveolar crest (Fig. 3-8F). These incisions follow the contour of the alveolar crest.
8. Scalers and curettes are used to remove the collar of tissue and scale and plane the exposed roots (Fig. 3-8G). Care should be taken to keep the healthy gingival fibers at the crest intact if possible. Irrigation is done only with sterile saline solutions.
9. When intraosseous defects are present, all fibers are removed to promote possible regeneration (Fig. 3-8H).
10. For proper flap adaptation, it may be necessary to remove some bone on the outer alveolar surfaces (osteoplasty) or to thin the flap further (Fig. 3-8I). *Note:* No mention is made in the original article of how much bone is to be removed in attempting flap adaptation. Proper flap adaptation with primary interproximal closure is critical; without it one will end up with "poor results with residual inflamed and deep periodontal pockets."
11. Interrupted sutures are used to adapt tissue tightly to teeth (Fig. 3-8J). Figure 3-8K shows that when suturing, a deep bite of tissue is not taken, so as to prevent interproximal buckling of margins. *Note:* This is sometimes difficult, if not impossible, with thin tissue. The procedure is outlined clinically in Figures 3-9 through 3-11.

Scaling, Root Planing, and Curettage

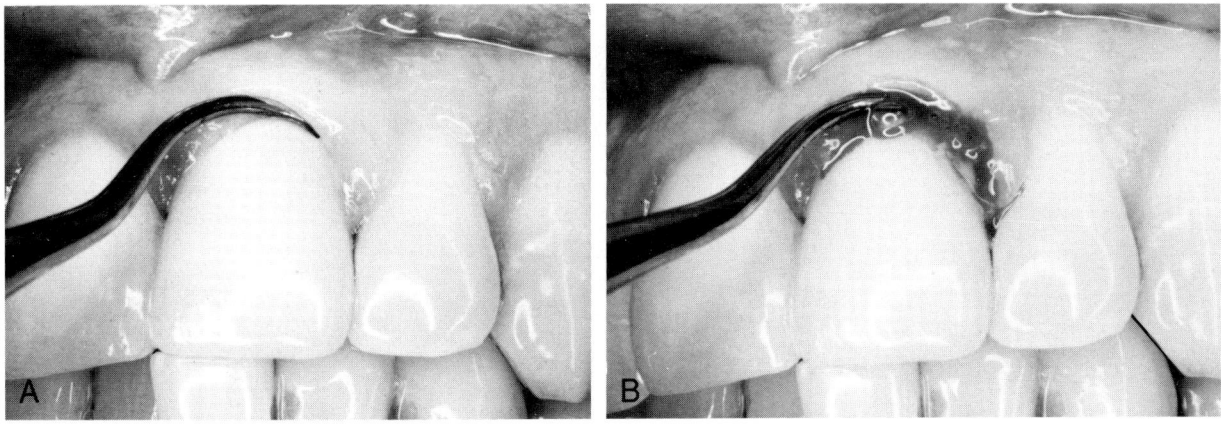

Fig. 3-1. Removal of Sulcular Tissue Wall. **A,** Scaler inserted. **B,** Removal of inflamed pocket wall.

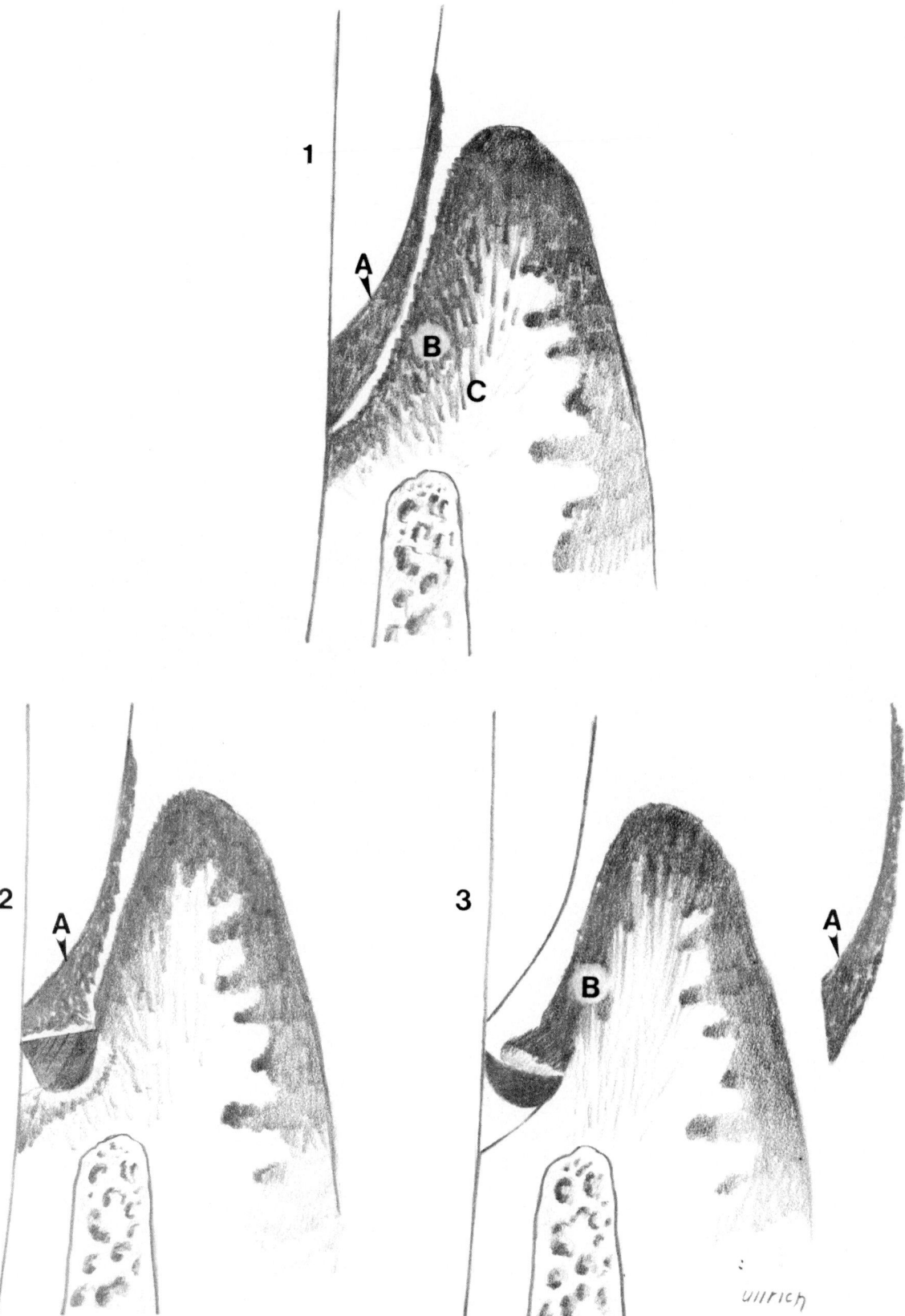

Fig. 3-2. Scaling and Curettage Technique. **1,** Represents the three zones that must be removed—Zone A: subgingival plaque and calculus; Zone B: sulcular epithelium and epithelial attachment; Zone C: inflamed connective tissue wall of pocket. **2,** Scaler in position to remove Zone A. **3,** Zone A removed and curette in position to remove Zone B.

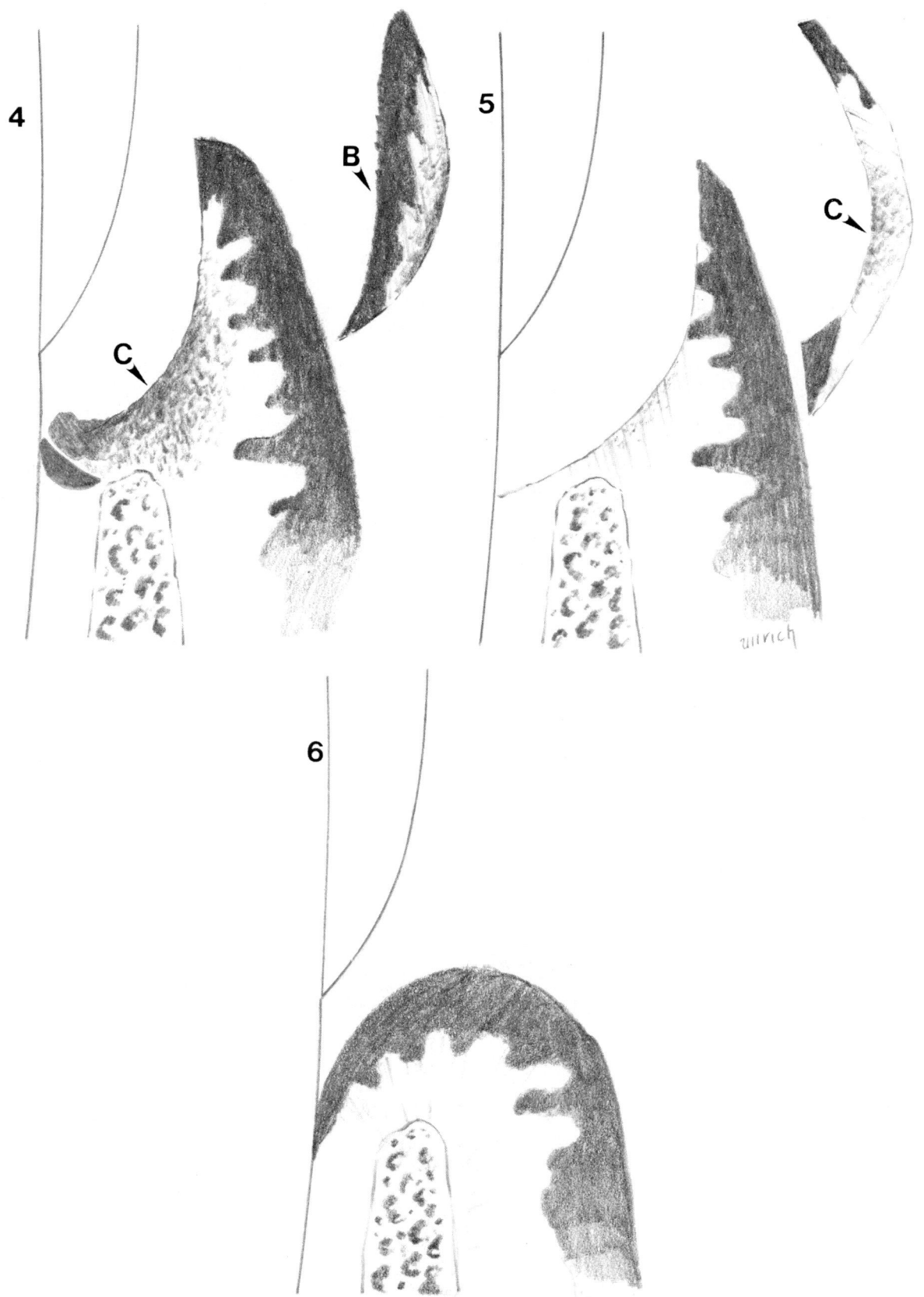

Fig. 3-2 (continued). **4,** Zone B removed and curette positioned to remove Zone C. **5,** Zone C removed and only healthy tissue remains. **6,** Healed tissue. Shrinkage has resulted in pocket elimination.

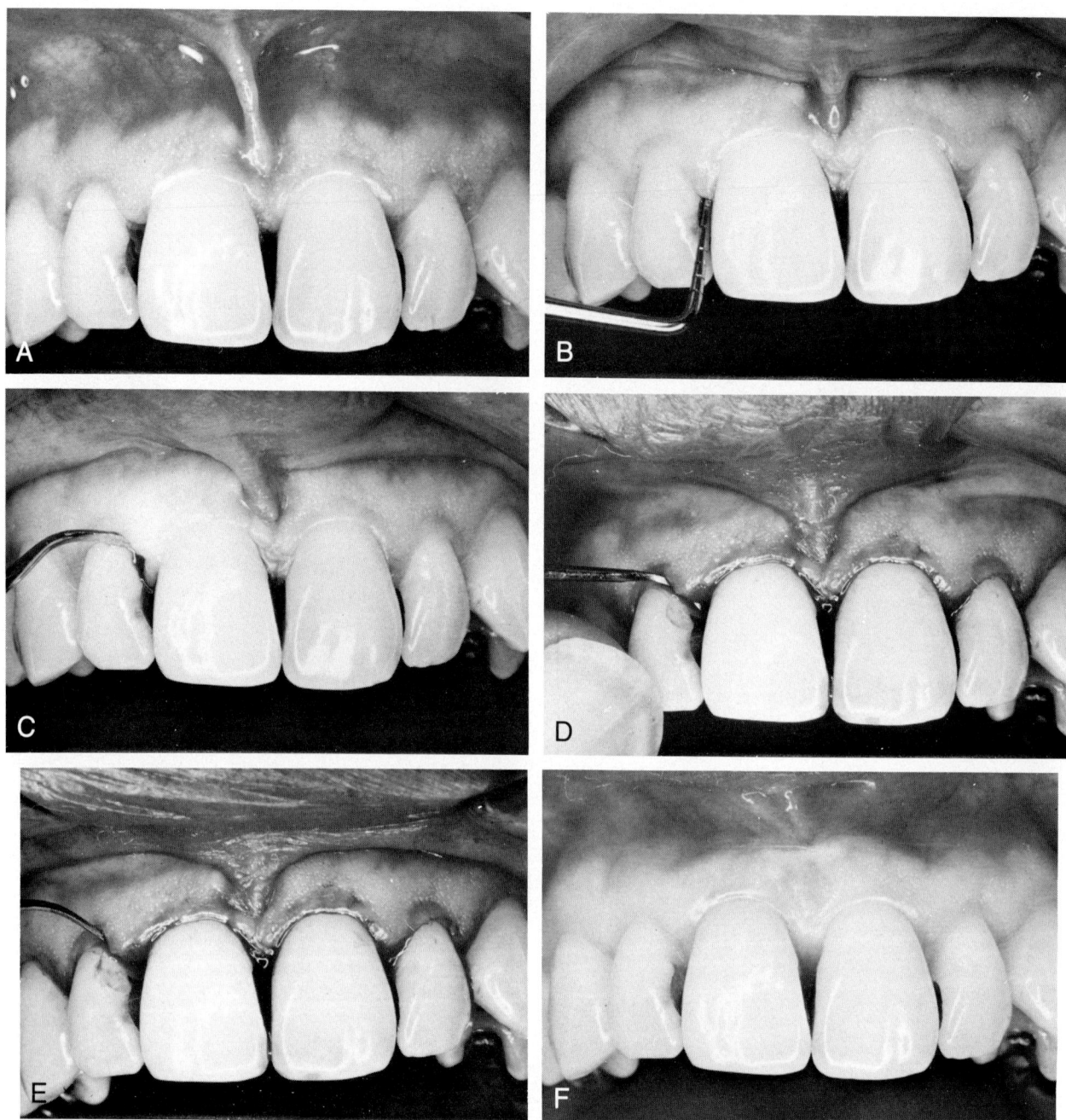

Fig. 3-3. Scaling and Curettage Procedure. **A,** Inflamed, enlarged edematous tissue. **B,** Probe showing pocketing of 3 to 5 mm. **C,** Curettage begun with open face of scaler toward the tissue. **D,** Scaling and root planing are begun with scaler inserted at 45° angle to tooth. **E,** Scaler moved in upward pulling motion. **F,** Two months after treatment. Note shrinkage of tissue and excellent contour.

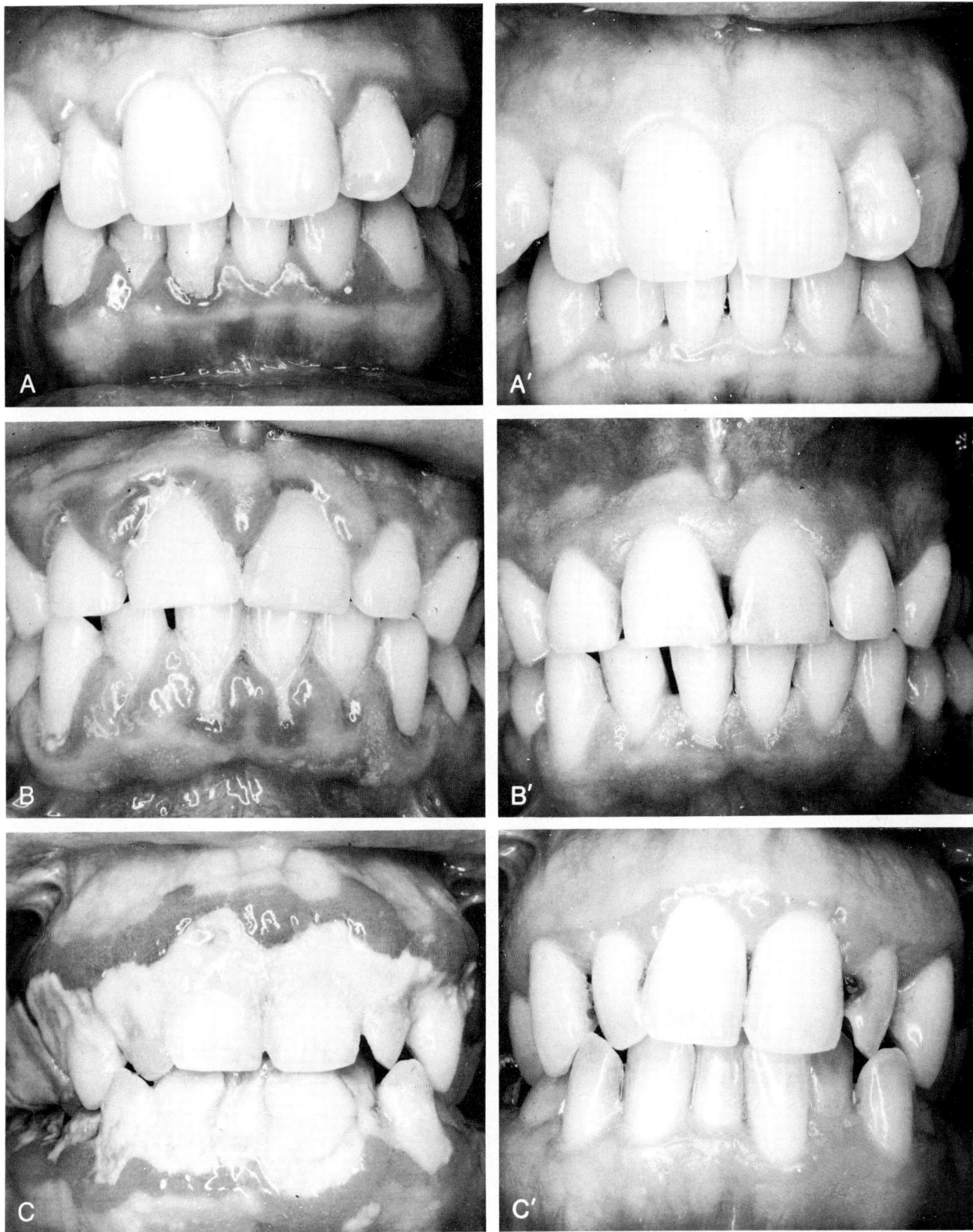

Fig. 3-4. Results obtainable with Scaling and Curettage. **A, B, C,** Before. **A′, B′, C′,** After.

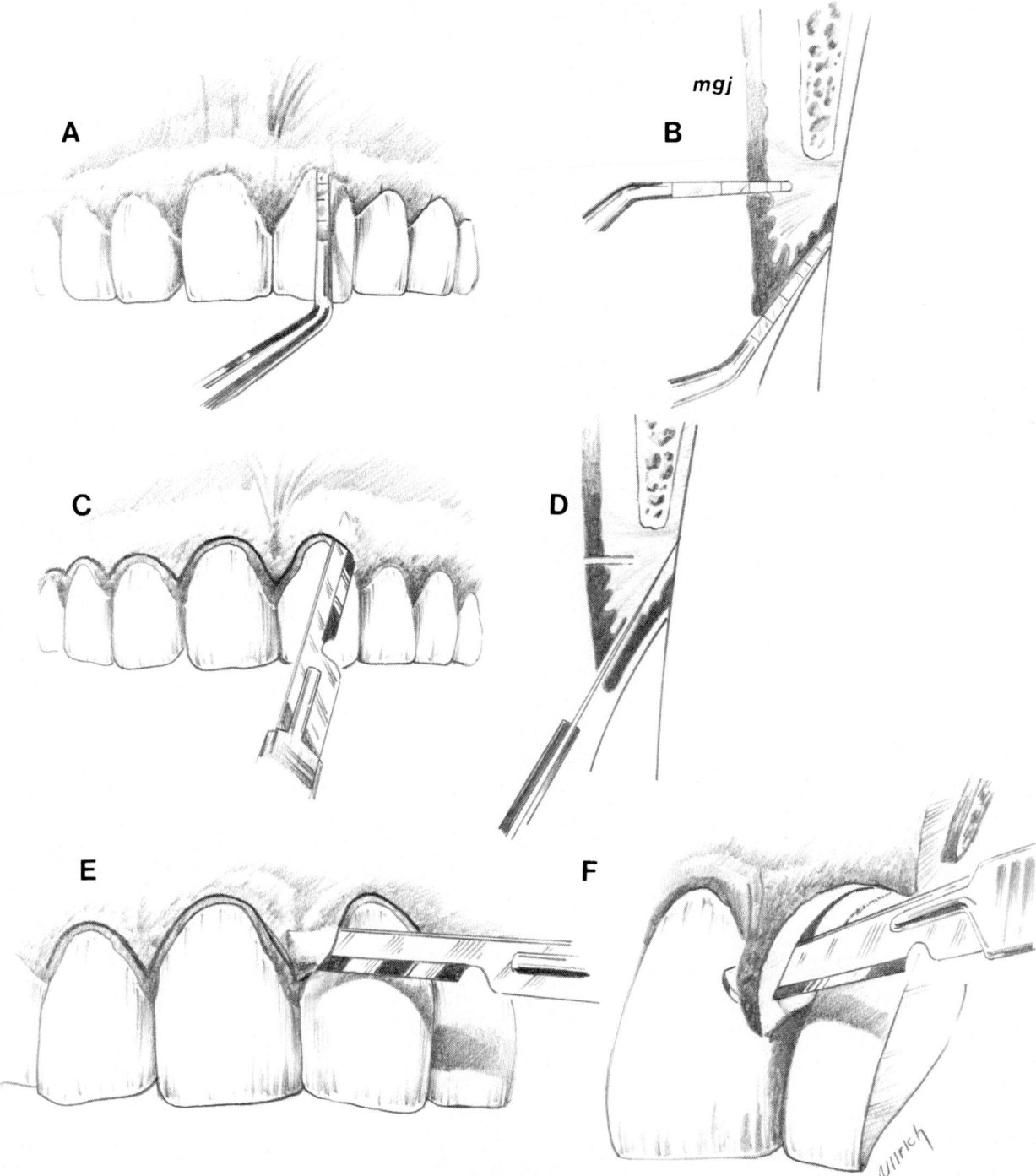

Fig. 3-5. Excisional New Attachment Procedure. **A, B,** Preoperative views showing suprabony pockets and an adequate zone of keratinized attached gingiva. **C,** A scalloped labial incision is made at the crest of the gingiva. **D,** The incision is carried down to the base of the pocket. **E, F,** Facial and cross-sectional (CX) views showing that the interproximal papillae are partially dissected to remove the thick triangular wedge of tissue. In effect, the papillae are treated as a partial-thickness flap.

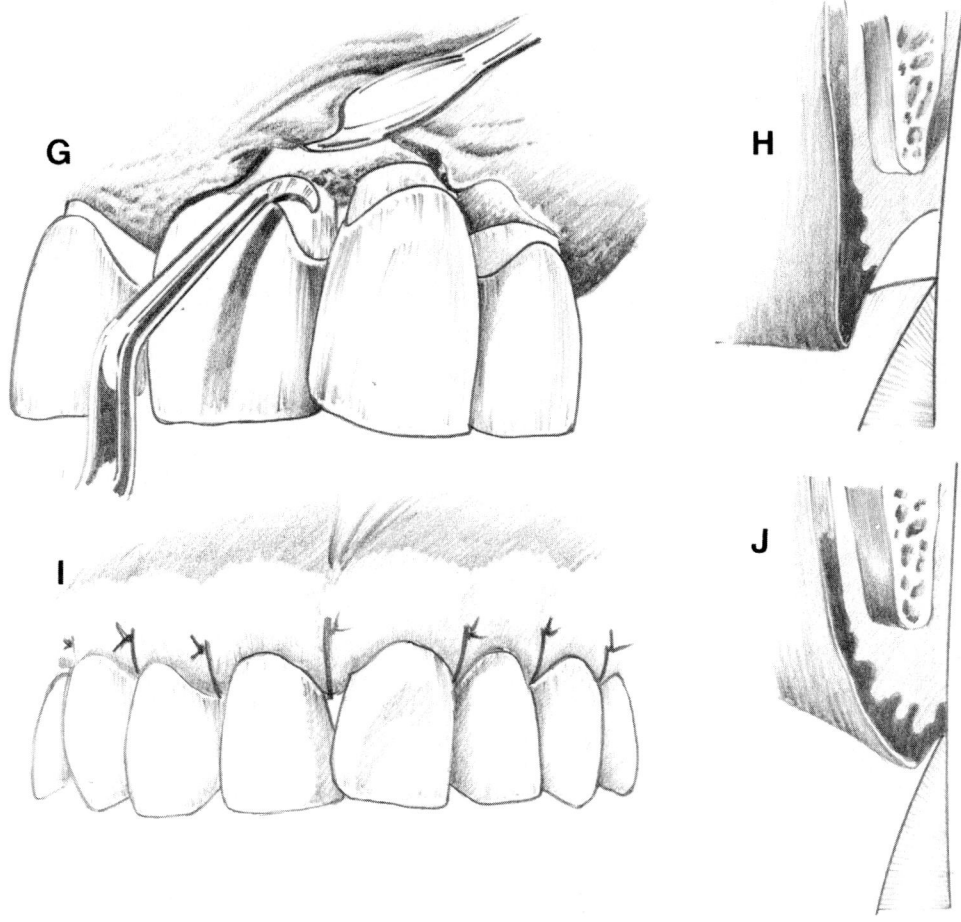

Fig. 3-5 (continued). **G,** The papillae are reflected slightly for access and the root is scaled and root planed. **H,** CX view showing the inflamed inner wall removed and the root scaled. **I,** Flap sutured at presurgical height. **J,** Healed tissue with pockets eliminated as a result of shrinkage and tight adaptation to the tooth.

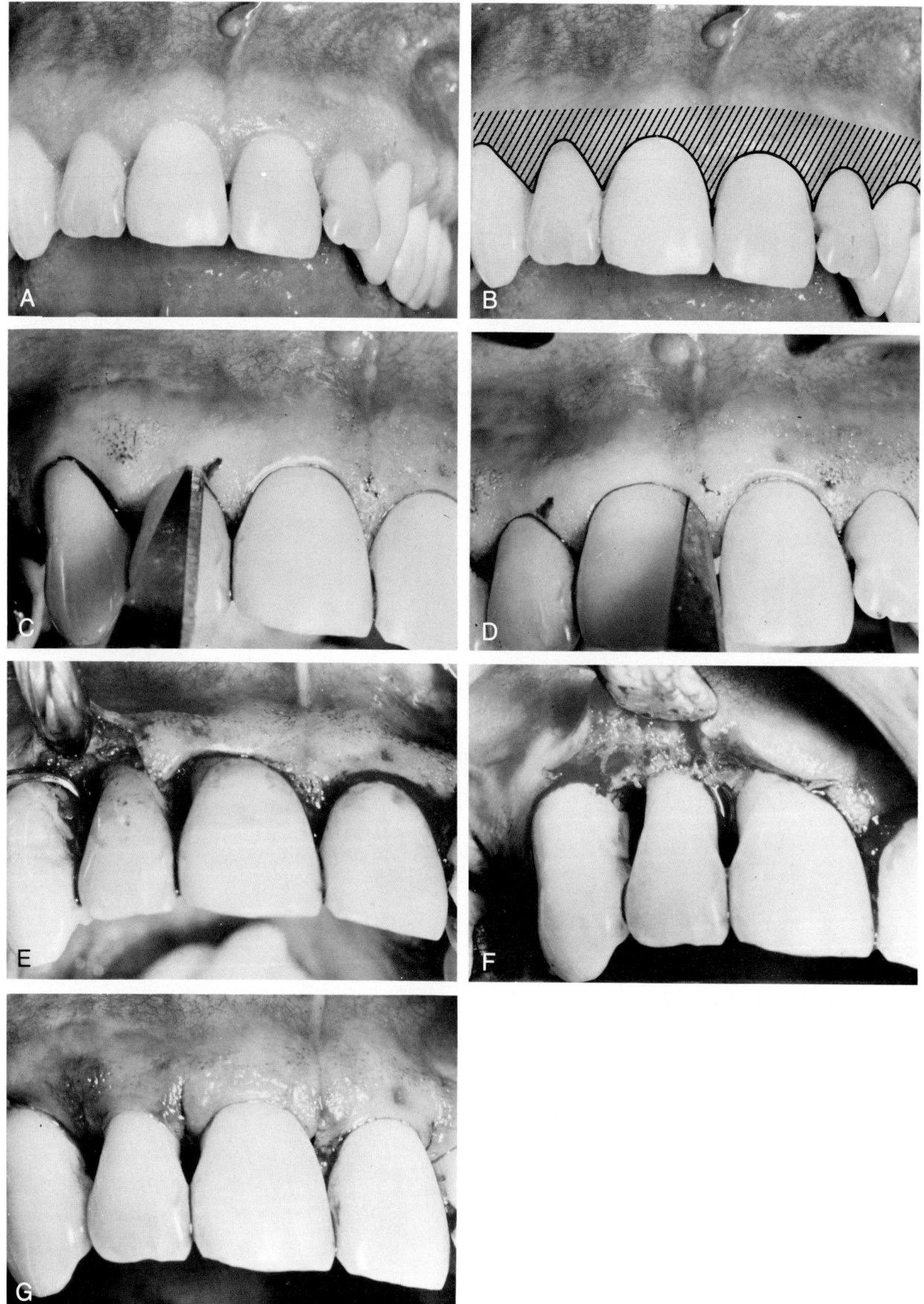

Fig. 3-6. Excisional New Attachment Procedure (E.N.A.P.). **A,** Before. **B,** Scalloped sulcular incision outlined. Lined portion shows that only a mini-flap is raised. **C,** Sulcular incision made to base of pocket with No. 11 blade. **D,** Continuation of incision interdentally. **E,** Flap reflected, exposing root; scaler inserted. **F,** Scaling completed and all granulation tissue removed. **G,** Interrupted suture placed.

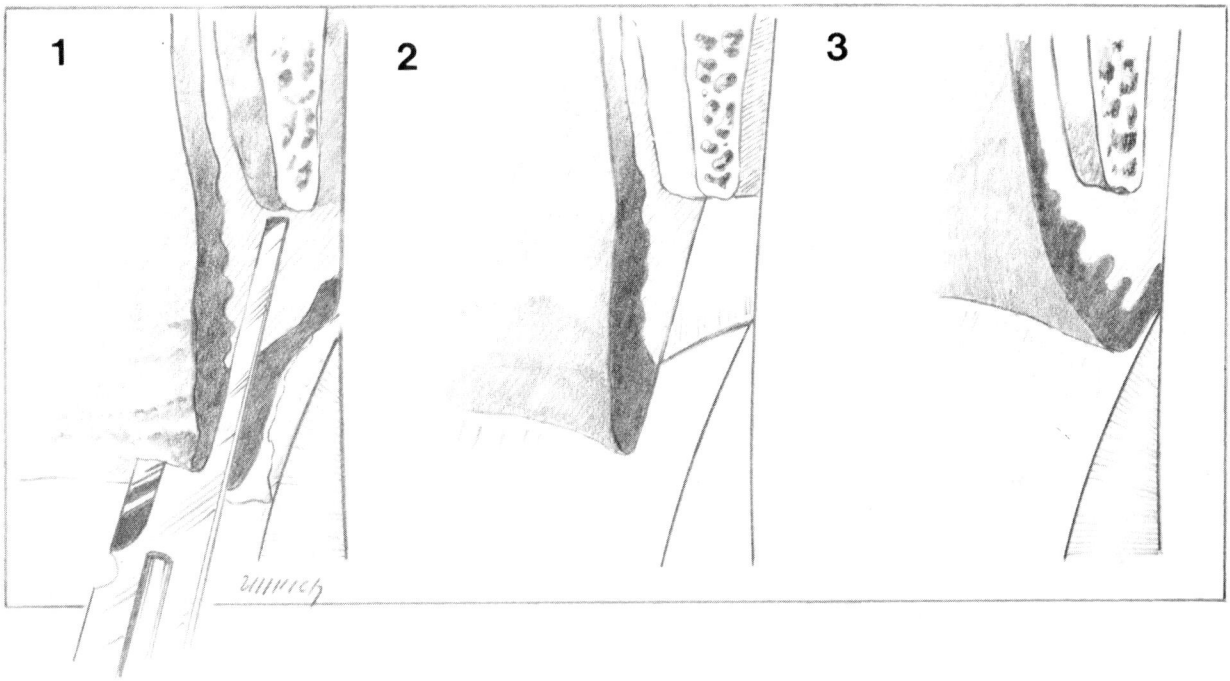

Fig. 3-7. Modification of E.N.A.P. **1,** Initial incision made to crest of bone instead of base of pocket. **2,** Inner wall removed down to crest of bone and periodontal ligament space. **3,** Healed tissue.

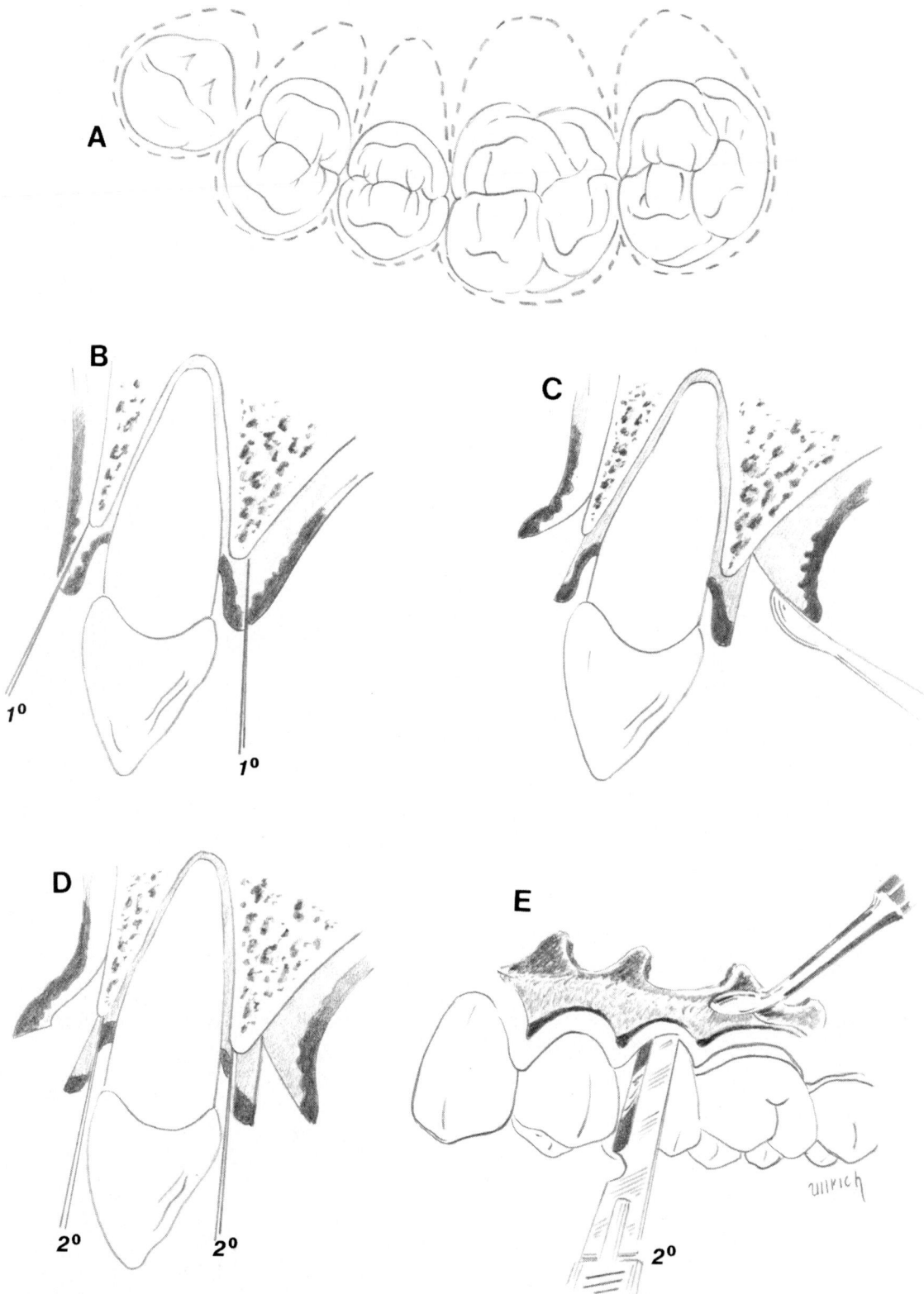

Fig. 3-8. Modified Widman flap. **A,** Outline of basic incision with exaggerated palatal scalloping to assure primary closure. **B,** Primary incisions made down to bone. **C,** The flap is reflected to expose only 2 to 3 mm of bone. **D,** A secondary sulcular incision is made to release the inner flap. **E,** Facial view, showing reflection of flap and secondary incision.

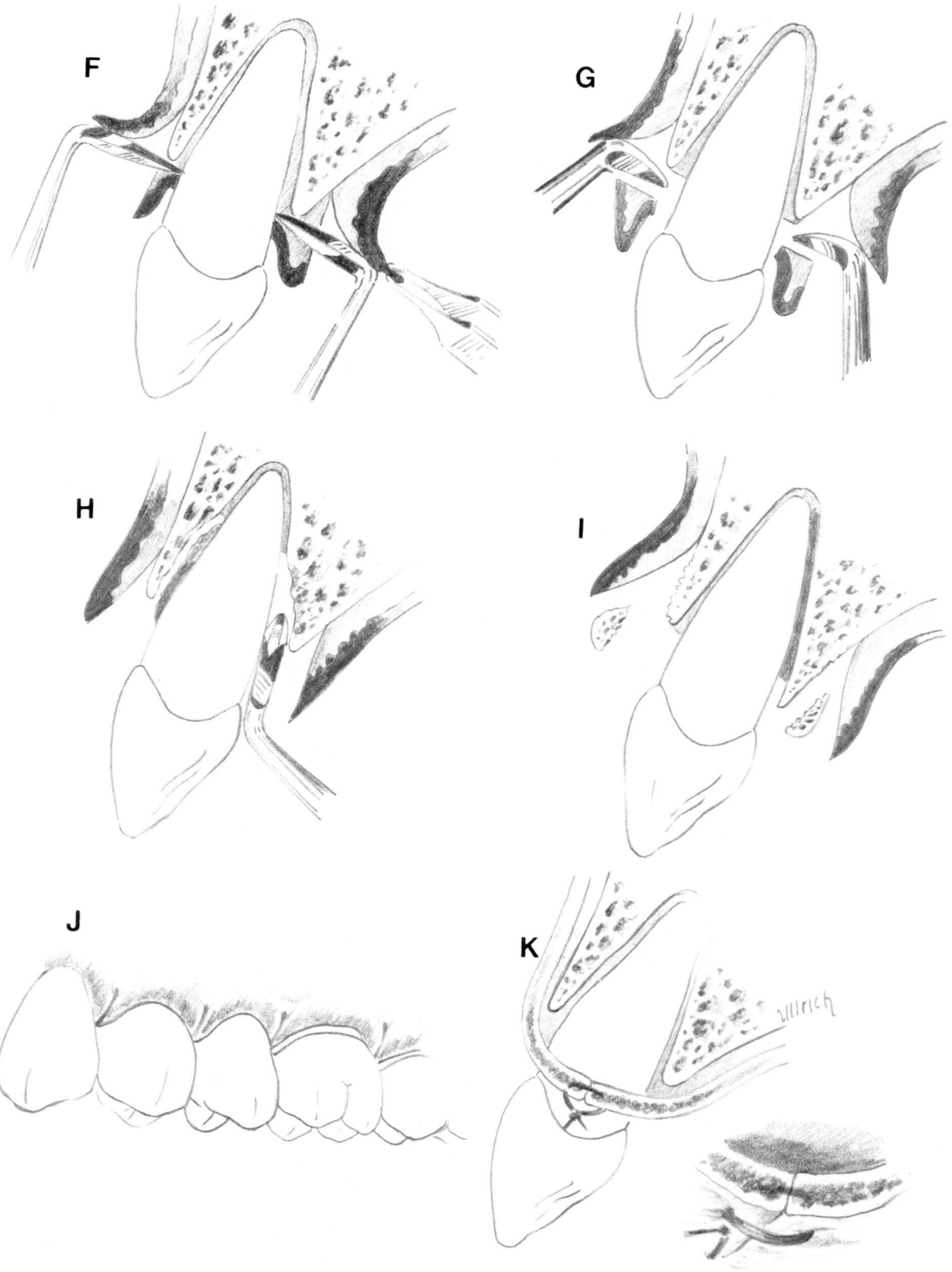

Fig. 3-8 (continued). **F,** A sharp periodontal knife is used to sever remaining collar of tissue above the crest of bone and loosen the tissue interproximally. **G,** Scalers are used to remove the inner flap. **H,** Intrabony defects are scaled and curetted if present. **I,** Osteoplasty is performed to remove bone ledges that inhibit flap placement. **J, K,** The flaps are sutured tightly without taking a deep bite of the tissue.

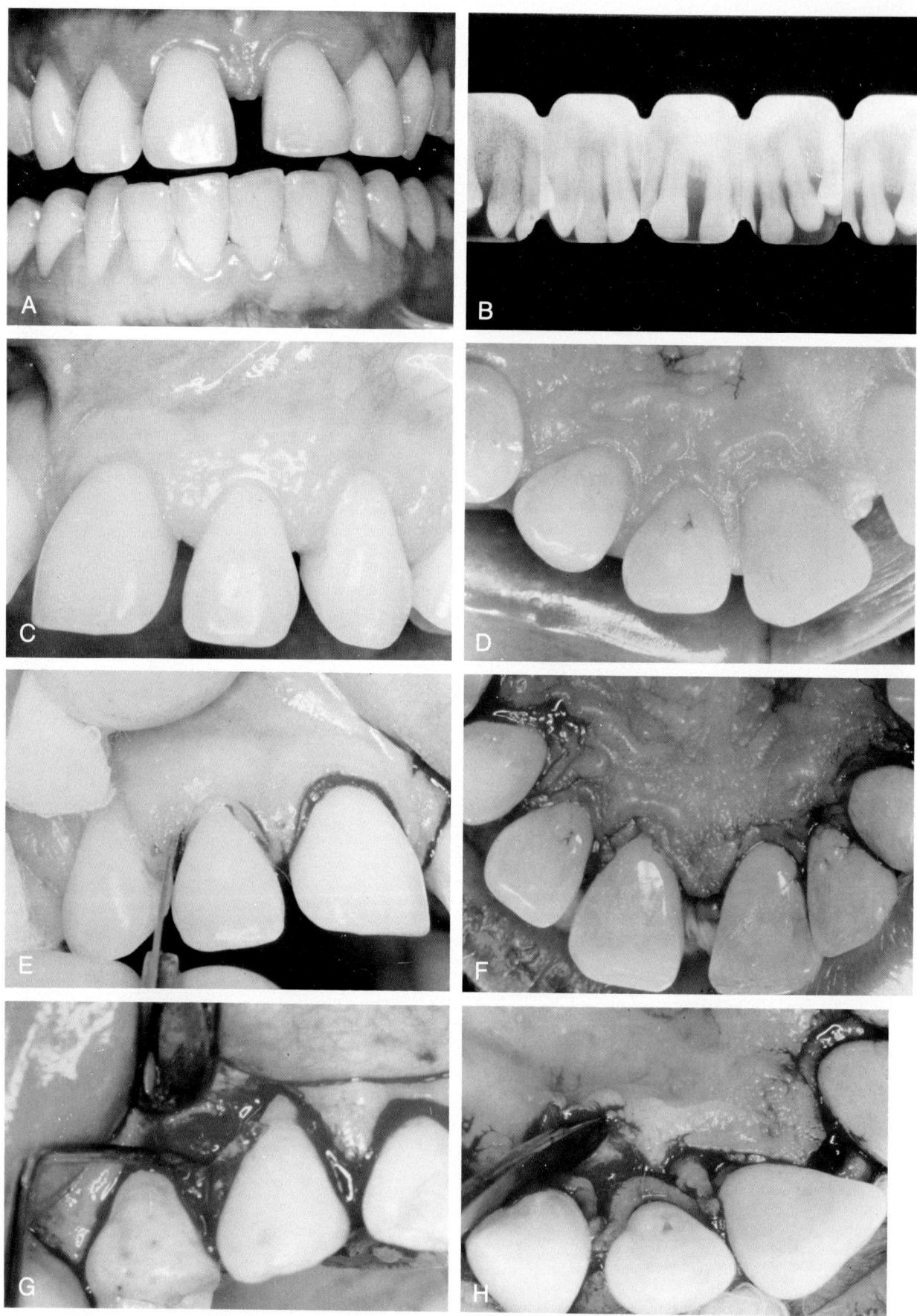

Fig. 3-9. Modified Widman flap. **A,** Before treatment. **B,** Pretreatment x-rays showing moderate bone loss. **C, D,** Close-up view of buccal and palatal tissue. **E,** Initial scalloped incision with maximum conservation of interproximal tissue. **F,** Palatal view after initial incisions. **G,** Mucoperiosteal flap reflected with horizontal cutting incision being made. **H,** Palatal view with flap reflected.

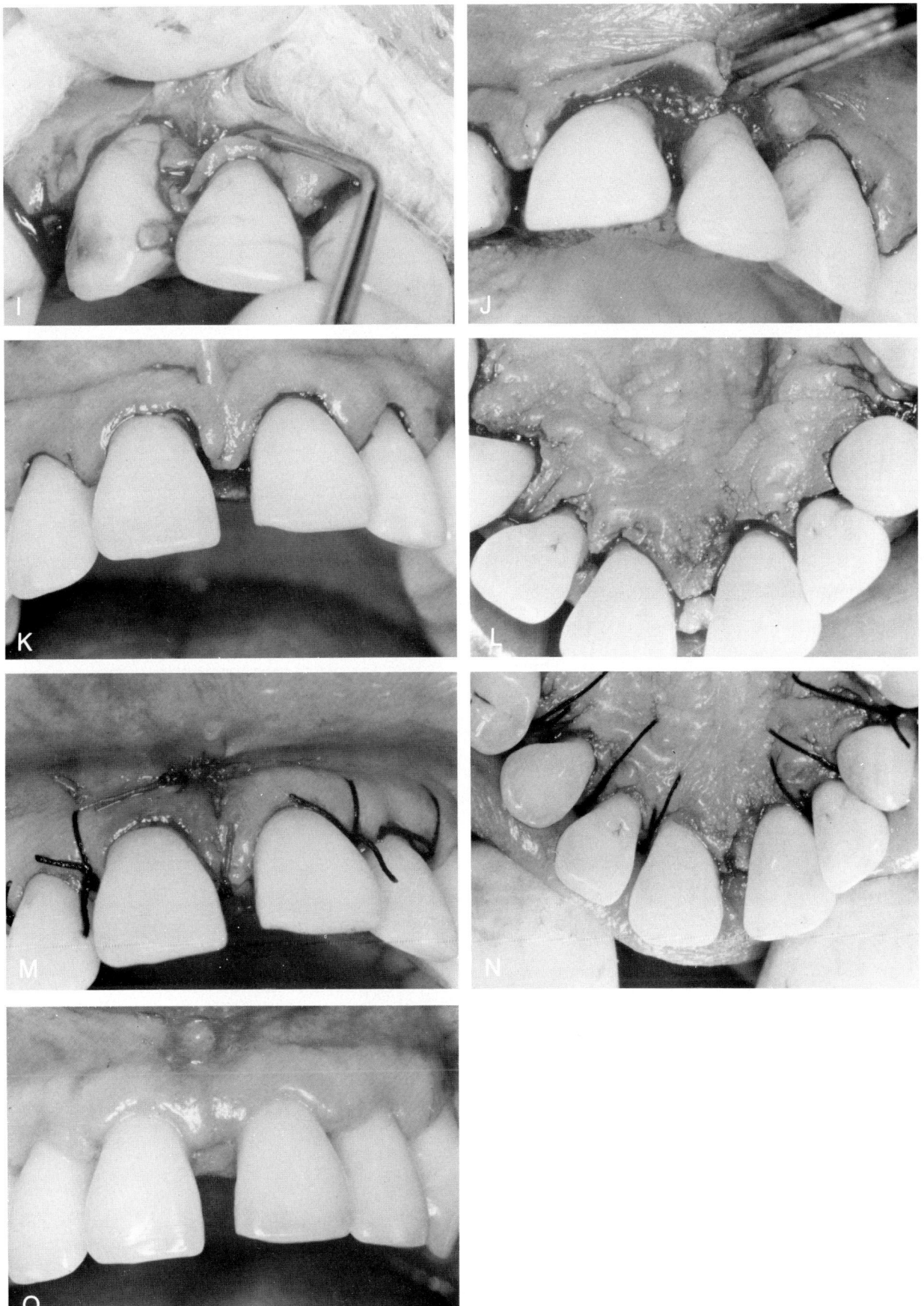

Fig. 3-9 (continued). **I,** Removal of secondary flap. **J,** Secondary inner flap removed and teeth sealed and root planed. Note that only 2 to 3 mm of bone have been exposed. **K, L,** Buccal and palatal views after completion of degranulation, scaling, and root planing. Note that maximum conservation of tissue will permit primary closure. **M, N,** Buccal and palatal views of completed interrupted suturing. **O,** Six weeks later. Note interproximal tissue craters. (Contributed by Giovanni Castellucci, Boston, MA).

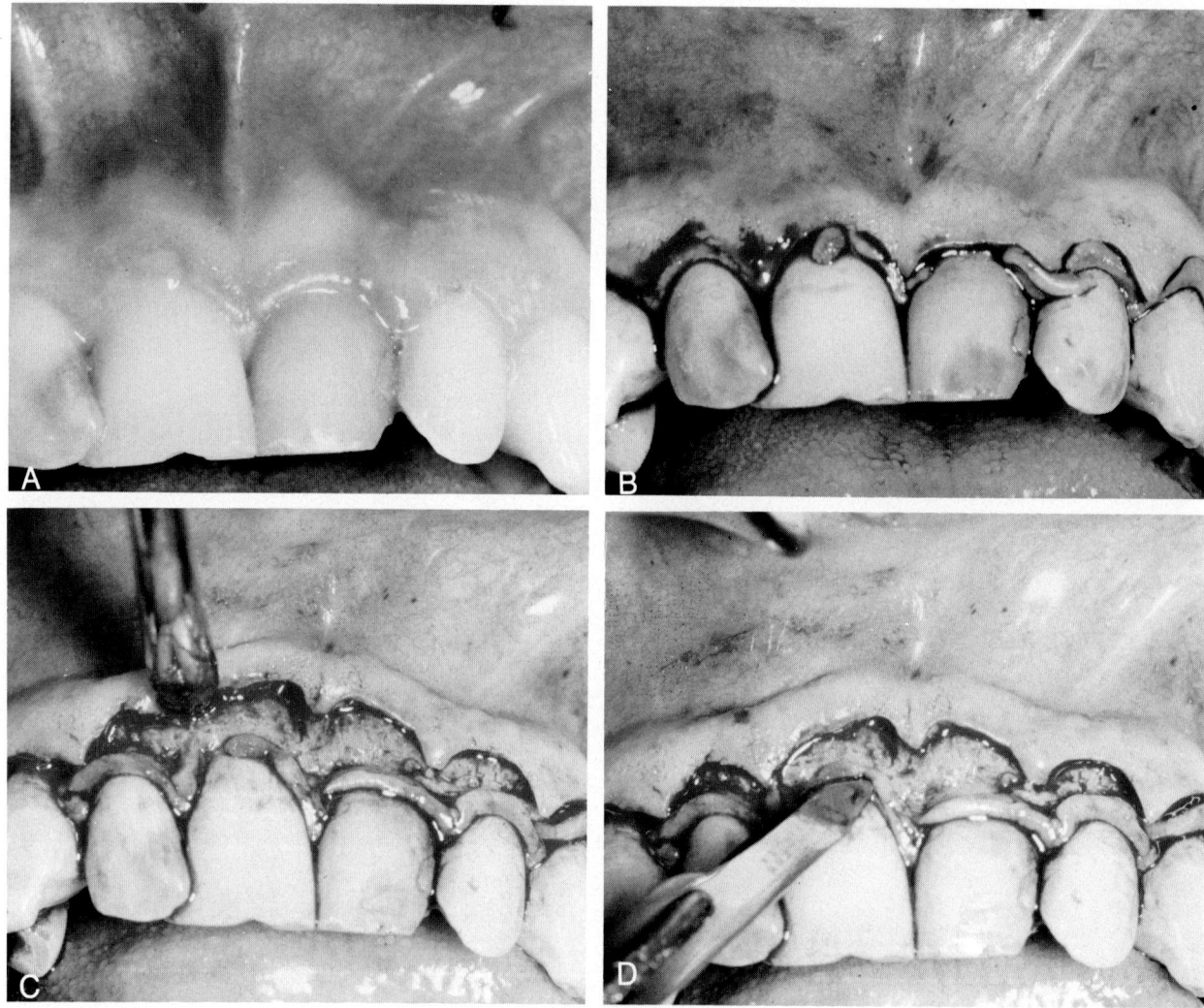

Fig. 3-10. Modified Widman Flap. **A,** Before treatment. **B,** Initial scalloped, inverse beveled incision completed. Note maximum conservation of interproximal tissue. **C,** Mucoperiosteal flap reflected to expose 2 to 3 mm of bone. **D,** Secondary sulcular incision.

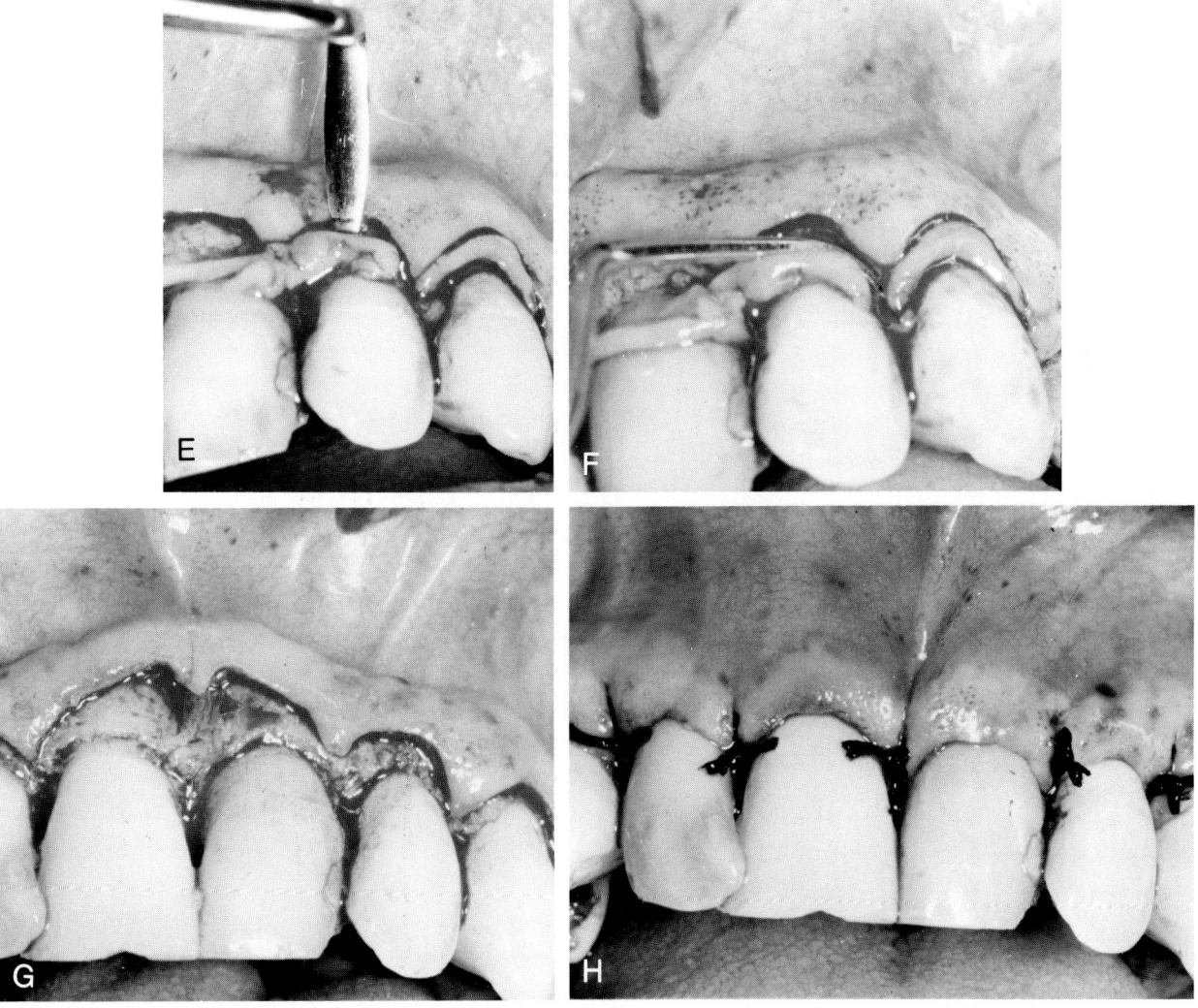

Fig. 3-10 (continued). **E,** Horizontal cutting incision to free secondary flap. **F,** Secondary flap being removed. **G,** Inner flap removed, and teeth scaled and root planed. **H,** Flap sutured with interrupted sutures.

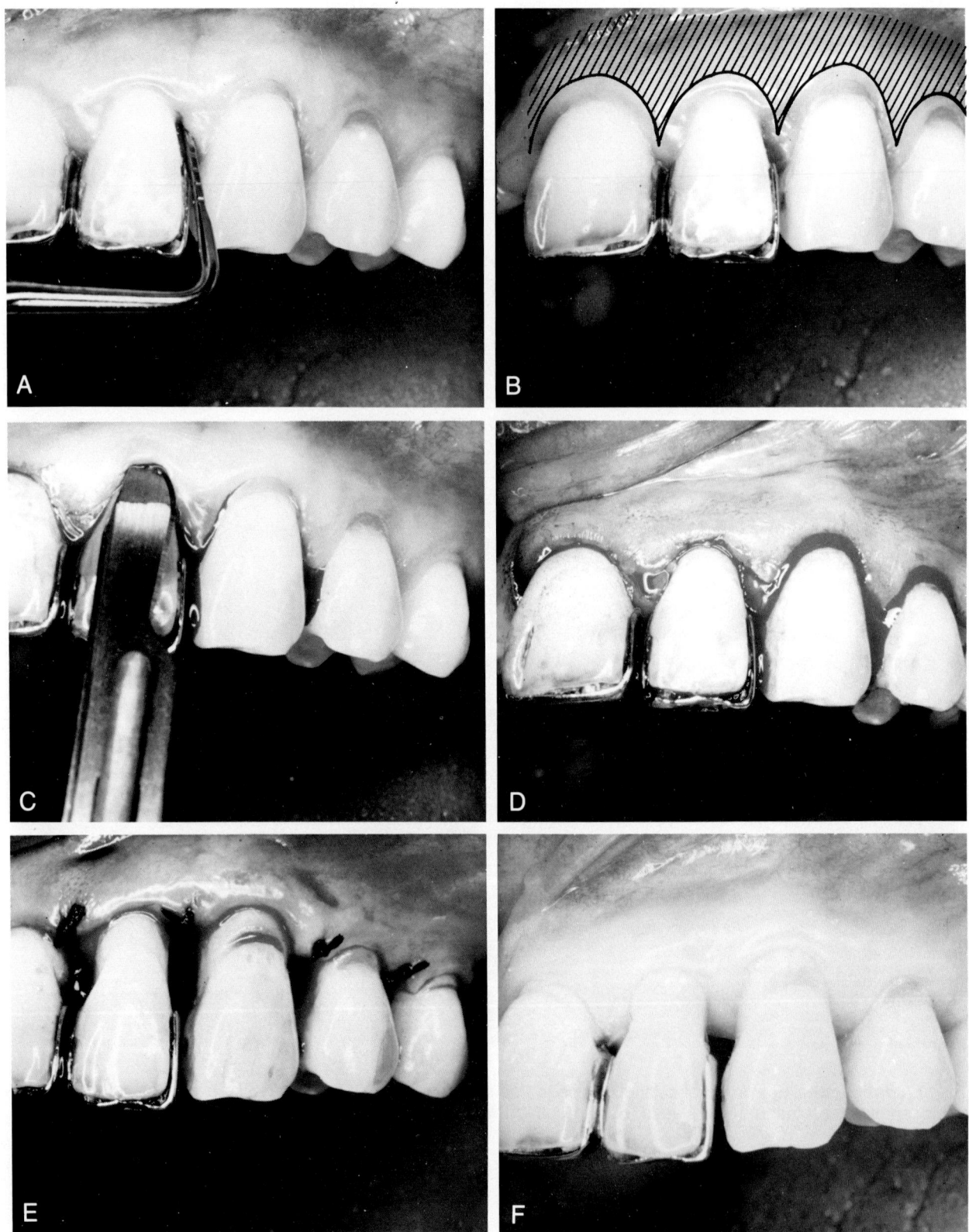

Fig. 3-11. Modified Widman Flap. **A,** Before treatment, with probe inserted showing moderate to deep pocketing. Note also enlarged edematous nature of tissue. **B,** Scalloped incision outlined with maximum conservation of interproximal tissue. **C,** Initial primary crestal, inverse beveled incision begun. **D,** Incisions completed. **E,** Secondary flap removed, scaling and curettage completed, and interproximal sutures placed. **F,** Ten months later; compare with A.

4

GINGIVECTOMY AND GINGIVOPLASTY

Gingivectomy is the excisional removal of gingival tissue for pocket reduction or elimination. The technique has, as its main advantages, simplicity and ease of mastery. *Gingivoplasty* is the reshaping of the gingiva to attain a more physiologic contour; a contour that allows a gradual rise of tissue interproximally and a fall on the labial and lingual surfaces. In gingivoplasty, the tissue is thinned interproximally to produce a more harmonious contour, with interproximal sluiceways for the easy passage of food. *Gingivectomy and gingivoplasty are usually performed at the same time.*

Rationale

1. Pocket elimination for root accessibility
2. Establish physiologic gingival contours

Indications

1. Suprabony pockets
2. An adequate zone of keratinized tissue
3. Pockets greater than 3 mm
4. When bone loss is horizontal and no need exists for osseous surgery
5. Gingival enlargements
6. Areas of limited access
7. Unesthetic or asymmetrical gingival topography
8. For exposure of soft-tissue impaction to enhance eruption
9. To facilitate restorative dentistry
10. To establish physiologic and gingival contours post acute necrotizing ulcerative gingivitis (ANUG) and flap procedures

Contraindications

1. An inadequate zone of keratinized tissue
2. Pockets that extend beyond the mucogingival line
3. The need for osseous resection or inductive techniques
4. Highly inflamed or edematous tissue
5. Areas of esthetic compromise
6. Shallow palatal vaults and prominent external oblique ridges
7. Treatment of intrabony pockets
8. Patients with poor oral hygiene

Advantages

1. Predictability
2. Simplicity
3. Ease of pocket elimination
4. Good access
5. Favorable esthetic results

Disadvantages

1. Healing by secondary intention
2. Bleeding postoperatively
3. Loss of keratinized gingiva
4. Inability to treat underlying osseous deformities

GINGIVECTOMY

Presurgical Phase

Presurgical preparation is carried out to reduce gross inflammation and remove local factors (calculus, plaque, or overhanging restorations). After initial healing, the zone of attached tissue can be assessed properly. At the time of operation, adequate local anesthesia is given. A vasoconstrictor should be used for control of hemorrhage, especially since healing is by secondary intention.

Under anesthesia, the pockets are probed to check their depth and make sure they do not extend beyond the mucogingival junction (Fig. 4-1A). By sounding, the osseous topography is determined and the need for osseous surgery determined (Fig. 4-1B).

Gingivectomy is contraindicated if osseous surgery is needed.

Pocket Marking

A *pocket marker* or *periodontal probe* is used to outline the base of the pockets with a series of small bleeding points (Fig. 4-1C). Three points (mesial, distal, and buccal) are marked on each buccal and lingual surface. These marks delineate the pocket wall to be removed.

The pocket marker is placed into the pocket and held parallel to the tooth. When the base of the pocket is reached, the tissue is marked (Fig. 4-1D). Once the bleeding points have been established, they form a dotted line that outlines the incision. The pocket marker must not be tilted or the incision will be too deep or too shallow (Fig. 4-1D).

Incisions

Incisions may be either *continuous* (Fig. 4-1E,H,I) or *discontinuous* (Fig. 4-1F,G). Both incisions are begun on the most terminal tooth and continued around until the incision is complete. No real differences exist between incisions except that one is an interrupted incision ending in the papillary area of each successive tooth until the incision is completed.

Incisions can be made with scalpels or gingivectomy knives, although the gingivectomy knife is easier to use because of the angulation and shape of the blade. The heel of the knife is used for the primary incision, which begins just apical to the bleeding points (Fig. 4-1J). The blade is held in such a manner that the incision is as close to the bone as possible for total pocket removal and production of a tissue bevel of 45°. The blade must pass fully through the tissue to the tooth.

An Orban or Kirkland interproximal knife is used to free the tissue interproximally. It is placed interdentally at a 45° angle both buccally and lingually until the tissue is freed (Fig. 4-1K,L). The knife also engages the tooth to free the tissue at the line angle. If the incisions have been made properly, the tissue can be removed in one strip. Figure 4-1M shows the correct and incorrect incision placements.

Once free, the tissue is removed by using a hoe or heavy scalers (Fig. 4-1N). Small scalers and curettes are now used for scaling and root planing to remove residual granulation tissue, calculus, and soft cementum (Fig. 4-1O).

GINGIVOPLASTY

The final contour of the tissue is established using scissors, tissue nippers, or diamond stones (Fig. 4-1P,Q). This final contouring, or *gingivoplasty*, is used to thin the tissue on the interradicular surfaces and establishes a more fluid contour. The healed tissue (Fig. 4-1R) will be thin, with a scalloped architecture that flows smoothly from the interdental areas onto the interradicular surfaces for easy passage of food.

The complete procedure is outlined clinically in Figure 4-2, and the results that can be attained are shown in Figure 4-3.

EDENTULOUS, RETROMOLAR, AND TUBEROSITY AREAS

The edentulous area between teeth is noteworthy only in that the incision should stretch the entire length of the space. Pockets tend to re-form if the incision is limited to an area adjacent to the teeth (Fig. 4-4).

The retromolar (Fig. 4-5) and tuberosity (Fig. 4-6) areas are blended with the buccal and lingual (palatal) incisions. In the retromolar area, gingivectomy is done only if there is adequate keratinized tissue distal to the tooth. The incision is flat or beveled to the base of the pocket.

COMMON REASONS FOR FAILURE

Wade (1954) outlined 15 reasons why gingivectomies fail, most of which are still valid today.
1. Unsuitable case selection. Cases with underlying osseous irregularities or intrabony defects
2. Incorrect pocket markings
3. Incomplete pocket elimination
4. Insufficient beveling of the incision
5. Failure to remove tissue tags, resulting in excessive (granulation) tissue
6. Failure to remove etiologic factors—calculus and plaque
7. Beginning or terminating the incision in a papilla

8. Failure to eliminate or control the predisposing factors
9. Inaccessible interdental spaces
10. Loose dressings
11. Lost dressings
12. Insufficient use of dressings
13. Failure to prescribe stimulators or rubber tipping for interproximal use
14. Failure to use stimulators or rubber tip
15. Failure to complete treatment

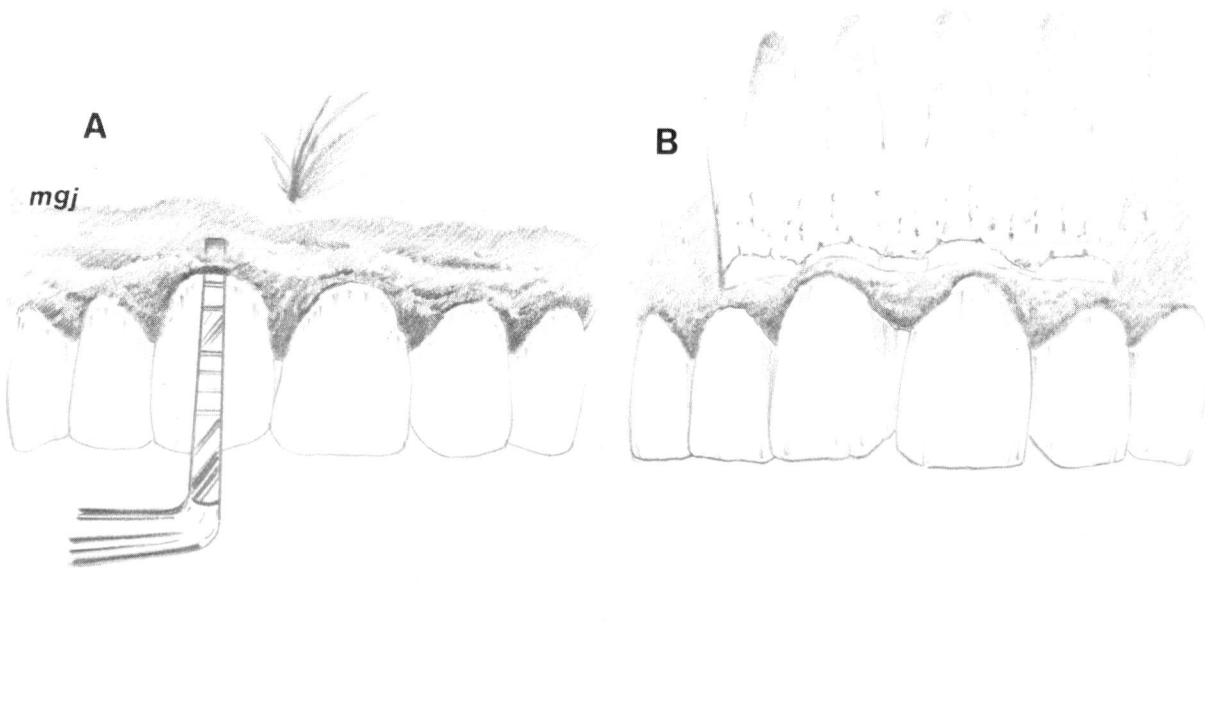
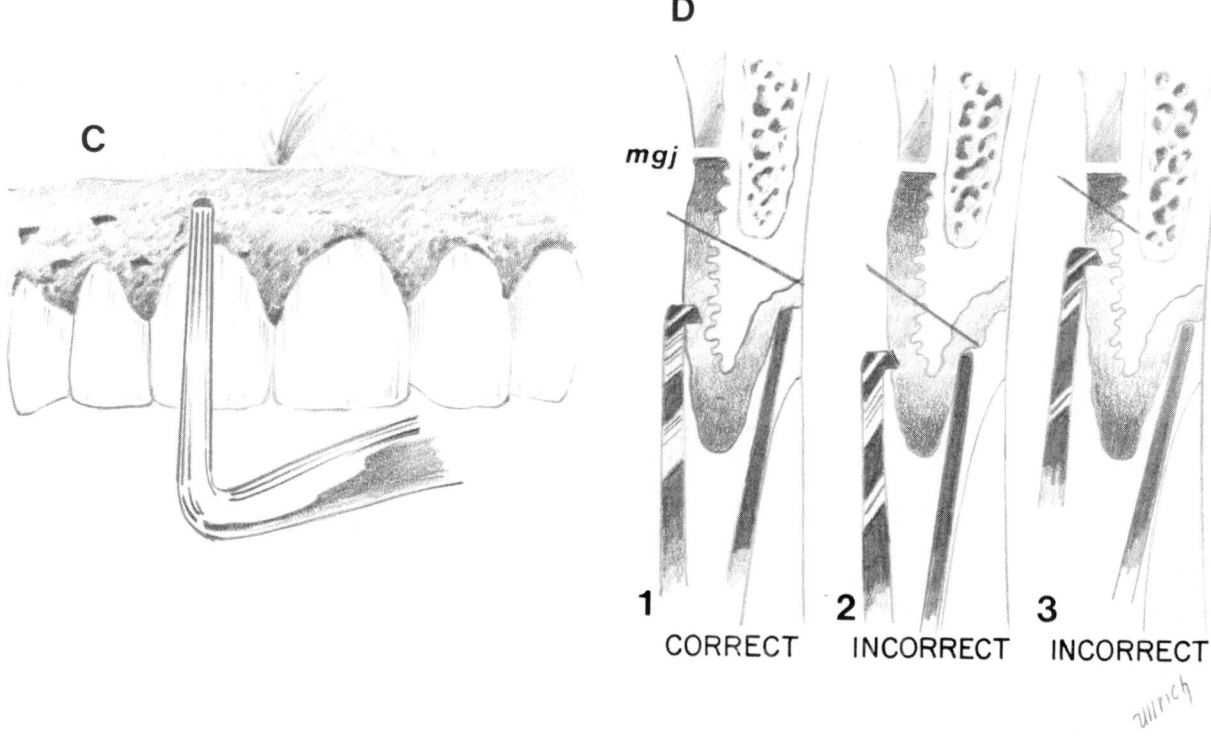

Fig. 4-1. Gingivectomy Technique. **A,** Represents enlarged gingival tissue with pocketing. **B,** Cutaway showing horizontal bone loss. **C,** Use of pocket markers to establish bleeding points for incisions outlined. **D,** Shows correct and incorrect placement of pocket markers and how incisions are affected: **1,** Correct marking with beveled incision to base of pocket; **2,** Incorrect shallow marking, resulting in incision above base of pocket; and **3,** Incorrect deep incision, resulting in bone exposure and possible removal of all attached gingiva.

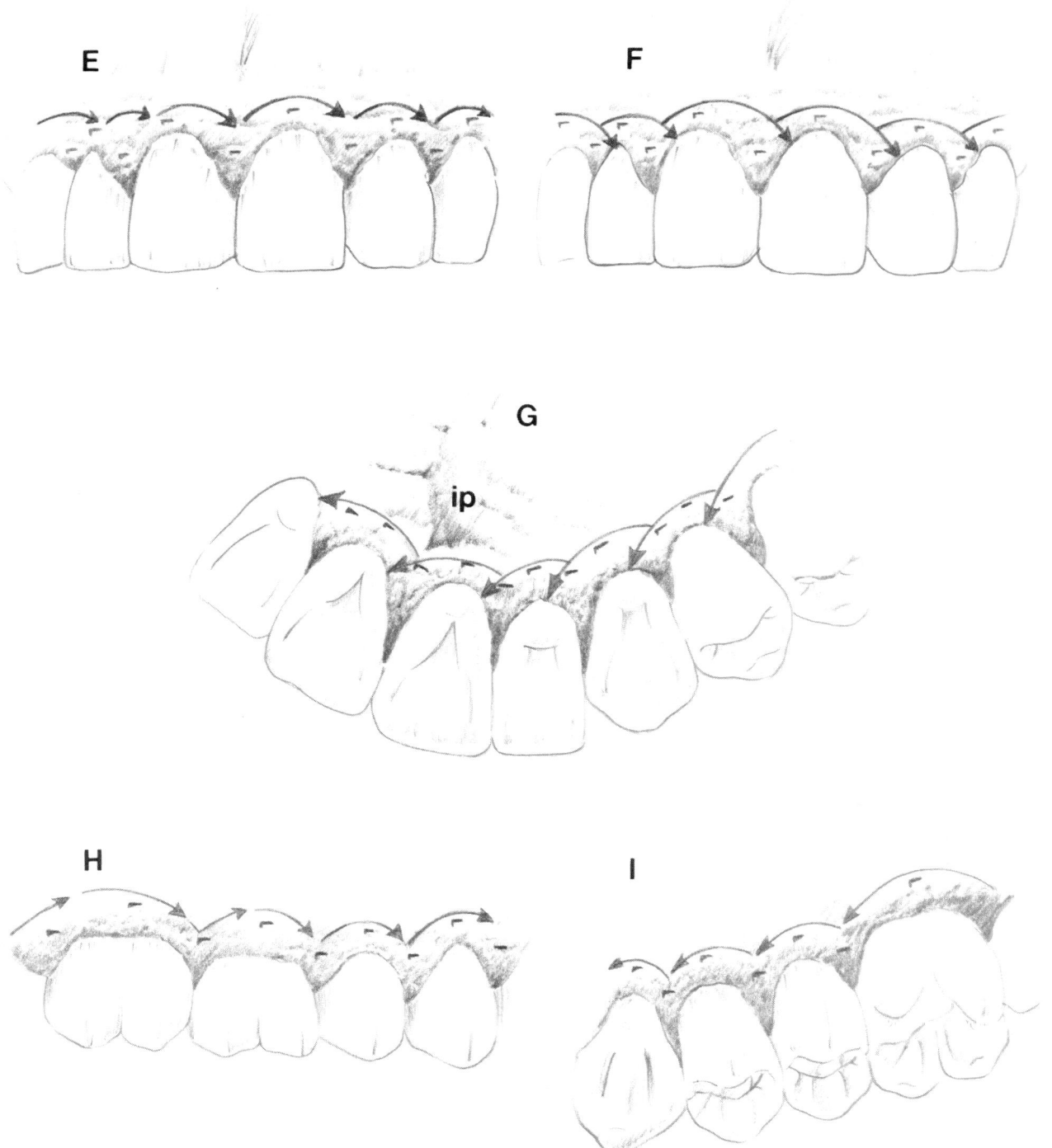

Fig. 4-1 (continued). **E,** Continuous incision on buccal aspect. Note how incisions follow outline of bleeding points. **F,** Discontinuous incision. **G,** Palatal incision. Note that the incisal papilla (ip) is outlined or avoided in this area. **H,** Continuous incision extending from tuberosity area onto the buccal aspect of teeth. **I,** Continuous incision on the palatal surface.

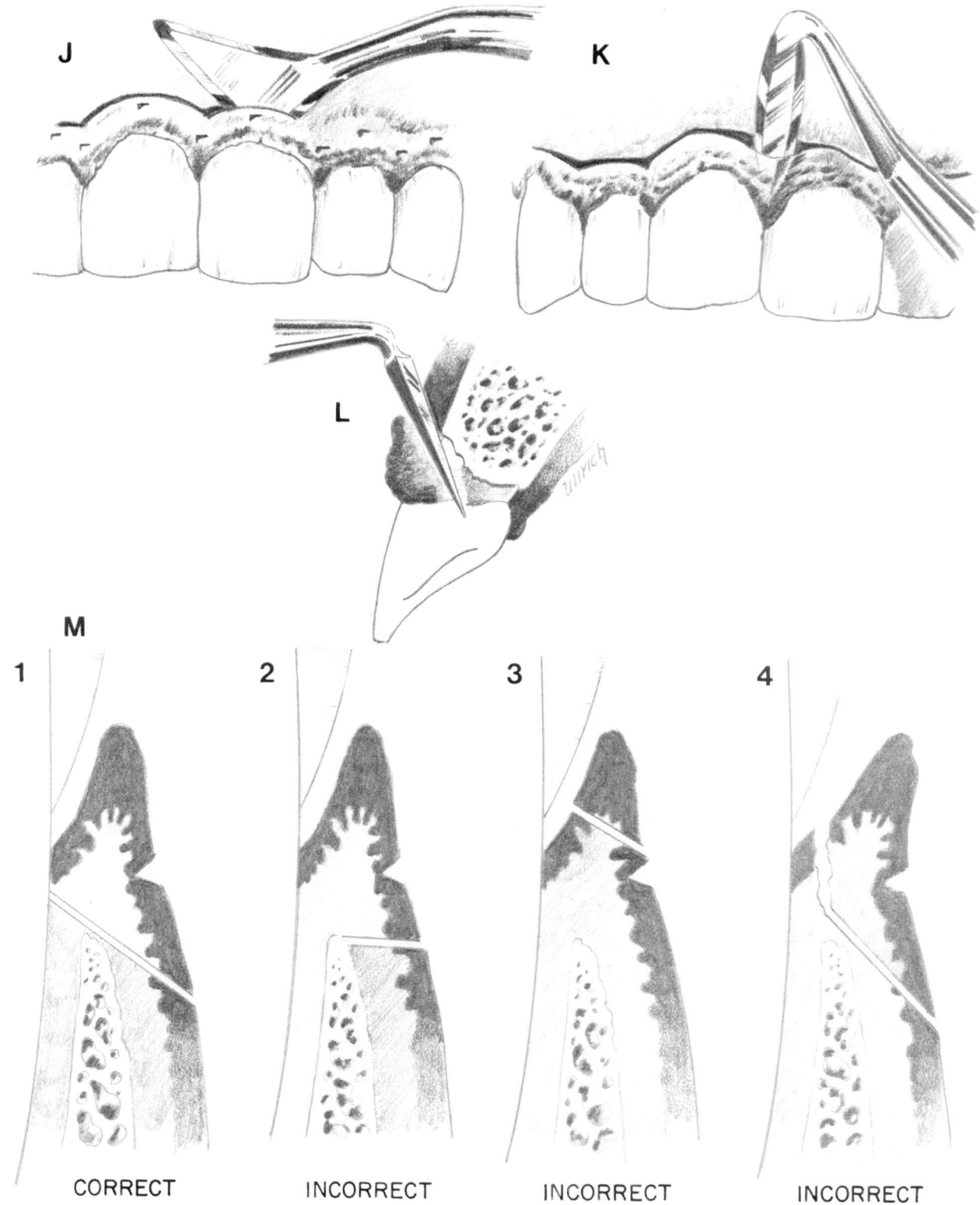

Fig. 4-1 (continued). **J,** Periodontal knife angulated at 45°, following continuous incision outline. **K,** Interproximal knife used to separate and detach tissue buccolingually. **L,** Proper angulation of interproximal knife to permit soft-tissue coverage. **M,** Incision. **1,** Correct incision beveled above bone to base of pocket; **2,** Incorrect incision; no bevel, and incision too deep, resulting in bone exposure; **3,** Incorrect shallow incision, resulting in failure to remove pocket; and **4,** Incomplete incision because of failure to carry incision to the tooth, resulting in ragged, torn tissue.

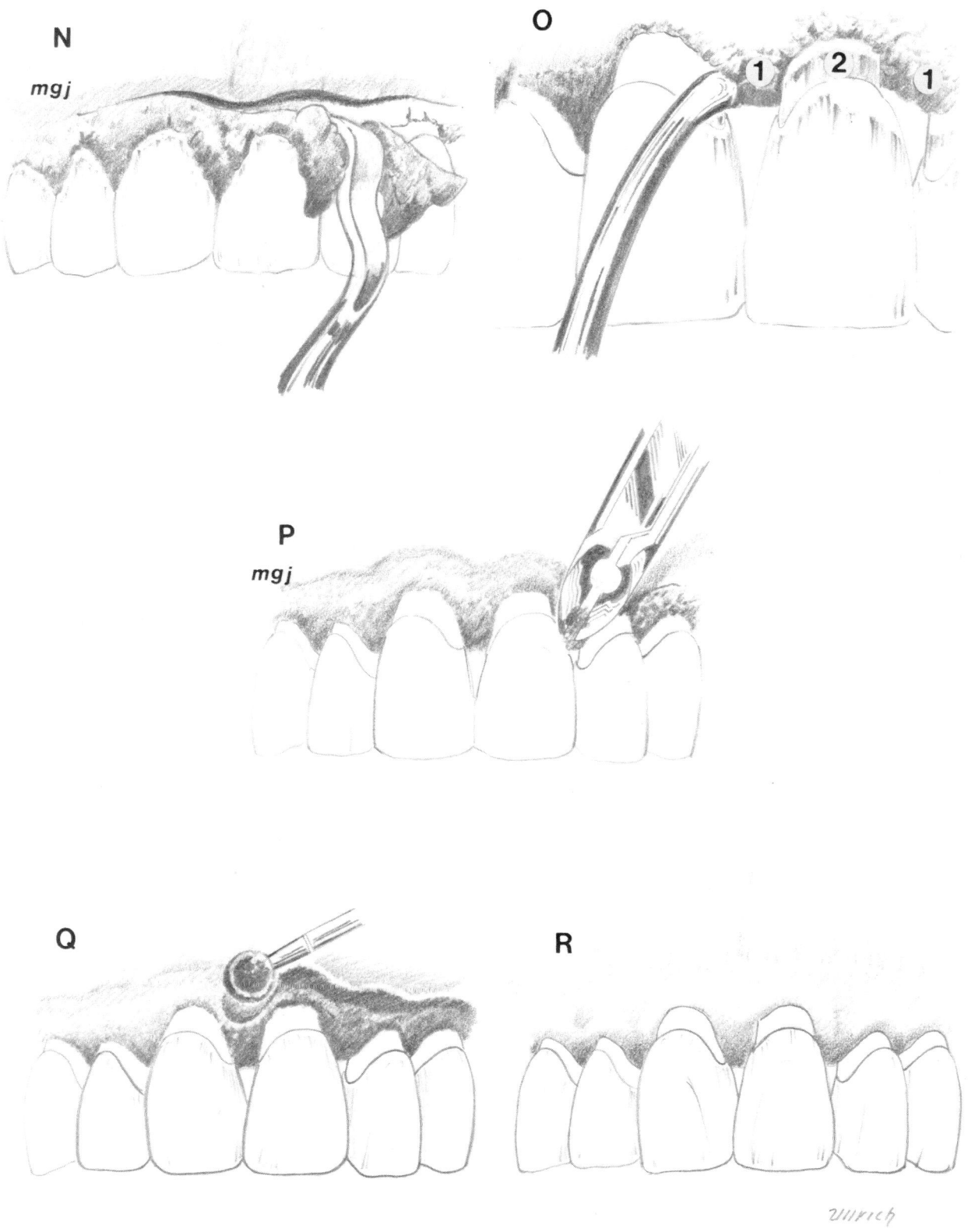

Fig. 4-1 (continued). N, Removal of excised tissue with hoe or heavy scalers. **O,** Scalers and curettes are now used to remove residual granulation tissue (1) and subgingival plaque and calculus (2). **P, Q,** Gingivoplasty is now completed using tissue nippers and diamond stones to establish a thin, even-flowing gingival architecture that has a scalloped outline rising interproximally to a conical shape. **R,** Final healed tissue.

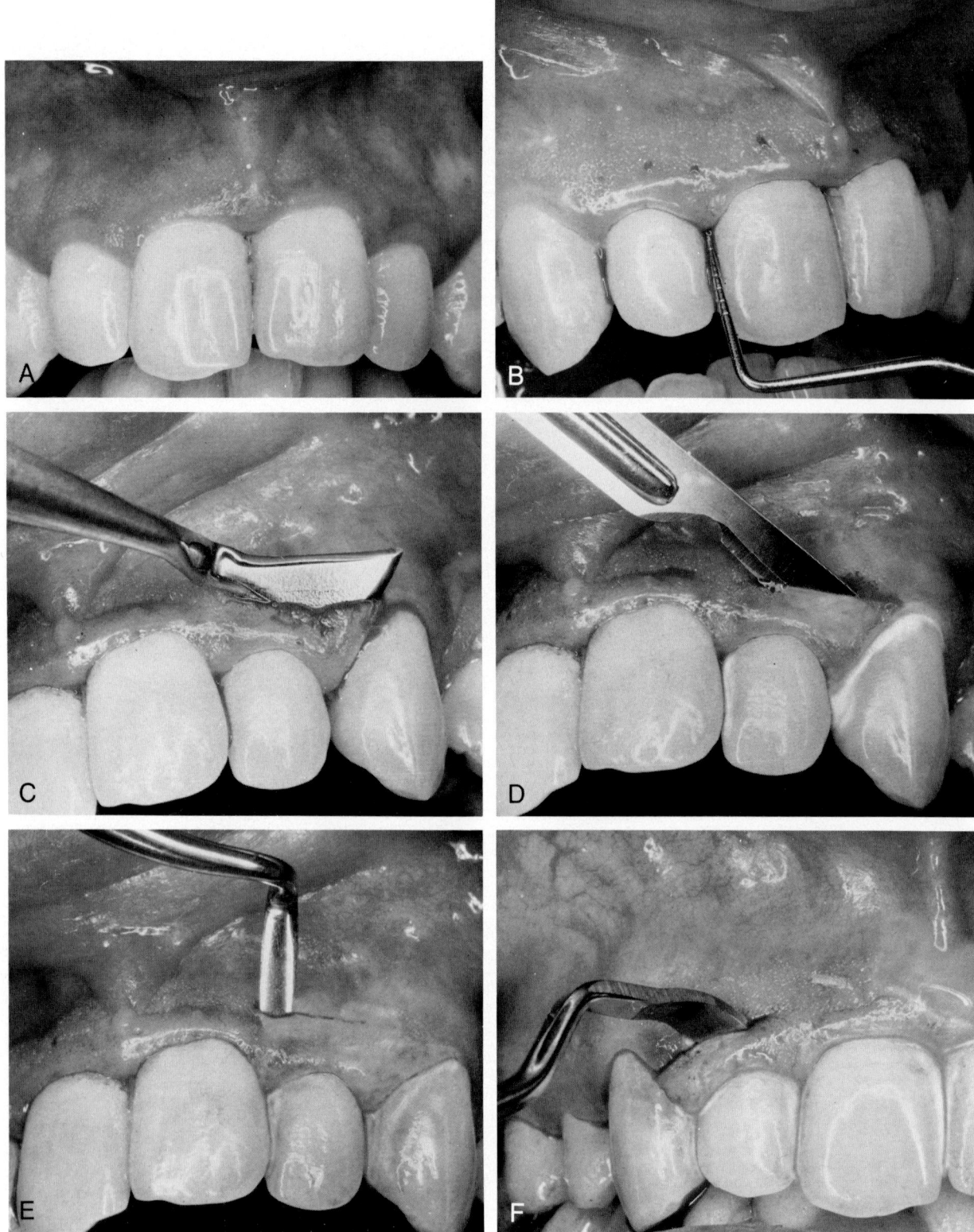

Fig. 4-2. Gingivectomy and Gingivoplasty Procedures. **A,** Before treatment. **B,** Bleeding points show marked pockets. Probe shows 4- to 5-mm pockets. **C,** Initial incision with periodontal knife angled at 45°. **D,** A No. 15 scalpel blade used for initial incision. **E,** Orban knife used to release interdental tissue. **F,** Heavy scalers used to remove incised tissue.

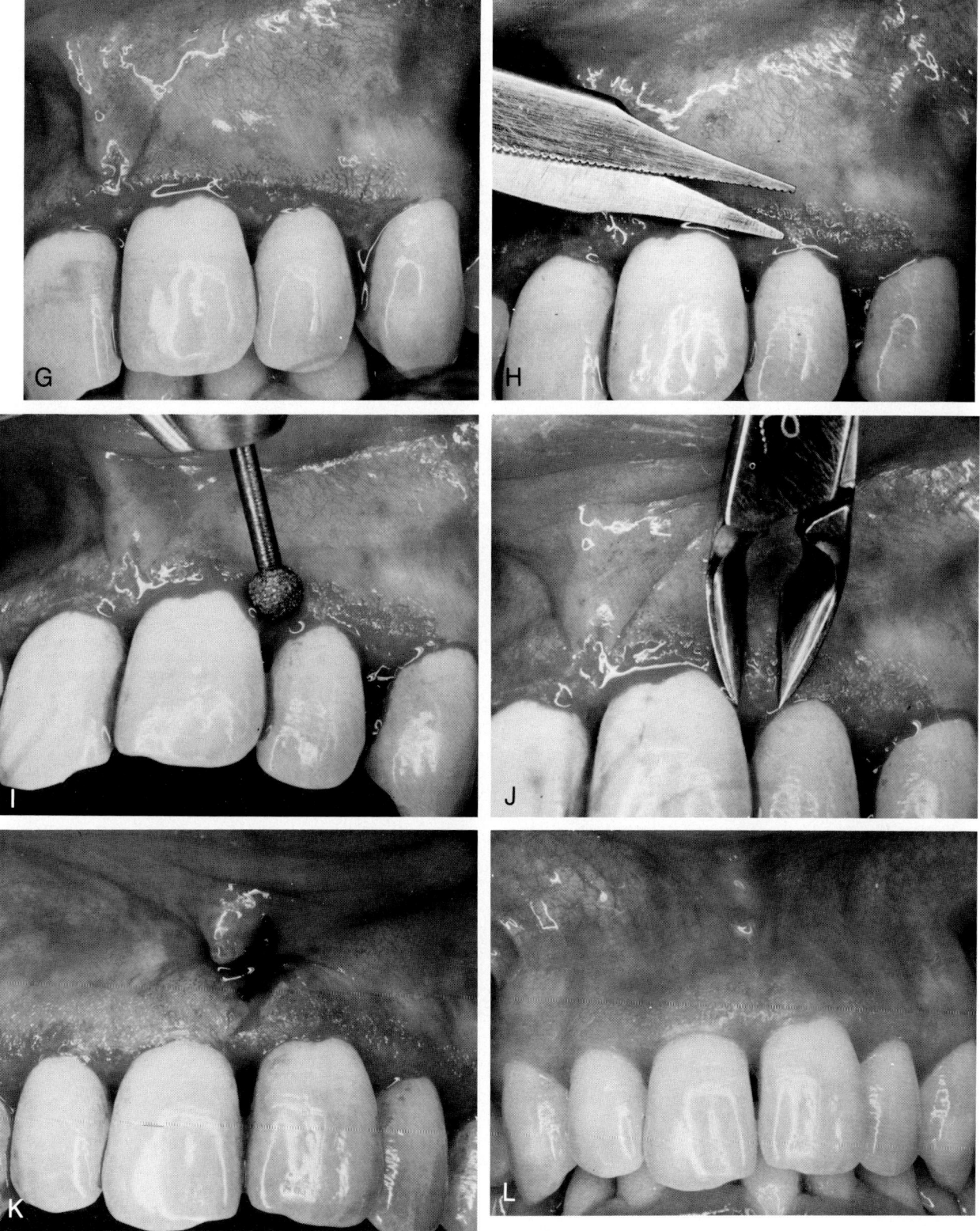

Fig. 4-2 (continued). G, Tissue removed. Note ledge of beveled tissue. **H,** Scissors used for reduction of ledge and gingivoplasty. **I,** Small diamonds are used to blend the tissue, especially interproximally on bulky tissue. **J,** Tissue nippers may be used for gingivoplasty. **K,** Completion of gingivoplasty. Note how tissue has been thinned and blended. **L,** Healed tissue 6 months later.

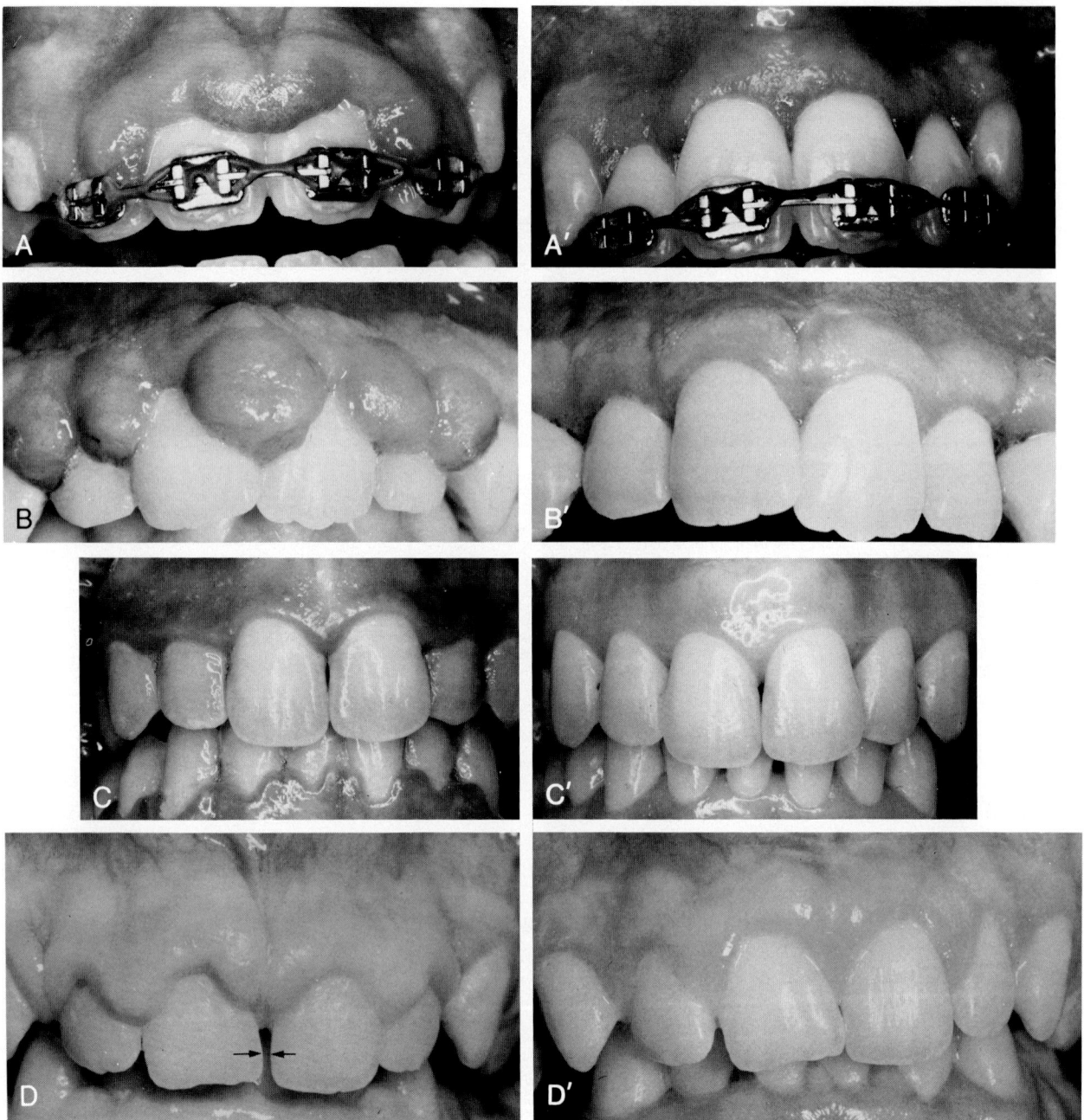

Fig. 4-3. Results obtained by gingivectomy. **A, B, C, D,** Before. **A', B', C', D',** After. Note how teeth have come together in D'.

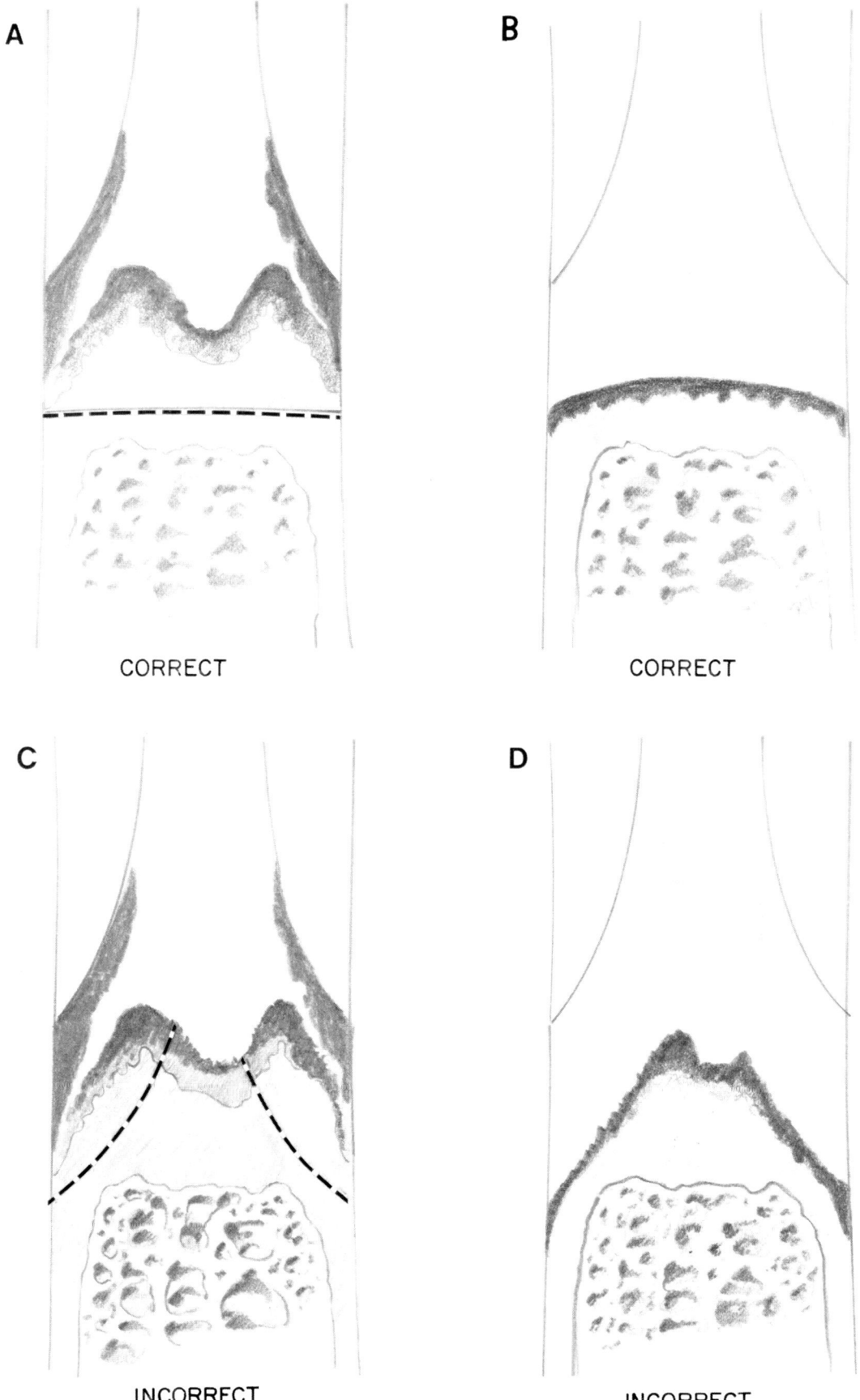

Fig. 4-4. Treatment of Edentulous Areas. **A,** Outline of correct incision to treat total edentulous space. **B,** Healed ridge with no residual pockets. **C,** Incorrect incision, which treats only pockets adjacent to teeth. **D,** Residual pockets or depressions remain after treatment.

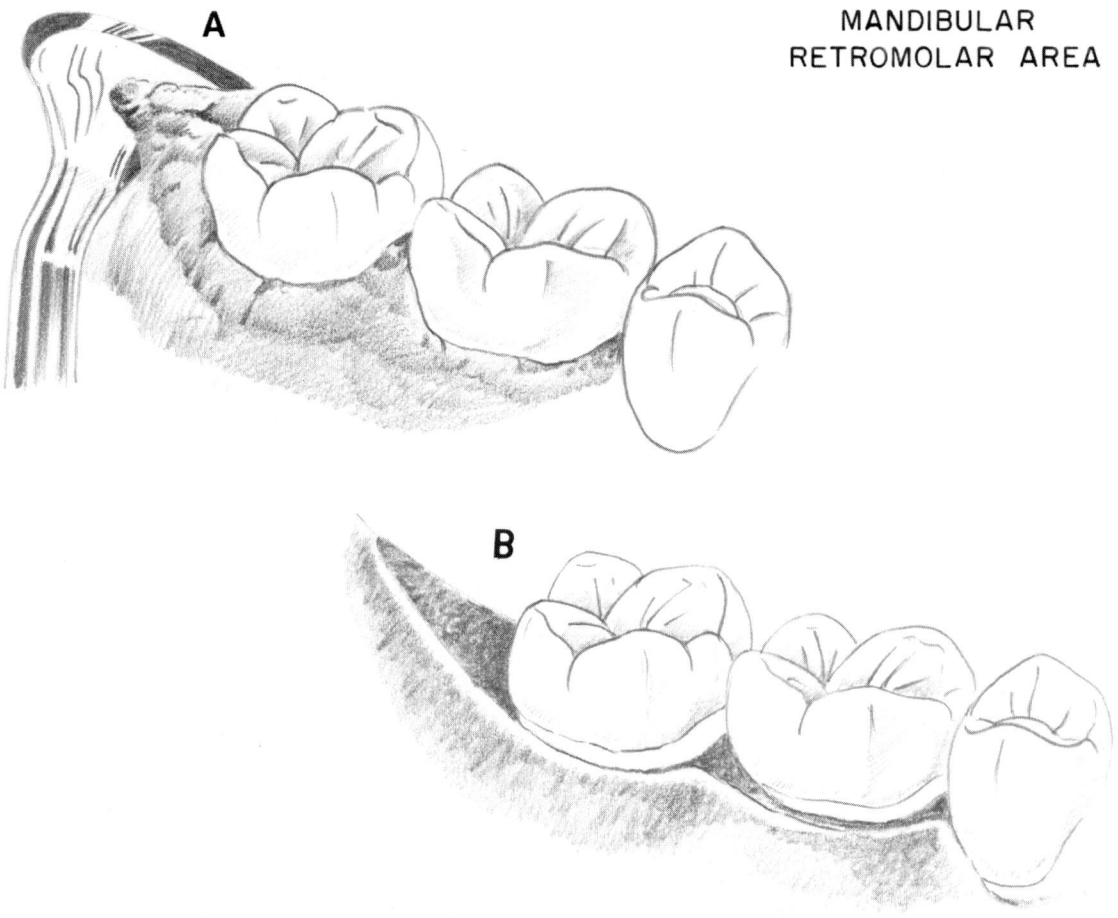

Fig. 4-5. Treatment of Mandibular Retromolar Area. **A,** A periodontal knife is used to blend the buccal and lingual incisions about the distal aspect of the last molar if enough keratinized attached gingiva is present. **B,** Retromolar area reduced and blended with other incisions.

Gingivectomy and Gingivoplasty

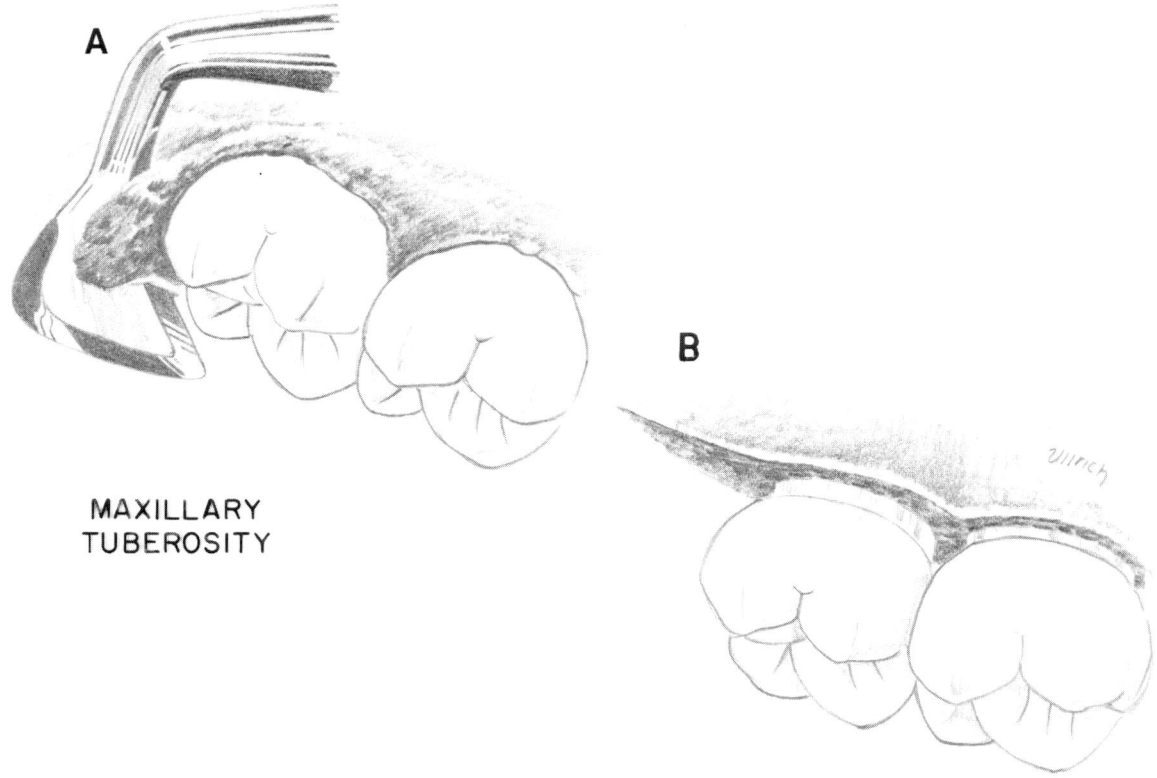

Fig. 4-6. Treatment of Maxillary Tuberosity. **A,** A periodontal knife is used to level and remove the tissue distal to the molars when no furcation involvement or osseous irregularities exist. **B,** Tuberosity tissue removed and blended with other incisions.

5

MUCOGINGIVAL SURGERY

Mucogingival surgical techniques are designed to provide a functionally adequate zone of keratinized attached gingiva (Friedman, 1962). These procedures, although not especially designed for pocket elimination or creation of proper physiologic form, may be combined with other procedures to obtain a healthy periodontal complex: a complex capable of withstanding the stresses of mastication, toothbrushing, trauma from foreign objects, tooth preparation associated with crown and bridge, subgingival restorations, orthodontics, inflammation, and frenulum pull.

No standard width of keratinized attached gingiva has been established. In people with good oral hygiene 1 mm or less may be sufficient for health (Lange and Loe, 1972; Miyasato et al., 1977; Hangorsky and Bissada, 1980; de Trey and Bernimoulin, 1980; Dorfman et al., 1980, 1982). Kirch et al. (1986), Wennström (1987), and Salkin et al. (1987) have shown that even a movable marginal tissue of alveolar mucosa can be maintained stable over a long period of time. Yet, it may be necessary to increase this zone of healthy tissue if it is to be subjected to the trauma of prosthetic treatment (Maynard and Wilson, 1979; Ericsson and Lindhe, 1984), orthodontic restoration (Maynard and Ochsenbein, 1975; Coatoam et al., 1981), frenulum pull (Gottsegen, 1954; Corn, 1964A; Gorman, 1967), or in instances of rapidly progressing recession (Baker and Seymour, 1976; de Trey and Bernimoulin, 1980).

TISSUE BARRIER CONCEPT

Goldman and Cohen (1979) outlined a "tissue barrier" concept for mucogingival surgery. They postulated that a dense collagenous band of connective tissue retards or obstructs the spread of inflammation better than does the loose fiber arrangement of the alveolar mucosa. They recommended increasing the zone of keratinized attached tissue to achieve an adequate tissue barrier (thick tissue), thus limiting recession as a result of inflammation. This view is "indirectly" supported by the findings of Kennedy et al. (1985) after recall evaluations of the unsupervised discontinued patients from their 6-year longitudinal study of free autogenous gingival grafts, as well as by the findings of Lindhe et al. (1973), Baker and Seymour (1976), Rubin (1979), and Lindhe and Nyman (1980).

In contrast to these findings, teeth possessing the least attached tissue (cuspids and bicuspids) are the least involved periodontally, whereas the incidence of disease is greatest on the lingual and palatal surfaces where the amount of keratinized tissue is greatest (Waerhaug, 1971). Furthermore, Wennström et al. (1981, 1982), Wennström and Lindhe (1983), and Kure et al. (1985) have shown that a free gingival unit supported by a loosely attached alveolar mucosa is not more susceptible to inflammation than is a free gingival unit that is supported by a wide zone of attached gingiva.

These procedures, therefore, should be used only where specifically indicated or where inflammation cannot be controlled. Wennström (1985) states, "A thin marginal tissue, in particular in the absence of underlying alveolar bone, will be at greater risk of recession since the plaque-induced inflammatory lesion may occupy and cause destruction of the entire connective tissue portion of the gingiva."

Hall (1977) noted several critical factors to be considered other than the mere lack of an adequate zone of attached gingiva:
1. Patient age
2. Level of oral hygiene

3. Teeth involved
4. Potential or existing esthetic problems
5. Existing recession with esthetic or sensitivity problems
6. The patient's dental needs
7. Previous dental treatment

GENERAL CONSIDERATIONS

Principles

1. Existing keratinized gingiva should always be maintained
2. Exposing bone to increase the zone of keratinized gingiva is contraindicated (Wilderman, 1964)
3. When an adequate zone of attached keratinized gingiva exists, vestibular depth is not a factor (Bohannan, 1963A)

Objectives

1. To create an adequate zone of attached keratinized gingiva
2. To eliminate pockets that extend beyond the mucogingival line
3. To eliminate muscle and frenulum pull
4. To deepen the vestibule
5. To cover denuded root surfaces for esthetics or hypersensitivity
6. To overcome the anatomic factors of tooth position, thin alveolar housing, and large prominent roots, which promote dehiscence and/or fenestration formation with gingival accession
7. To minimize recession during orthodontic movement
8. To overcome the trauma of prosthetic or restorative dentistry requiring subgingival placement
9. To stabilize and maintain a healthy mucogingival complex
10. To correct areas of progressive gingival recession
11. To correct ridge deformities and undercuts

CLASSIFICATION OF PROCEDURES

The surgical methods available for correction of mucogingival problems are as follows:
1. Periodontal Flaps—Positioned and Repositioned
   a. Full-thickness (mucoperiosteal; modified, apically positioned)
   b. Flap curettage
   c. Partial-thickness (apically positioned)
   d. Curtain procedure
2. Free Soft-Tissue Autografts
   a. Grafting for root coverage
   b. Connective tissue pedicle graft
   c. Ridge augmentation for esthetics
3. Subepithelial Connective Tissue Graft
4. Laterally Positioned Pedicle Flaps (partial-thickness, full-thickness)
   a. Edentulous ridge modification
   b. Oblique rotated pedicle flap
   c. Periosteally stimulated pedicle flap
   d. Partial-full-thickness pedicle flap
   e. Submarginal incisions
   f. Coronally positioned flap
5. Double Papilla Laterally Positioned Flap
   a. Horizontal lateral sliding papillary flap
   b. Rotated or transpositional rotated flap
6. Frenulectomy and Frenulotomy

PERIODONTAL FLAPS—POSITIONED AND REPOSITIONED

The periodontal flap, *apically positioned or repositioned (unpositioned), full-thickness (mucoperiosteal), or partial-thickness (mucosal),* is the most widely used technique in periodontics today. It is used to eliminate pockets, increase the zone of attached tissue, and relocate frenula. The full-thickness flap is used when osseous (resective or inductive) techniques are indicated. The partial-thickness flap is indicated for mucogingival problems as well as in areas where dehiscences or fenestrations may exist and bone must be protected (see Table 1-2).

Full-Thickness (Mucoperiosteal) Flap

The full-thickness flap procedure, as practiced today in periodontics, does not use a simple full-thickness flap but rather a *partial-full-thickness flap.* This is a result of the inverse beveled incision described by Friedman (1964A), in which the marginal tissue and papillae are thinned or partially dissected by the initial incision.

This thinning incision eliminates thick gingival margins and papillae with large triangular pieces of interdental tissue. A thick tissue would be difficult, if not impossible, to trim properly once the flap has been raised and freed. Close approximation of the tissue to both tooth and bone would also be difficult, with a resultant bulbous or ledging-type tissue upon healing.

Goldman et al. (1982) noted the use of a partial-full-partial-thickness positioned flap or *tertiary* flap. The flap is identical to that already described except that once an adequate amount of bone has been exposed, sharp dissection is again employed. The advantage to this lies mainly in the ability to use periosteal sutures for proper flap positioning.

Indications

1. Pockets that extend beyond the mucogingival junction
2. Areas of minimal keratinized gingiva
3. Inductive or resective osseous surgery required
4. Enhance cleansibility
5. Facilitate restorative procedures
6. Unesthetic or asymmetrical gingival topography

Advantages

1. Pocket elimination
2. Preservation of existing keratinized gingiva
3. Ability to perform inductive or osseous resective procedures
4. Relocation of frenulum
5. Primary-intention healing
6. Access to roots for definitive scaling and root planing
7. Flaps can be positioned apically, coronally, or unpositioned

Disadvantages

1. Cannot be combined with other procedures to increase the zone of keratinized gingiva without exposure of bone
2. Moderate degree of difficulty
3. Should not be used in presence of thin periodontium where dehiscences or fenestrations may exist
4. Apical positioning may increase root exposure and sensitivity and cause cosmetic and phonetic problems, especially anteriorly

Contraindications

1. Esthetic considerations
2. Inadequate keratinized gingiva
3. Teeth having a poor prognosis: excessive mobility, poor crown/root ratio, advanced attachment loss

Incision Placement

Proper placement of the initial or primary inverse beveled incision is critical when the amount of keratinized gingiva is limited. Friedman (1964A) classified incision placement based on the amount of keratinized attached tissue present.

Class I Keratinized gingiva is more than adequate; use of *labial or buccal incision* placed 1 to 3 mm from crest of gingiva; flap apically positioned to cover 1 to 2 mm cementum (Fig. 5-1A).

Class II Keratinized gingiva is adequate; use of *crestal incision*; flap apically positioned to crest of bone (Fig. 5-1B).

Class III Keratinized gingiva inadequate; use of *sulcular incision*; flap apically positioned 1 to 2 mm below crest of bone to increase zone of keratinized gingiva (Fig. 5-1C). *Note:* A partial-thickness flap is indicated here.

Procedure

With the patient under anesthesia the area is probed to determine pocket depth (Fig. 5-2A) and underlying osseous topography (Fig. 5-2B). The need for a full-thickness flap is indicated when pockets extend to or below the mucogingival junction and osseous surgery is needed.

Vertical incisions are used to outline the surgical site and are made at the mesial or distal line angles of the terminal teeth. These incisions should extend 3 to 4 mm into the alveolar mucosa and down to the bone to allow proper flap reflection.

A primary scalloped, inverse beveled thinning incision is made 1 to 2 mm on the labial or buccal aspect of the gingival tissue (Fig. 5-2C), thus preserving the remaining keratinized gingiva. In Figure 5-2D, the primary inverse beveled incision is carried down to the crest of the bone.

The papilla, because of its greater interproximal tissue bulk, must be thinned during the initial incision. If this is not done, the papilla will have a large triangular piece of tissue that will make later close tissue adaptation difficult. Once free, the papilla is difficult, if not impossible, to thin properly. In Figure 5-2E and F, the initial inverse beveled incision partially dissects or splits the papilla, making it a partial-thickness flap.

A secondary incision is made about the necks of the teeth from the base of the sulcus to the crest of the bone (Fig. 5-2G,H). This loosens or frees the inner secondary flap, making removal of the tissue collar easier (Fig. 5-2I).

The periosteal elevator is now placed at the terminal end of the flap, and while pressing against the bone, the flap is raised (Fig. 5-2J). Once the flap is lifted off the bone, the elevator is directed from the side, *always pressing against the bone*, to raise the remaining portion of the flap. Tearing of the flap is common when a dull elevator is used or a sharp one is not maintained against the bone.

With the flap raised, scaling, root planing, degranulation, and osseous surgery are completed (Fig. 5-2K).

The flap can be positioned apically or coronally or

unpositioned, depending on the preference of the operator. Interrupted or continuous sutures may be used, although sling sutures permit better flap placement (Fig. 5-2L). Pocket elimination is achieved only by apically positioning the flap.

The procedure is shown clinically in Figures 5-3 and 5-4.

Modified Apically Positioned Full-Thickness Flap

The modified flap procedure uses no vertical incisions. Although generally indicated for the posterior area as an extension of the distal wedge operation, the modified flap may be used anywhere.

Procedure

1. The area is probed for pocket depth and underlying osseous topography (Fig. 5-5A).
2. The primary incision is continued anteriorly from the distal wedge incision with a No. 15 scalpel blade (Fig. 5-5B).
3. At the anterior extension of the flap, no vertical incision is made. Instead, the tissue is undermined and blended into the sulcus of the next tooth. A No. 15 scalpel blade is worked under the mucosal tissue on the facial aspect of the last tooth (Fig. 5-5C). This permits adequate tissue drape so that a vertical incision becomes unnecessary. Adequate tissue drape may also be achieved by extending the flap one tooth beyond the surgical area.
4. After completion of the secondary incision, the flap is raised with a periosteal elevator and the secondary inner flap is removed with heavy scalers (Fig. 5-5D).
5. The teeth are scaled and root planed, and osseous surgery is completed (Fig. 5-5E).
6. The suturing is completed with continuous or interrupted sutures (Fig. 5-5F).

The procedure is shown clinically in Figures 5-6 and 5-7.

Common Mistakes

1. Figure 5-8A shows correct and incorrect placements for the incision. Incisions made over the radicular or facial surface may result in excessive bone loss with dehiscence or fenestration formation. The papilla should be taken full and not split, permitting greater ease of handling and suturing.
2. Figure 5-8B shows an inverse beveled incision, which incorrectly removes all keratinized gingiva.
3. Figure 5-8C shows poor flap design, with a narrow constricted base that may compromise blood supply and result in flap necrosis.
4. Figure 5-8D shows *mouse-holing*, which results from inadequate extension or release of the flap, limiting access and visibility and creating excessive tension at the margins.
5. Figure 5-8E shows excessive bone exposure because of poor flap adaptation, resulting in bone loss.
6. Figure 5-8F depicts poor suturing technique, resulting in the flap's being pulled too high onto the enamel. This, in effect, replaces the pockets and causes a loss of the existing keratinized attached gingiva.

Flap Curettage

In 1976, Ammons and Smith outlined a technique for achieving reattachment and regeneration, using a full-thickness flap for access and visibility to the roots for scaling and root planing. They further sought to maximize the existing periodontal support and, at the same time, reduce or eliminate periodontal pockets.

Flap curettage involves no more than an apically positioned full-thickness flap with or without vertical incisions. It includes thorough scaling, root planing, and debridement, but no osseous surgery.

Olsen et al. (1985), in their 5-year review of apically repositioned flaps with and without osseous surgery, found that those areas treated with osseous surgery had significantly less bleeding and less postoperative pocketing. Neither treatment produced a gain in attachment.

Apically Positioned Partial-Thickness Flap

The technique for partial-thickness flaps uses a sharp dissection parallel to the bone, leaving a periosteal covering in an attempt to protect the underlying bone, eliminate pockets, reduce postoperative pain, and shorten healing time (Ariaudo and Tyrell, 1960; Hileman, 1960).

Indications

1. Areas of thin periodontium or prominent roots where dehiscences or fenestrations may be present.
2. A need to increase the zone of keratinized gingiva

Advantages

1. Eliminate pockets
2. Protect underlying bone (i.e., donor site of pedicle flap)
3. Can be combined with other mucogingival procedures to increase the zone of keratinized gingiva

4. Permit periosteal suturing for flap stabilization and exact positioning

Disadvantages

1. Cannot be used for osseous surgery without resulting in a ragged, torn periosteum
2. High degree of difficulty to perform
3. Secondary-intention healing

Procedure

Figure 5-9A depicts diagnostic probing and preoperative evaluation to determine the amount of keratinized gingiva and the presence of bony dehiscences or fenestrations (Fig. 5-9B) prior to surgery.

A good rule of thumb to use in deciding whether a partial-thickness flap should be used is as follows: *If the roots of the teeth can be palpated or visualized through the tissue, then a partial-thickness flap should be used.* This ability to palpate the roots through the tissue has been termed the *washboard effect* and is generally representative of a thin periodontium with underlying dehiscences or fenestrations (see Figs. 9-7 and 9-9).

With a No. 15 blade, two incisions are made: a straight vertical incision and a scalloped horizontal incision, *neither one* of which is made down to the bone (Fig. 5-9C). In Figure 5-9D, the scalpel blade is held parallel to the bone as the scalpel is moved apically toward the mucogingival junction. This provides the initial separation of the flap. *The incision should maximize the maintenance of the existing keratinized gingiva.*

Figure 5-9E shows how the remainder of the flap is sharply dissected. While applying gentle tension, the surgeon, using rat-tail tissue pliers, reflects the flap adjacent to the vertical incision outward. A No. 15 scalpel blade is placed into the vertical incision and moved toward the mucogingival junction. The flap peels away from the underlying bound-down periosteum. The scalpel should always be kept in close proximity to the bone to prevent flap perforation.

Flap dissection should be carried out in an apico-occlusal direction not in an occlusoapical direction (Fig. 5-9F), because the tissue at the mucogingival junction is firmly bound down. This fact often results in flap perforation as a result of the scalpel blade accidentally slicing buccally instead of moving apically when dissection is attempted from the occlusal direction.

The gingival tissue above the crest of the bone is removed by first making an incision perpendicular to the teeth with a gingivectomy knife or No. 15 scalpel blade (Fig. 5-9G,H), then using sharp scalers and curettes, making sure to leave intact the fibers at and just above the bony crest (Fig. 5-9I,J).

Periosteal sutures (4-0 or 5-0 silk or gut) are used to stabilize and position the flap (Fig. 5-9K,L).

The zone of attached gingiva can be increased by apically positioning the flap below the crest of bone. The amount of keratinized attached gingiva gained this way is unpredictable and will generally be equal to about 50% of the exposed area.

The procedure is shown clinically in Figures 5-10, 5-11, and 5-12.

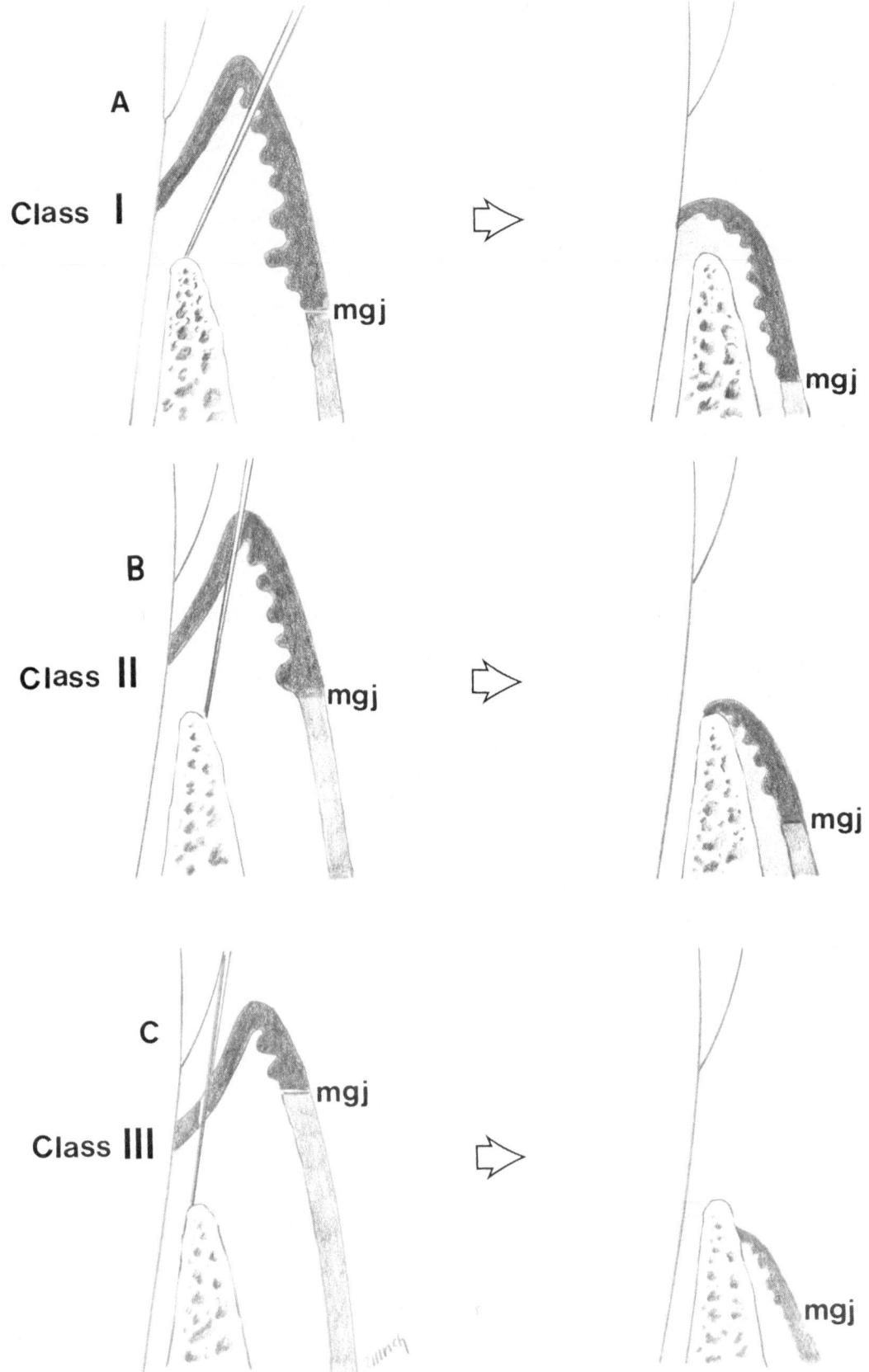

Fig. 5-1. Classification of Incision Placement Based on Presence of Existing Keratinized Gingiva. **A,** Class I. More than adequate keratinized tissue; initial incisions buccal to crest of gingiva and apically positioned to cover bone. **B,** Class II. Adequate keratinized tissue; initial incision at crest of gingiva, and flap positioned only to crest of bone. **C,** Class III. Minimal or inadequate keratinized gingiva; sulcular incision and flap positioned apically to below crest of bone to increase keratinized gingiva. *Note:* A partial-thickness flap is indicated here.

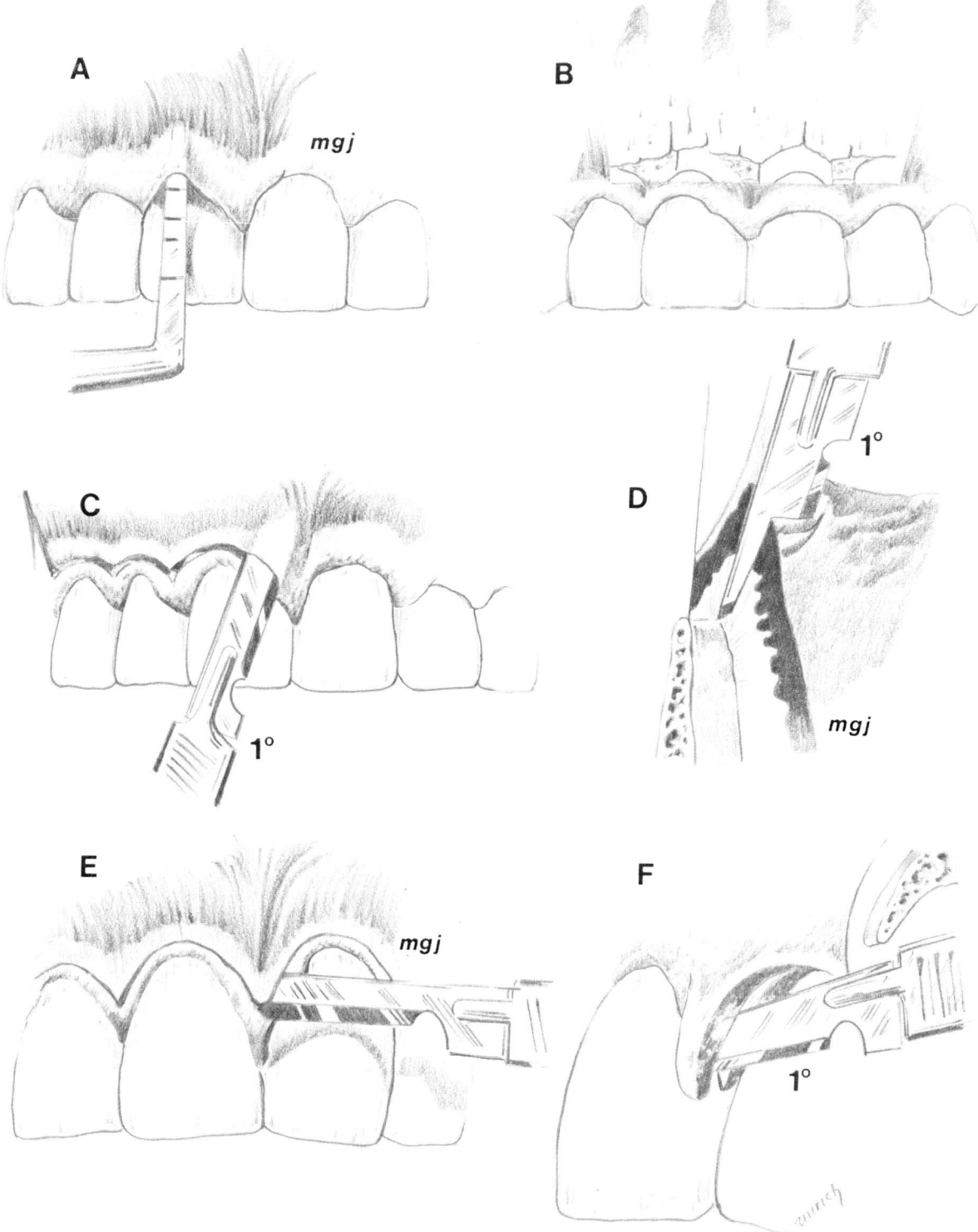

Fig. 5-2. Full-Thickness Apically Positioned Mucoperiosteal Flap. **A,B,** Deep pockets and bone loss with pockets probing to the mucogingival junction (mgj). **C,D,** Primary inverse scalloped, beveled incision made down to the crest of bone. This primary incision thins the tissue. Vertical incisions are used to outline the flap. **E,F,** The papilla is dissected to create a partial-thickness flap and thus remove the thick triangular wedge of interproximal tissue.

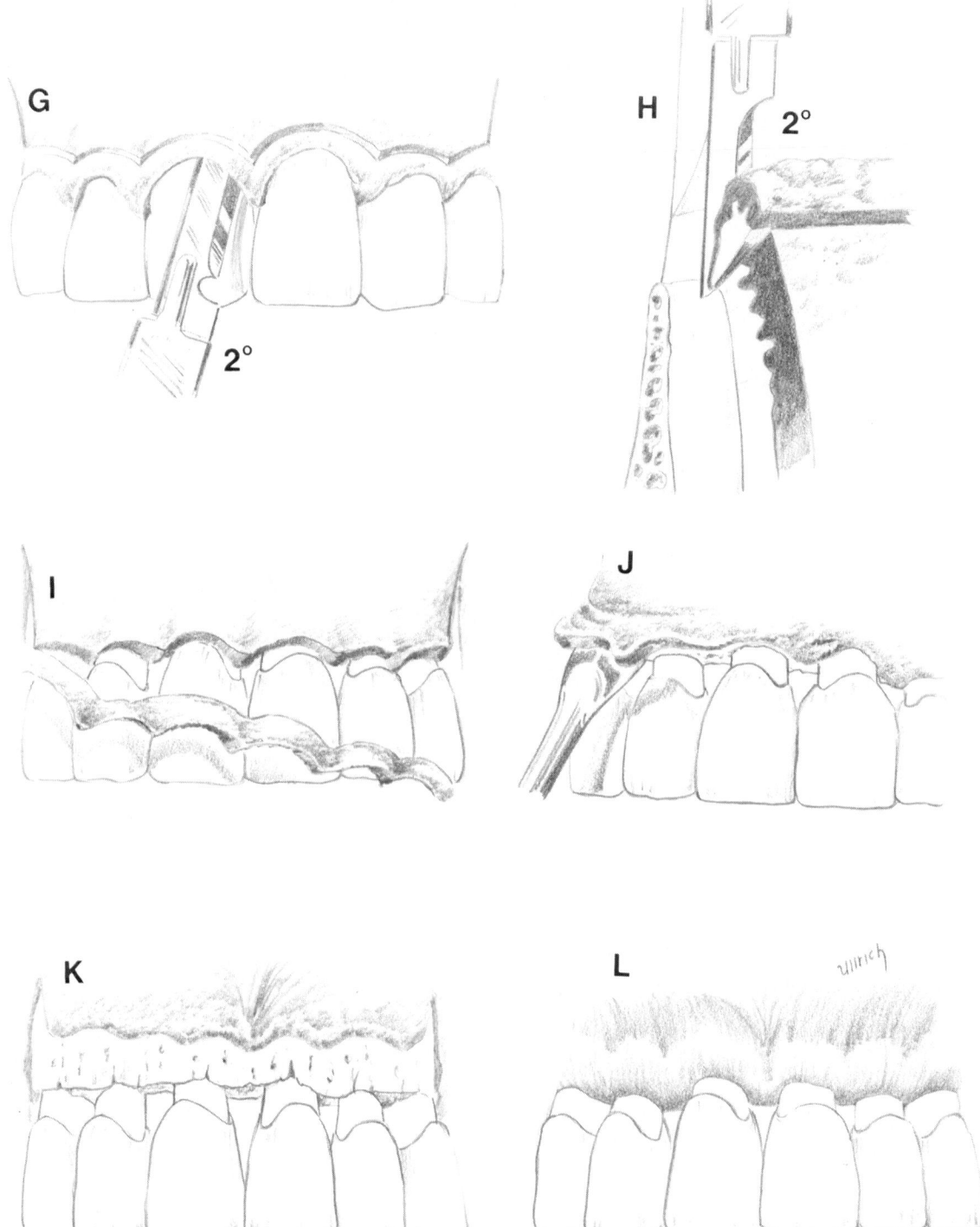

Fig. 5-2 (continued). **G,H,** A secondary sulcular incision down to the crest of bone frees the inner flap of tissue. **I,** Scalers are used to remove the inner flap of tissue. **J,** The flap is raised with a periosteal elevator. **K,** Osseous resective measures are implemented. **L,** The flap is apically positioned to the crest of bone and sutured. Final healing shown.

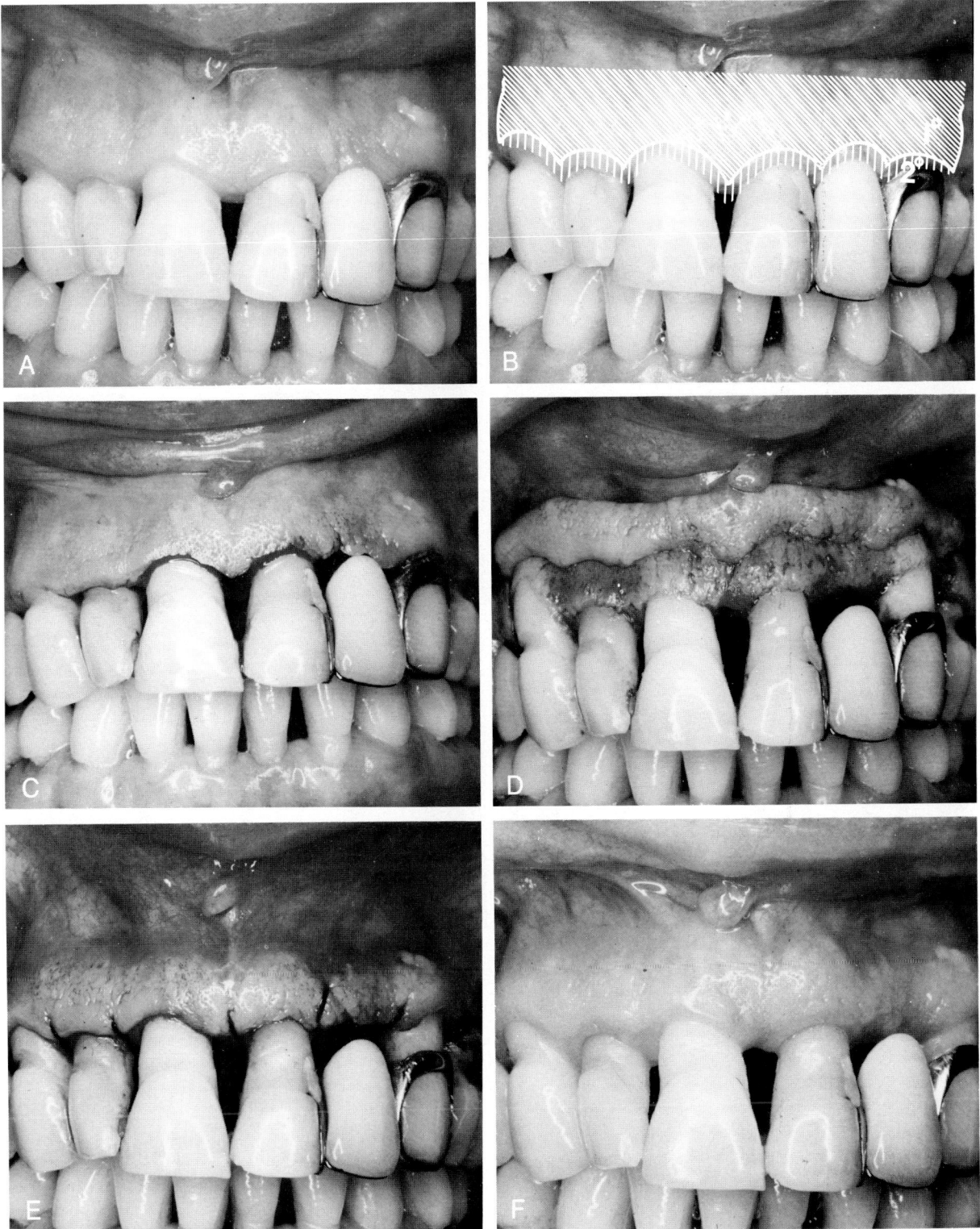

Fig. 5-3. Apically Positioned Mucoperiosteal Flap. **A,** Before. **B,** Incisions outlined: scalloped inverse beveled incisions and bilateral vertical incisions: primary (1°) and secondary (2°) flaps. **C,** Removal of secondary inner flap. **D,** Flap reflected. **E,** Flap apically positioned. Vertical incision permits adequate apical positioning. **F,** Five months later. Note excellent contour and preservation of keratinized gingiva.

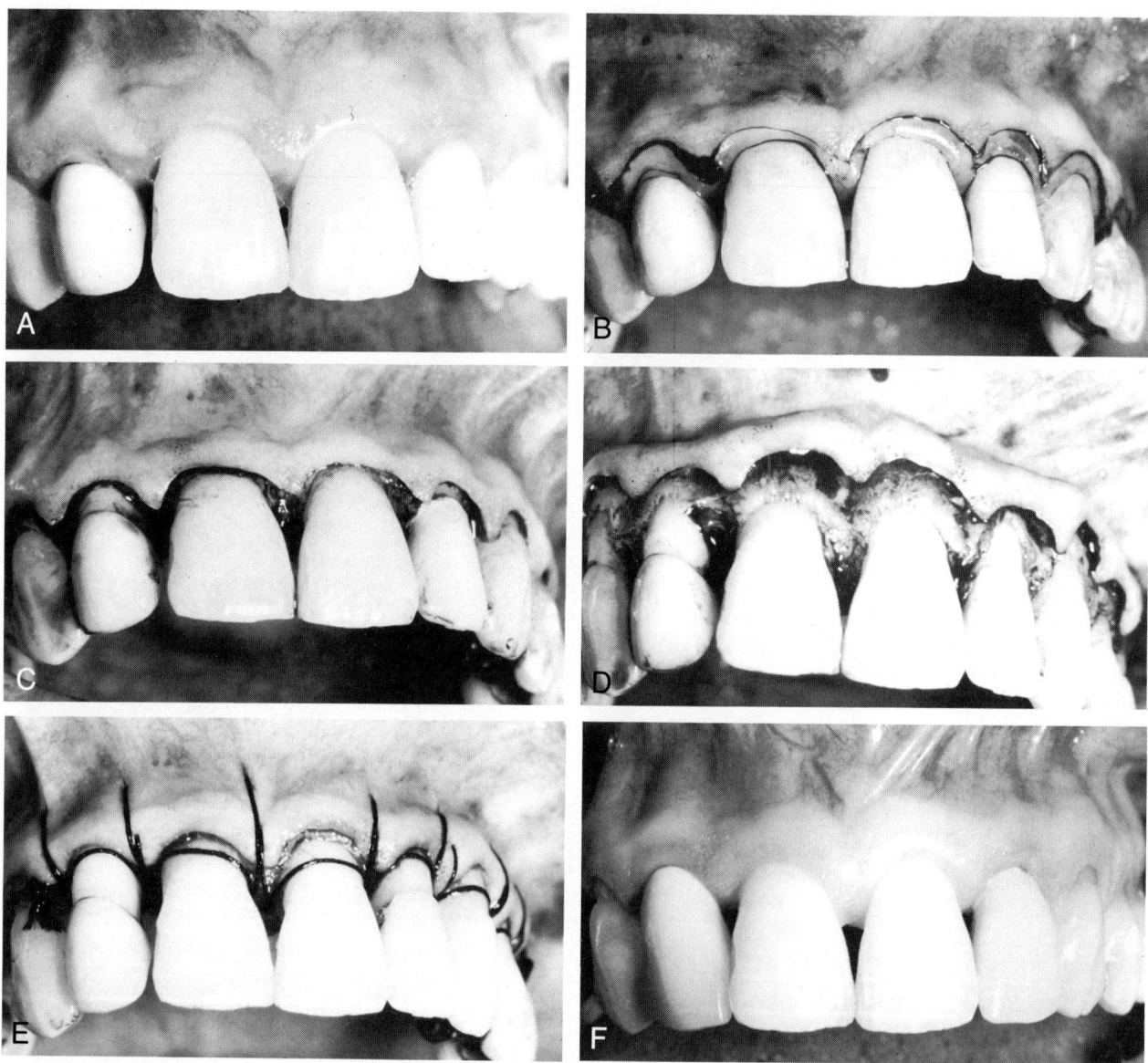

Fig. 5-4. Apically Positioned Mucoperiosteal Flap. **A,** Before surgery. **B,** Primary scalloped incision completed. **C,** Secondary inner flap removed. **D,** Flap reflected. **E,** Periosteal suspensory suturing completed. **F,** Case completed 5 years later.

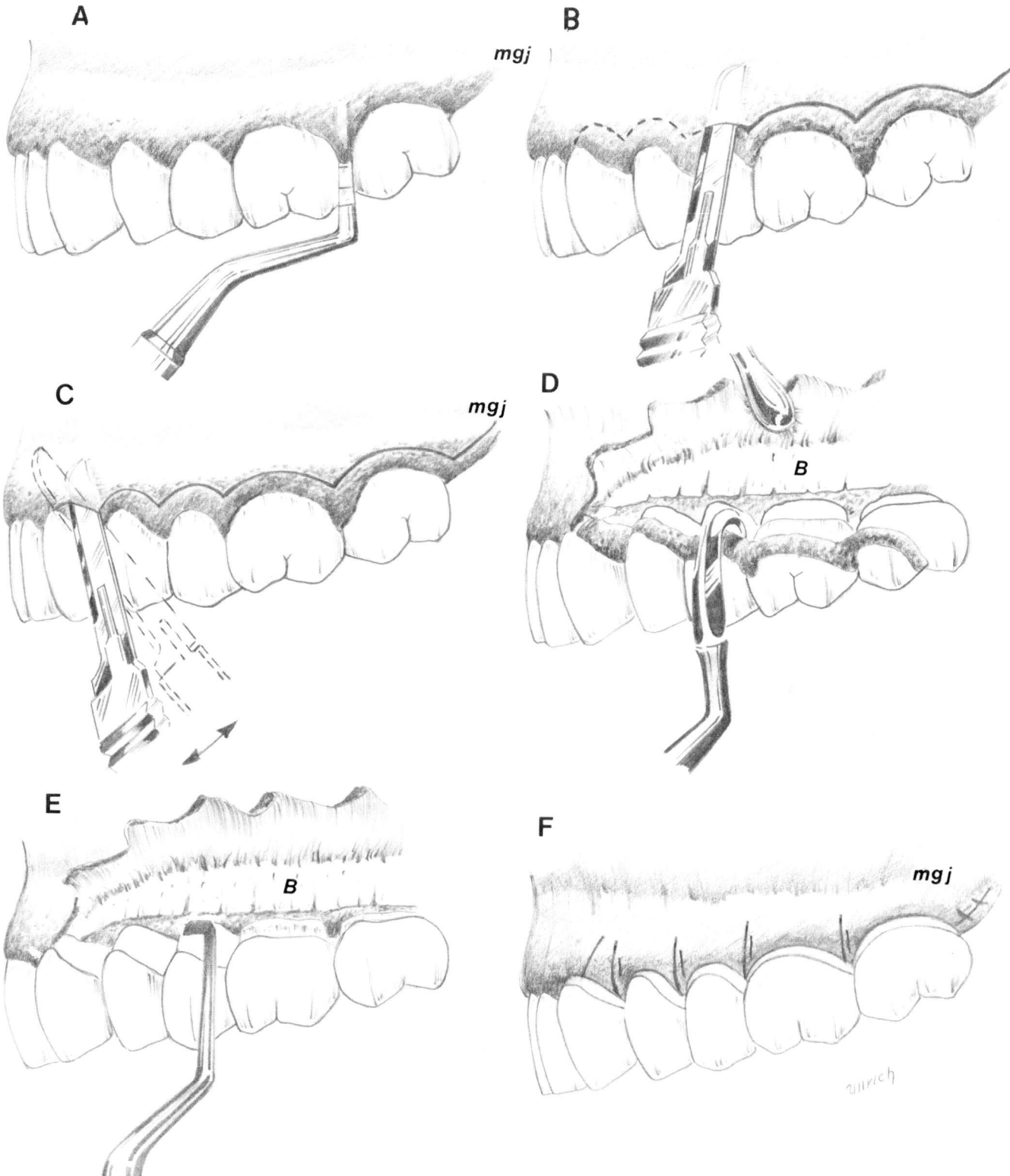

Fig. 5-5. Modified Flap Procedure. **A,** Deep pockets probed at or below the mucogingival junction (mgj). **B,** A scalloped, inverse beveled incision with no vertical incisions continued from the distal wedge. Maximum conservation of keratinized gingiva is attempted. **C,** For proper reflection, the flap is undermined at its most anterior extension. This permits adequate drape without the use of vertical incisions. **D,** The flap is reflected and the secondary flap is removed. **E,** Scaling and osseous surgery are carried out. **F,** The flap is apically positioned and sutured.

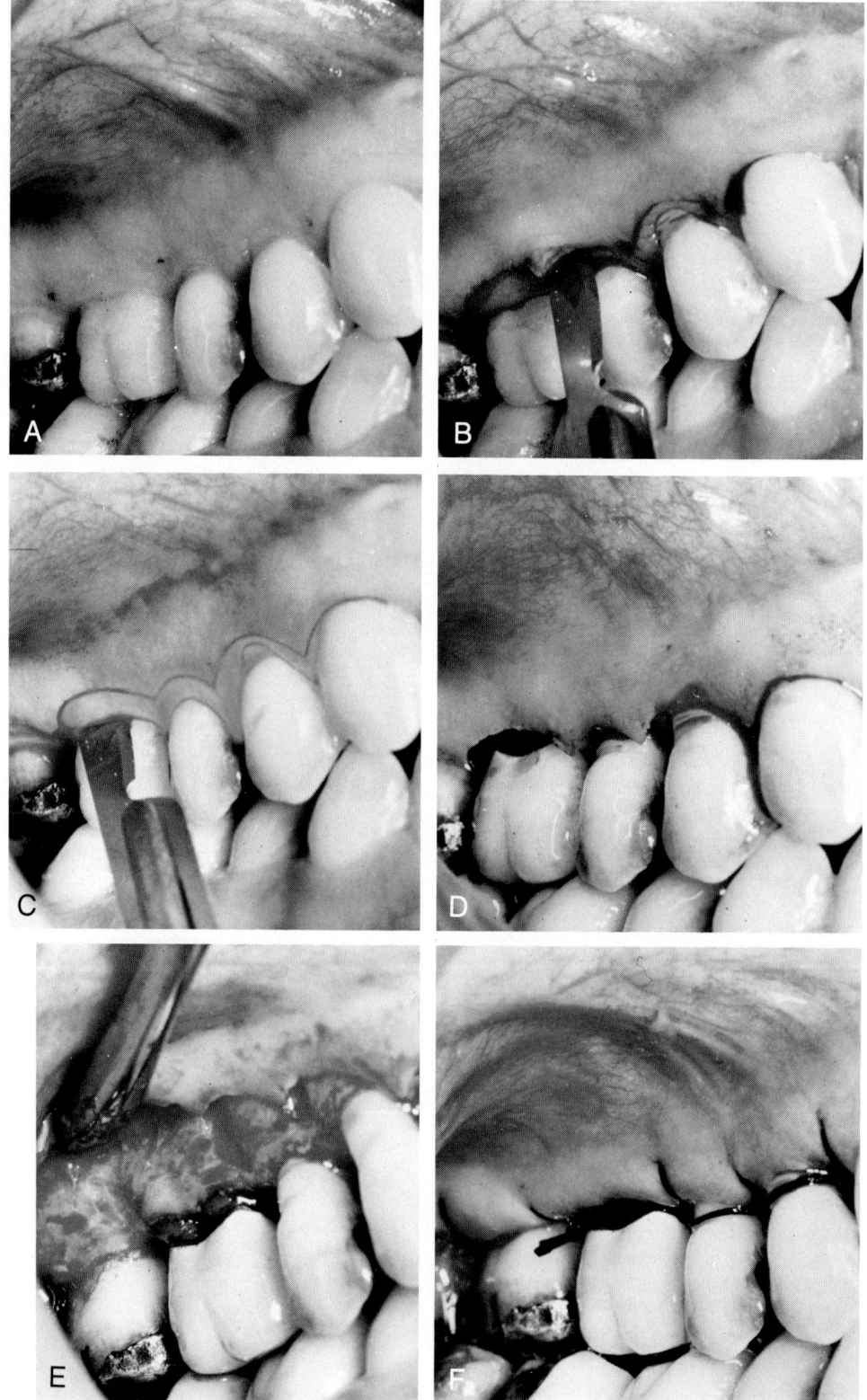

Fig. 5-6. Modified Apically Positioned Mucoperiosteal Flap. **A,** Before treatment. **B,** Primary inverse beveled, scalloped incision to thin the tissue. **C,** Secondary or sulcular incision used to free the secondary or internal flap. **D,** Secondary flap removed. **E,** Flap reflected and osseous surgery completed. **F,** Flap positioned apically and sutured.

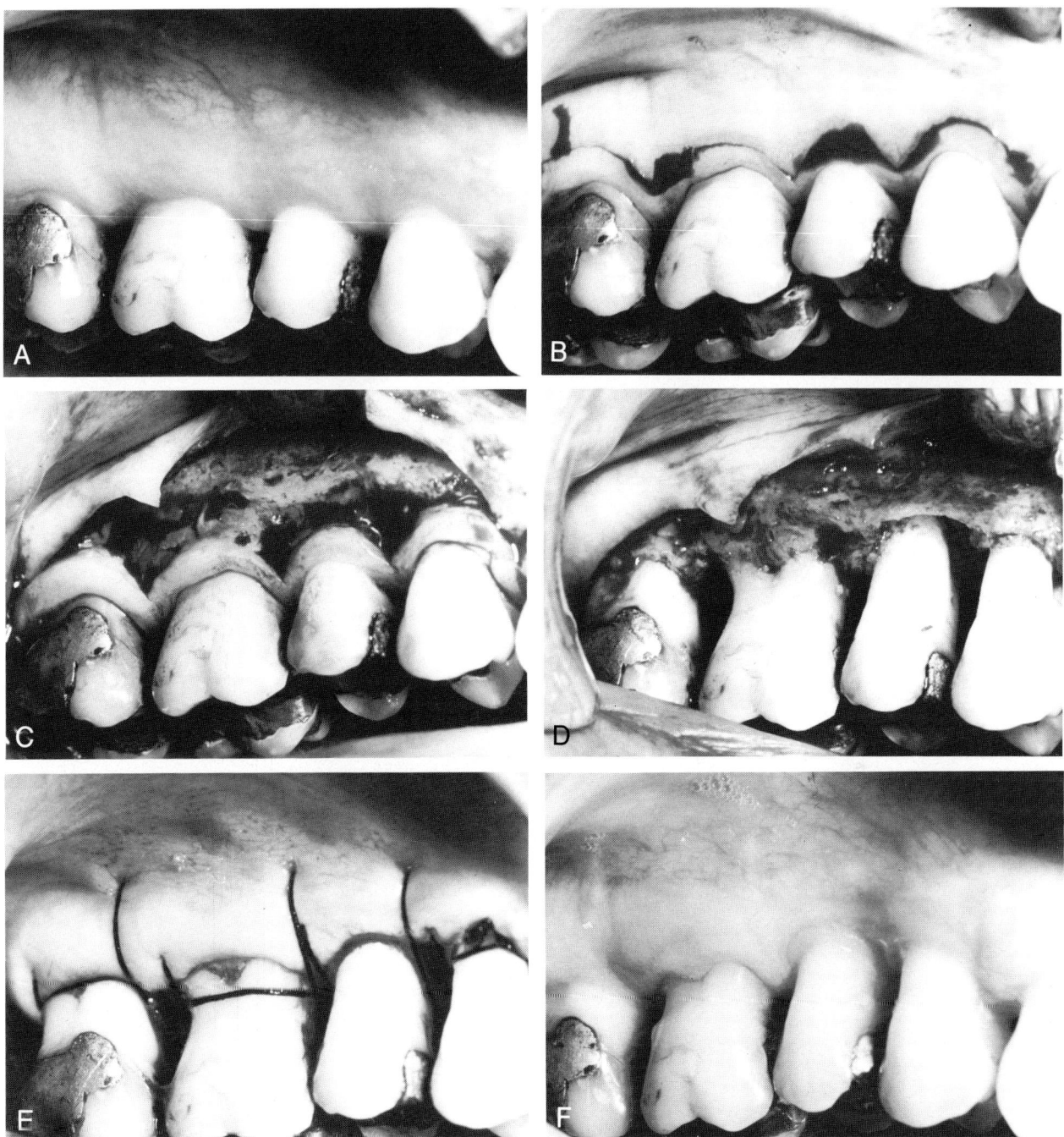

Fig. 5-7. Modified Apically Positioned Flap. **A,** Before treatment. **B,** Primary inverse beveled, scalloped incision to thin tissue. **C,** Primary flap reflected. **D,** Secondary flap reflected and area scaled and debrided. **E,** Vertical mattress periosteal continuous sling suture. **F,** Four years later. Note excellent adaptation and maintenance of tissue contours.

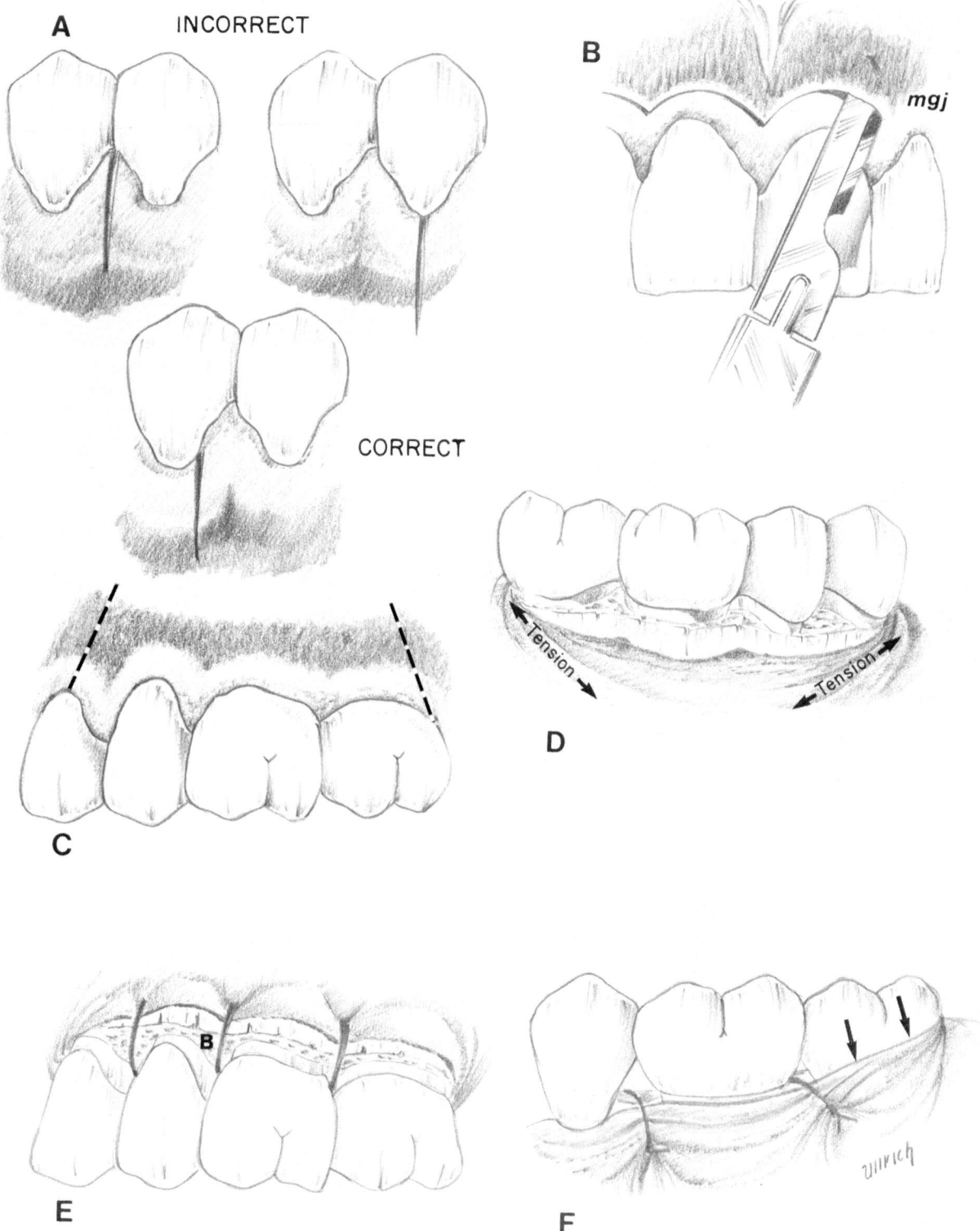

Fig. 5-8. Mistakes in Flap Design. **A,** Correct and incorrect placement of vertical incisions. Vertical incisions are always made at the line angles of the teeth and include the full papillae, not on the facial surface but in the middle of the papillae. **B,** Initial inverse beveled incision removes all attached gingiva. **C,** Vertical incisions make base of flap too narrow and may compromise blood supply. **D,** Excessive tension is placed on flap because of poor extension. **E,** Excessive bone exposed owing to drop of flap. **F,** Flap pulled too high onto tooth, replacing pockets.

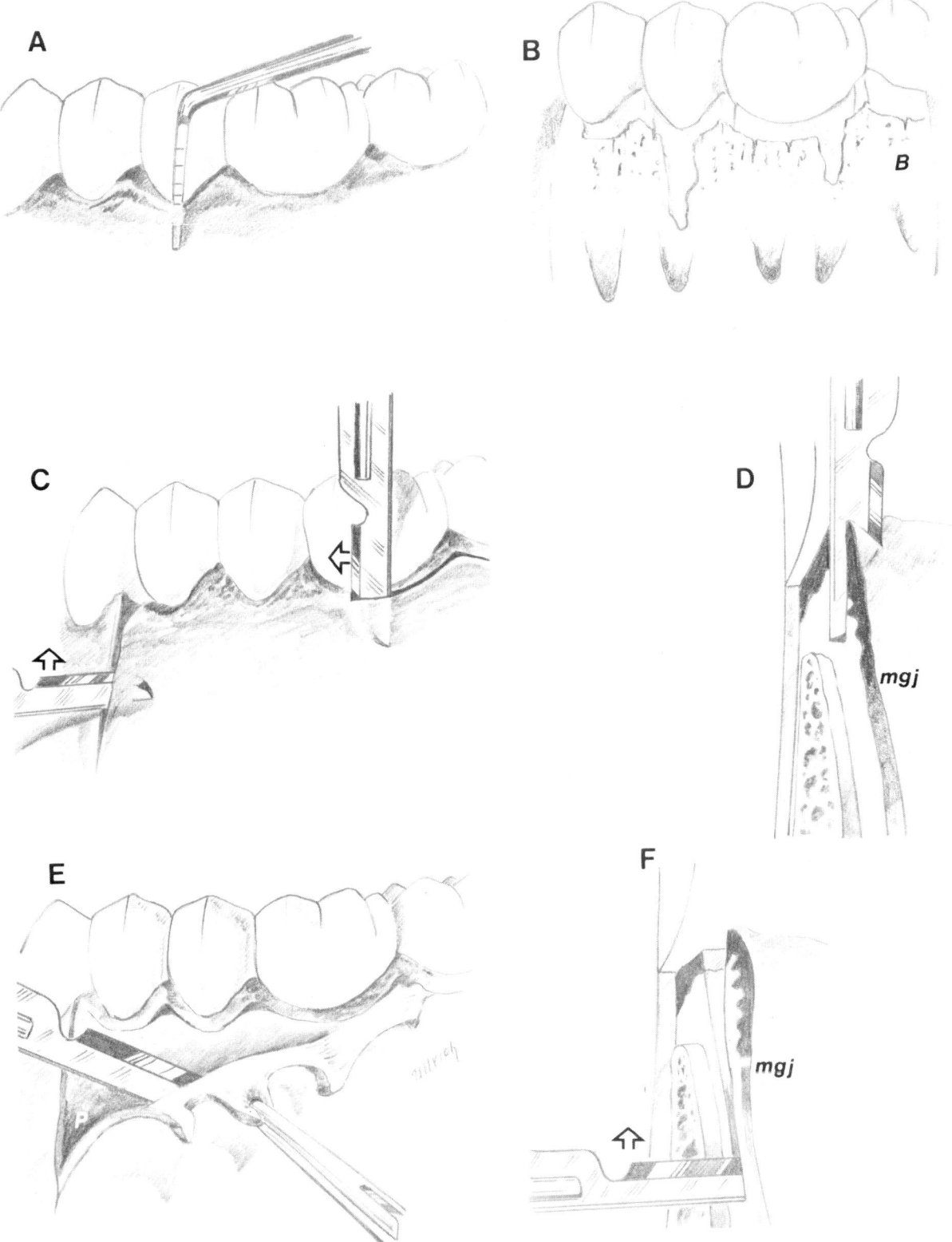

Fig. 5-9. Partial-Thickness Flap. **A,** Minimum amount of attached keratinized tissue present; ability to probe beyond the mucogingival junction. **B,** Cutaway showing thin periodontium with dehiscences and fenestrations. **C,** Initial vertical incision and horizontal incisions are made. **D,** Shows that incisions are not made down to bone. **E,F,** The flap is dissected from an apico-occlusal direction as tension is applied to the flap with tissue pliers.

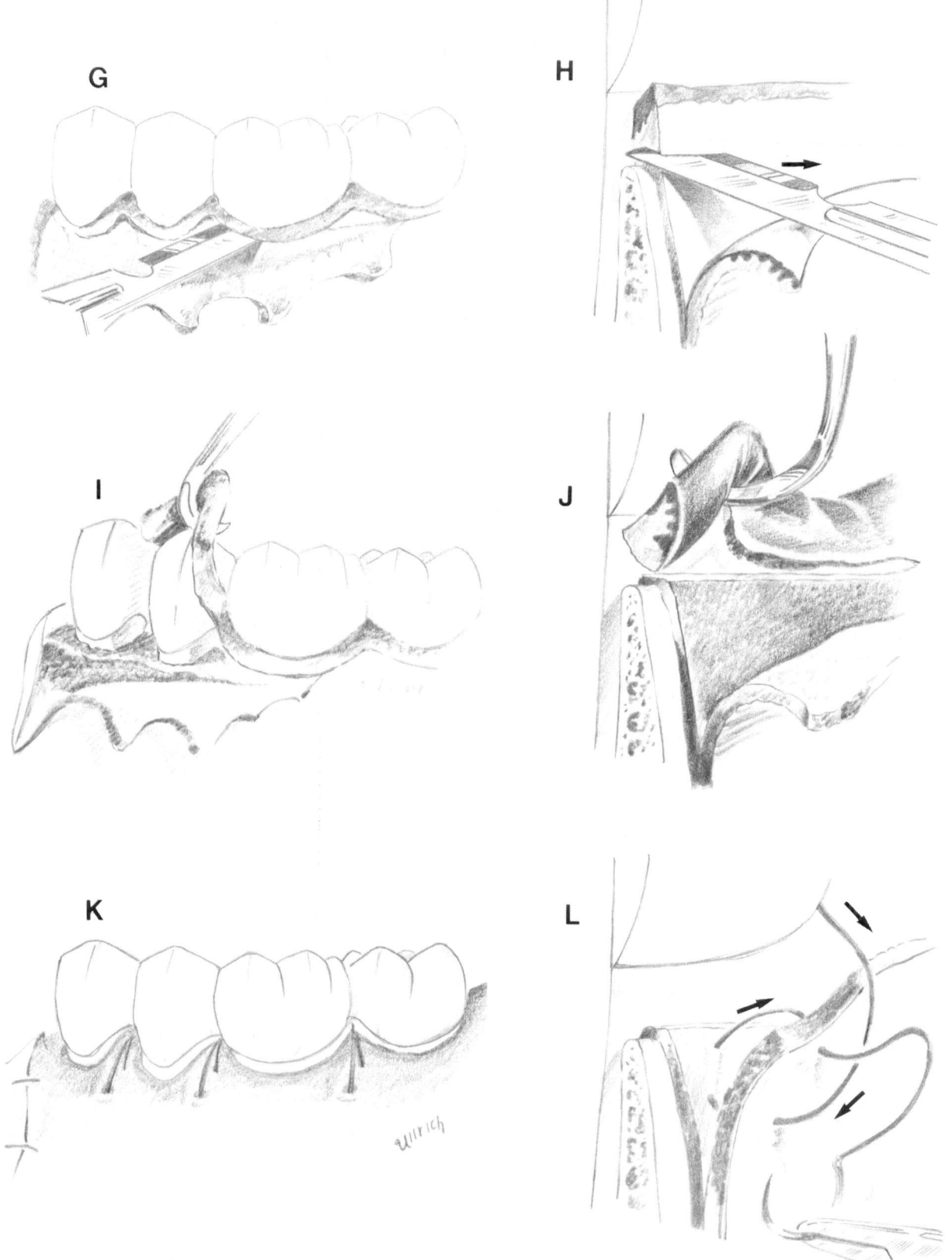

Fig. 5-9 (continued). **G,H,** A horizontal incision is made just above the crest of bone to permit removal of the inner flap. **I,J,** Scalers and curettes are now used to remove the inner flap and residual granulation tissue. **K,L,** Periosteal sutures permit exact flap placement at or below the crest of bone. A more apical placement is used if necessary to increase the zone of attached gingiva.

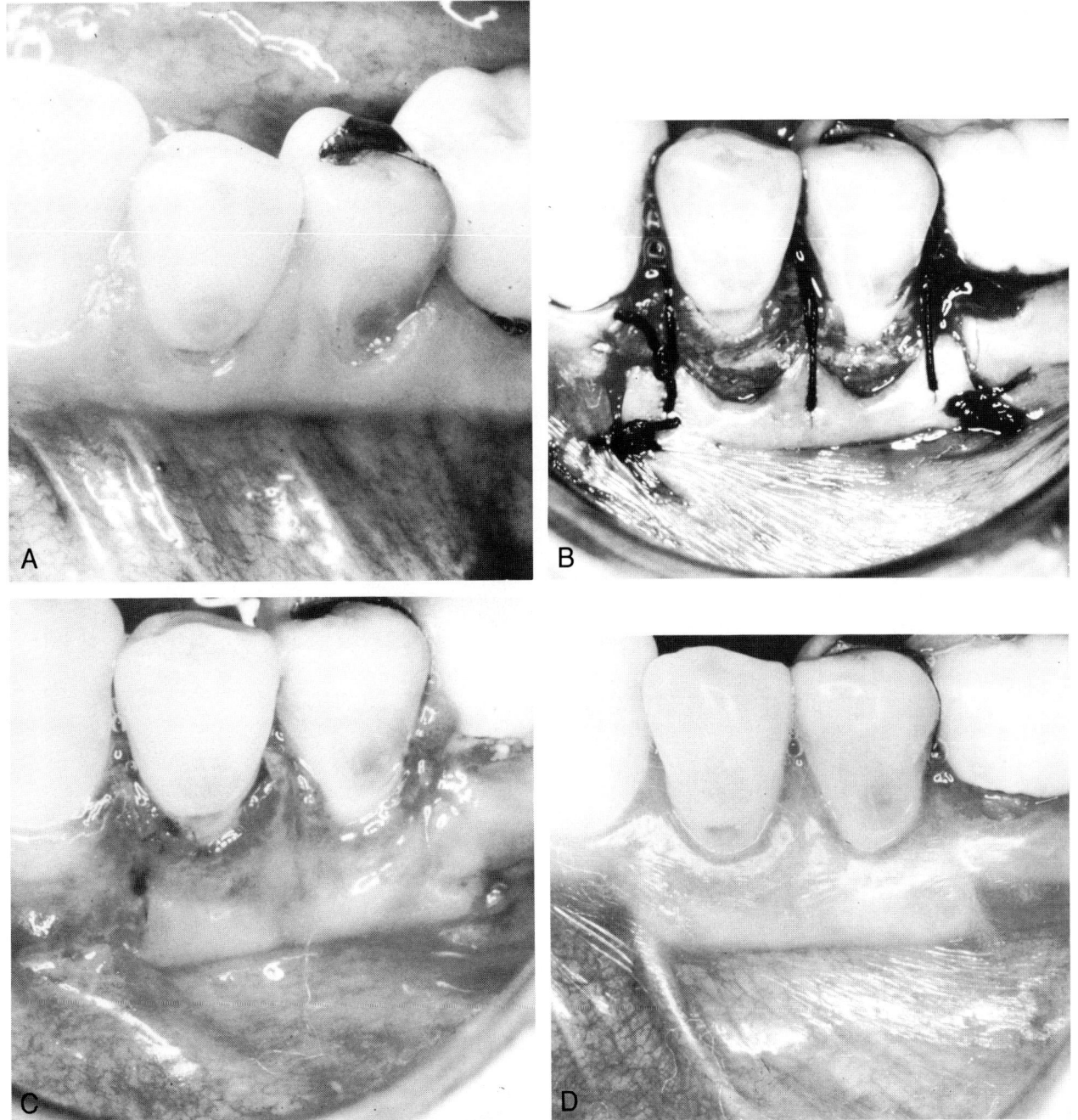

Fig. 5-10. Apically Positioned Partial-Thickness Flap. **A,** Before treatment. **B,** Partial-thickness flap apically positioned by simple suspensory suture. **C,** One week later. **D,** Two months later. Note apical displacement of mucogingival junction and increased zone of keratinized gingiva.

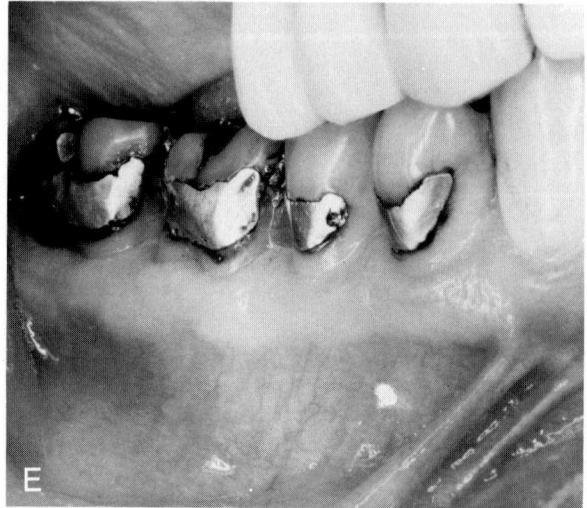

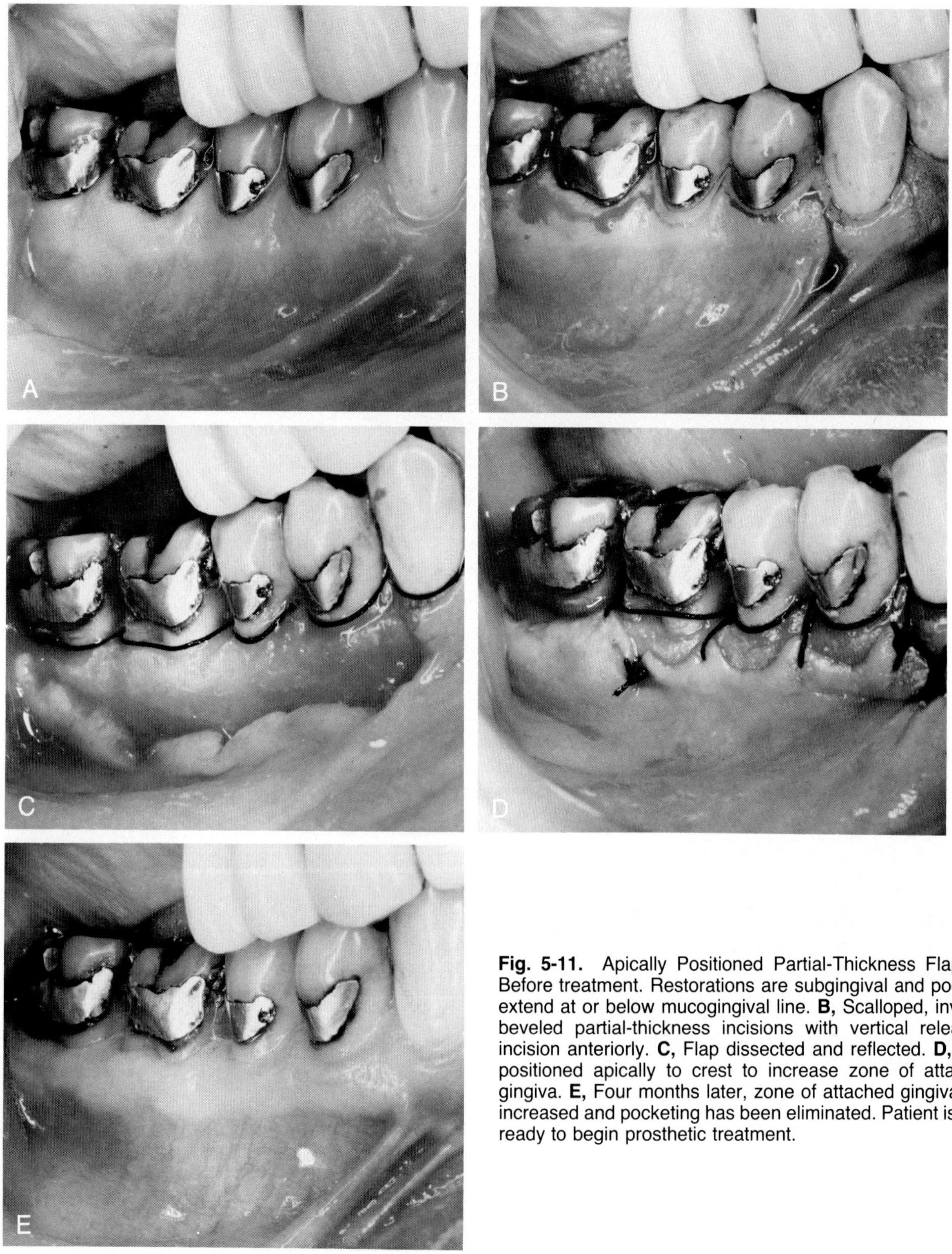

Fig. 5-11. Apically Positioned Partial-Thickness Flap. **A,** Before treatment. Restorations are subgingival and pockets extend at or below mucogingival line. **B,** Scalloped, inverse beveled partial-thickness incisions with vertical releasing incision anteriorly. **C,** Flap dissected and reflected. **D,** Flap positioned apically to crest to increase zone of attached gingiva. **E,** Four months later, zone of attached gingiva has increased and pocketing has been eliminated. Patient is now ready to begin prosthetic treatment.

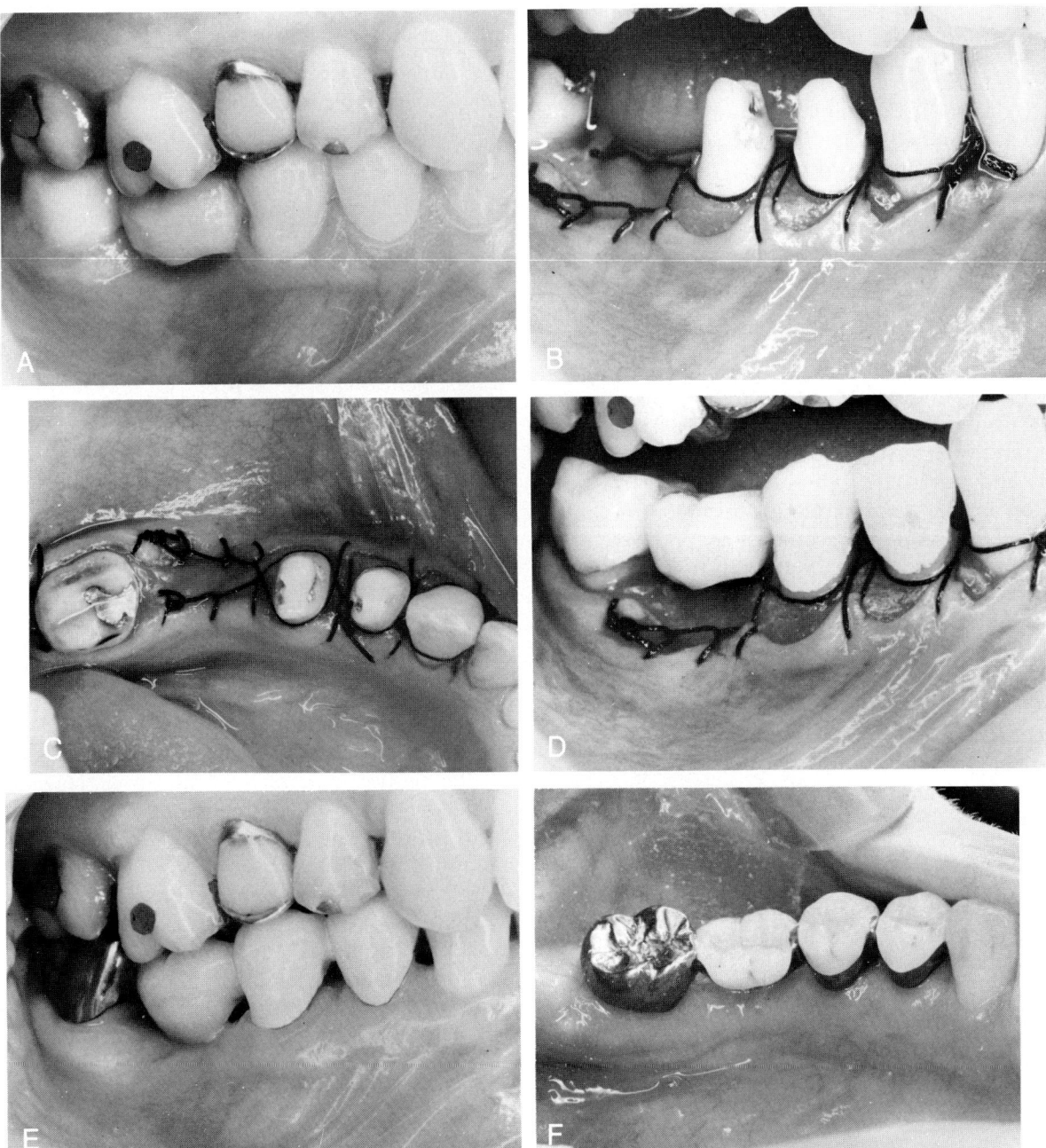

Fig. 5-12. Apically Positioned Partial-Thickness Flap for Crown Lengthening Prior to Prosthetics. **A,** Before treatment. Note margins are subgingival and the attached gingiva is inadequate. **B,** Partial-thickness flap positioned apically to crest of bone to increase zone of attached gingiva. **C,** Occlusal view showing the mucoperiosteal flap on the lingual aspect for osseous correction of small defects and pocket elimination. **D,** Temporary bridge replaced. Note adequate tooth structure visible below crown margins. Adequate *biologic width* established. **E,F,** Six months later, case complete. Note open embrasures and margins at or above gingival crest. (Prosthetics done by Dr. Bernard Croll, New York.)

FREE SOFT-TISSUE AUTOGRAFT

The free soft-tissue graft is the most widely used, most predictable technique for increasing the zone of attached gingiva. It is a highly versatile procedure, with such unlimited potential, either solely or in conjunction with other procedures, that there is a tendency to overuse. It is simple enough, while requiring a moderate degree of technical expertise, that it is within the scope of the general dentist.

Historical Background

Published reports on gingival grafting began appearing in the American literature in the 1960s: Bjorn (1963), King and Pennel (1964), Cowan (1965), Nabers (1966B), and Haggerty (1966). Yet, it was not until Sullivan and Atkins (1968) published their classic trilogy of articles on indications, techniques, and wound healing that grafting became popular. So complete were their articles that, with the exception of certain modifications, the principles and techniques outlined then are still valid today.

1. Gargiulo and Arrocha (1967) used gingivectomy tissue as donor tissue.
2. Pennel et al. (1969) developed the submarginal technique and supplemental combined use of periosteal fenestration.
3. Karring et al. (1972, 1974) showed that the connective tissue determines the nature of graft tissue and described the use of connective tissue autografts.
4. Dordick et al. (1976) placed grafts directly on bone for a firmer attachment.
5. Carvalho et al. (1982) used a periosteal pedicle as an aid in root coverage.
6. Holbrook and Ochsenbein (1983) demonstrated a refined suturing technique for root coverage.
7. Ellegaard et al. (1974) used free gingival grafts to retard epithelial migration over osseous grafts.

Advantages

1. High degree of predictability
2. Simplicity
3. Ability to treat multiple teeth at the same time
4. Can be performed when keratinized gingiva adjacent to the involved area is insufficient
5. As the first step in a two-stage procedure for attaining root coverage
6. As a single step for attaining root coverage

Disadvantages

1. Two operative sites
2. Compromised blood supply
3. Lack of predictability in attempting root coverage
4. Greater discomfort
5. Poor hemostasis
6. Retention of graft

Procedure

Preparation of Recipient Site

Anesthesia is obtained by local infiltration with a 30-gauge needle, using 1:100,000 epinephrine. Concentrations of 1:50,000 are generally unnecessary unless hemostasis is a problem. Furthermore, in giving anesthesia, an attempt should be made not to distort the mucosal tissue with excessive anesthetic, which may make preparation of the recipient site more difficult.

The surgical site is carefully examined to determine whether root coverage will be attempted. If root coverage is to be attempted, then epithelial denudation of the marginal and papillary tissue is necessary. If not, then only a submarginal incision is used.

Figure 5-13A shows a tooth with gingival recession and a minimal amount of attached tissue. Figure 5-13B gives a cross-sectional view of the same areas.

Prior to making the first incision, tension is placed on the tissue by retracting the lip or cheek. This retraction (Fig. 5-13C,D) generally lifts the mucosal tissue off the bone and up to or near the mucogingival junction. This is made possible by the loose underlying alveolar submucosal tissue.

A No. 15 scalpel blade is used to make the first incision while the tissue is still being retracted. The incision is usually begun at the distal end of the surgical site, with the blade held nearly parallel to the alveolar process. A small stab incision is made at or just below the mucogingival junction (Fig. 5-13E,F). The mucosal tissue immediately separates and retracts as a combined result of the tension and loose elastic nature of this tissue. The blade continues to be drawn in a mesial direction for the full length of the incision (Fig. 5-13G).

Once the incision is completed, sharp dissection with the scalpel blade is continued apically to separate the remaining alveolar mucosa from the firmly bound-down periosteum. The periosteal bed would be overextended in an occlusoapical direction to compensate for primary and secondary shrinkage of the graft during healing. It is generally extended 6 to 8 mm except where anatomically limited (e.g., by the mental nerve, external oblique ridge, or zygomatic arch).

An alternative method for preparation of the recipient site uses small vertical incisions to outline the surgical area. The vertical incisions are then connected with a horizontal incision at the mucogingival junction. Often, the mucosal flap is sutured at the base of the vestibule.

In the mandibular bicuspid area, special care must be given to preventing damage to the mental nerve. For this reason, LaGrange curved scissors are sometimes recommended for separating the alveolar connective tissue and reflecting the mucosa. Visualization of the branches of the mental nerve through tissue will limit apical extension of the bed.

Figure 5-13H shows the mucosal flap reflected with a submarginal incision. A small band of alveolar mucosa is still present between the periosteal bed and the keratinized attached gingiva. If this is not removed, a red band of bound-down alveolar mucosa will be permanently established between new and old tissue (Fig. 5-13E). Scissors or tissue nippers may be used to remove this residual band of alveolar mucosa (Fig. 5-13I). In Figure 5-13J, the final blending of tissue up to the mucogingival junction is complete.

In Figure 5-13K, scissors are used to remove all residual muscle and connective tissue fibers from the periosteal bed. A periodontal knife may also be used in a pushing motion apically to remove fiber and extend the periosteal bed apically. High-speed, round diamond stones or tissue nippers (Fig. 5-13K) are used to complete the epithelial denudation if this is desired. Some epithelial denudation is desirable to allow some overlap of the graft and keratinized tissue even if root coverage is not a primary goal.

Even though suturing the mucosal flap apically is unnecessary, it is often done for hemostasis and greater stability. Chromic gut sutures are recommended for apical suturing because tissue overgrowth is common at 1 week, making removal of sutures difficult. Suturing can be either interrupted or continuous.

The final step is determining graft size. This is best accomplished with a tin foil template cut to the correct size and shape and fitted first at the recipient site (Fig. 5-13L). A periodontal probe can also be used, once familiarity and confidence with the technique are developed.

A moistened saline sponge is placed over the recipient bed for hemostasis and protection.

Preparation of Donor Tissue

Site selection and thickness of donor tissue will vary according to individual operator preference and the intended purpose and function of the graft tissue.

GRAFT THICKNESS. Graft thickness was originally outlined and classified by Sullivan and Atkins (1968 A and B), who also determined the viability of the graft and its ability to withstand functional stress. Figure 5-14 shows the various thicknesses of palatal tissue they outlined. It is now generally accepted that a thin or intermediate-thickness graft is best for increasing the zone of keratinized attached gingiva, whereas a thick or full-thickness graft is recommended for root coverage and ridge augmentation procedures.

Thin or intermediate-thickness grafts of approximately 0.5 to 0.75 mm are the ideal thickness for increasing the zone of keratinized attached gingiva (Soehren et al., 1973) and at the same time producing a result that is esthetically pleasing. Grafts of this thickness undergo minimal *primary contraction* because of the small amount of elastic fibers (Orban, 1966).

On the other hand, they do undergo a good deal of *secondary contraction* of approximately 25 to 45% (Ratertschak et al., 1979; Seibert, 1980; Ward, 1974) as a result of cicatrization, which binds the graft to the underlying bed (Barsky et al., 1964). *This shrinkage can be compensated for by making the graft appropriately wider at the time of operation.*

Thick or full-thickness grafts of 1.25 to 2 mm or greater are indicated for root-coverage and ridge-augmentation procedures. They are thick enough to sustain themselves over avascular root surfaces, while thinning without splitting, until the *plasmatic diffusion* can be effective. They also tend to create an unesthetic patch-like graft; they have greater *primary contraction* owing to the large amount of elastic fibers (Davis and Kitlowski, 1931), but minimal *secondary contraction* because of the thicker lamina propria (Barsky et al., 1964). The greater primary contraction tends to delay revascularization by closing down the blood vessels (Davis and Davis, 1966).

OBTAINING GRAFT TISSUE. Donor tissue although obtainable from various sites—edentulous ridge, tuberosity area, gingivectomy tissue—is most often secured from palatal tissue. The area of choice is the *gingival zone* distal to the anterior ruga on the posterior portion of the palate (Fig. 5-13M). This has the widest gingival zone with the least amount of submucosa (Fig. 5-13N). The submucosal tissue is fatty anteriorly and glandular posteriorly.

If excessive fat or glandular tissue is taken as part of the graft, it may inhibit *graft-take* by reducing plasmatic diffusion. This is usually not a problem with thin or intermediate-thickness grafts of 0.5 mm to 1 mm, but with thicker grafts of 1.5 mm to 2 mm, which are used for root coverage, it may present a problem. On the other hand, Miller (1985B) advocated leaving a thin submucosal layer to assure adequate thickness and theorized that it may act as a barrier to the cells of the periosteum, thus permitting population by cells of the periodontal ligament and increasing potential root coverage. As shown in

Figure 5-13,O the palate has been anesthetized with xylocaine 1:50,000 for control of pain and hemorrhage. The tin foil template is placed close to the marginal area and outlined with a No. 15 scalpel blade.

The incision is begun along the occlusal aspect of the palate with a No. 15 scalpel blade held nearly parallel to the tissue. A beveled *access incision* (Sullivan and Atkins, 1968A) is sometimes recommended for achieving the desired graft thickness. Once the incision on the occlusal aspect is complete, the blade is continued apically, lifting and separating the graft as it moves through the tissue toward the apical border. *Note that, in directing the blade apically, special care should be given to maintaining an even thickness and not taking too deep a wedge.*

It is necessary to release the most anterior vertical incision prior to detaching the graft apically (Fig. 5-13P). Once that is done, tissue pliers are used to retract the graft distally as it is being separated apically and dissected, until the graft is totally freed (Fig. 5-13Q).

The freed graft is placed on a gauze moistened with saline until needed. The palate is then sutured with chromic gut or silk to assure hemostasis (Fig. 5-13R). Most postoperative problems are the result of bleeding from the palate and not from the recipient site.

More recently, a microfibrillar collagen hemostat (MCH) has been used for donor site coverage to achieve hemostasis. The MCH is supplied in two forms—a shredded fluff (Avitene) and a nonwoven web (Collestat, Avitene). The shredded form is much more difficult to work with than the sponge form. Both prevent oozing from the exposed connective tissue of the palate (Stein et al., 1985; Saroff et al., 1980).

GRAFT PREPARATION. The underside or nonepithelial side of the graft is inspected for any glandular or fatty tissue remnants (Fig. 5-13S). The thickness of the graft is also checked to make sure it is generally smooth and uniform. If necessary, the graft, while on the moistened gauze, is trimmed of fat and glandular and excessive tissue using a new No. 15 scalpel blade (Fig. 5-13T). Care should be taken not to overthin and perforate the graft.

The graft should now be brought to the patient's mouth and checked for proper size and shape. The final shaping is usually done with scissors, outside the mouth and on a wet gauze.

Suturing is begun by holding the graft with Corn pliers and passing a suture through it (Fig. 5-13V); whether silk or gut sutures are used does not matter. The graft is now returned to the mouth, where the suturing is continued. A *Castroviejo* needle holder facilitates suturing. It is also helpful to have the assistant hold the graft in place with a small round instrument as the first suture is being placed. This prevents the lifting and movement of the graft that is common on the first one or two sutures.

If a thick or full-thickness graft has been utilized, a horizontal stretching suture should be used to overcome the effects of primary contraction (Sullivan and Atkins, 1968A). This stretching suture allows the blood vessels within the graft to open, permitting early diffusion of fluids.

The final placement of the graft will be either at the mucogingival junction (Fig. 5-13W), if a submarginal incision was performed, or on the denuded epithelial tissue (Fig. 5-13X), if root coverage was attempted (for variations of this procedure, see Holbrook and Ochsenbein, 1983; Carvalho et al., 1982).

The procedure is depicted clinically in Figures 5-15, 5-16, and 5-17.

Common Reasons For Graft Failure

1. The most common cause for the failure of grafts is their use for root coverage. If the denuded root defect is small enough, the collateral circulation will be adequate to support bridging. On the other hand, when prominent roots with relatively wide areas of root exposure are grafted, two-point collateral circulation is insufficient for graft support. As a result, the center of the graft thins and becomes necrotic, the graft splits and ultimately fails (Fig. 5-18A).
2. Proper graft adaptation to the underlying periosteum is important. After suturing, slight pressure is applied to the graft with gauze moistened with saline for 5 minutes to permit fibrin clot formation and prevent bleeding. Bleeding will result in a hematoma under the graft with subsequent necrosis (Fig. 5-18B).
3. To permit adequate transfusion of the graft, it has been recommended that all fat and glandular tissue be removed prior to suturing to prevent possible necrosis and/or inadequate take (Fig. 5-18C). Even though the need for this has been questioned, it is still generally accepted procedure.
4. Graft movement as a result of inadequate or insufficient suturing will surely result in failure because no plasmatic diffusion will occur (Fig. 5-18D).
5. The final failure is often seen only after the graft has healed. The clinical appearance is acceptable, but the graft is totally movable when probed. This is a failure of technique and results from not removing all loose connective tissue

and muscle fibers from the periosteal bed prior to placement and not making sure that the bed is firmly attached to the underlying bone.

Recipient Modification

Graft stabilization and fixation are primary objectives of therapy. In an attempt to achieve more predictable stabilization, various modifications have been advocated.

Full-Thickness Recipient Site

The use of a full-thickness flap for placement of graft directly onto bone has been advocated for achieving greater graft stability (Dordick et al., 1976). It is advocated only where the alveolar housing is thick enough to prevent excessive bone resorption with its resultant dehiscence and/or fenestration formation. Seibert (1980) recommended the use of a full-thickness flap only in the mandibular molar areas where the periosteum is not firmly bound down and is easily lifted off the bone.

The general consensus is that this technique need not be used if proper care is taken with the periosteal bed technique. Furthermore, healing is delayed with this technique, with a chance of necrosis or infection.

PROCEDURE. A No. 15 scalpel blade is used to make an incision at the mucogingival junction down to the bone (Fig. 5-19A and B). The flap is reflected by blunt dissection and sutured apically, thus exposing the bone (Fig. 5-19C and D).

All other aspects of preparation of the donor area are the same (i.e., epithelial denudation, removal of the remainder of alveolar mucosa, etc.). *Note: **This technique is not recommended for use when attempting root coverage. It is also not recommended when the periodontium is thin and the roots are palpable through the tissue.***

Vertical Osseous Clefts

To overcome the negative aspects of total bone exposure, the technique has been modified further to permit preparation of the periosteal bed with vertical interradicular openings for bone exposure (Fig. 5-20,1). This has the main advantage of preventing excessive bone resorption over the radicular surfaces. The amount of additional retention achieved is questionable.

Periosteal Separation

In this procedure, periosteal fenestration (Corn, 1962; Robinson, 1961) is used at the base of the periosteal bed for apical scarring and greater graft stabilization (Fig. 5-20,2). The separation is achieved using a No. 15 scalpel blade at the base to make a horizontal incision down to the bone. The incision is widened by blunt dissection, exposing 1 to 2 mm of bone. Apical suturing of the mucosal flap is optional.

This procedure achieves little additional graft stability when the donor site is prepared properly; also, it is limited in the mandibular premolar area because of the mental nerve. Morman et al. (1979) also pointed out that, since the gingival blood supply is in an apico-occlusal direction and not a mesiodistal direction, this procedure may also compromise the blood supply.

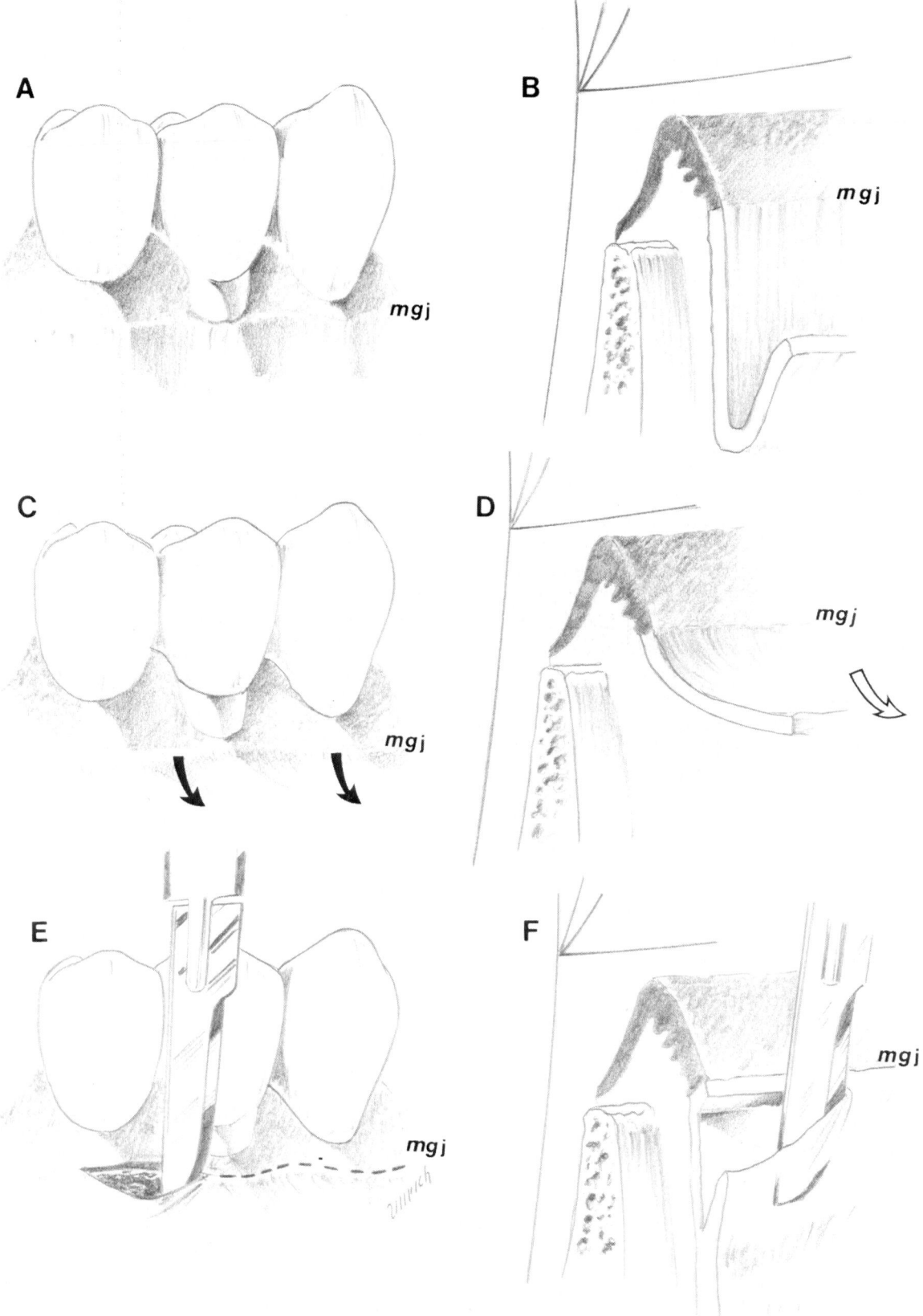

Fig. 5-13. Free Soft-Tissue Autograft. **A,** Preoperative view, showing recession and lack of attached keratinized gingiva on bicuspid. **B,** Cross section (CX) of bicuspid with recession and lack of attached gingiva. **C,D,** Facial and CX views display the effects of tension applied to tissue. Note that the tension raises the mucosal tissue off the bone. **E,F,** Initial stab incision just at or below mucogingival junction (mgj) with blade held parallel to the bone.

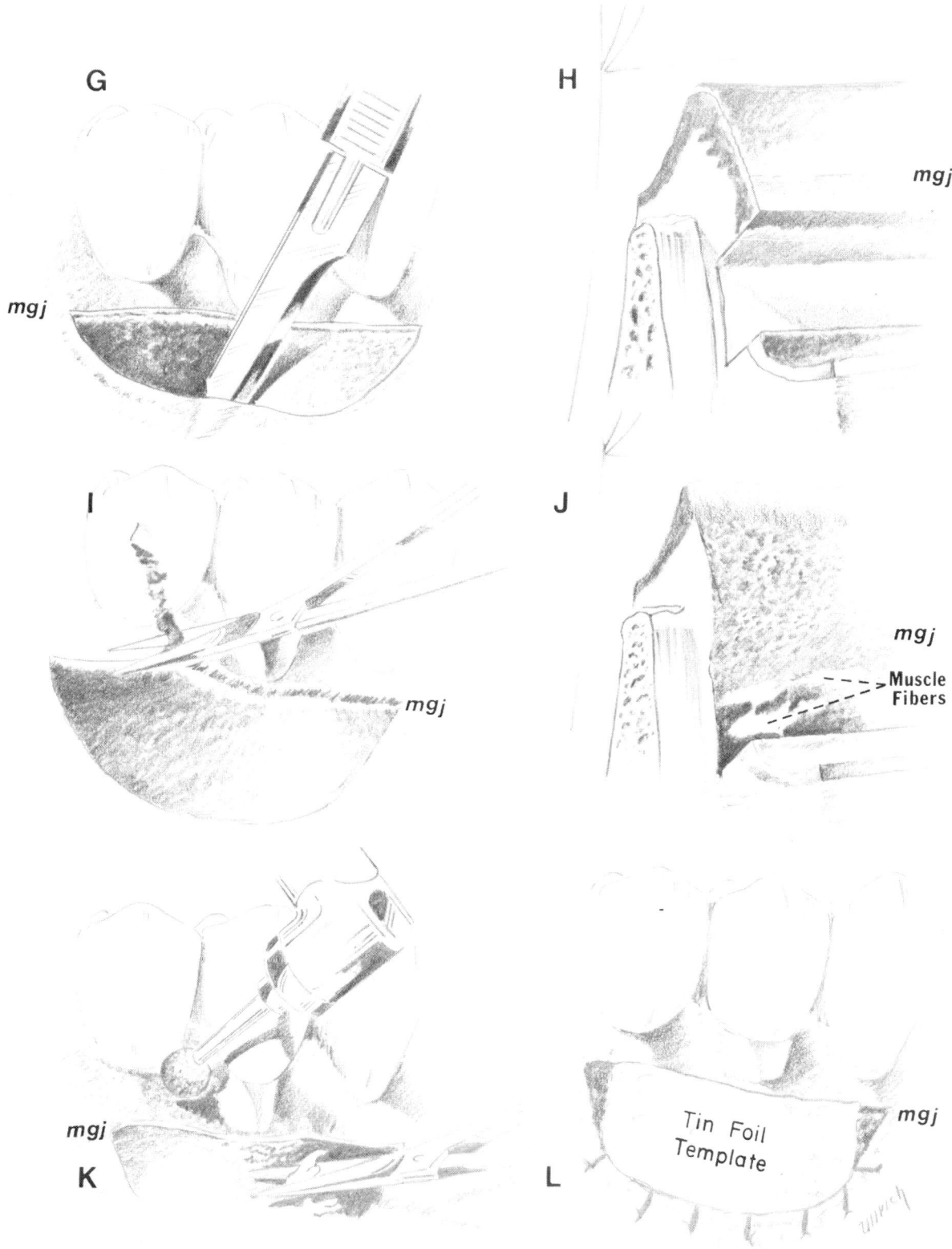

Fig. 5-13 (continued). **G,** Continuation of incisions both horizontally and apically. **H,** CX, showing tissue reflected, leaving a periosteal bed. **I,** Removal of residual alveolar mucosa at mgj. **J,** CX shows *blending* of prepared periosteal bed with coronal attached gingivae and removal of residual alveolar mucosa. **K,** Final removal of muscle and connective tissue fibers from periosteal bed as well as *blending* of incisions. **L,** Tin foil template used to help establish size of donor tissue.

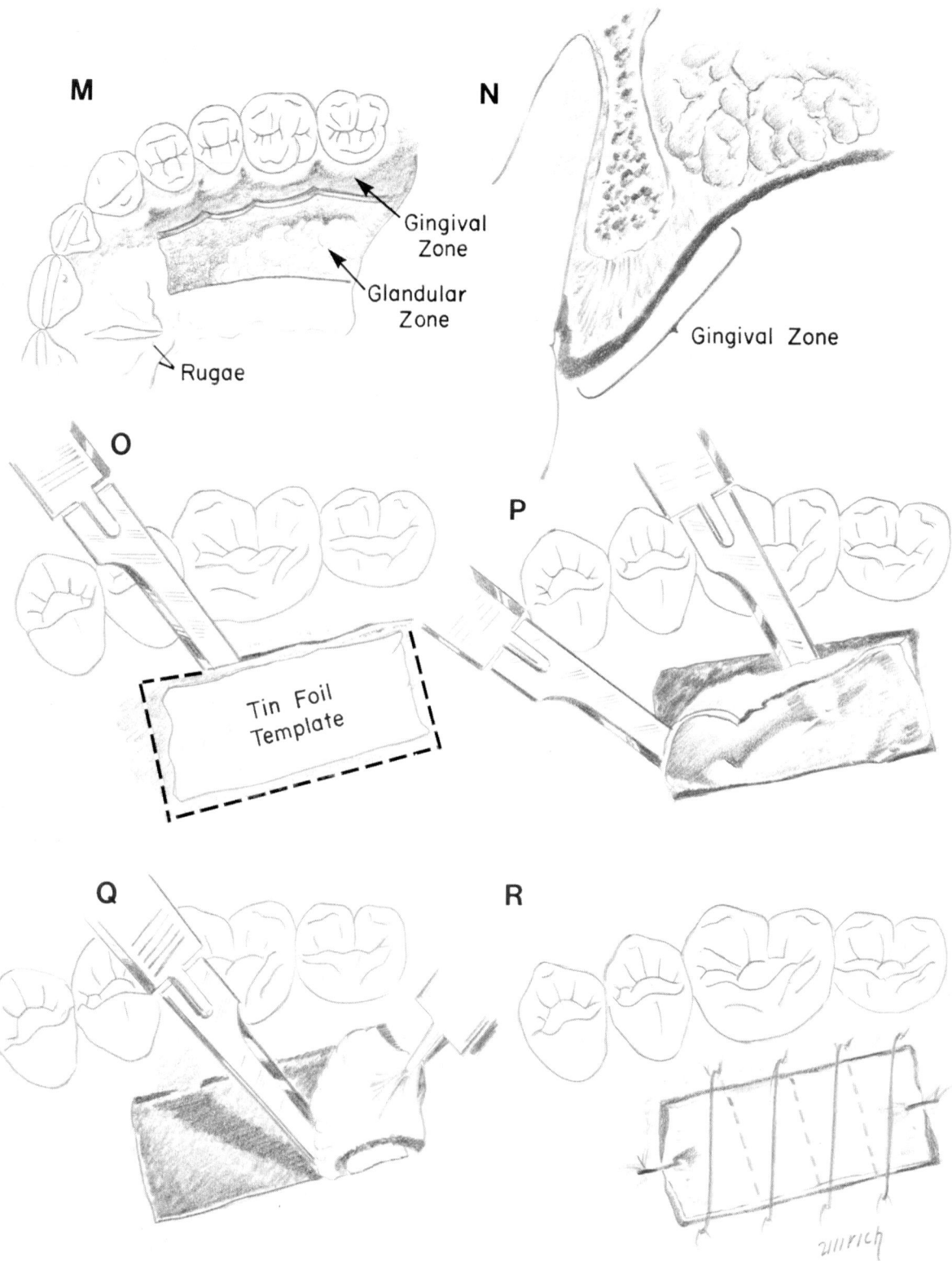

Fig. 5-13 (continued). M, Represents various zones of palate from which donor material may be selected. **N,** CX enlargement of posterior gingival zone from which material is usually selected. **O,** Outlining of graft from previously sized tin foil template. **P,** Partial-thickness dissection of graft. **Q,** Use of tissue pliers to reflect graft tissue as it is being dissected. **R,** Graft removed and palate sutured for hemostasis.

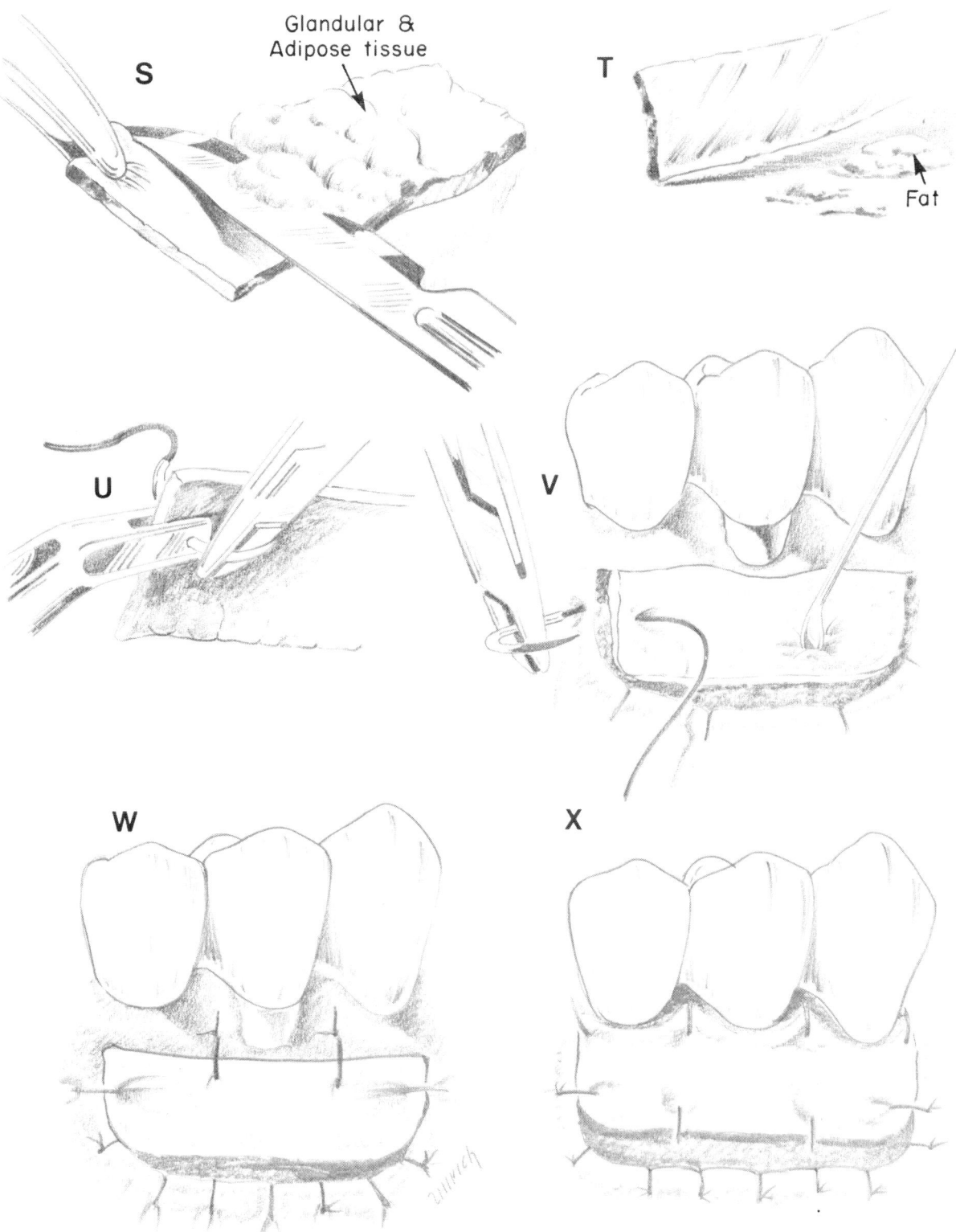

Fig. 5-13 (continued). **S,** Use of sharp scalpel blade to remove any fat or glandular tissue and to reduce underlying tissue irregularities. **T,** Graft smoothed. **U,** Initial suture placed in graft. **V,** Stabilization of graft during suturing phase. **W,** Graft placed below recession and sutured in position. Note apical suturing of mucosal flap, which is optional. **X,** Coronal positioning for root coverage.

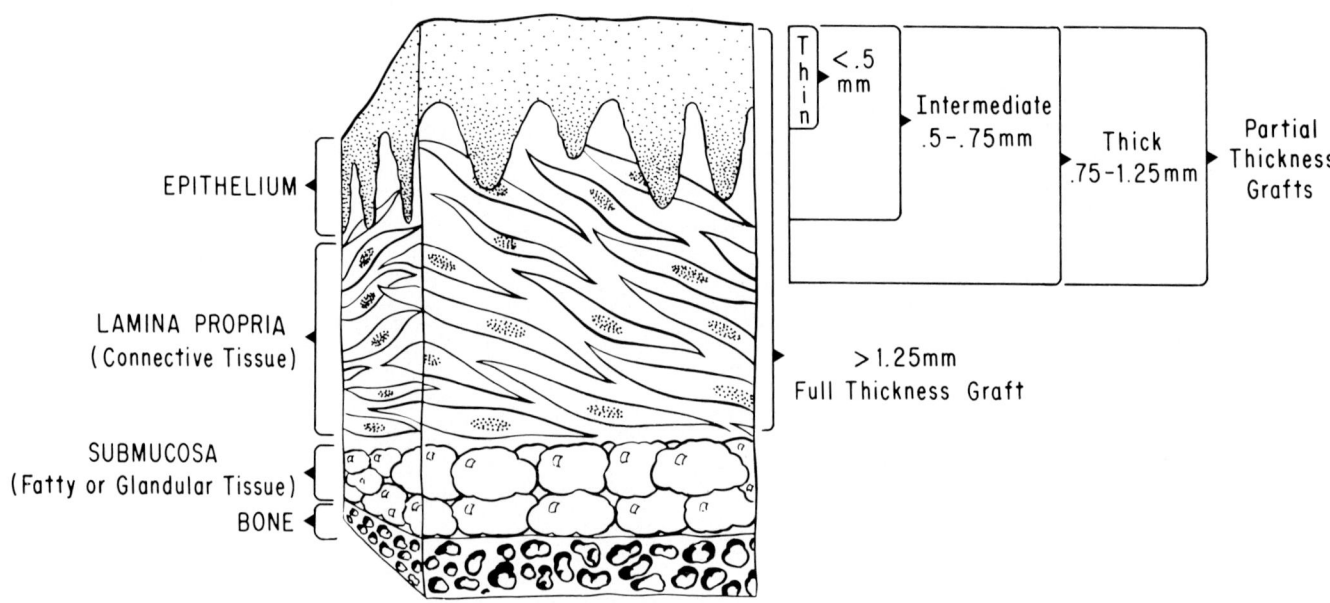

Fig. 5-14. Diagrammatic Representation of Palatal Tissue. Illustration of partial- and full-thickness soft-tissue grafts of various thicknesses.

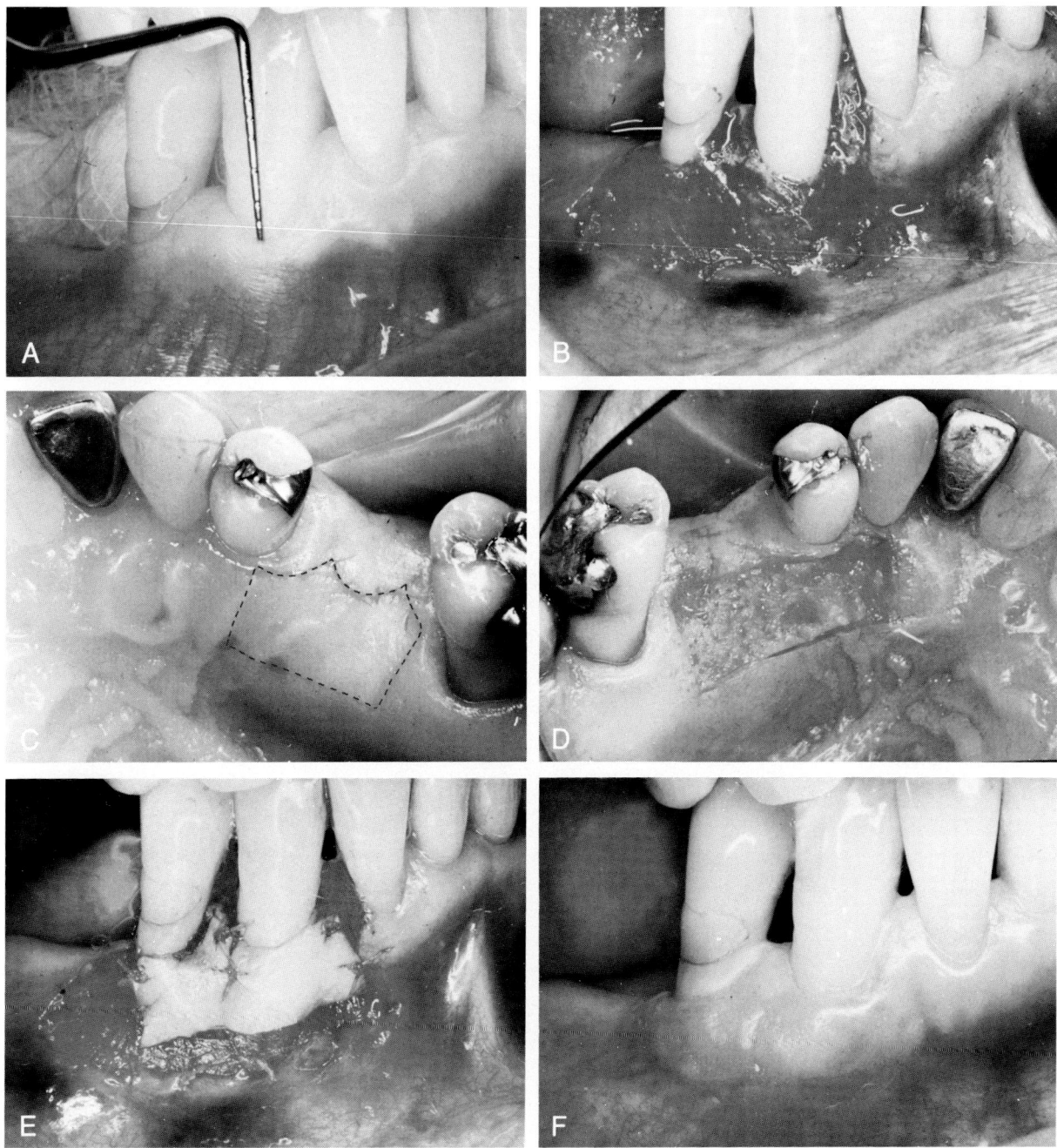

Fig. 5-15. Free Soft-Tissue Autograft. **A,** Before, with probe showing minimal attached tissue. **B,** Mucosal flap reflected and sutured apically with periosteal bed prepared. **C,** Graft outlined on palate. **D,** Graft removed. **E,** Graft sutured. **F,** Six months later, amount of keratinized attached gingiva is significantly increased.

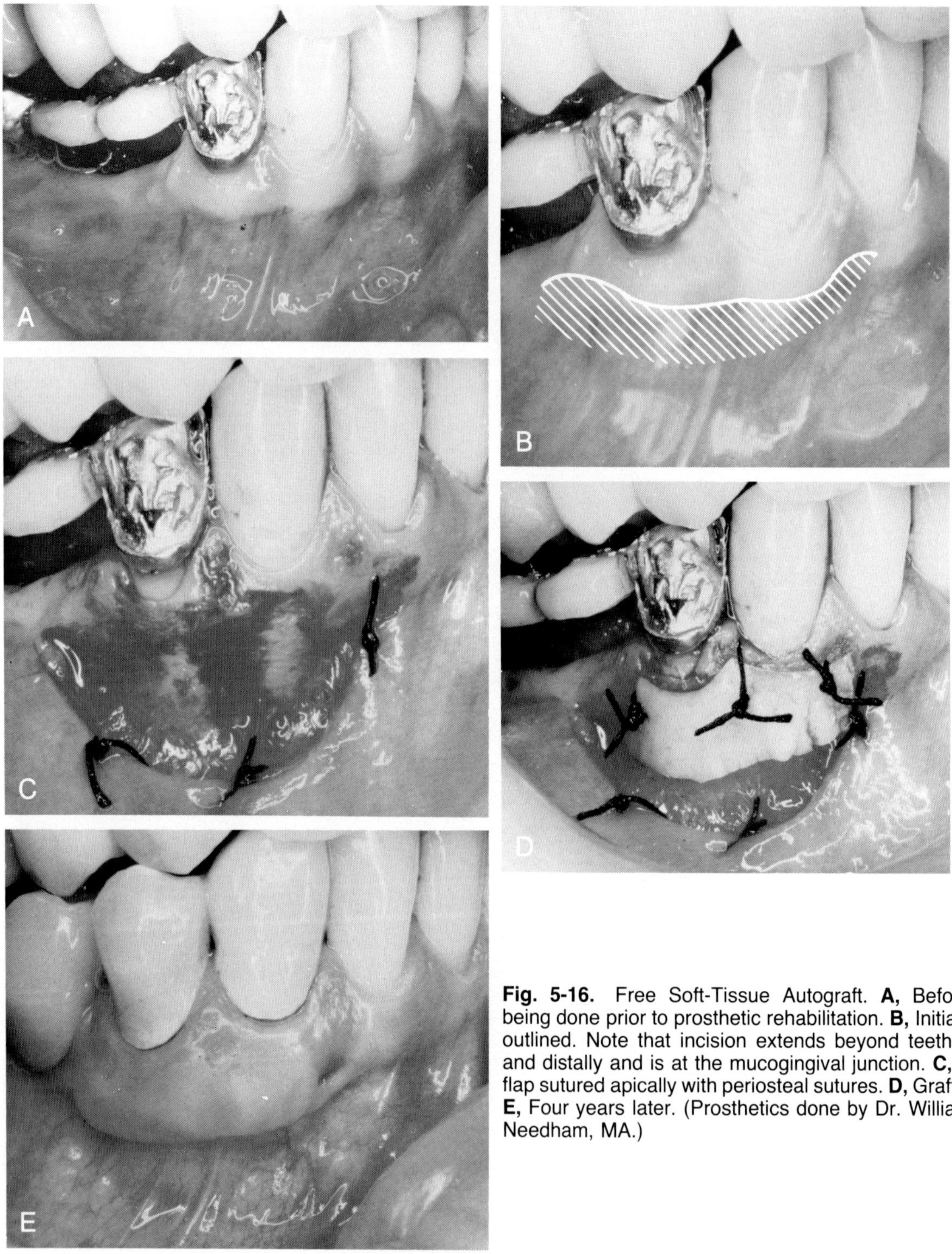

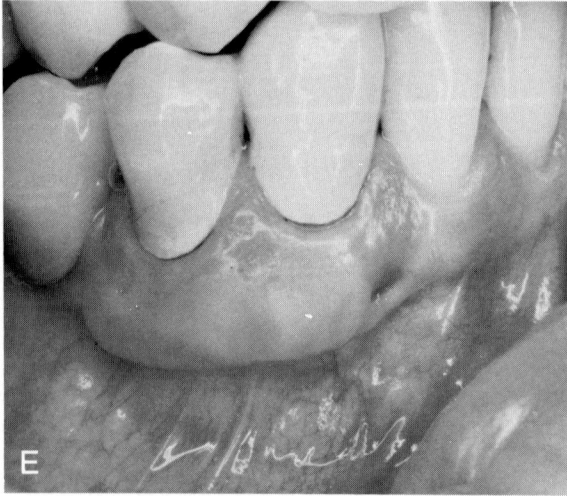

Fig. 5-16. Free Soft-Tissue Autograft. **A,** Before. Graft being done prior to prosthetic rehabilitation. **B,** Initial incision outlined. Note that incision extends beyond teeth mesially and distally and is at the mucogingival junction. **C,** Mucosal flap sutured apically with periosteal sutures. **D,** Graft sutured. **E,** Four years later. (Prosthetics done by Dr. William Irving, Needham, MA.)

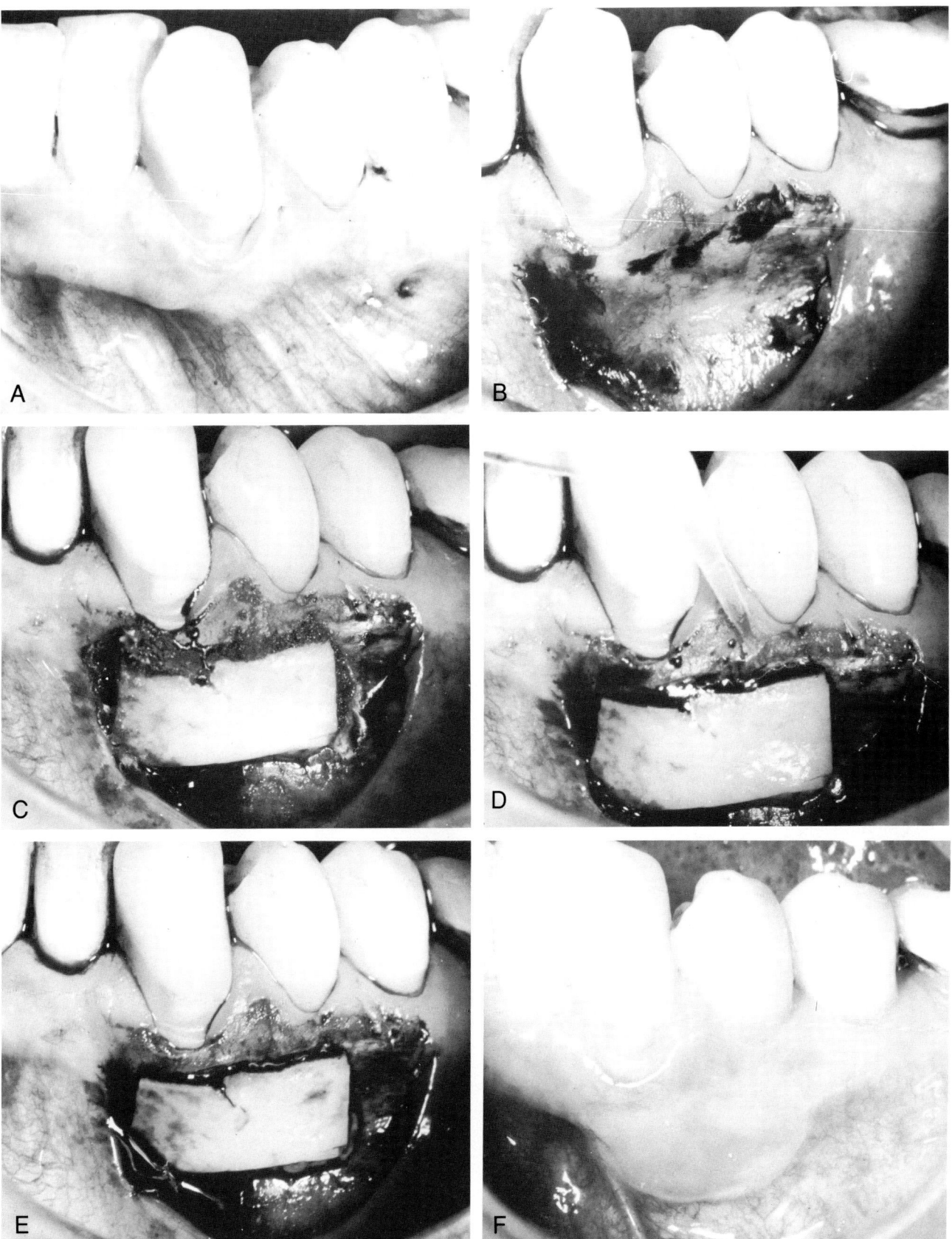

Fig. 5-17. Free Soft-Tissue Autograft with Cyanoacrylate. **A,** Before treatment. **B,** Periosteal bed prepared. **C,** Autograft positioned. **D,** Micropipet with cyanoacrylate. **E,** Graft stabilized with cyanoacrylate. **F,** Two months later.

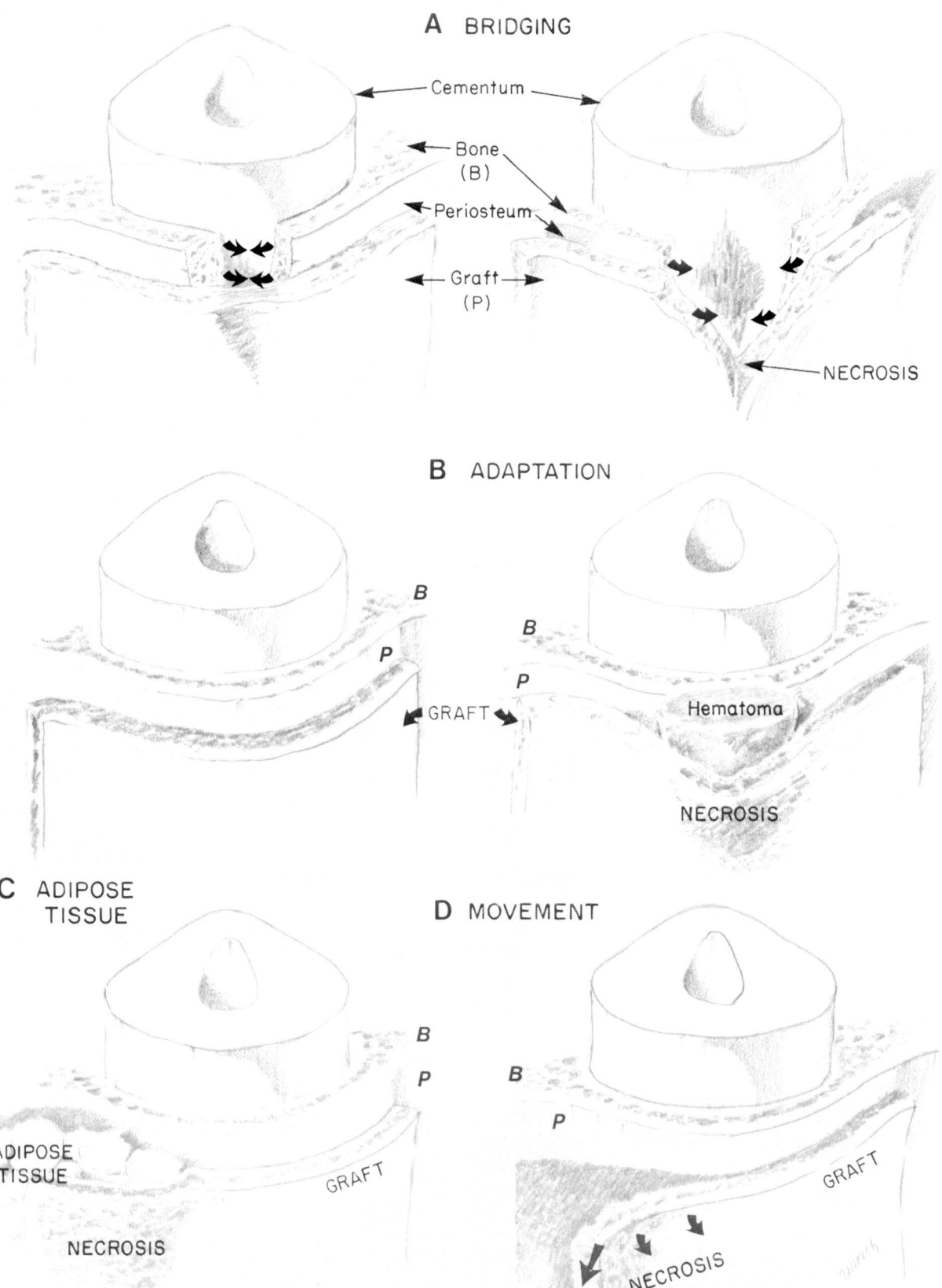

Fig. 5-18. Reasons for Graft Failure. **A,** If the area of exposed root to be covered is small, blood vessels of the periosteum will maintain graft vitality (left). Graft necrosis occurs when the blood vessels from the periosteum cannot bridge the gap (right). **B,** Close graft-periosteum adaptation (left) will prevent hematoma formation (right) and graft necrosis. **C,** Residual fatty or glandular tissue may prevent graft take. **D,** Movement of graft because of poor stabilization will result in failure.

Mucogingival Surgery

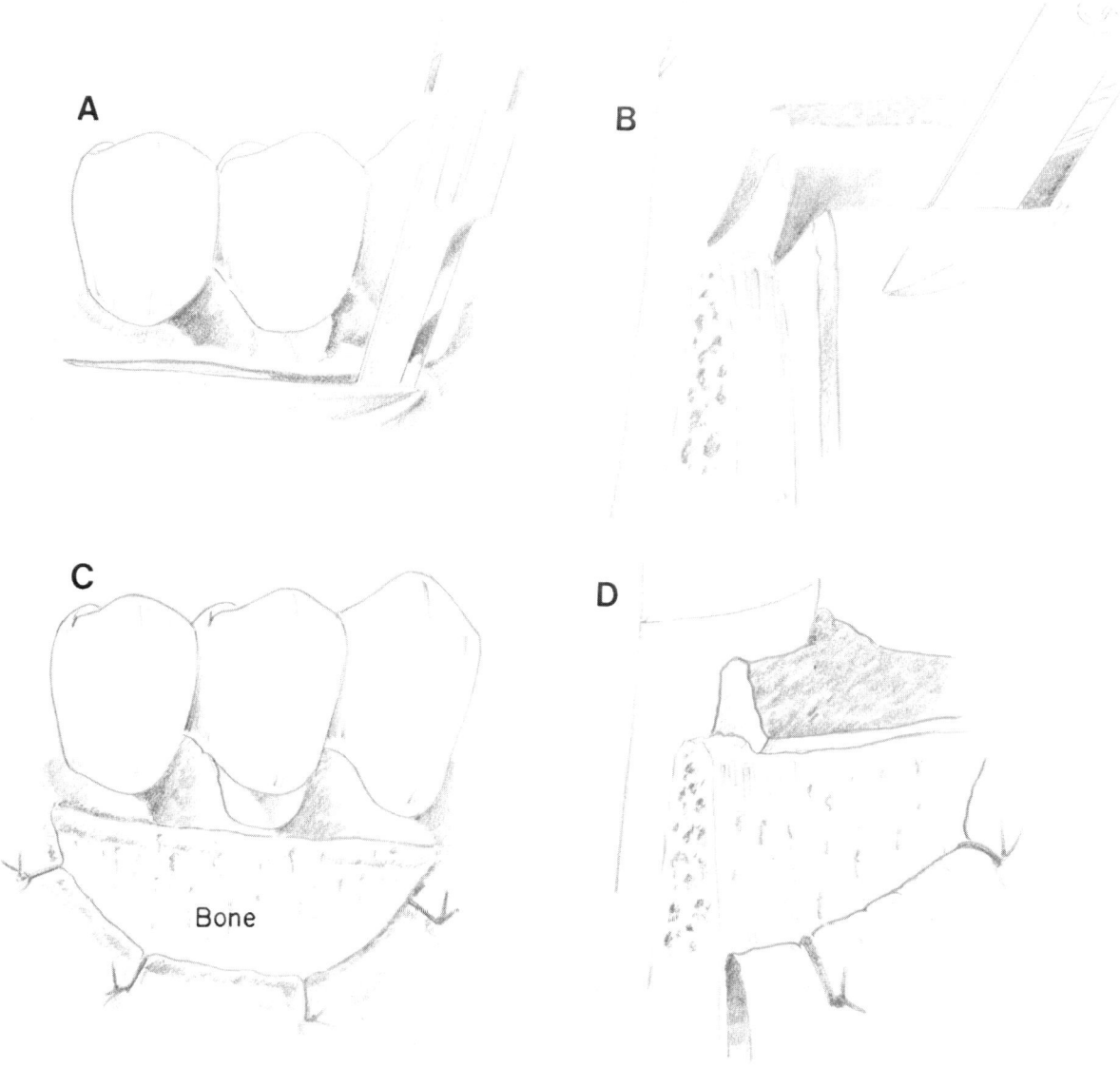

Fig. 5-19. Modification of Recipient Bed for Graft Placement. **A,B,** Facial and side views showing that a full-thickness mucoperiosteal flap is reflected. **C,D,** Apical suturing of mucosal flap and exposure of bone.

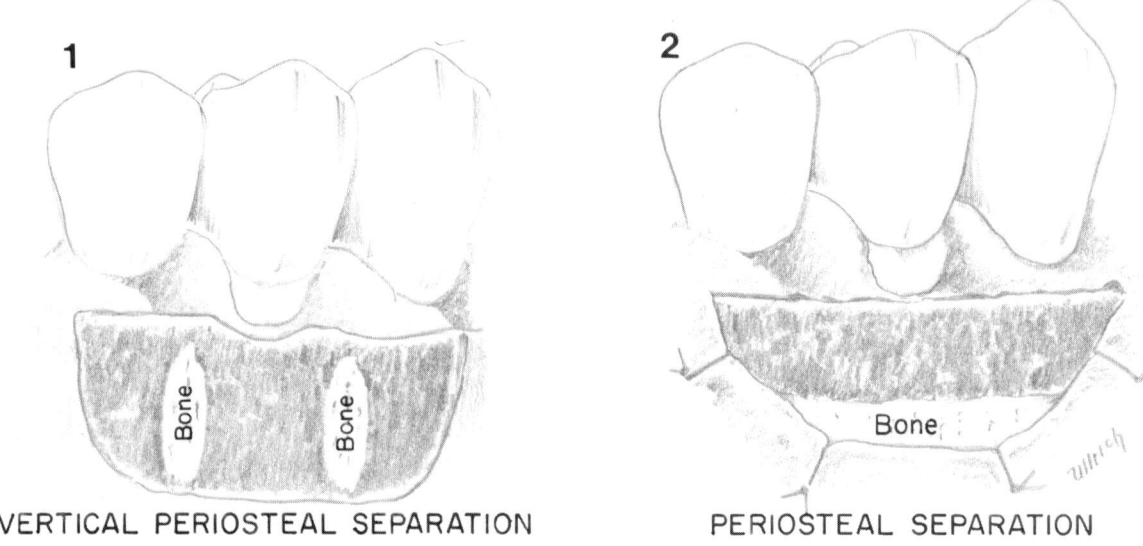

Fig. 5-20. Modification of Recipient Bed for Graft Placement. **1,** Vertical interradicular bone exposure to enhance graft take without exposure of bone over the radicular surfaces. **2,** Periosteal separation to bind down apical areas and prevent shrinkage or movement.

LATERALLY POSITIONED PEDICLE FLAPS

Historical Review

In 1956, Grupe and Warren developed an original and unique procedure called the *sliding flap operation* for covering an isolated exposed root (Fig. 5-21A). It involved moving a full-thickness flap to the mucogingival junction, after which a partial-thickness flap was raised. To prevent donor site recession, Grupe in 1966 modified this to a submarginal incision on the donor site (Fig. 5-21B). Staffileno (1964) solved this problem by using a partial-thickness flap to protect the donor site from recession. Corn (1964B) further modified this by adding a *cutback* incision to release tension (Fig. 5-21C). He also took the pedicle from the edentulous ridge. Dahlberg (1969) used engineering principles with the *rotated pedicle flap,* which did not require a cutback incision (Fig. 5-21D). Goldman and Smukler in 1978 added the *periosteally stimulated* flap and a *partial-full rotated* flap in 1983, which allowed a full-thickness flap to cover the denuded root surface and a partial-thickness flap to cover the exposed bone (Fig. 5-21E).

Advantages

1. One surgical site
2. Good vascularity of the pedicle flap
3. Ability to cover a denuded root surface

Disadvantages

1. Limited by the amount of adjacent keratinized attached gingiva
2. Possibility of recession at the donor site
3. Dehiscence or fenestrations at the donor site
4. Limited to one or two teeth with recession

Contraindications

1. Presence of deep interproximal pockets
2. Excessive root prominences
3. Deep or extensive root abrasion or erosion
4. Significant loss of interproximal bone height

Basic Procedure

All pedicle flaps are variations of the basic procedural techniques outlined below.

Preparation of Recipient Site

Figure 5-22 graphically shows one tooth with recession extending beyond the mucogingival junction and with no remaining attached gingiva. The basic incisions over the denuded root (a,b,c) and the anticipated flap outline (d,e,f) are depicted in Figure 5-22B.

The first step prior to the start of surgery is root planing to remove softened cementum and to reduce or eliminate prominent convexity of the root. *Citric acid* (pH 1.0) *is burnished in with a moistened cotton pledget for 3 to 5 minutes if root coverage is to be attempted.* The citric acid is used to help detoxify the exposed root and expose the embedded connective tissue fibers. This exposure of tissue fibers may permit *linkage* (Stahl and Tarnow, 1985).

A No. 15 scalpel blade is used to make a *V-shaped* incision about the denuded root, removing the adjacent epithelium and connective tissue (Fig. 5-22C). In the case of deep labial pockets and associated frenula, the apex of the V-shaped incision is extended far and wide enough apically to remove them (Fig. 5-22C and D). It is also important that the V-shaped incision is *beveled out* (bi) on the opposite side from the donor area, permitting overlap and increased vascularity for the donor tissue in this area (Fig. 5-22D). Finally, all tissue remnants are removed from the area before the root is planed.

Preparation of Donor Site

Figure 5-22B outlines the incision (d,e,f) that will be used for the donor flap. *The donor flap as shown should be at least 1½ times the size of the recipient area to be covered and 3 to 4 times longer than it is wide.*

A partial-thickness flap is begun with a scalloped, inverse beveled incision at the gingival crest, using a No. 15 scalpel blade. The incision extends from the V-shaped incision to the vertical incision (Fig. 5-22E). *This incision is not made down to the bone.* The horizontal incision is stopped at the mucogingival junction. All of the interproximal papillae are partially dissected, thinned, and maintained.

A vertical incision is now made with a No. 15 scalpel blade at the donor site, but *it is not made down to bone.* It is extended far enough apically into the mucosal tissue to permit adequate mobility of the flap. The base of the flap must be wide, but not wider than the coronal portion, to permit adequate vascularity. The scalpel blade is inserted into the vertical incision apical to the mucogingival line (Fig. 5-22F). The blade is moved in a coronal direction as tension is placed on the flap with tissue pliers, permitting easy separation. The flap is sharply dissected, making sure to carefully preserve all of the interproximal papillae.

Preparation of Pedicle Flap

The flap is raised and reflected forward. A No. 15 scalpel blade is used to further free and smooth the underlying side from residual muscle and connective tissue fibers (Fig. 5-22G). *The flap should be free enough to permit movement to the recipient site with no tension.*

If a full-thickness pedicle flap were raised using

blunt dissection, the flap would still have to be freed on its underlying side (Fig. 5-22H). Note that, except for the use of the full-thickness flap, all other stages are similar.

When attempting to position the pedicle flap over the recipient site, if tension is encountered, a *cutback* or releasing incision will be required to dissipate the tension (Fig. 5-22J).

Figure 5-22K and L show the finished case. The pedicle flap is positioned coronally 1 to 2 mm onto the enamel of the recipient tooth or to the maximum height that the interproximal tissue will allow. The concept that the maximum height for gaining coverage is determined by the interproximal tissue height has sometimes been termed the *peak theory*. Suturing is done with 4-0, 5-0, or 6-0 silk or gut suture. All sutures are interrupted except for a sling suture used to pull the papillae interproximally and hold the tissue tightly against the neck of the tooth. It is sometimes helpful to hold the pedicle with Corn suture pliers for the first one or two sutures or until the flap is stabilized adequately.

Note that the only exposed areas are the interradicular spaces between the teeth and not the facial surfaces. This helps to prevent recession at the donor site, and in a full-thickness pedicle flap, will prevent excessive bone resorption. Further, note the overlap of the pedicle with the *beveled-out* portion of the V-shaped incision.

The procedure is depicted clinically in Figures 5-23, 5-24, and 5-25.

Common Reasons For Failure

1. Figure 5-26A represents one of the more common errors of tension at the base of the distal incision. This is easily corrected by use of a releasing or *cutback* incision.
2. Figure 5-26B represents the worst type of mistake, a pedicle that is too narrow. There is no correction for this, and failure is almost assured. The basic rule is for a *pedicle or donor flap to be at least 1½ times as wide as the recipient bed*.
3. Figure 5-26C is a common fault of the full-thickness flap that results in exposure of bone over the radicular surface. This permits bone loss, fenestration and/or dehiscence formation. The right side of Figure 5-26D is representative of the type of bony defects found on the radicular surface of a thin periodontium. Full-thickness flaps are contraindicated in the presence of a thin periosteum.
4. Figure 5-26D depicts poor stabilization and mobility of the flap. Movement prevents intimate contact between tooth and flap and generally results in failure.

Edentulous Ridge Modification

This procedure is similar to that for laterally positioned pedicle flaps in all respects except that, if the edentulous area is long enough, more teeth may be treated and the amount of keratinized donor tissue may be increased by operating more lingually or palatally to the ridge.

Figure 5-27A shows a molar with recession on the mesiobuccal root adjacent to an edentulous area.

Figure 5-27B shows the basic outline of the incisions and a probe extending beyond the mucogingival junction. In making the V-shaped incision (a,b,c), the surgeon takes care not to involve the furcation area and extends the incision down far enough apically to remove any pockets. Instead of a straight vertical incision, more of an oblique incision is made in the donor area. This permits more of a *rotated* pedicle flap and creates minimal need for a *cutback* releasing incision.

In Figure 5-27C, a No. 15 scalpel blade has been used to make a V-shaped incision and remove a wedge. The initial incision is carried along the crest of the ridge as a partial-thickness incision (Fig. 5-27D). A full-thickness pedicle flap is often used over the edentulous area because of the regenerative ability of the bone and the lack of adjacent teeth.

Figure 5-27E and F represent situations in which the zone of keratinized gingiva is adequate in one (E) and inadequate in the other (F). In the case of the inadequate zone, the incision will have to be made on the lingual (palatal) aspect of the ridge to increase the amount of keratinized tissue. The dotted lines in both represent the partial-thickness incision.

The pedicle is dissected with a No. 15 scalpel blade being moved in an apico-occlusal direction (Fig. 5-27G); once split, it is reflected forward and freed from underneath using the same scalpel blade (Fig. 5-27H).

In Figure 5-27I the flap is reflected and a *beveled-out* incision is added to the fixed recipient portion of the V-shaped incision to permit overlapping of the donor pedicle. Figure 5-27J shows a full-thickness pedicle flap.

Figure 5-27K and L show the sutured pedicle in place. Note that, when the oblique incision at the donor area is properly executed, no cutback incision is required.

The procedure is depicted clinically in Figures 5-28, 5-29, and 5-30.

Oblique Rotated Pedicle Flap

Dahlberg (1969) designed incisions for pedicle flaps based on a center of rotation about an axis at the base of the vertical donor incision. This permitted the pedicle to be moved over the donor site without tension and without the need for releasing incisions.

Figure 5-31A shows the outline of the incisions. The donor flap is outlined by two incisions, one of which also forms part of the V-shaped incision. Each incision is made at an oblique angle. The two vertical incisions are carried apically far enough that the apex of the V-shaped incision extends distal to the recipient site, and the base of the donor incision extends to the distal line angle of the next tooth.

The incisions, V-shaped and oblique, are made with a No. 15 scalpel blade, and the flap is dissected as described earlier (Fig. 5-31B).

The pedicle is then rotated over the recipient site with no tension and sutured in place (Fig. 5-31C).

Periosteally Stimulated Pedicle Flap

To enhance the chance of root coverage, Goldman and Smukler (1978) thought of using a stimulated periosteum, one which was in an activated state.

As shown in Figure 5-32A, a sharp instrument or 25-gauge needle is used to make sharp penetrations through the gingivae that firmly engage the underlying bone. This is carried out under anesthesia 17 to 21 days prior to surgery to slightly damage the periosteum and induce healing. The theory is that healing activates primordial cells capable of bone and cementum formation.

Figure 5-32B shows the lifting of a full-thickness pedicle flap 17 to 21 days later. The flap is placed over the recipient site and sutured (Fig. 5-32C).

Partial-Full-Thickness Pedicle Flap

In an effort further to enhance root coverage, Goldman et al. (1982) introduced a technique that had the advantage of allowing placement of a full-thickness flap over the denuded root surface and at the same time permitting coverage of the exposed donor site with periosteum.

Figure 5-33A and B show the area of recession as well as the outline and removal of the V-shaped incision, using a No. 15 scalpel blade.

The variation in technique comes in the next step. The pedicle flap is begun at least two teeth away from the recipient site (Fig. 5-33C). A partial-thickness flap is used over the tooth farthest away. This part of the procedure is similar to that already outlined.

When approaching the approximating tooth, the No. 15 scalpel blade is directed toward the bone and in an apico-occlusal direction, cutting into the periosteum. This allows a full-thickness flap to be raised by blunt dissection with a sharp periosteal elevator (Fig. 5-33D).

Figure 5-33E shows the flap reflected to illustrate the partial-full-thickness design. Note the *beveled-out* area of the V-shaped incision.

In Figure 5-33F, the flap is sutured in place, and only the periosteally covered area is left exposed.

The clinical procedure is shown in Figure 5-34.

Submarginal Incisions

This type of incision can be used for all procedures provided that an adequate width (25 mm) of keratinized gingiva is present at the donor site. This will permit leaving a small collar of tissue about the necks of the teeth in order to prevent recession at the donor site, thus facilitating use of a full-thickness pedicle flap if desired. In Figure 5-35A, the basic problem is outlined. In Figure 5-35B, the flap has been raised (in this case, a partial-full-thickness pedicle) and the V-shaped incision has been removed. The flap is rotated over the recipient site and sutured below the submarginal incision (Fig. 5-35C).

The procedure is depicted clinically in Figures 5-36 and 5-37.

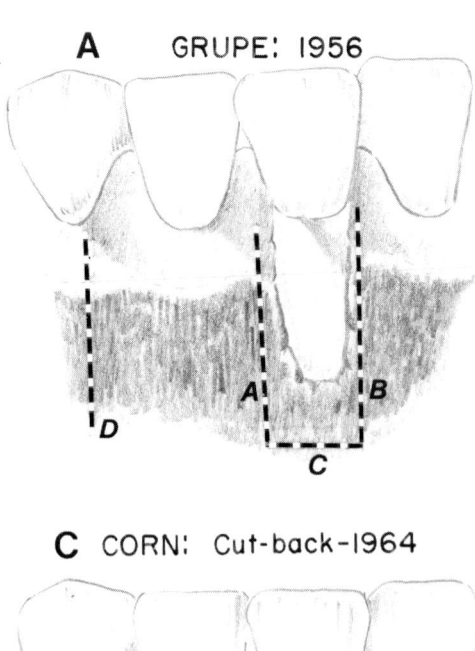
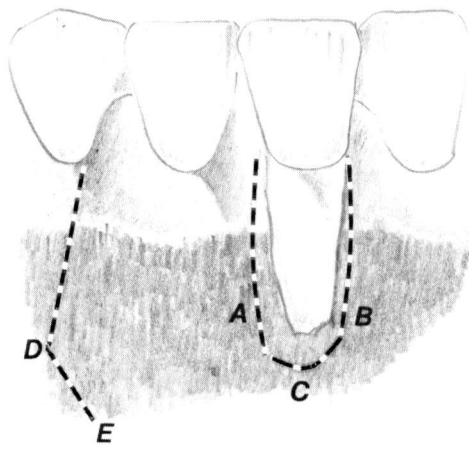
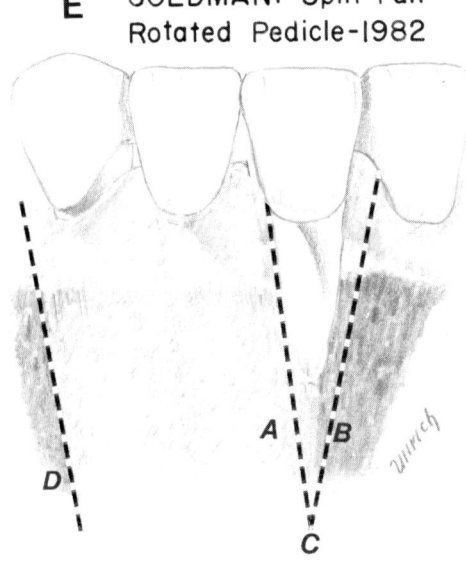
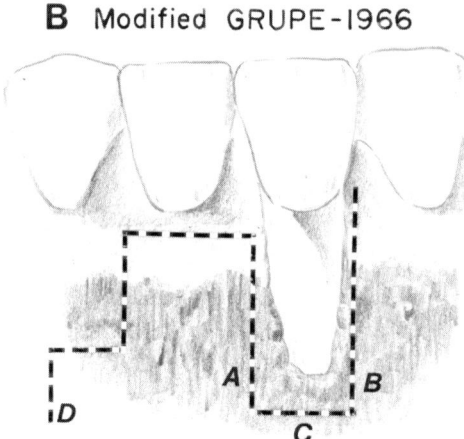
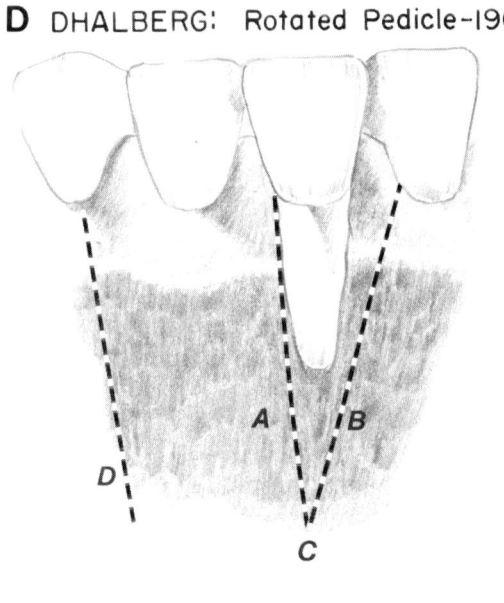

Fig. 5-21. Historical Outline of Laterally Positioned Flap Design. **A,** Original Grupe design. **B,** *Submarginal* incision placement to prevent recession at donor site. **C,** *Cutback* releasing incision for tension release. **D,** *Rotated* pedicle flap permitting placement without need for cutback incision. **E,** Use of more than one tooth to permit periosteal placement over exposed root without bone exposure (stimulated or nonstimulated).

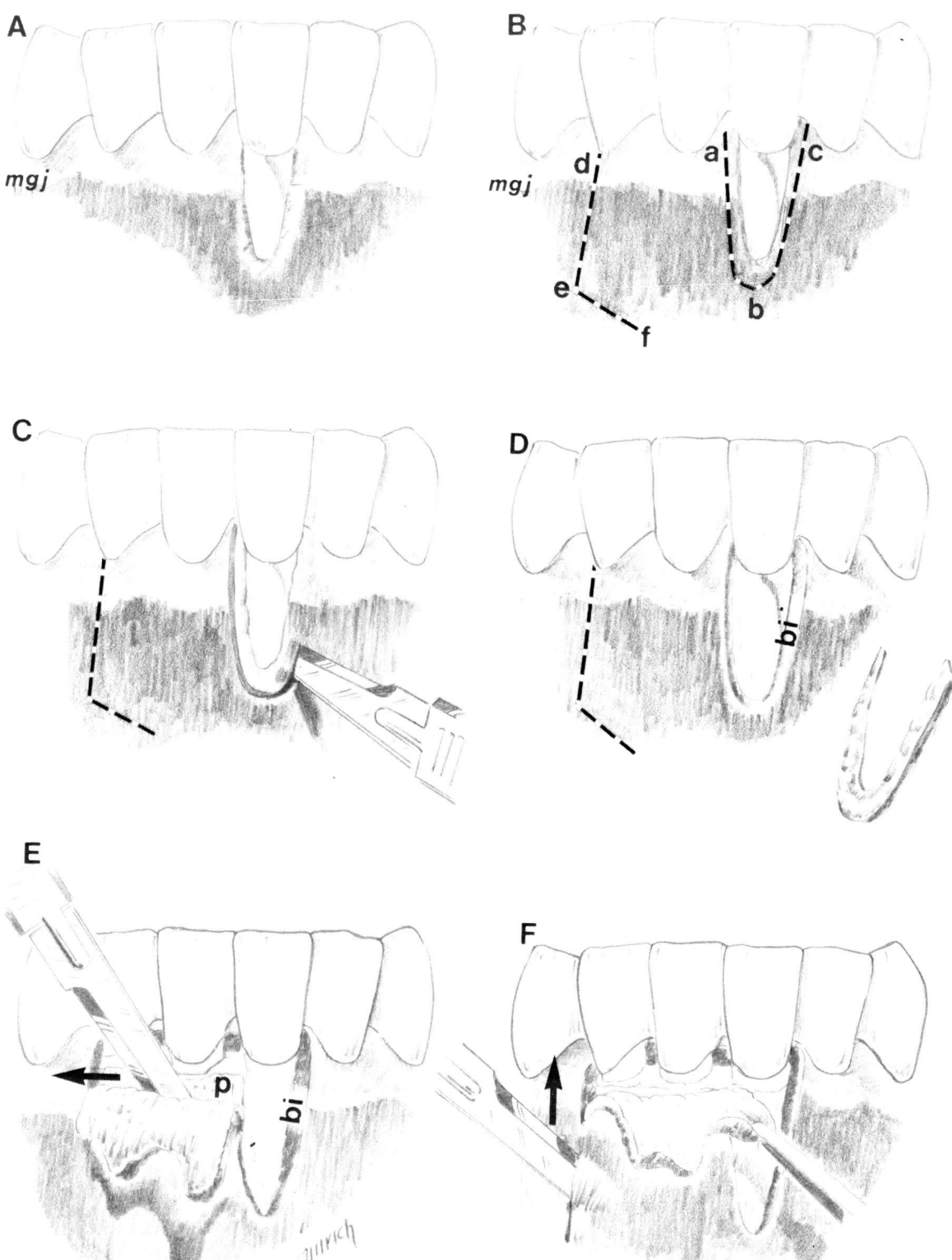

Fig. 5-22. Laterally Positioned Pedicle Flap. **A,** Preoperative view of root exposed as a result of recession and lack of attached gingiva. **B,** Basic incisions are outlined. **C,** *V-shaped* incision is made about exposed root. **D,** *V-shaped* incision removed. Note beveled incision (bi) on the opposite side of the donor area to permit overlap of flap. **E,** Coronal portion of pedicle flap begun. **F,** Final dissection of pedicle is in an apico-occlusal direction.

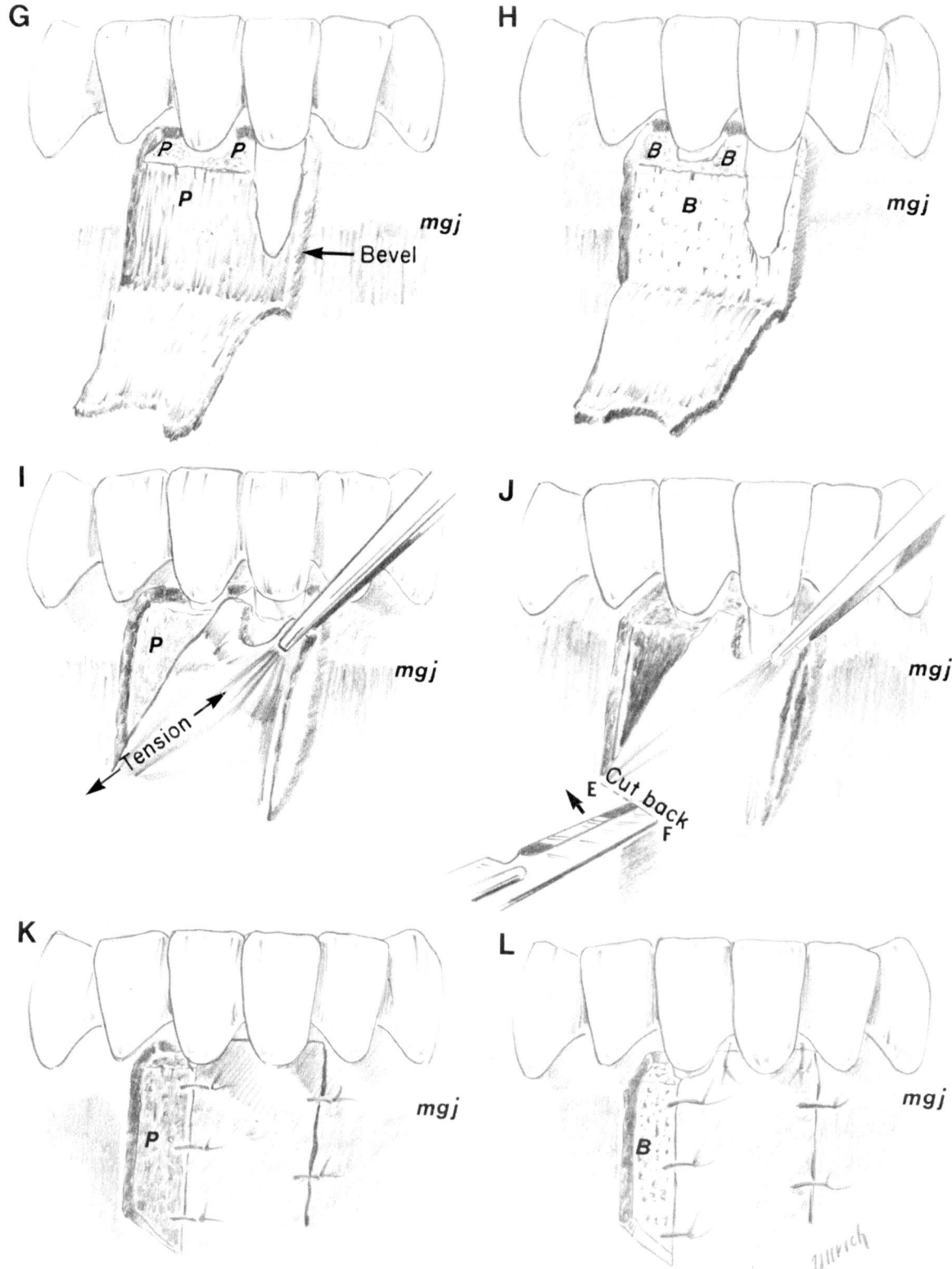

Fig. 5-22 (continued). **G,** Pedicle flap is released and reflected, exposing underlying periosteum (P). **H,** If a full-thickness pedicle flap were raised, the underlying bone (B) would have been exposed. **I,** Tension is placed on the pedicle when positioning is attempted. **J,** The cutback or releasing incision is now made (E–F). **K,** Partial-thickness pedicle is sutured with periosteum covering bone. **L,** Example of full-thickness pedicle flap with bone exposure.

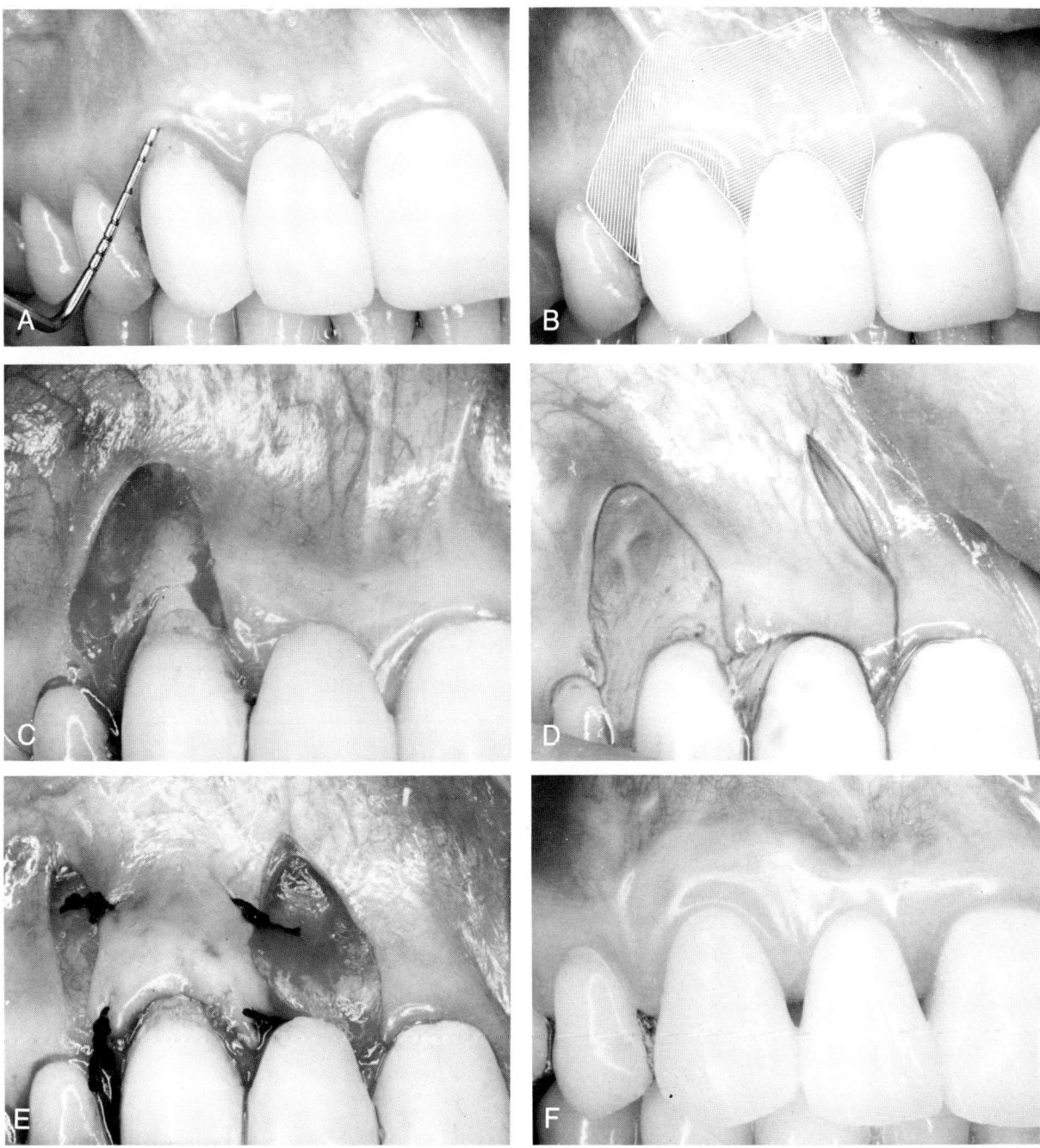

Fig. 5-23. Partial-Thickness Laterally Positioned Flap. **A,** Before treatment. Probe in place, showing no attached gingiva. **B,** Incisions outlined: *V-shaped* incision (1) and pedicle flap (2), which will be moved distally. **C,** V-shaped incision completed and wedge removed. Note beveled out portion of incision permitting adequate overlap. **D,** Pedicle flap incisions completed. Note angulation of incisions toward recipient site. **E,** Pedicle flap sutured. Note total lack of tension. **F,** Two years later. Note significant increase in attached gingiva. (Prosthetics done by Dr. William Irving, Needham, MA.)

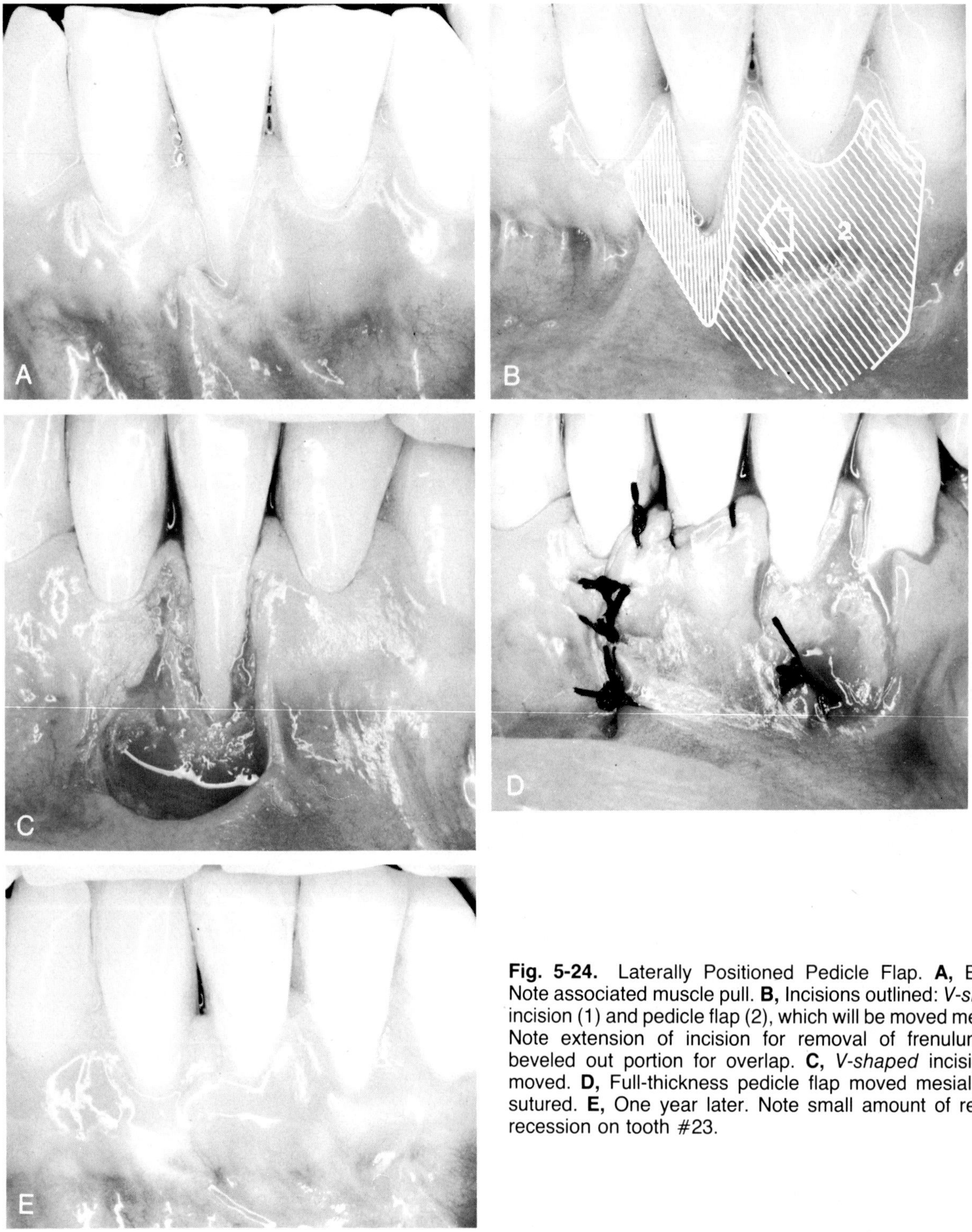

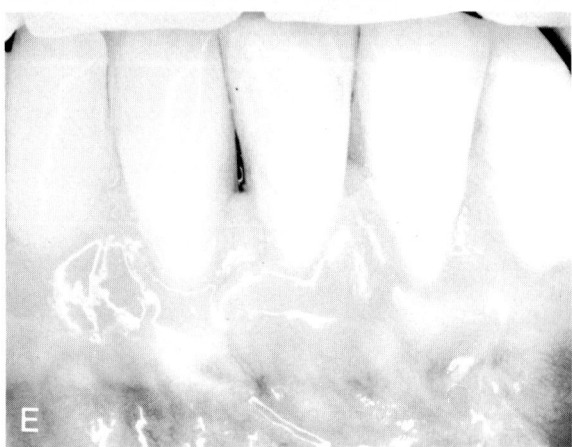

Fig. 5-24. Laterally Positioned Pedicle Flap. **A,** Before. Note associated muscle pull. **B,** Incisions outlined: *V-shaped* incision (1) and pedicle flap (2), which will be moved mesially. Note extension of incision for removal of frenulum and beveled out portion for overlap. **C,** *V-shaped* incision removed. **D,** Full-thickness pedicle flap moved mesially and sutured. **E,** One year later. Note small amount of residual recession on tooth #23.

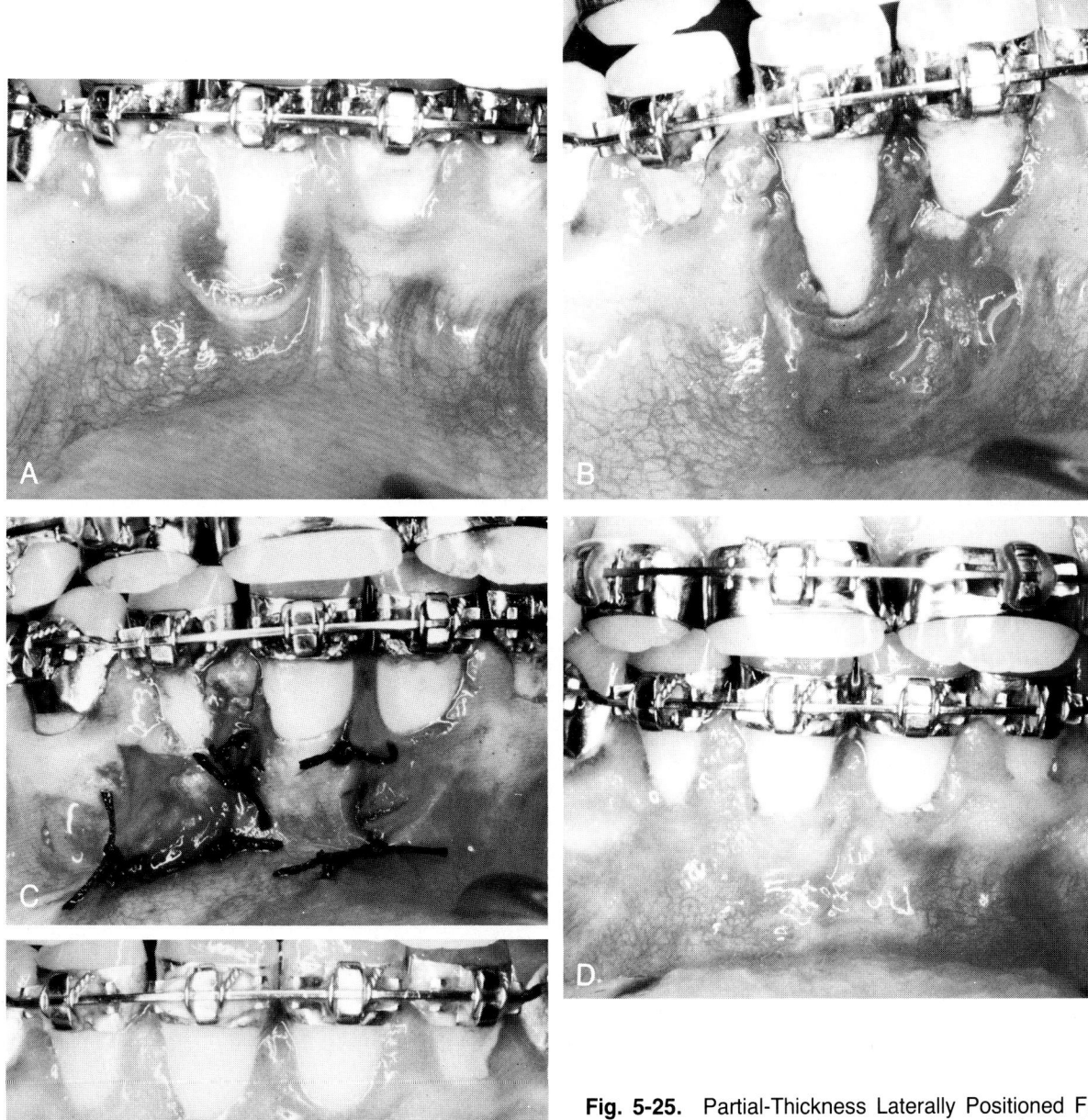

Fig. 5-25. Partial-Thickness Laterally Positioned Flap. **A,** Before. Recession has occurred during orthodontic therapy. **B,** Recipient site prepared. **C,** Submarginal laterally positioned pedicle sutured. **D,** Three weeks later. **E,** Two months later. Compare with A and B.

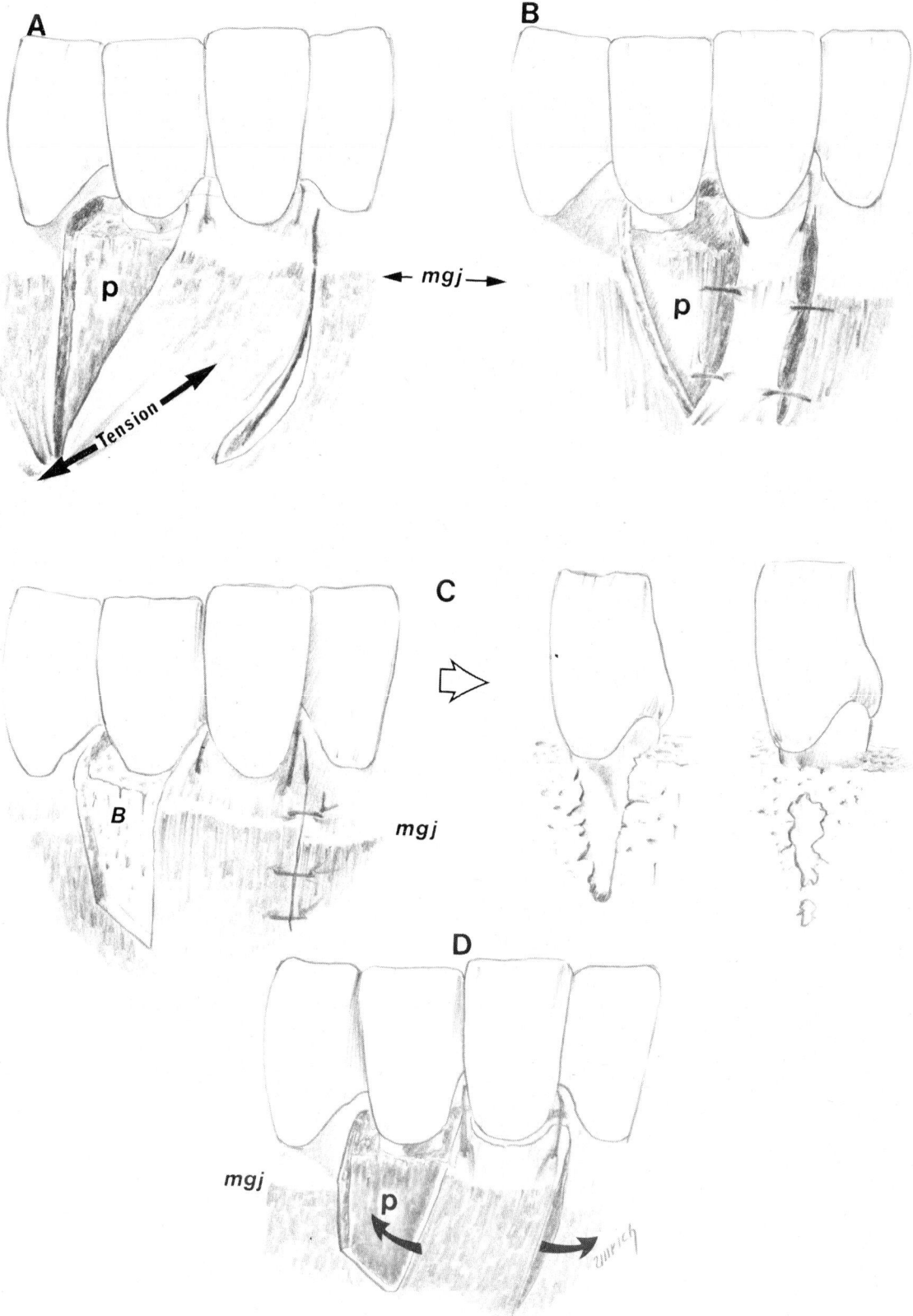

Fig. 5-26. Reasons for Pedicle Flap Failure. **A,** Inadequate stabilization because of tension. **B,** Pedicle flap too narrow. **C,** Bone exposed (right), resulting in dehiscence or fenestration formation. **D,** Excessive movement because of poor stabilization.

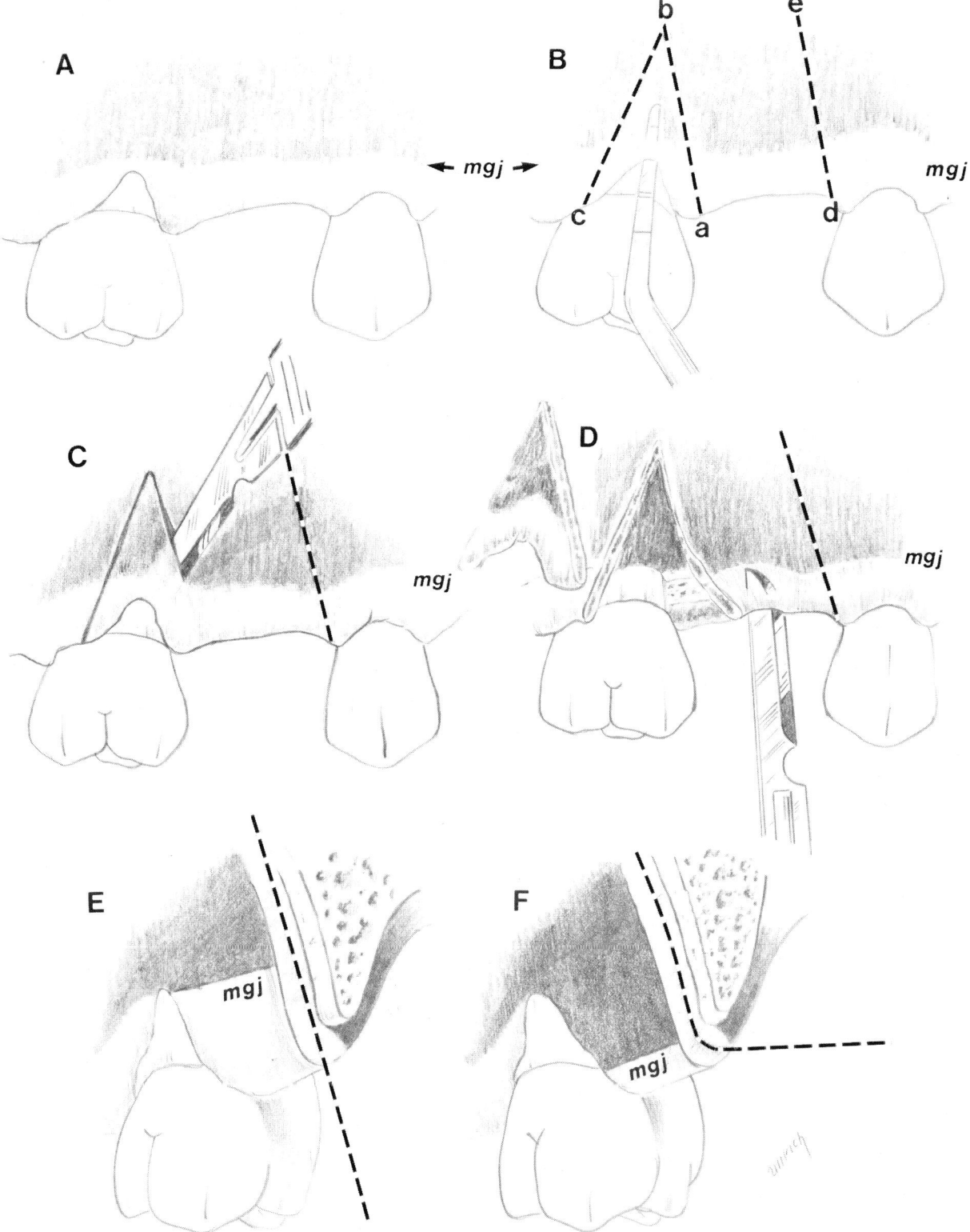

Fig. 5-27. Laterally Positioned Rotated Pedicle Flap from Edentulous Ridge. **A,** Preoperative view of molar with recession and no attached keratinized gingiva. **B,** Outline of incisions: a,b,c, is *V-shaped* incision; d,e, is oblique, flap-releasing incision. Probe shows a lack of attached gingiva. **C,** The V-shaped incision is begun. **D,** With the removal of the V-shaped incision, a partial-thickness pedicle flap is raised. **E,F,** Dotted lines outline incision for pedicle flap in the presence of adequate (E) or inadequate (F) zones of keratinized gingiva.

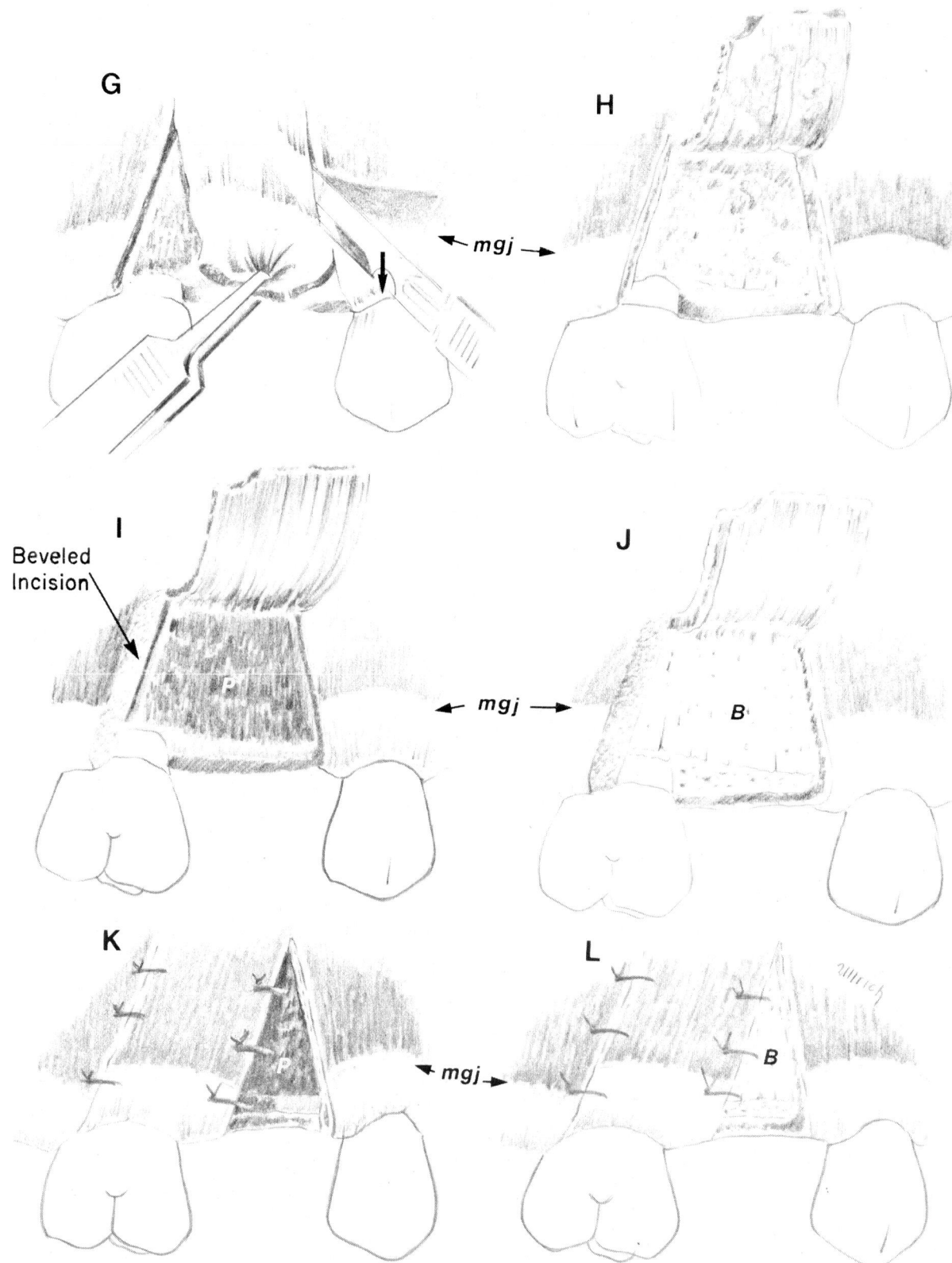

Fig. 5-27 (continued). **G,** Dissection of the partial-thickness pedicle flap is completed in an apico-occlusal direction. **H,** Flap reflected. **I,** A bevel is placed on the distal side of the V-shaped incision to permit flap overlap. **J,** Represents a full-thickness pedicle flap. **K,L,** Represent sutured flaps of partial- and full-thickness designs, respectively. (P, periosteum; B, bone.)

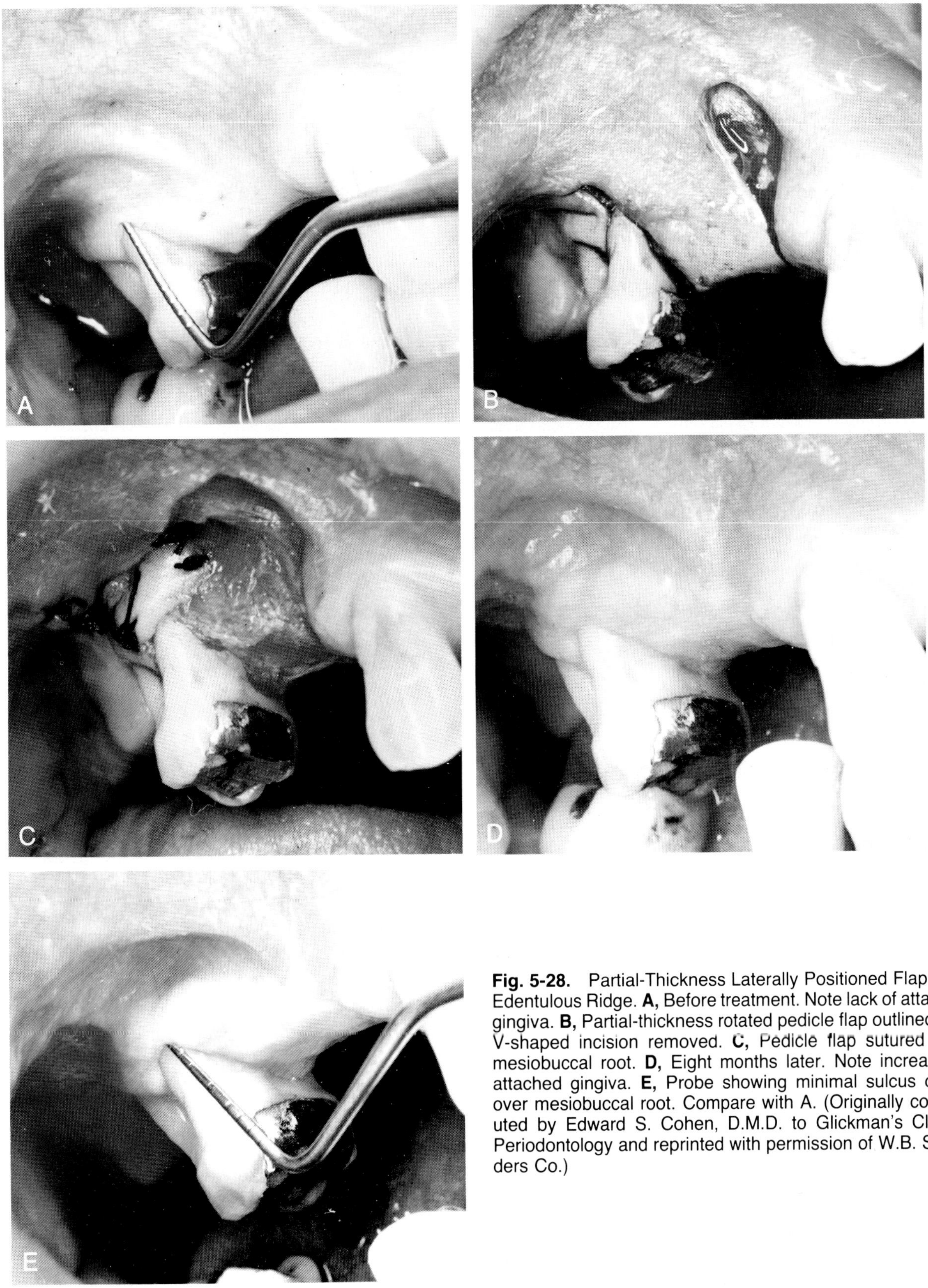

Mucogingival Surgery

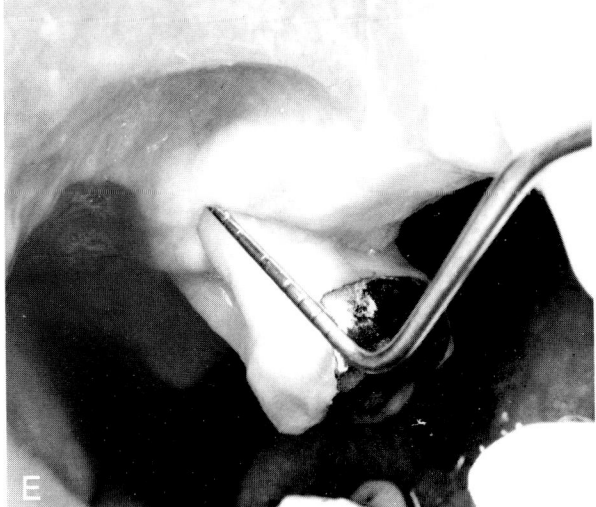

Fig. 5-28. Partial-Thickness Laterally Positioned Flap from Edentulous Ridge. **A,** Before treatment. Note lack of attached gingiva. **B,** Partial-thickness rotated pedicle flap outlined and V-shaped incision removed. **C,** Pedicle flap sutured over mesiobuccal root. **D,** Eight months later. Note increase in attached gingiva. **E,** Probe showing minimal sulcus depth over mesiobuccal root. Compare with A. (Originally contributed by Edward S. Cohen, D.M.D. to Glickman's Clinical Periodontology and reprinted with permission of W.B. Saunders Co.)

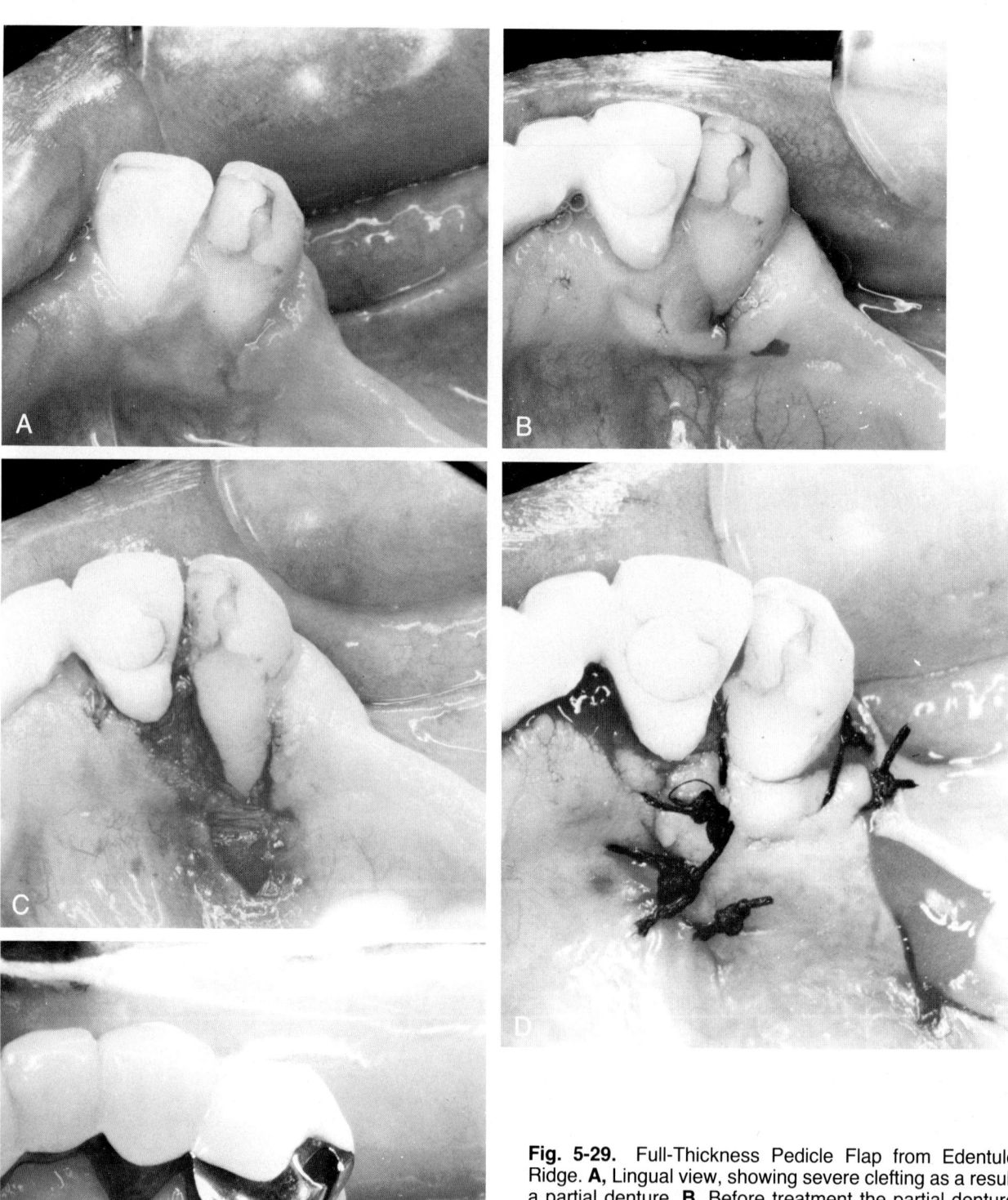

Fig. 5-29. Full-Thickness Pedicle Flap from Edentulous Ridge. **A,** Lingual view, showing severe clefting as a result of a partial denture. **B,** Before treatment the partial denture is removed and a temporary bridge inserted. **C,** V-shaped wedge removed at recipient site. **D,** Full-thickness pedicle flap reflected and sutured in place. **E,** Three years later. Note excellent result. (Prosthetics done by Dr. Paul McDonald, Foxboro, MA.)

Mucogingival Surgery

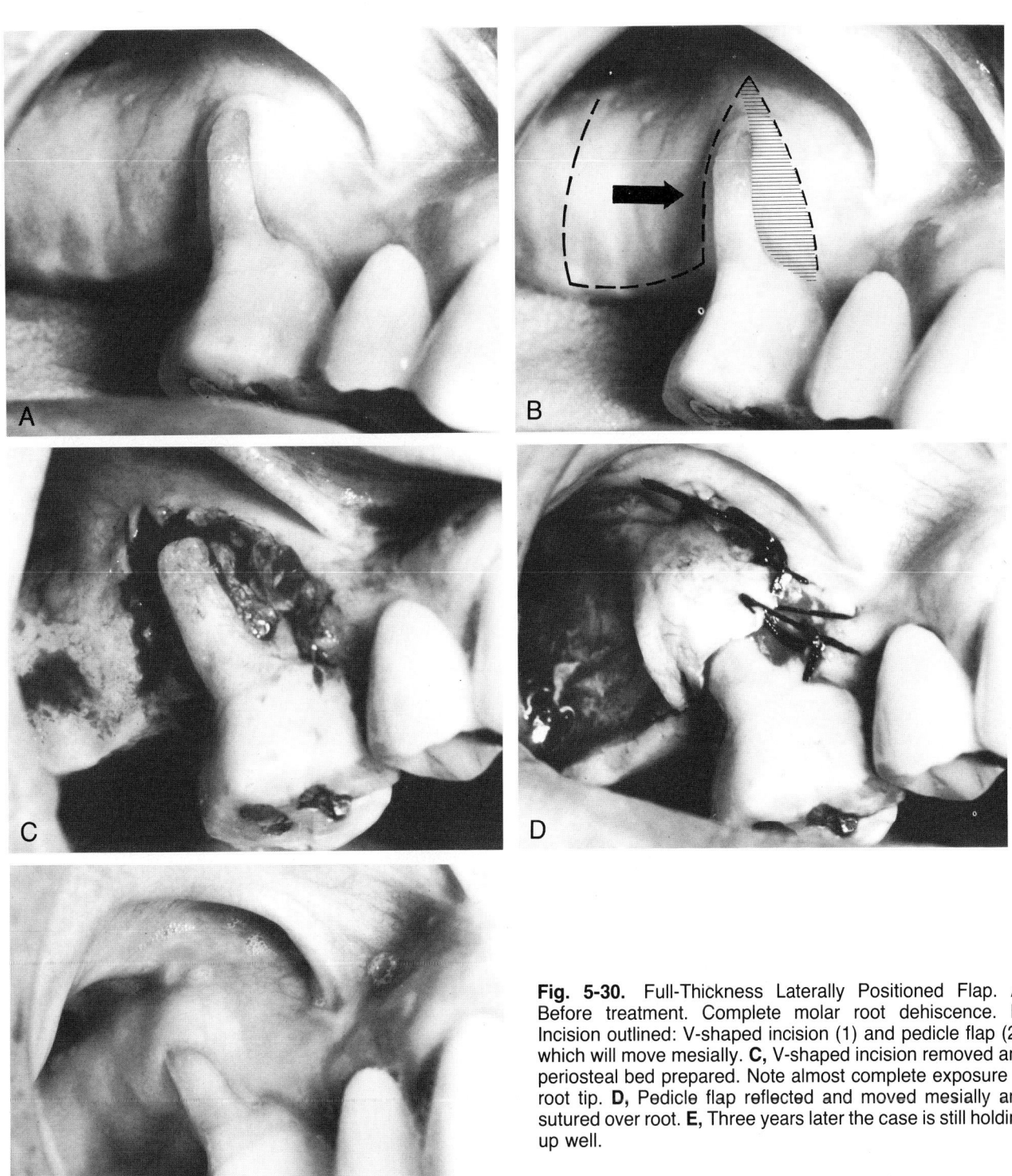

Fig. 5-30. Full-Thickness Laterally Positioned Flap. **A,** Before treatment. Complete molar root dehiscence. **B,** Incision outlined: V-shaped incision (1) and pedicle flap (2), which will move mesially. **C,** V-shaped incision removed and periosteal bed prepared. Note almost complete exposure of root tip. **D,** Pedicle flap reflected and moved mesially and sutured over root. **E,** Three years later the case is still holding up well.

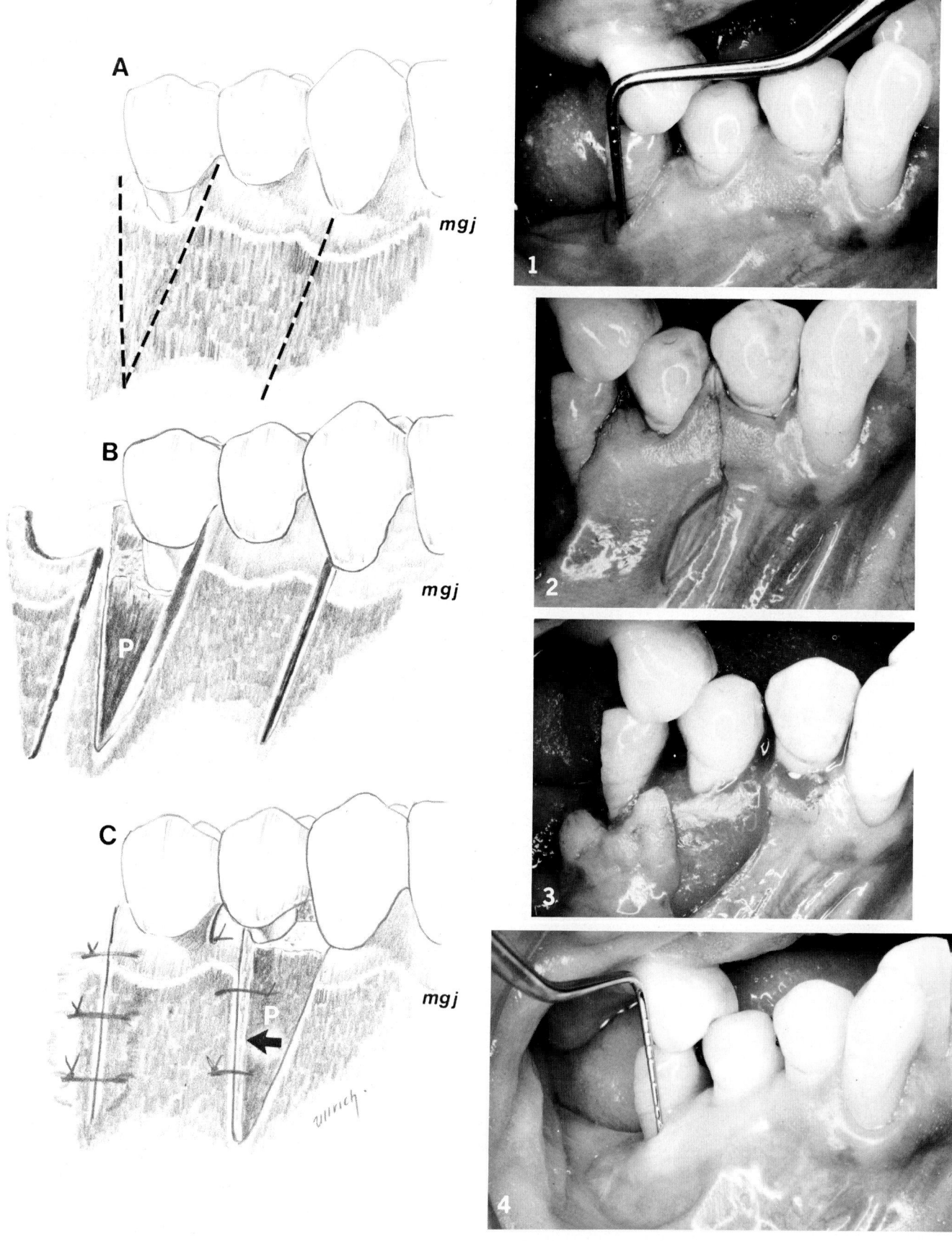

Fig. 5-31. Oblique Rotated Pedicle Flap. Diagrammatic View: **A,** V-shaped incision and pedicle flap outlined. **B,** Incisions completed and V-shaped incision removed. Note obliquely angled donor flap. **C,** Pedicle flap rotated over tooth. Clinical View: **1,** Preoperative clinical view with probe in place. Pockets extend beyond the mucogingival line. **2,** Incisions outlined. **3,** Pedicle flap rotated. Note complete lack of tension. **4,** Seven months later. Note increase in attached gingiva.

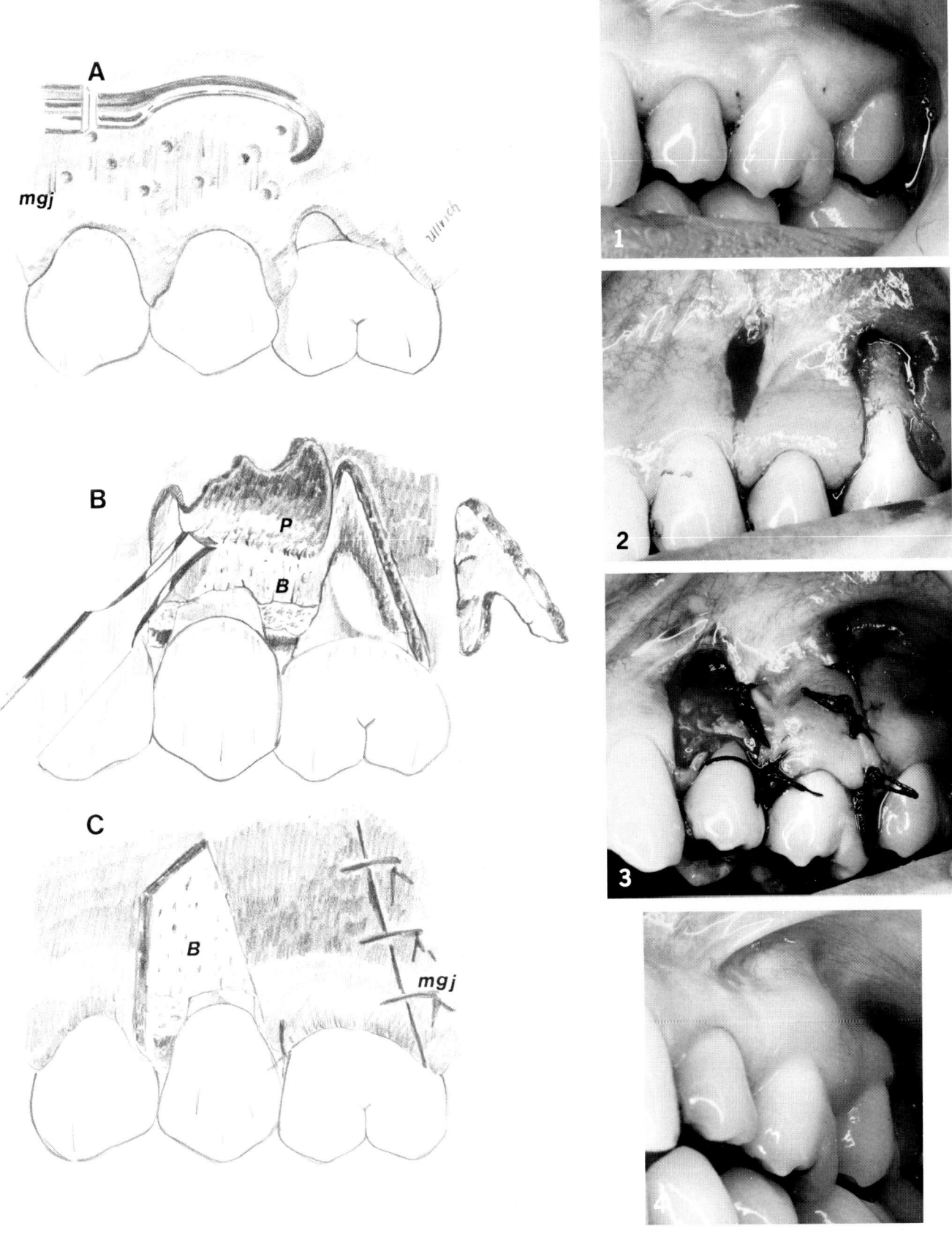

Fig. 5-32. Periosteally Stimulated Pedicle Flap. Diagrammatic View: **A,** Periosteal stimulation 17 to 21 days prior to surgery. **B,** Full-thickness pedicle flap raised and bone (B) exposed. **C,** Pedicle flap sutured in position with bone (B) exposed on recipient site. Clinical View: **1,** Before surgery, 21 days after stimulation. **2,** Incisions completed and V-shaped incision removed. **3,** Full-thickness flap reflected and sutured over recipient site. **4,** Six months later, total root coverage with minimal recession at donor site.

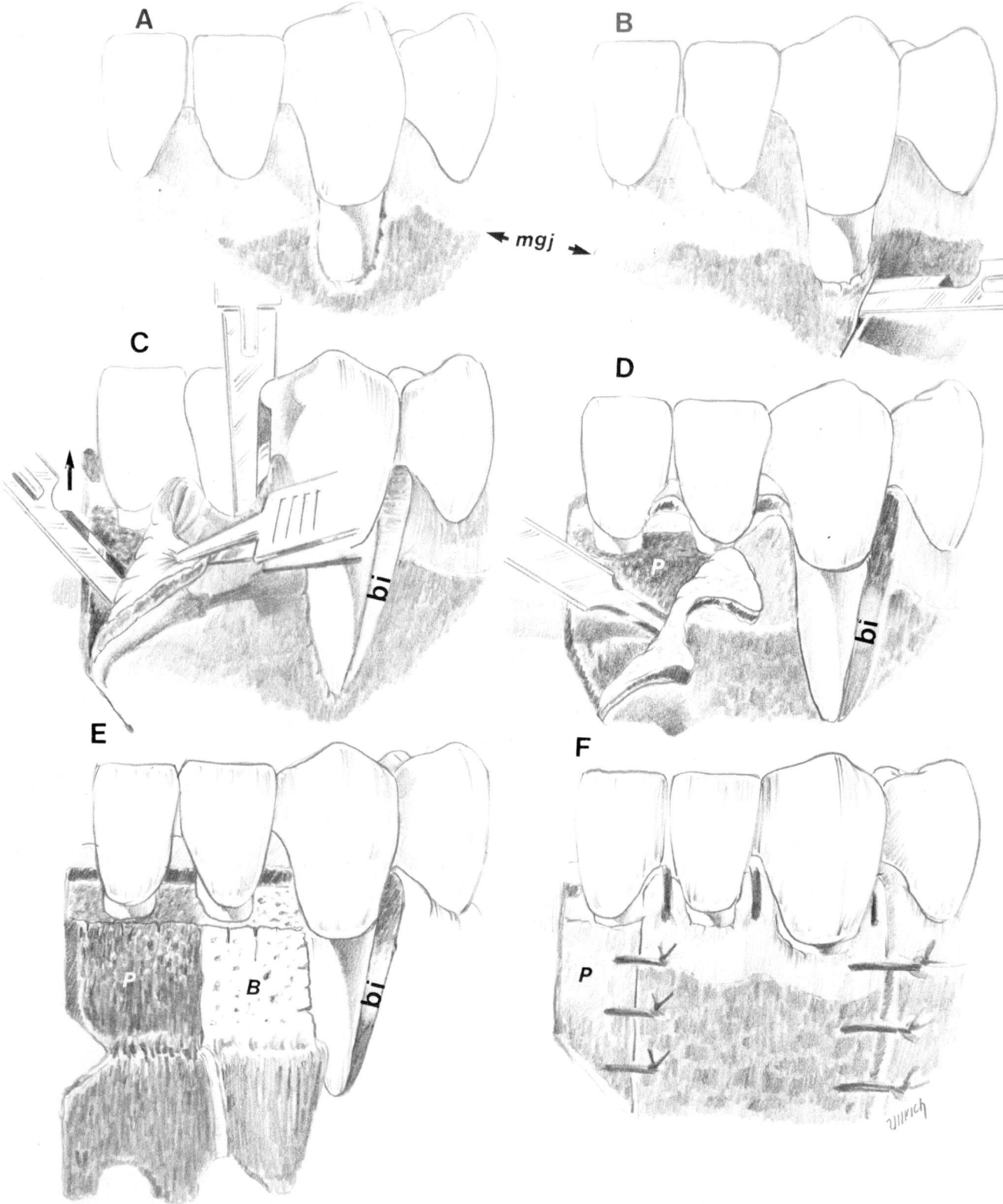

Fig. 5-33. Partial-Full-Thickness Pedicle Flap. **A,** Initial view. **B,** V-shaped incision over exposed root begun. **C,** V-shaped beveled incision (bi) completed and partial-thickness flap begun. **D,** Partial-thickness flap portion completed and full-thickness flap begun (P, periosteum; B, bone). **E,** Partial-full-thickness flap raised. **F,** Flap sutured with overlap of beveled incision.

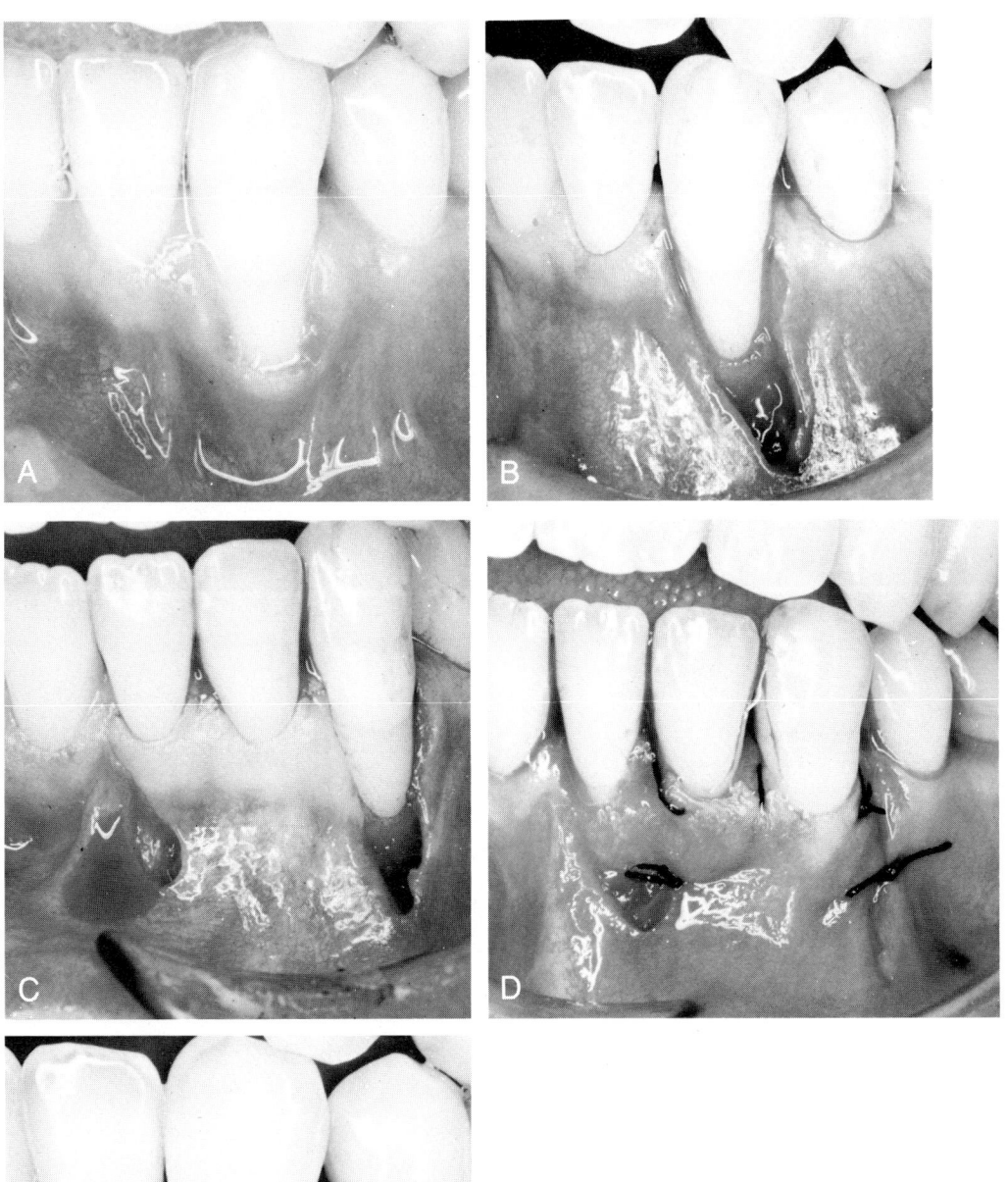

Fig. 5-34. Partial-Full-Thickness Laterally Positioned Flap. A, Before treatment. B, *V-shaped* incision completed at recipient site. C, Partial-full-thickness pedicle flap outlined. D, Flap rotated over recipient site. E, Seven months later. Compare with A.

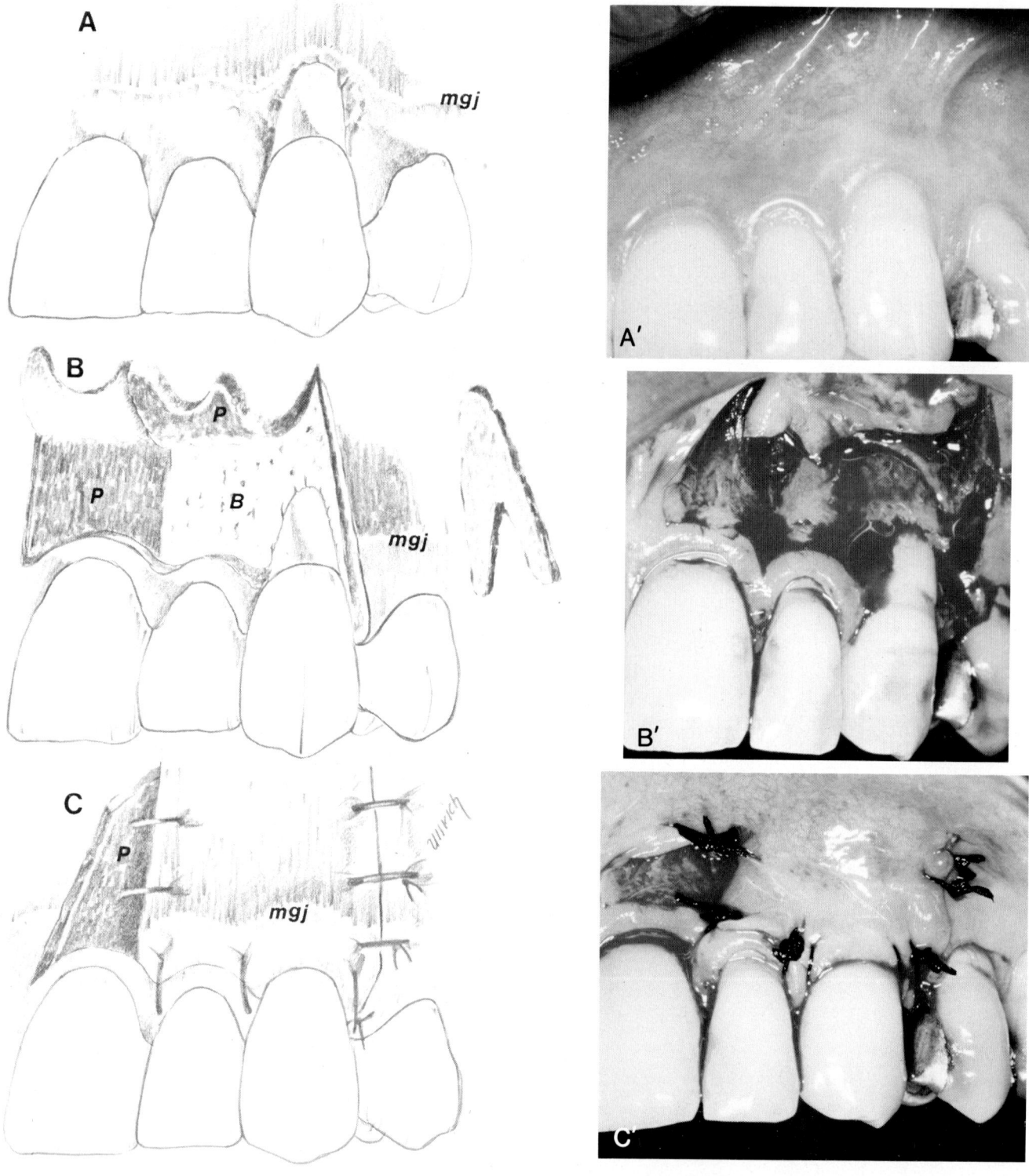

Fig. 5-35. Submarginal Partial-Full-Thickness Pedicle Flap. **A,A'**, Preoperative views of cuspid tooth with recession. **B,B'**, Partial-full-thickness flap reflected and V-shaped incision removed. **C,C'**, Pedicle flap sutured in position for root coverage. Note use of cutback incision for release of tension.

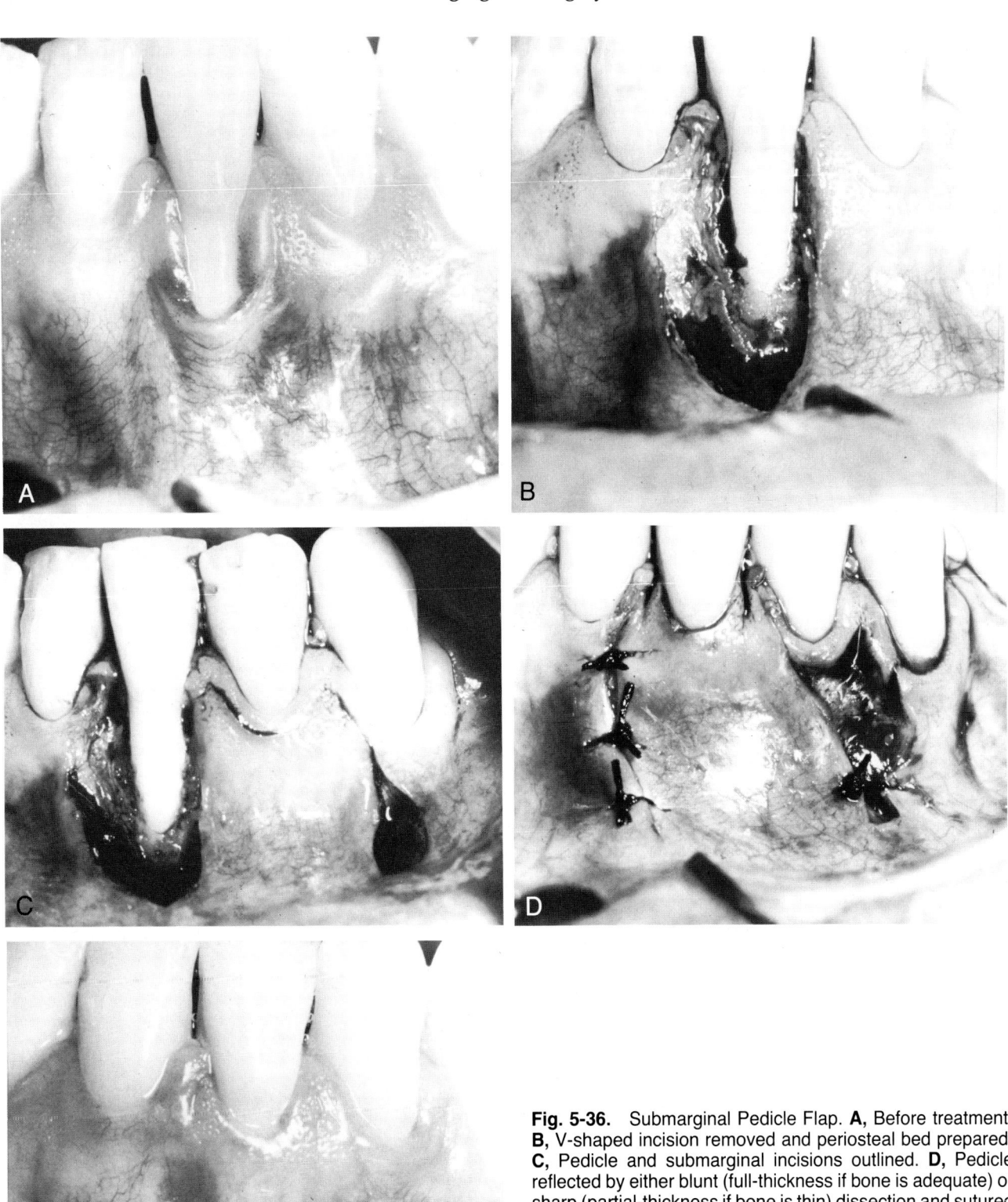

Fig. 5-36. Submarginal Pedicle Flap. **A,** Before treatment. **B,** V-shaped incision removed and periosteal bed prepared. **C,** Pedicle and submarginal incisions outlined. **D,** Pedicle reflected by either blunt (full-thickness if bone is adequate) or sharp (partial-thickness if bone is thin) dissection and sutured laterally. **E,** Four year later note excellent result with no shrinkage at the donor site.

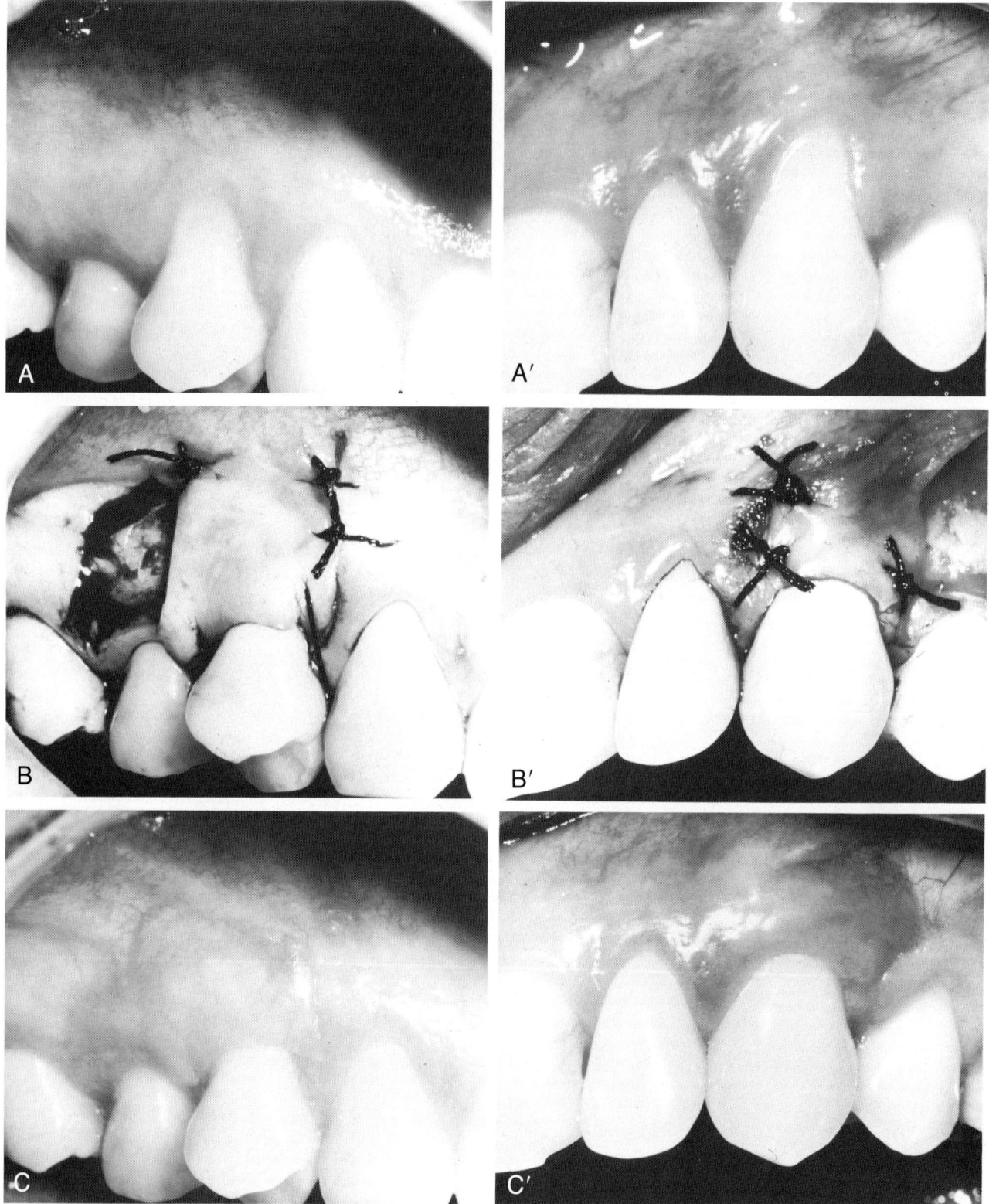

Fig. 5-37. Full-Thickness Submarginal Pedicle Flaps. **A,A′,** Before treatment. **B,B′,** Full-thickness submarginal pedicle flaps reflected, moved mesially, and sutured. **C,C′,** Cases completed. Note excellent results without recession at donor sites.

DOUBLE PAPILLA LATERALLY POSITIONED FLAPS

This procedure, first described by Wainberg as the *double lateral repositioned flap* (see Goldman et al., 1964), was refined by Cohen and Ross (1968) as the *double papilla flap*. It is designed to achieve an adequate zone of attached keratinized gingiva and/or coverage of a denuded root surface by joining two interdental papillae.

Indications

1. When the *interproximal papillae* adjacent to the mucogingival problem are *sufficiently wide*
2. When the *attached gingiva* on an approximating tooth *is insufficient* to allow for a laterally positioned flap
3. When periodontal pockets are *not* present

Advantages

1. The risk of loss of alveolar bone is minimized because the interdental bone is more resistant to loss than is radicular bone.
2. The papillae usually supply a greater width of attached gingiva than can be gotten from the radicular surface of a tooth.
3. The clinical predictability of this procedure is fairly good.

Disadvantage

The primary disadvantage of this procedure is in having to join together two small flaps in such a way that they act as a single flap.

Procedure

The mucogingival junction is the line of demarcation between the coronally attached gingiva and the oral mucosa below (Fig. 5-38A). When the periodontal probe is inserted, note that it extends 1 mm beyond the mucogingival line (Fig. 5-38B); therefore, that 1 mm of marginal tissue is not attached to the root surface.

The surgical incisions are outlined in Figure 5-38B by dotted lines. The lateral releasing incisions will be made at the mesiofacial and distofacial line angles of the adjacent teeth and should not encroach upon the radicular surfaces of the approximating teeth because this will expose radicular bone. A V-shaped incision will be made to remove a wedge of gingiva over the root.

This incision should extend far enough apically into the mucosa to prevent bunching of the tissue when the flaps are brought together. Horizontal incisions will be made across the tops of the papillae to allow better placement of the flap.

Using a No. 15 scalpel blade, the V-shaped incision is made and extended to the depth of, but not including, the periosteum (Fig. 5-38C). The V-section is then removed and the root surface is thoroughly scaled (Fig. 5-38D). Note that the periosteum (P) has been retained.

Once the horizontal incisions are made across the tops of the papillae (Fig. 5-38E), the tissue is grasped with rat-tail tissue pliers and gently lifted, as it is separated from the underlying tissue by means of a No. 15 scalpel. Care must be exercised to prevent lifting the periosteum off the bone or accidentally puncturing or severing the flap.

The tissue at the mucogingival line is more firmly bound and is easier to separate from the mucosal side. Therefore, to completely release the flap, the scalpel blade is inserted into the base of the lateral releasing incision and moved in an apico-occlusal direction (Fig. 5-38F) until the flaps are lifted off the periosteum (P or G—the periosteum overlying the bone coronal to the mucogingival junction) (Fig. 5-38G).

A full-thickness mucoperiosteal flap is occasionally used as a modification by which the underlying bone (B) is exposed (Fig. 5-38H). It is indicated when periosteal retention is difficult because of a mobile tissue base, but it is not the treatment of choice.

The tissue is now grasped with Corn tissue pliers and the suture needle is passed through the outer surface of the first papilla (Fig. 5-38I) and on through the undersurface of the second papilla (Fig. 5-38J). Coaptation of the double papilla flap is accomplished using 4-0, 5-0, or 6-0 silk or chromic gut suture with a P-3 atraumatic needle.

Special care must be taken to ensure that there is no separation of the flaps. Removal of the outer epithelium on one flap, allowing the two papillae to overlap with contact on their connective tissue surfaces, may be used to prevent separation.

Complete fixation of the flaps is accomplished by both sling and periosteal sutures (Fig. 5-38K). If a full-thickness mucoperiosteal flap is used (Fig. 5-38L), the lack of underlying periosteum permits only a sling suture, which makes movement and resultant failure possible.

Digital pressure is now applied for 5 minutes to aid initial adherence of the flaps to the underlying periosteum and to prevent the formation of a blood clot.

The complete procedure is shown clinically in Figures 5-39 and 5-40.

Variation for Root Coverage

Sometimes an isolated tooth has a denuded root surface that may or may not present a mucogingival problem. In this instance, it is sometimes desirable to try specifically to achieve root coverage for either esthetic or prosthetic considerations.

The primary factor to consider is whether the papillae have an adequate amount of tissue; if the procedure fails, the tooth should still be left with a functional zone of attached tissue. Therefore, there must be enough attached tissue to (1) cover the denuded root surface, and (2) cover part of the periosteum over the root.

In the illustrated and clinical examples, note the loss of gingiva on the facial aspect of the cuspid tooth (Fig. 5-41A and A'). Note also that a mucogingival problem is present only in the illustration (Fig. 5-41). The incisions (e.g., lateral releasing or V-shaped) are accomplished in the same manner as described earlier (Fig. 5-41B and B'). Once the papillae have been freed, the teeth are thoroughly root planed to remove any calculus and necrotic cementum present, and the flaps are then brought together and sutured (Fig. 5-41C and C'). Note that the flaps are actually brought 1 mm onto the enamel. This is to allow for shrinkage of the flaps as healing occurs. More importantly, note that the zone of attached tissue is wide enough to cover both the root surface and the periosteum adequately.

The complete clinical example is seen in Figure 5-42.

Common Reasons For Failure

1. Adequate suturing is necessary to ensure proper healing in the desired position. Without adequate closure of the double papilla flap, separation can occur with possible nonunion of the component flaps. This is the most frequent cause of failure (Fig. 5-43A).
2. The utilization of full-thickness flaps as opposed to the recommended split-thickness flap can lead to surgical failure if, after raising the full-thickness flap, dehiscence or fenestration of the osseous support is present. The failure will be unsightly exposure of the root surface (Fig. 5-43B).
3. For the double papilla flap procedure to be successful, it is imperative that adequate attached gingiva be available in the papillary area for transfer. Proper evaluation of the donor areas should be made prior to surgery so that another procedure may be done if necessary (Fig. 5-43C).
4. Proper placement of the flap on the periosteal bed is necessary to ensure success of the procedure. Note that the attached gingiva is placed only over the root surface and not over part of the periosteum. If the attached gingiva does not take on the root surface, the whole procedure will fail (Fig. 5-43D).
5. Adequate fixation of the flaps to the underlying periosteum is necessary to prevent shifting of the component flap tissues and the formation of a blood clot. Two sutures should be made at the base of the flaps to ensure fixation in the case shown in Figure 5-43E.
6. In the patient shown in Figure 5-43F, two additional sutures placed at the coronal aspect of the flaps but not at the base would have been the preferred procedure.

Horizontal Lateral Sliding Papillary Flap

Hattler (1967) outlined the use of a papillary flap for increasing the zone of keratinized attached gingiva. The procedure involves the movement of adjacent interdental papillae to the facial surfaces of teeth. Unlike the double papilla flap procedure, which brings two papillae together, only single papillae are used.

The main limiting factor is the need for a broad interdental papilla.

The technique is outlined in Figure 5-44.

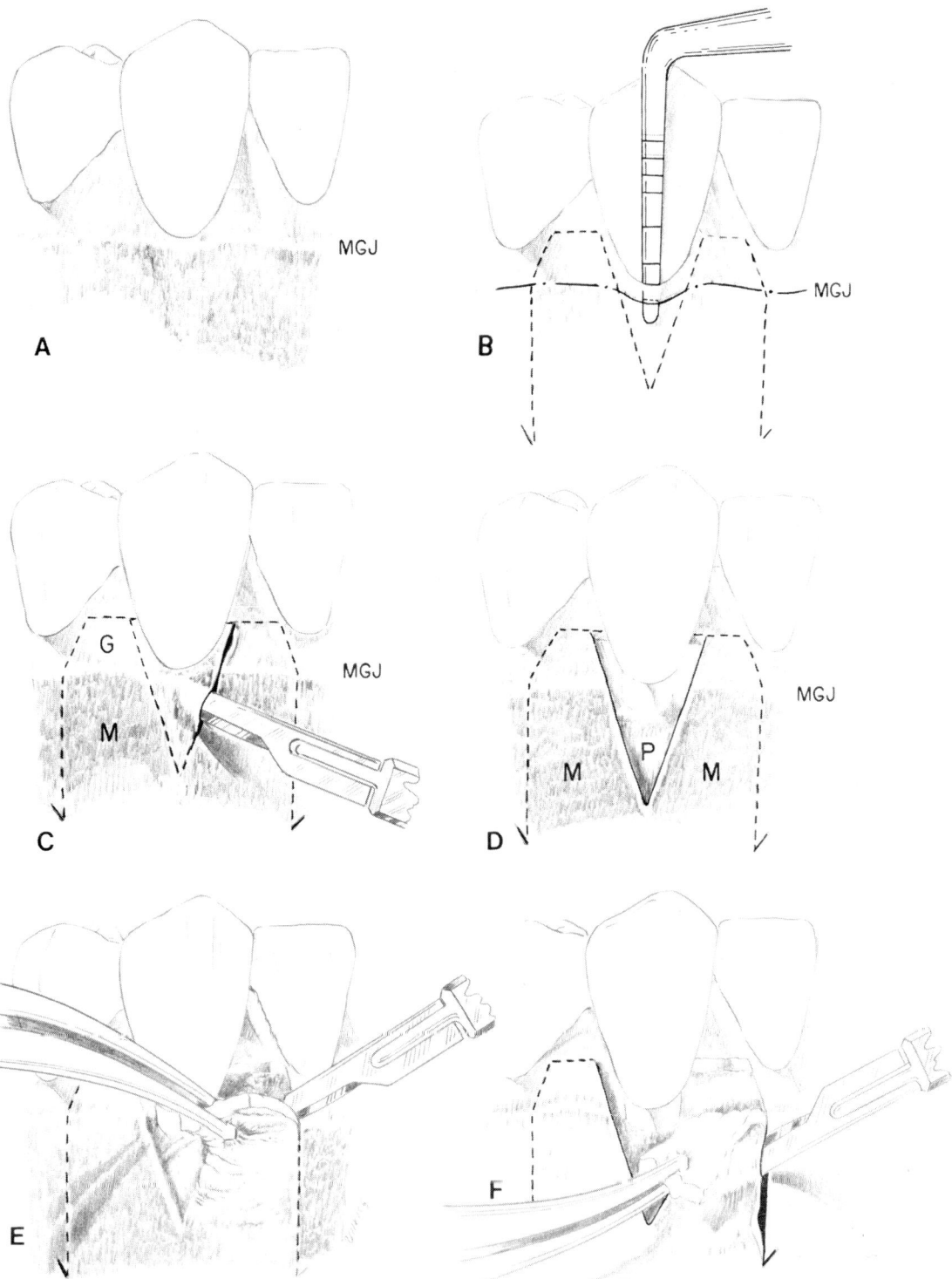

Fig. 5-38. Double Papilla Flap. **A,** Before. **B,** Incisions outlined and probe in place showing mucogingival problem. **C,** *V-shaped* incision begun. **D,** V-shaped wedge removed. **E,** Papillary flaps begun with occlusal aspect. **F,** Papillary flap completed with dissection in an apico-occlusal direction.

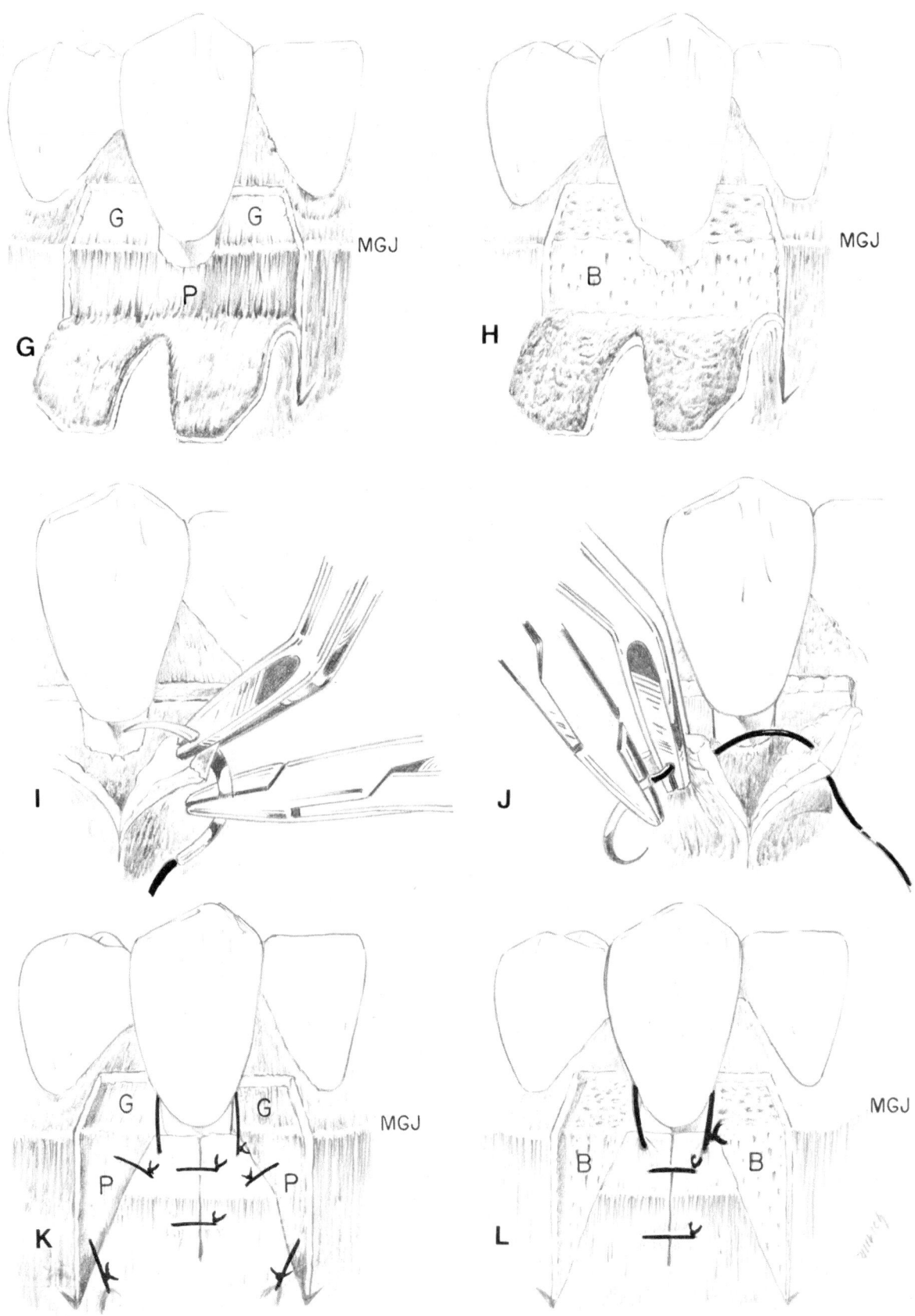

Fig. 5-38 (continued). **G,** Papillary flaps reflected with periosteum (P and G) left. **H,** Full-thickness papillary flaps reflected. **I,** Papilla held with Corn tissue pliers as suturing is begun. **J,** Initial suture passed through papilla. **K,** Double papilla flap sutured and stabilized. **L,** Final suturing of full-thickness double papilla flap.

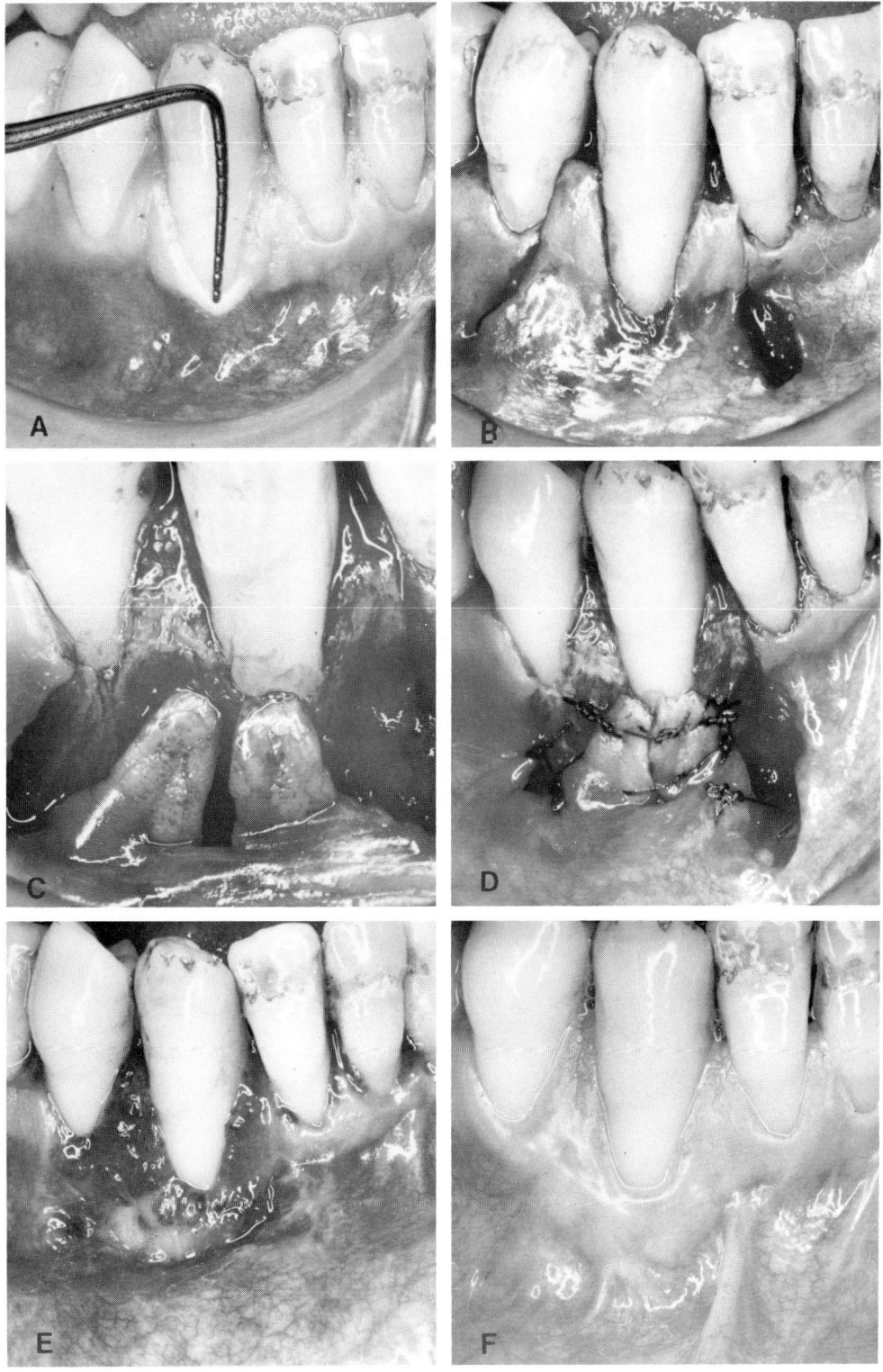

Fig. 5-39. Double Papilla Flap. **A,** Before. Probe showing a total lack of attached keratinized gingiva. **B,** Initial incisions and V-shaped incision complete. **C,** Papillae positioned for increasing the zone of attached keratinized gingiva only. **D,** Papillae sutured. **E,** One week later. **F,** Six months later.

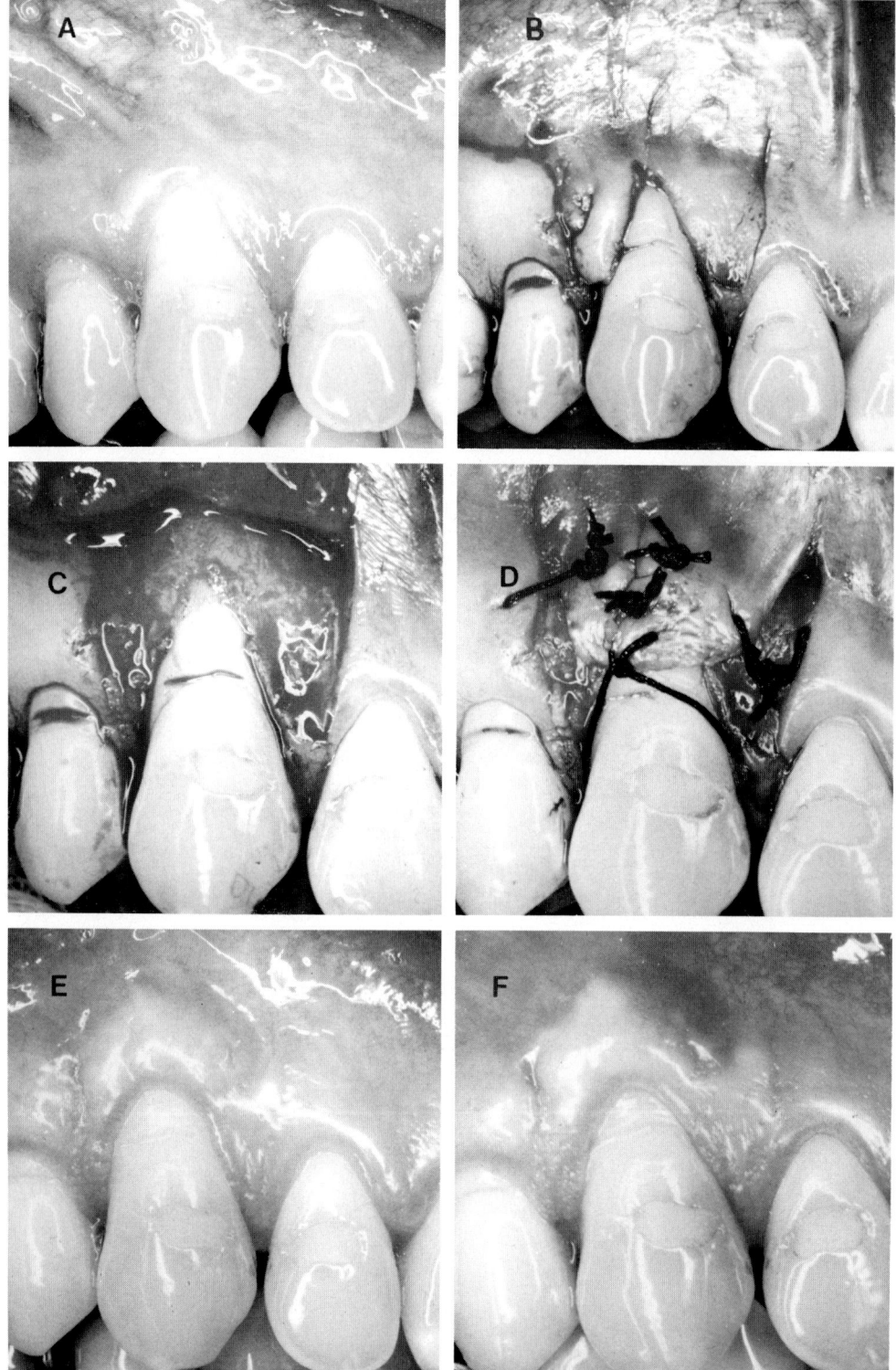

Fig. 5-40. Double Papilla Flap. **A,** Before. **B,** Incisions outlined. **C,** Partial-thickness double papilla flap reflected. **D,** Double papilla flap sutured. **E,** Three months later. **F,** Four years later. Note increase in attached keratinized gingiva; compare with A.

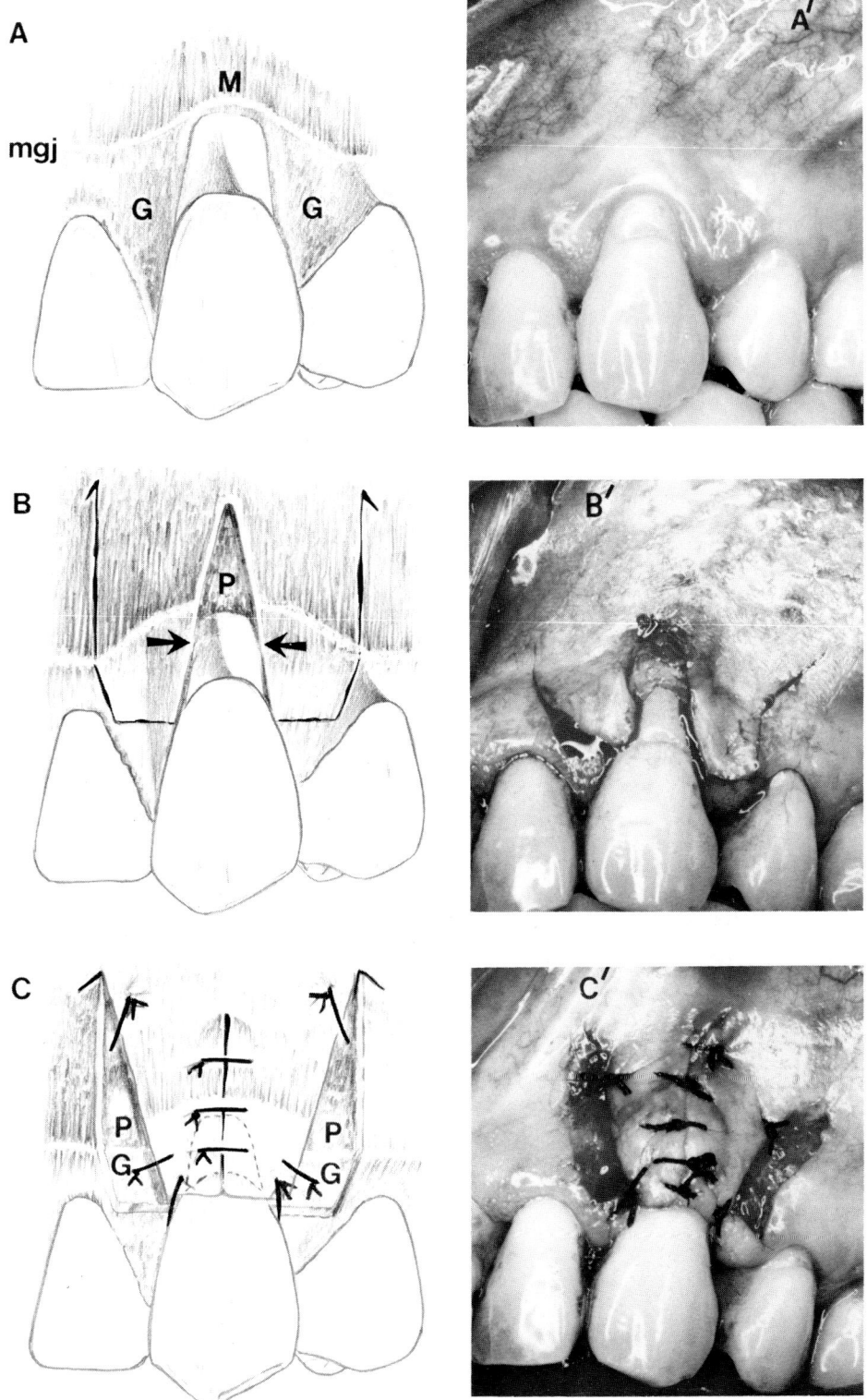

Fig. 5-41. Double Papilla Modification for Root Coverage. **A,A′,** Before; cuspid shows recession. **B,B′,** Incisions completed and V-shaped wedge of tissue removed. **C,C′,** Double papilla flap suture. Note overlap onto enamel and close approximation of papillae.

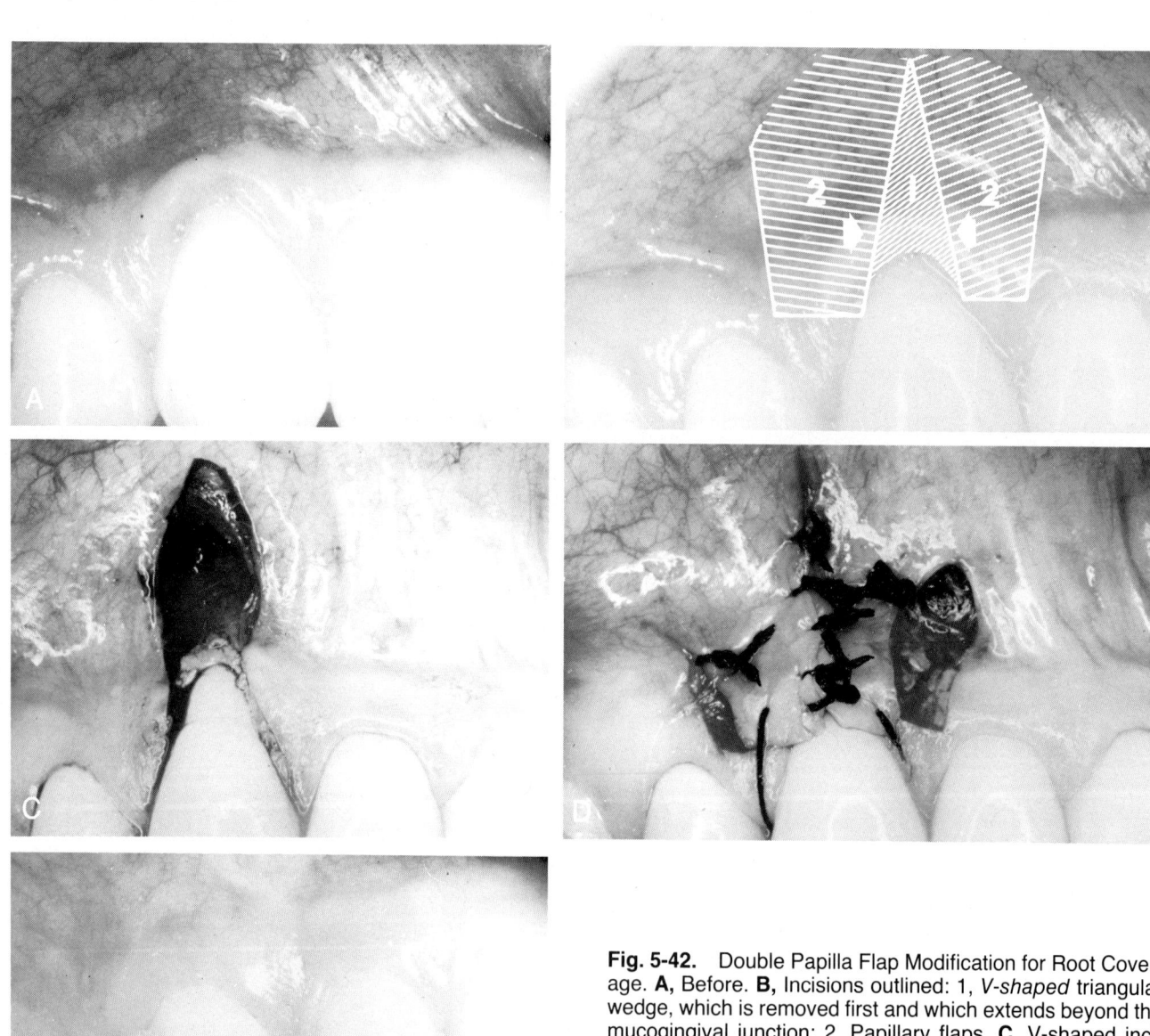

Fig. 5-42. Double Papilla Flap Modification for Root Coverage. **A,** Before. **B,** Incisions outlined: 1, *V-shaped* triangular wedge, which is removed first and which extends beyond the mucogingival junction; 2, Papillary flaps. **C,** V-shaped incision completed. **D,** Papillary flaps sutured. **E,** Six years later. Compare with A and C.

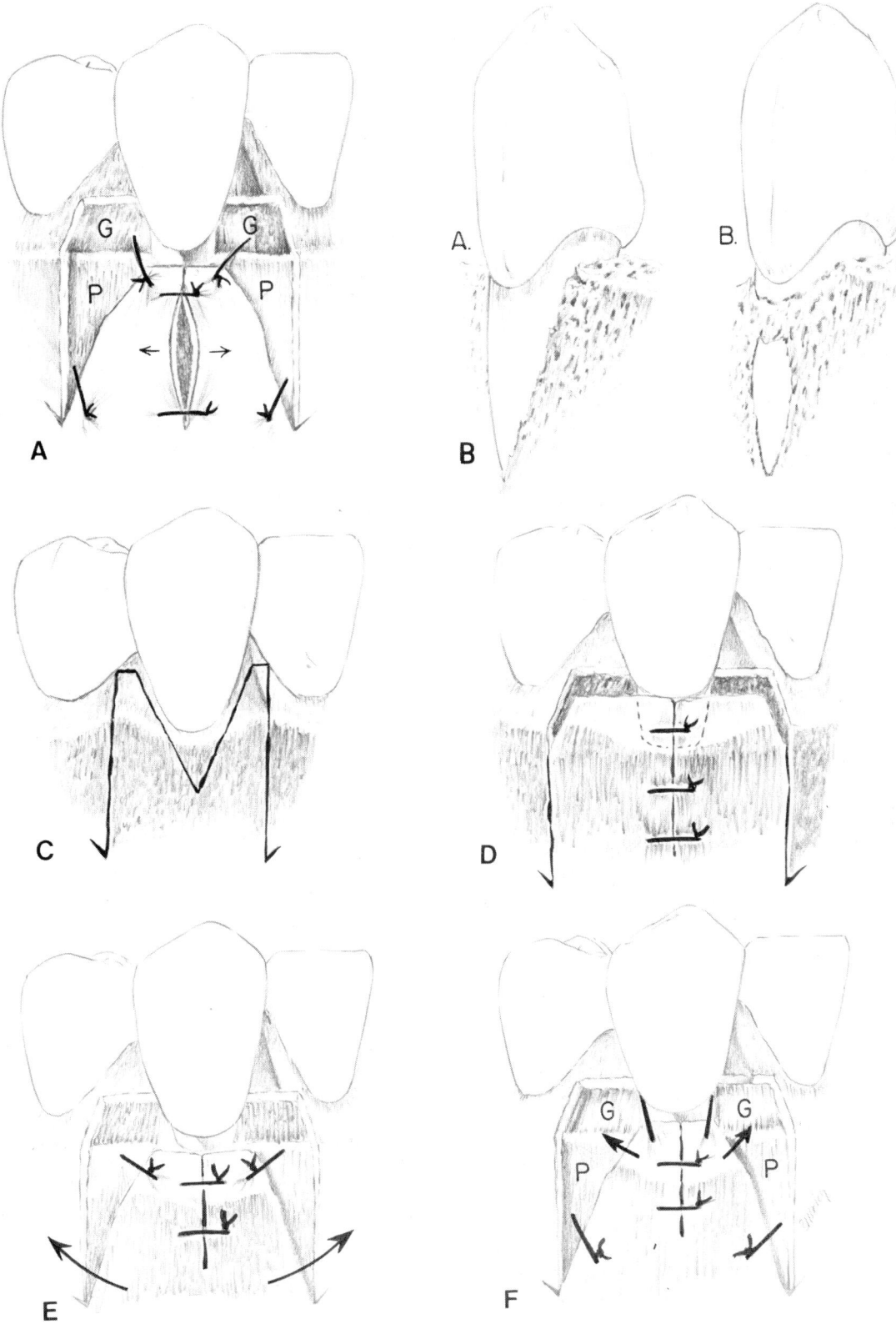

Fig. 5-43. Double Papilla Flap—Reasons for Failure. **A,** Separation of papillae as a result of inadequate suturing. **B,** Formation of dehiscence (A) or fenestration (B) with use of full-thickness flaps. **C,** Narrowness of papilla. **D,** Inadequate keratinized tissue present for root coverage. **E,F,** Flap movement because of inadequate stabilization.

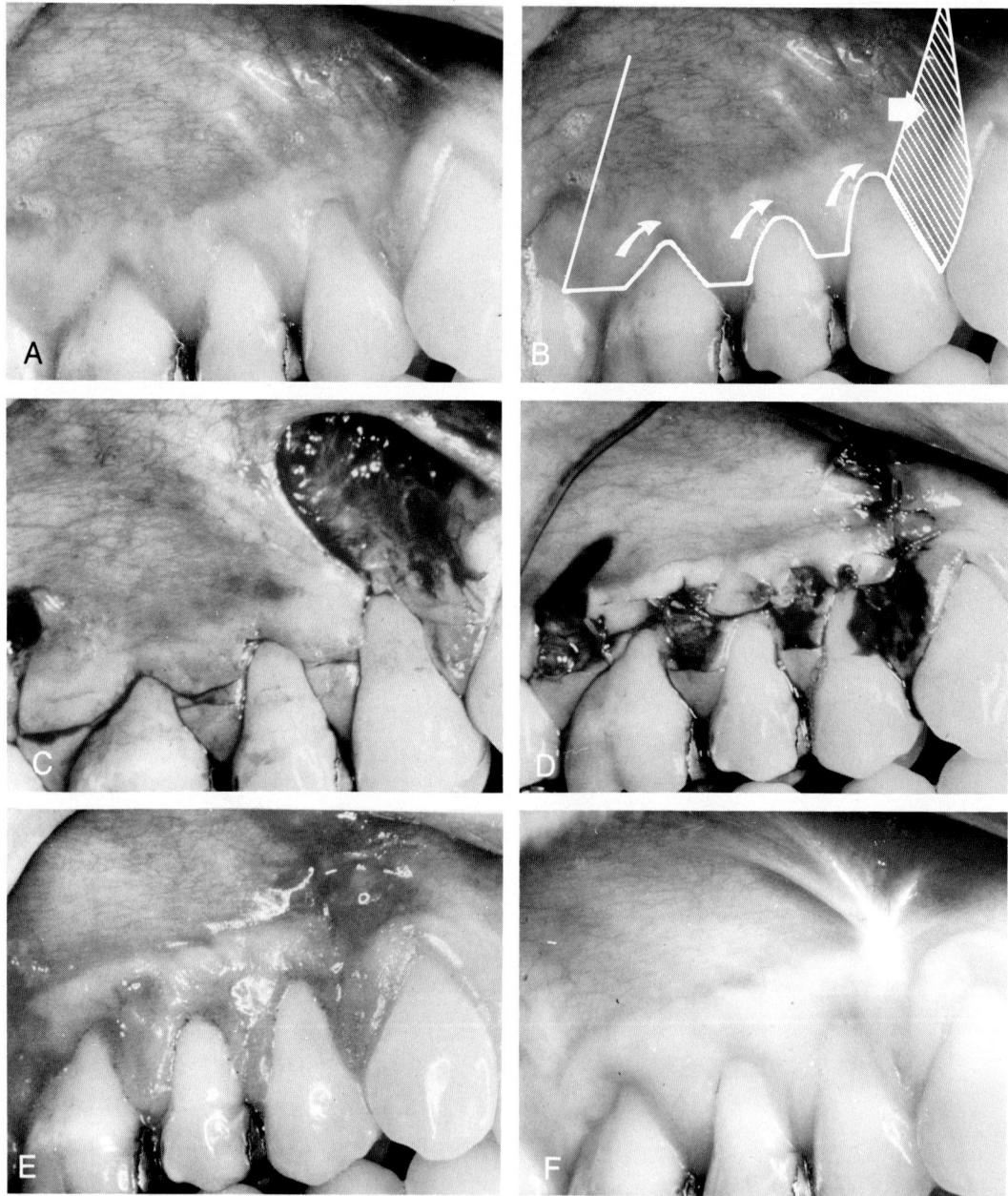

Fig. 5-44. Horizontal Sliding Papillary Flap. **A,** Before; note minimal attachments on molar and bicuspids. **B,** Flap incisions outlined. **C,** V-shaped incision removed and incisions outlined. **D,** Pedicle papillary flap rotated to buccal aspect of teeth and held with periosteal sutures. **E,** Three weeks later. **F,** Four months later. Note significant increase in attached gingiva.

FRENULECTOMY (FRENECTOMY) AND FRENULOTOMY (FRENOTOMY)

The frenulum is defined as a small band or fold of mucosal membrane that attaches the lips and cheeks to the alveolar process and that limits their movements. When the frenulum is abnormal, in that it becomes capable of initiating periodontal disease by retracting healthy gingival margins, it must be removed. If an abnormal frenulum is left in place, it can result in the following (Corn, 1964A):

1. Gingival recession
2. Diastema formation
3. Accumulation of debris by reflection and opening of the sulcus

The frenulum must also be removed when it is so thick and wide that it may interfere with toothbrushing, thus promoting inflammation and periodontal breakdown, or with orthodontic movement.

Frenulotomy is the simple excisional release of the frenulum from the apex of its insertion to its base and down to the alveolar process. *Frenulectomy* is the complete removal of the frenulum, including its attachments to the underlying alveolar process. Frenulectomy and frenulotomy can be performed separately as *localized* procedures or in conjunction with other procedures to increase the zone of attached gingiva.

Procedure

The frenulectomy procedure is outlined in Figure 5-45.

Frenulotomy Procedure

Frenulectomy is rarely needed. A frenulotomy will more than serve if done thoroughly and completely, even in extreme cases. It will also be less traumatic.

With the patient under adequate anesthesia, the surgeon releases the frenulum using the following procedure. Starting at the apex and using a No. 15 scalpel blade, the surgeon releases each side individually. The incisions at the base are extended adequately to allow proper tapering of the flap.

All tissue tags are removed. The periosteum over the alveolar process is *scored* with the scalpel blade but not removed. This disrupts any residual muscle fibers and promotes scarring.

The remaining alveolar mucosa just below the attached gingiva is removed. The underside of the lip is sutured closed with interrupted chromic gut sutures and then sutured down at the base. *Adequate suturing makes it impossible for the frenulum to re-form.*

The frenulotomy procedure is outlined in Figures 5-46, 5-47, and 5-48.

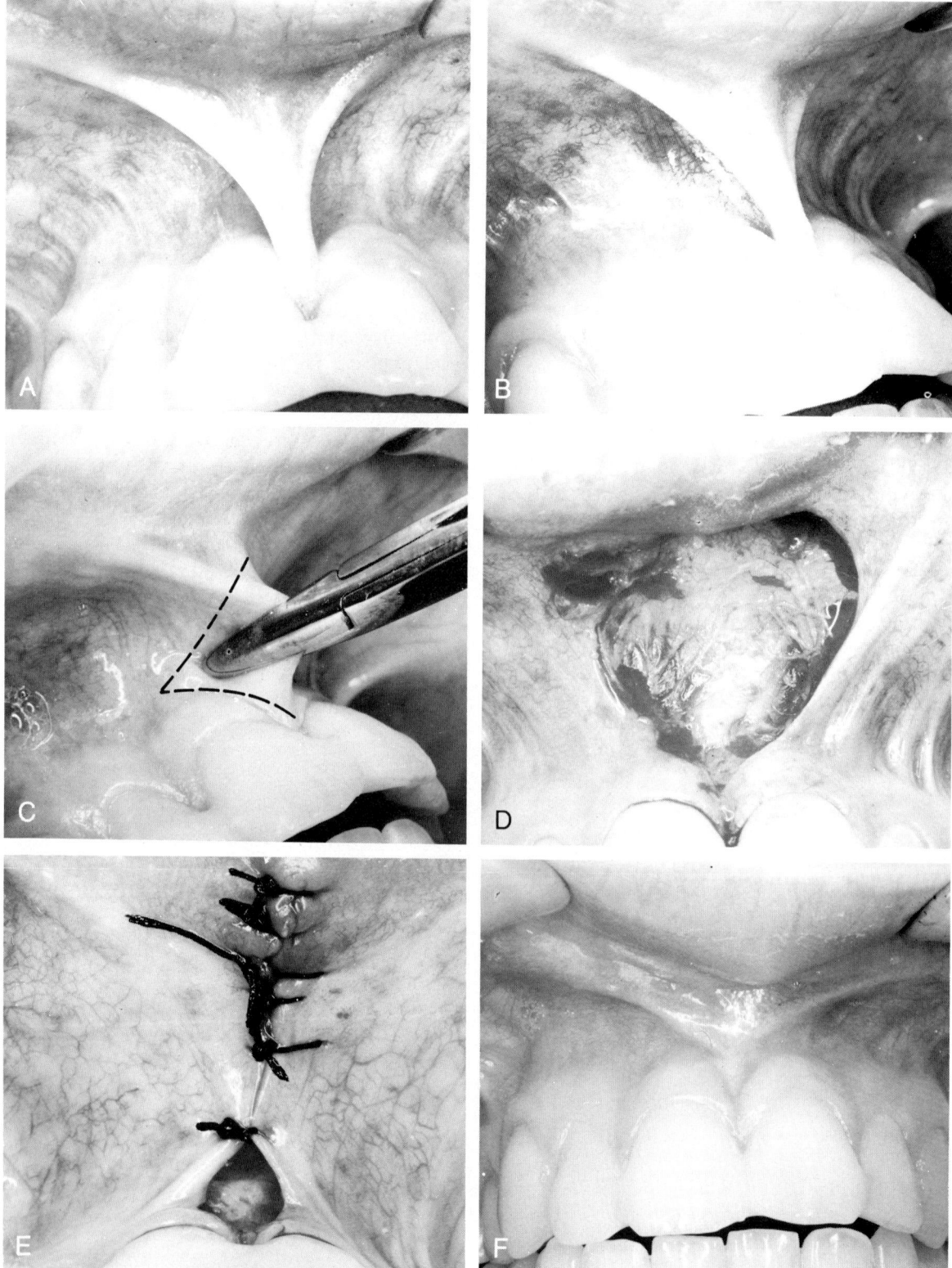

Fig. 5-45. Frenulectomy (Frenectomy). **A,** Before. **B,** Side view before. Note how high frenulum attaches incisally. **C,** Hemostat holding frenulum. Note outline of incisions for excision of frenulum. **D,** Incisions completed and frenulum removed. **E,** Tissue sutured. **F,** Case completed 6 months later.

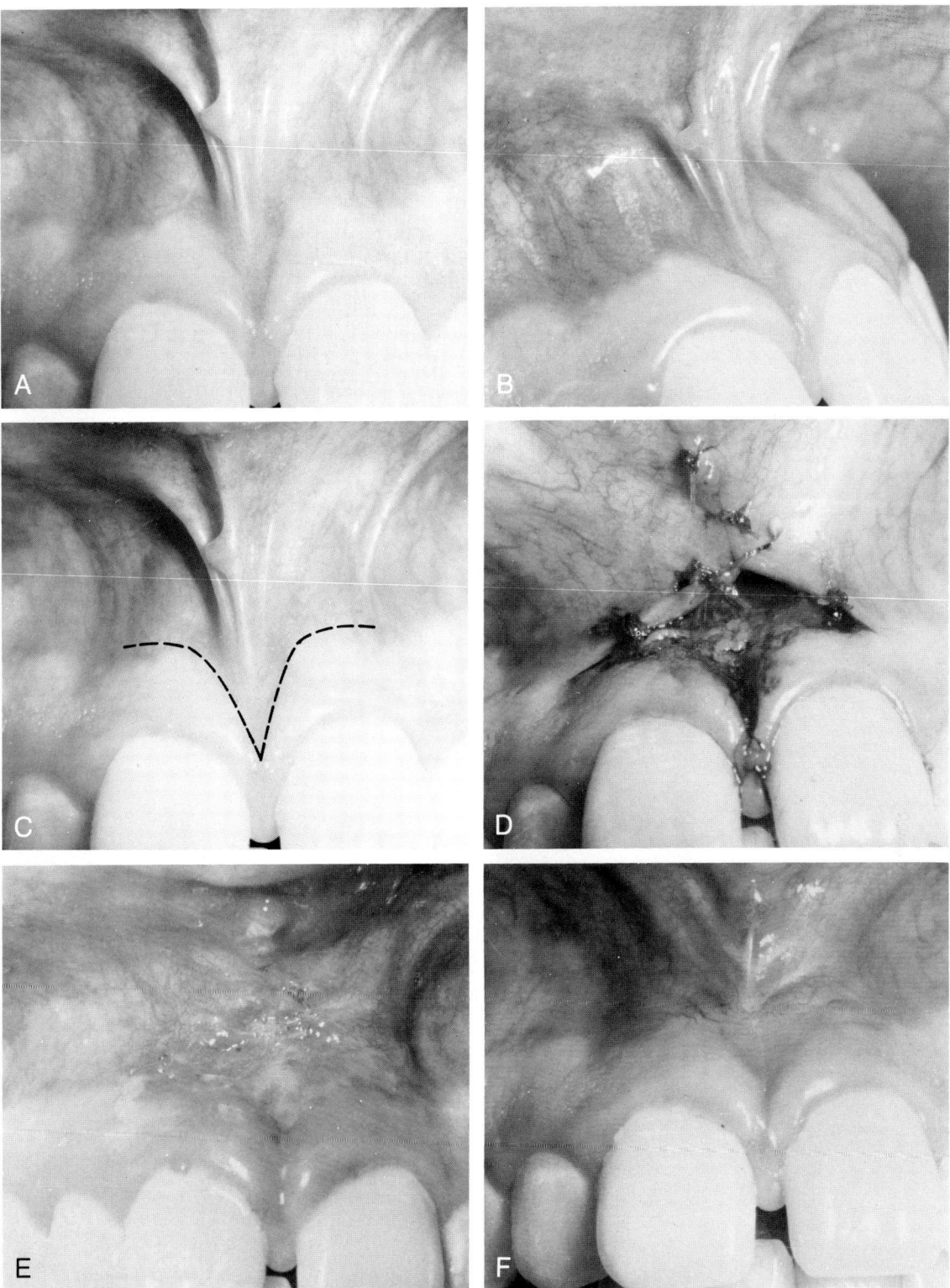

Fig. 5-46. Frenulotomy (Frenotomy). **A,** Before. **B,** Side view showing broad, high attachment of frenulum. **C,** Releasing incisions outlined. **D,** Flap sutured; note almost primary closure of incision, which will minimize trauma. **E,** One week later. **F,** Ten weeks later.

Mucogingival Surgery

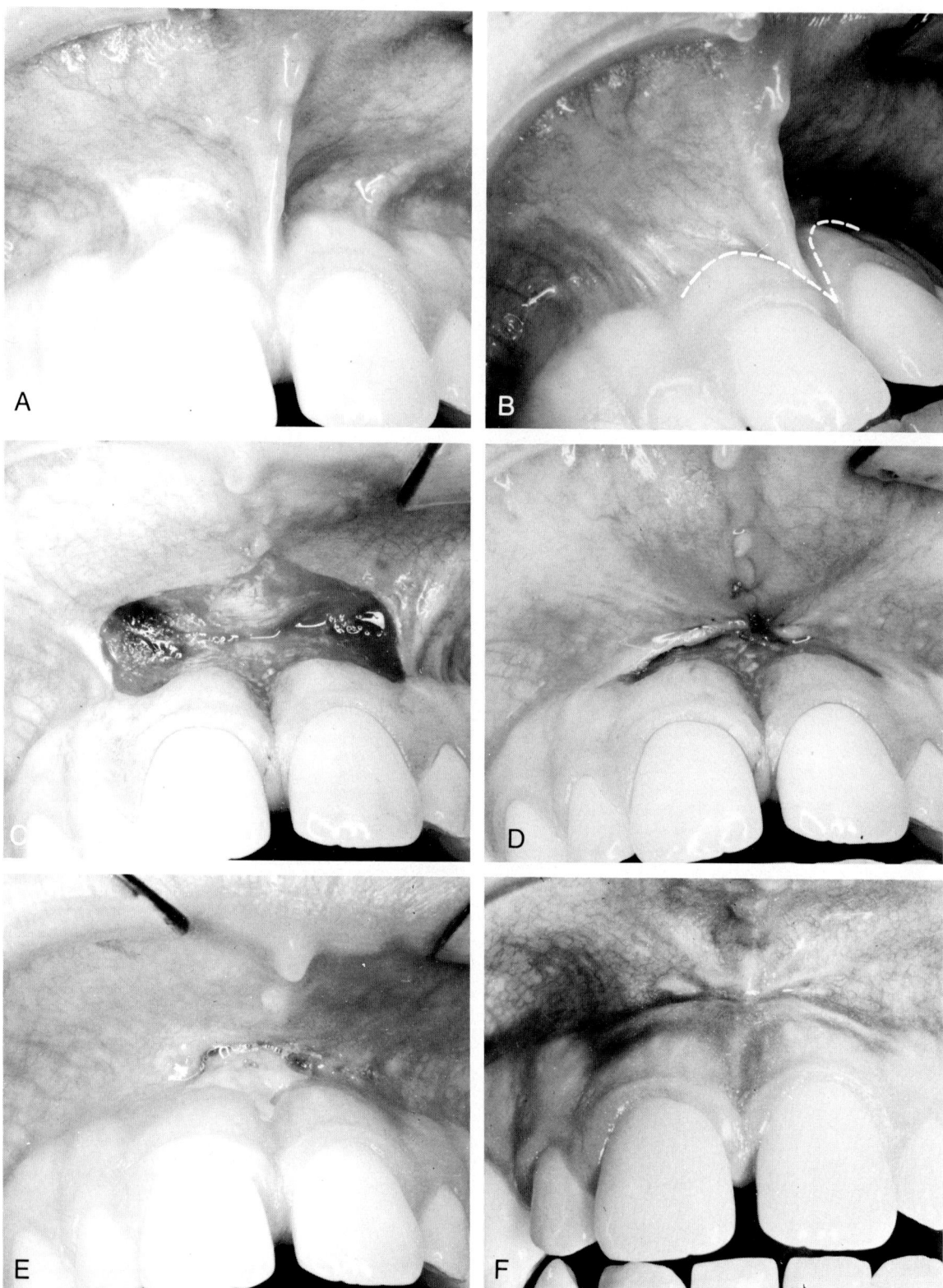

Fig. 5-47. Frenulotomy (Frenotomy). **A,** Before. **B,** Side view with outline of incision for release of muscle. **C,** Tissue release. Note broad release of tissue even without total excision of tissue. **D,** Tissue suture with almost primary closure to reduce trauma and prevent muscle reattachment. **E,** One week later. **F,** Five months later. The result is excellent.

Mucogingival Surgery

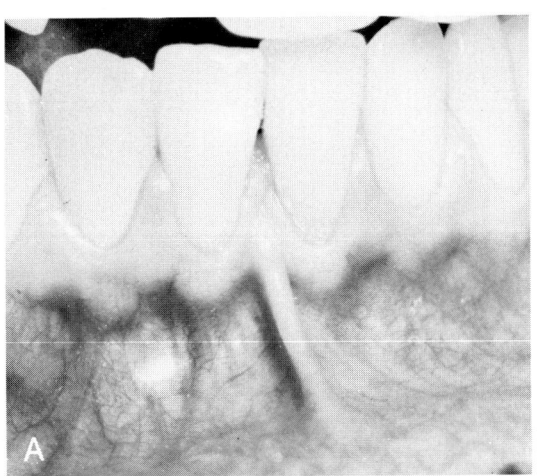
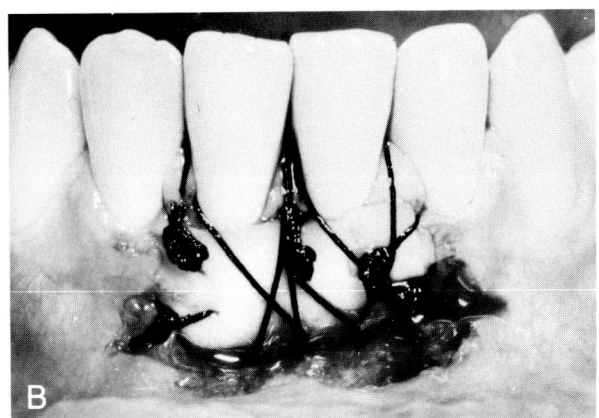
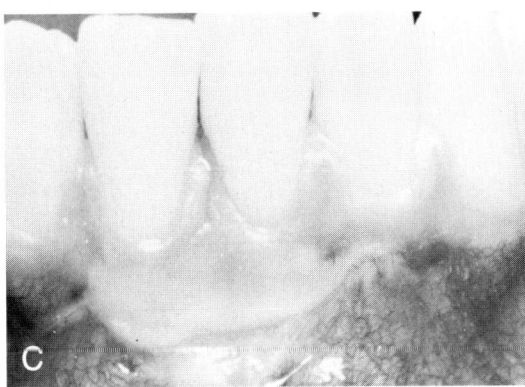

Fig. 5-48. Frenulotomy (Frenotomy). **A,** Frenulum and associated mucogingival problem. **B,** Excision of muscle and placement of free soft-tissue autograft. **C,** Case completed, frenulum removed, and mucogingival problem corrected. Note increased width of attached keratinized tissue.

6

PALATAL FLAPS

The palate, unlike other areas, is composed mainly of dense collagenous connective tissue. This fact precludes the palatal tissue from being positioned apically, laterally, or coronally. Therefore, surgical techniques are required that allow the tissue to be thinned and apically positioned at the same time.

Historical Review

The palatal flap procedure historically involved reflecting a full-thickness flap to gain access to the underlying bone and remove necrotic and granulomatous tissue. It was not until Ochsenbein and Bohannan (1963, 1964) described a palatal approach for osseous surgery that precise palatal surgical techniques were described and developed.

Figure 6-1, shows the outline of the three types of palatal flap designs: (A) full-thickness flap, (B) modified partial-thickness flap, and (C) partial-thickness palatal flap. The objective and result of all three are the same—a thin, even-flowing gingival architecture that closely approximates the underlying bone (Fig. 6-1D).

Ochsenbein and Bohannan, in comparing the palatal and buccal approaches to osseous surgery, noted the following advantages, disadvantages, and indications of the palatal approach.

Advantages of Palatal Approach

1. Esthetics
2. Easier access for osseous surgery
3. Wider palatal embrasure space
4. A naturally cleansing area
5. Less resorption because of thicker bone

Disadvantages of Buccal Approach

1. Esthetics
2. Close root proximity
3. Possible involvement of the buccal furcation
4. Thin plate of bone overlying the maxillary molars where dehiscences and fenestrations may be present

Indications

1. Areas that require osseous surgery
2. Pocket elimination
3. Reduction of enlarged and bulbous tissue

Contraindications

The palatal approach procedure is contraindicated when a broad, shallow palate does not permit a partial-thickness flap to be raised without possible damage to the palatal artery.

Diagnostic Probing

Before beginning the operation, but after adequate administration of anesthetic, periodontal probing or *sounding* for the underlying osseous topography is indicated (Easley, 1967). This is especially important on the palate, where frequently the tissue is enlarged and bulbous with underlying heavy bony ledges and exostoses. These exostoses frequently occur in second and third molar areas (Fig. 6-2).

Sounding permits one to discriminate between dense fibrotic tissue and enlarged tissue resulting from the osseous irregularities (Fig. 6-3). Furthermore, because palatal tissue cannot be positioned, failure to access the underlying topography adequately often results in a flap that is either too long or too short. Tissue thickness is one of the determining factors for incision placement—*the thicker the tissue, the more exaggerated the scalloping of the incision.* A more exaggerated incision would also be needed if extensive osteoplasty was needed for reduction and removal of heavy bony ledges and exostoses.

The various tissue-bone relationships and the anticipated incisions are reviewed in Figure 6-4. Note that, even though the tissue appears to be the same in all instances and the results may be the same, the incisions vary according to the underlying osseous topography.

PARTIAL-THICKNESS PALATAL FLAP

This technique was developed by Staffileno (1969A) to overcome some of the problems of extensive gingival resection and to facilitate treatment of palatal osseous defects, which until then was approached cautiously.

Advantages

1. Minimal trauma
2. Rapid healing
3. Ease of palatal tissue manipulation
4. Establishment of favorable gingival contours

The partial-thickness palatal flap is a procedure that requires a high degree of technical skill and one that should be attempted only after some advanced training because the palatal artery can be damaged.

Presurgical Phase

With the patient under adequate anesthesia, the operator sounds for the underlying osseous topography. This is very important because the flap cannot be positioned after the initial incision. A short flap will result in bone exposure and a long flap will have to be trimmed, which is difficult and leaves thick marginal tissue.

The thicker the tissue, the more exaggerated the scalloping of the incision. For this reason, the exact thickness of the tissue must be determined at the start. *Underlying osseous irregularities and osseous resection techniques must also be anticipated.*

Once all the factors have been taken into account, the exact placement of the incision is determined (Fig. 6-5A). A sounding will not only help to determine the amount of scalloping required, but also the length and degree of tapering of the incision in an occluso-apical direction to allow proper positioning and adaptation of the flap (Fig. 6-5A'). ***This is much more difficult than it appears.***

Surgical Phase

The primary incision is made with a No. 15 (usually) or No. 12 (if access is limited) scalpel blade. It is usually begun at the margin of the last tooth in the tuberosity area as an extension of the distal wedge procedure. It is continued forward, using a scalloped, inverse beveled, partial-thickness incision to create a thin partial-thickness flap (Fig. 6-5B,B').

The blade of the scalpel should always be kept on the vertical height of the alveolus. This prevents unnecessary involvement or cutting of the palatal artery.

When the tissue is thick, bulbous, or enlarged, it is often difficult, if not impossible, to make this first incision all the way down to the bone. The incision will have to follow the contour of both the tissue and underlying osseous topography.

Once the initial part of the primary incision has been completed, the tissue may be retracted with rat-tail pliers for completion of the incision (Fig. 6-5C,C'). Upon completion, the scalpel blade is directed toward the bone to *score* it at the base of the flap. This separates the periosteum in this area and permits easy removal of the secondary flap from bone. Without this scoring, it is more difficult to remove the secondary inner flap and generally results in a torn, ragged periosteal tissue with many tags.

A secondary sulcular incision is now completed both facially and interproximally, using a No. 15 or No. 12 scalpel blade down to the crest of the bone (Fig. 6-5D,D'). This incision frees the coronal aspects of the inner or secondary flap, permitting removal.

Ochsenbein chisels (Nos. 1 and 2) are now used from both the occlusal and apical extensions of the flap to completely free and remove the secondary inner flap (Fig. 6-5E,E'). The No. 1 chisel is directed from the occlusal direction against the bone, lifting off or separating the periosteum of the secondary inner flap from the bone. The No. 2 chisel is placed in the scoring incision at the base of the primary thinning incision, and, directing it occlusually, is used to remove the secondary inner flap. If the periosteum has not previously been scored, this procedure will be more difficult and leave a torn, ragged periosteum. A Friedman rongeur may also be used to remove the secondary inner flap.

Once the secondary inner flap has been removed and all necessary scaling and root planing and osseous surgery have been completed, the flap is allowed to fall back against the bone, and it is then sutured. If design was proper, the flap will be at the crest of the bone with the scalloped papillae positioned interproximally, permitting primary closure (Fig. 6-5F,F'). Either interrupted or suspensory sutures can be used.

It is important to note that the inner 2° flap of connective tissue that has been removed can now be trimmed and used for a free connective-tissue autograft (Edel, 1974) or as part of a subepithelial connective-tissue graft (Langer and Colagna, 1980; Langer and Langer, 1985).

The procedure is shown clinically in Figures 6-6 and 6-7.

MODIFIED PARTIAL-THICKNESS PALATAL FLAP

Ochsenbein in 1958, and Ochsenbein and Bohannan in 1963 described this technique, but it was not until 1965 that it became popularized by Prichard. It has also become known as the *ledge-and-wedge technique*.

This is a two-stage procedure that is technically easier than the single-step partial-thickness palatal flap. It has as its main disadvantage the fact that healing interdentally is by secondary intention. This fact precludes the use of this procedure with such procedures as the modified Widman flap, E.N.A.P., osseous grafting, and any others that require primary closure.

This procedure also requires a certain degree of technical skill or the palatal artery can be damaged easily.

Presurgical Phase

With the patient under adequate anesthesia, sounding is carried out to determine the underlying osseous topography, pocket depth, and thickness of the tissue. This stage is not as critical as it is in the single-stage procedure because the first-stage gingivectomy incision will allow visualization of tissue thickness.

Surgical Phase

Stage I: Gingivectomy

It is not necessary to mark the base of the pockets with pocket markers. A periodontal probe may be used to estimate pocket depth (Fig. 6-8A,A'). A periodontal knife is used to resect the tissue above the crest of bone (Fig. 6-8B,B'). Unlike the basic gingivectomy technique, *no bevel is placed*. A tissue ledge is established to allow visualization of tissue thickness and permit easier placement of the primary palatal incision (Fig. 6-8C,C').

Sometimes it may *not* be desirable to make the gingivectomy incision down to the base of the pocket, especially on thicker tissue. When such tissue is thinned and falls back against the bone, it will be short of the bony crest. This can result in excessive bone exposure and a good deal of postoperative discomfort.

A scalloped-type gingivectomy incision has sometimes been advocated to achieve interproximal primary closure. This is not recommended because the results are not satisfactory and primary closure is not attained.

Stage II: Partial-Thickness Flap

Once the gingivectomy procedure is complete, the remainder of the procedure is similar to that already described for the partial-thickness palatal flap.

A primary partial-thickness thinning incision is now completed down to the bone (Fig. 6-8D,D'). ***This incision stays within the vertical height of the alveolus to avoid involvement of the palatal artery.*** A *scoring* incision is used at the base of the flap to permit periosteal release of the secondary inner flap. A secondary incision about the necks of the teeth and interproximally is completed down to the crest of bone (Fig. 6-8D,D'). Ochsenbein chisels (Nos. 1 and 2) or a Friedman rongeur is used for occlusal and apical release of the secondary inner flap (Fig. 6-8E,E') and exposure of bone. Scaling, root planing, and osseous resection procedures are carried out, and the flap is sutured with interrupted or continuous sling sutures at or just above the crest of bone (Fig. 6-8F').

The procedure is shown clinically in Figures 6-9 and 6-10.

Common Mistakes

1. The short flap. This generally is the result of too deep a primary incision, gingivectomy to the crest of bone of a thick tissue, or use of a beveled gingivectomy (Fig. 6-11A). This results in delayed healing and increased patient discomfort.
2. Poor marginal flap adaptation caused by incomplete thinning of the tissue. The margin of the flap stands away from the tooth when the flap is replaced (Fig. 6-11B). This can be corrected either by additional thinning of the inner flap surface close to the base of the original incision or by more osteoplasty. Careful examination will reveal the problem.
3. Incision beyond the vertical height of the alveolus, bringing the scalpel blade in close proximity to the palatal artery (Fig. 6-11C). Cutting the palatal artery can be especially dangerous near its exit point from the greater palatine foramen.
4. Extension beveling or thinning of tissue on a low, broad palate invites damage to the palatal artery (Fig. 6-11D).

5. Tissue placement high onto the teeth results in poor adaptation and recurrent pocket formation. This can be corrected by proper trimming at the time of flap placement prior to suturing (Fig. 6-11E); this is usually accomplished with scissors or scalpel blade. It often results in a thick, heavy margin.

DISTAL WEDGE

The retromolar area of the mandible and the tuberosity area of the maxilla offer unique problems for the clinician. They generally have enlarged tissue, unusual underlying osseous topography, and in the case of the retromolar area, a fatty, glandular, mucosal-type tissue. Historically, while periodontal surgical techniques were being developed for all other areas, development in this one area remained stagnant, and gingivectomy was the treatment of choice. This problem was first addressed by Robinson in 1963 and later by Kramer and Schwartz (1964), but it was Robinson's classic article on "The Distal Wedge Operation" (1966) that outlined the indications and treatment procedures still used today.

The distal wedge operation overcame the shortcomings, of the gingivectomy procedure, which did not allow treatment of irregular osseous deformities or access to the maxillary distal furcation area.

Advantages

1. Maintenance of attached tissue
2. Access for treatment of both the distal furcation and underlying osseous irregularities
3. Closure by a mature thin tissue, which is especially important in the retromolar area
4. Greater opening and access when done in conjunction with other flap procedures. The main limitation is only one of access or anatomy (e.g., ascending ramus or external oblique ridge)

Wedge Designs

1. Triangular
2. Square, parallel, or H-design
3. Linear or pedicle

Size, shape, thickness, and access of the tuberosity or retromolar area determine treatment procedures.

Triangular Design

This requires an adequate zone of keratinized tissue and can be used in a very short or small tuberosity.

A triangular incision is made distal to the last molar, using a No. 12 or No. 15 scalpel blade (Fig. 6-12A). Using scalers, hoes, or knives, the triangular wedge of tissue is removed (Fig. 6-12B). The walls of the wedge are thinned or undermined, using scalpel blades to allow proper adaptation to the underlying bone. In Figure 6-12C and D we see the outline of the incisions, removal of the secondary wedges, and reflection of the flap for bone exposure. Periosteal elevators are used to reflect the flap. It is sometimes necessary to use small releasing incisions at the apex of the incision to relieve tension (Fig. 6-12A,a,b). Once the osseous corrective procedures have been completed, the teeth scaled, root planed, and flushed of debris, primary closure is done by interrupted sutures (Fig. 6-12E,F).

A small area adjacent to the tooth usually is not completely closed and heals by secondary intention.

Square, Parallel, or H-Design

This technique allows conservation of keratinized tissue and maximum closure. It also provides greater access to the underlying bony topography and the distal furcation. It is indicated where the tuberosity is longer.

Using a No. 15 blade, two parallel inversely beveled thinning incisions are made. They begin at the distal end of the edentulous area and are continued to the tooth (Fig. 6-13A,B). Two more incisions are made to free the flaps, one in the sulcus adjacent to the tooth and the other at the terminal end of the operative field (Fig. 6-13A). The blade is directed toward the buccal and palatal aspects of the edentulous ridge as the incisions are made.

Periosteal elevators are used to raise the flaps buccally and lingually or palatally. Kirkland or Orban knives may be used to remove the wedge of tissue down to the bone (Fig. 6-13C,D). After the bone is exposed, and the necessary osseous surgery and scaling and root planing have been completed (Fig. 6-13E), interrupted sutures are used for closure (Fig. 6-13F).

The retromolar area often has minimal keratinized tissue, and the tissue is often mucosal glandular tissue for which gingivectomy cannot be used. The wedge is the only possible way to thin and reduce the tissue in this area.

The procedures are outlined clinically in Figures 6-14, 6-15, and 6-16.

PALATAL APPROACH TO IMPLANT PLACEMENT

To avoid the difficult healing with vestibular incisions and at the same time provide adequate implant coverage, especially when augmentation procedures are required, Langer and Langer (1990) recommended a palatal approach.

Advantages

1. The use of overlapping flaps prevents flap opening and implant exposure
2. Facilitates healing and reduces postoperative trauma

Procedure

1. A horizontal incision is made 5 to 6 mm apical to the crest of the ridge with a No. 15 blade (Fig. 6-17A).
2. The horizontal incision is extended apically with a No. 15 blade held parallel to the vertical height of the palate. A partial-thickness flap is raised (Fig. 6-17B).
   Note: All incisions are kept on the vertical height of the alveolus to avoid damaging the palatal artery.
3. The blade is now used to score the periosteum apically for flap release.
4. Internal vertical releasing incisions are made at the terminal end of the horizontal incisions, which are carried onto the buccal surface. The outer epithelial portion of the flap need not be incised.
5. Oschenbien chisels or large hoes are now employed for reflection of the inner flap (Fig. 6-17C).
6. The implant(s) is placed (Fig. 6-17D).
7. The flap is repositioned (Fig. 6-17E).
8. Vertical and/or horizontal mattress sutures are used for flap closure and stabilization. Mattress sutures will minimize clot formation by pulling the flaps tightly against the bone and to each other (Fig. 6-17F).

The clinical procedure is depicted in Figure 6-18.

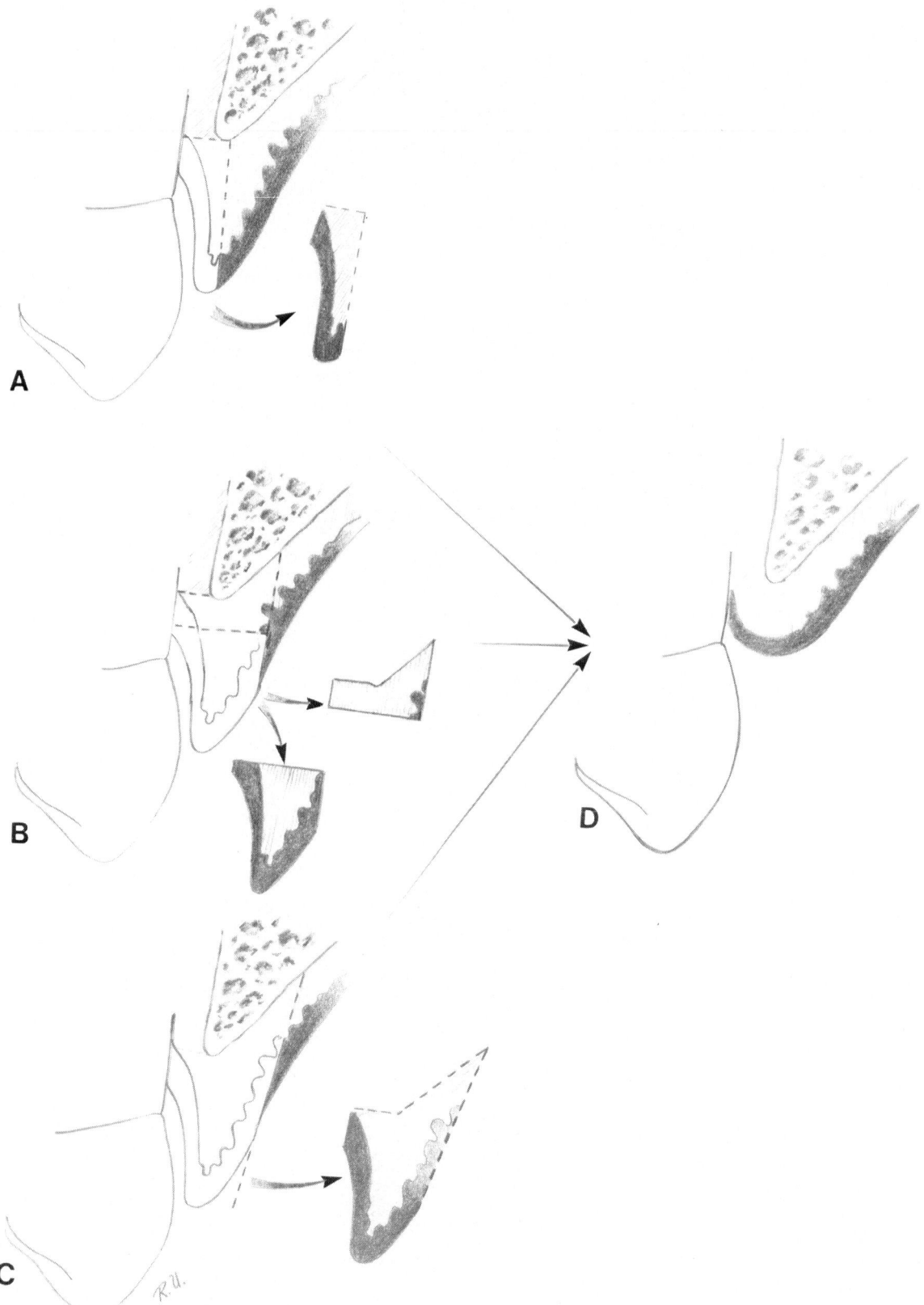

Fig. 6-1. Outline of Basic Palatal Flap Techniques. **A,** *Full-thickness* palatal flap used predominantly on thin palatal tissue. **B,** Modified partial-thickness *ledge-and-wedge* flap for thicker palatal tissue. **C,** *Partial-thickness* primary flap for thicker palatal tissue. **D,** Ideal result that should be achieved whichever technique is used.

Palatal Flaps

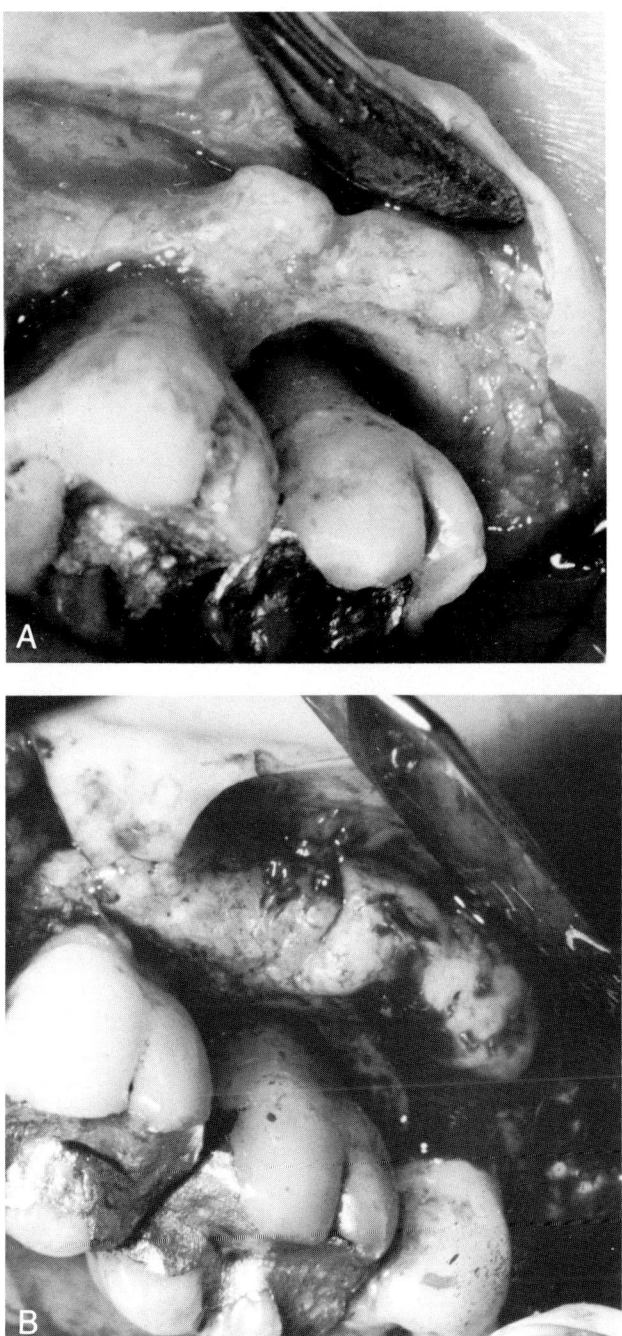

Fig. 6-2. Palatal Exostosis. Usually found in second and third molar areas.

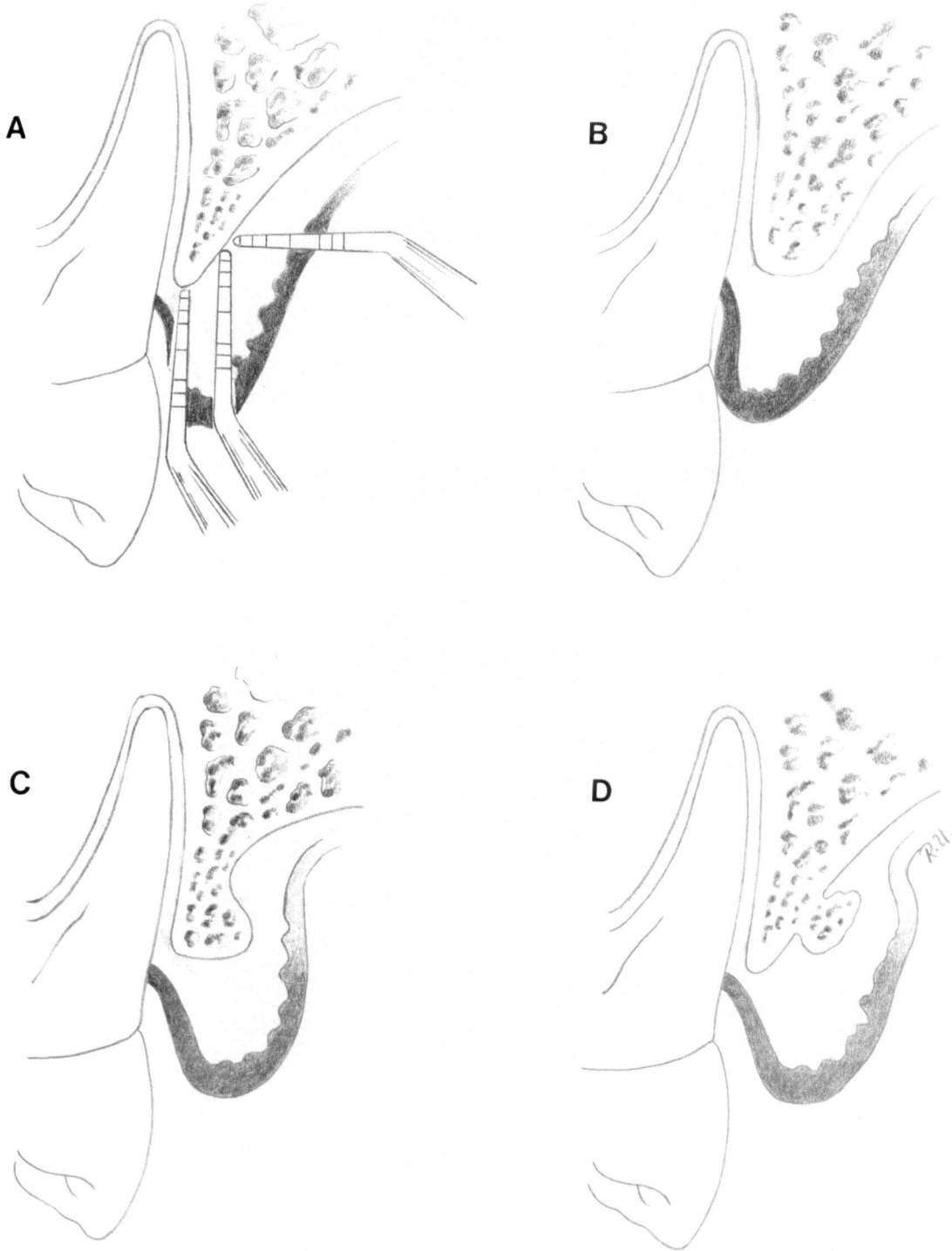

Fig. 6-3. Periodontal *Sounding* for the Underlying Osseous Topography and Common Osseous Irregularities. **A,** Periodontal probes inserted both vertically and apically not only to determine osseous defects interproximally but also to determine thickness and height of alveolar bone and the presence of irregularities. **B,** Thick bony margins. **C,** Heavy bony margins. **D,** Exostoses.

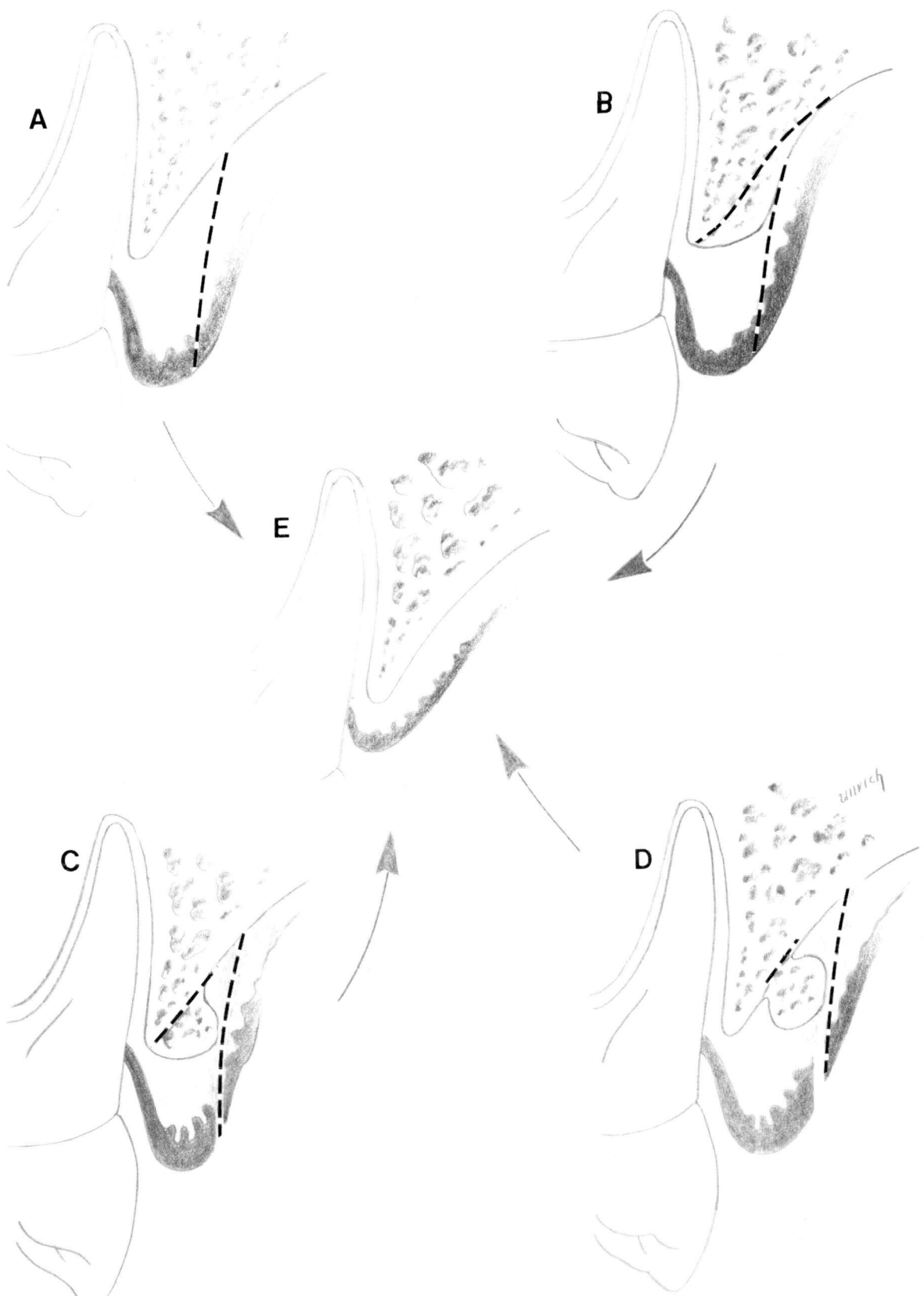

Fig. 6-4. Variations in Tissue-Bone Relationships. Note that, even though the palatal tissue is the same, the incision varies with changes in the underlying osseous topography and the nature and extent of the osseous contouring required. The dotted lines indicate flap design and osseous recontouring required in each instance to achieve an ideal form. **A,** Tissue enlargement only. **B,** Thickened palatal bone. **C,** Heavy bone margins. **D,** Exostoses. **E,** Final ideal form that should be attained by all.

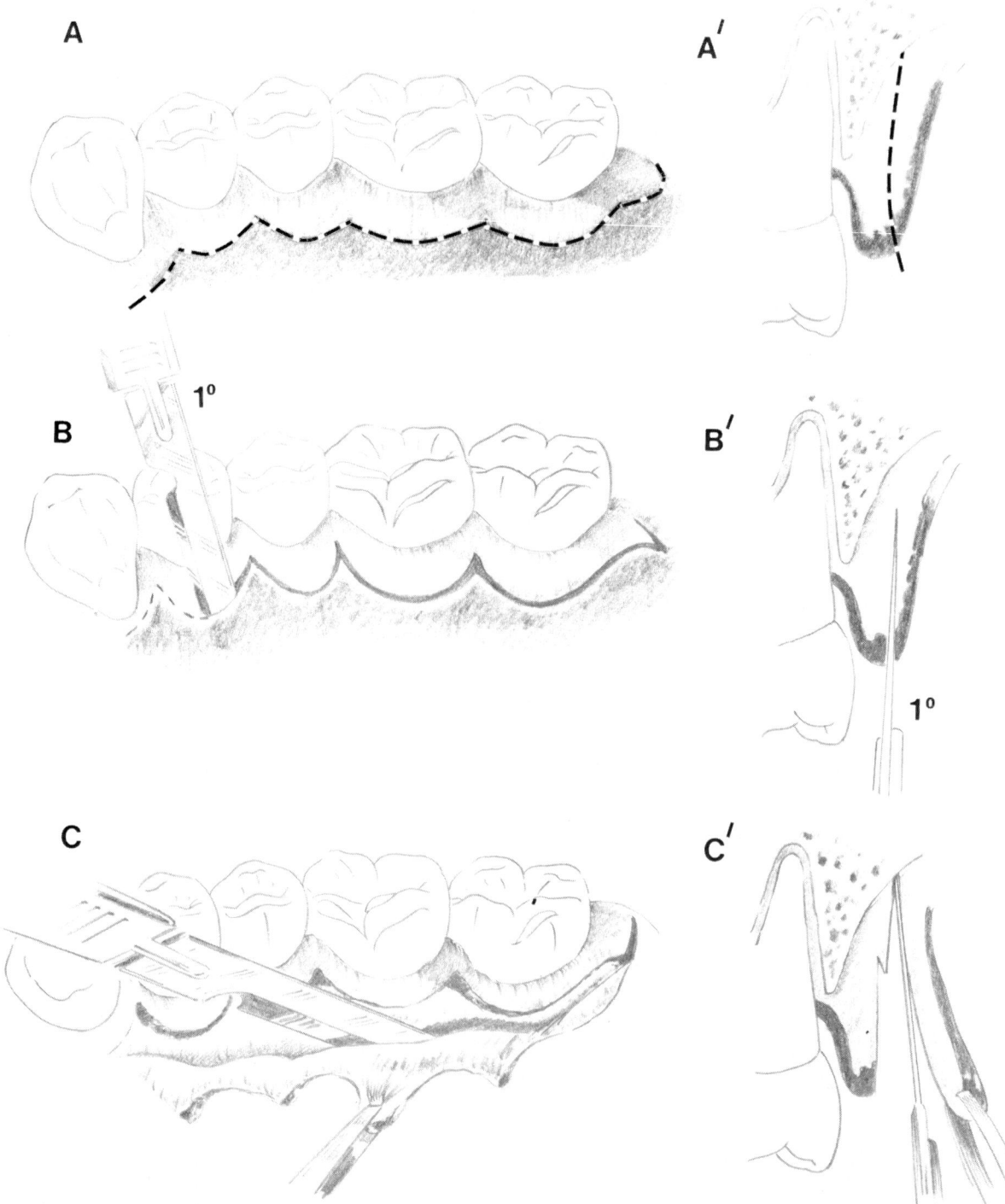

Fig. 6-5. Primary Partial-Thickness Palatal Flap. **A,** Outline of primary initial scalloped incisions on palate. **A′,** Cross-sectional (CX) view of primary thinning incision. **B,** Primary scalloped incision is begun. **B′,** CX view shows that in thick palatal tissue it is not always possible to go straight down to the bone. **C,C′,** Tissue pliers may be used to reflect the palatal flap as the incision is carried down to the bone, severing the periosteum at the base. *Note:* The **primary incision** is used **both to thin and shorten the flap at the same time.**

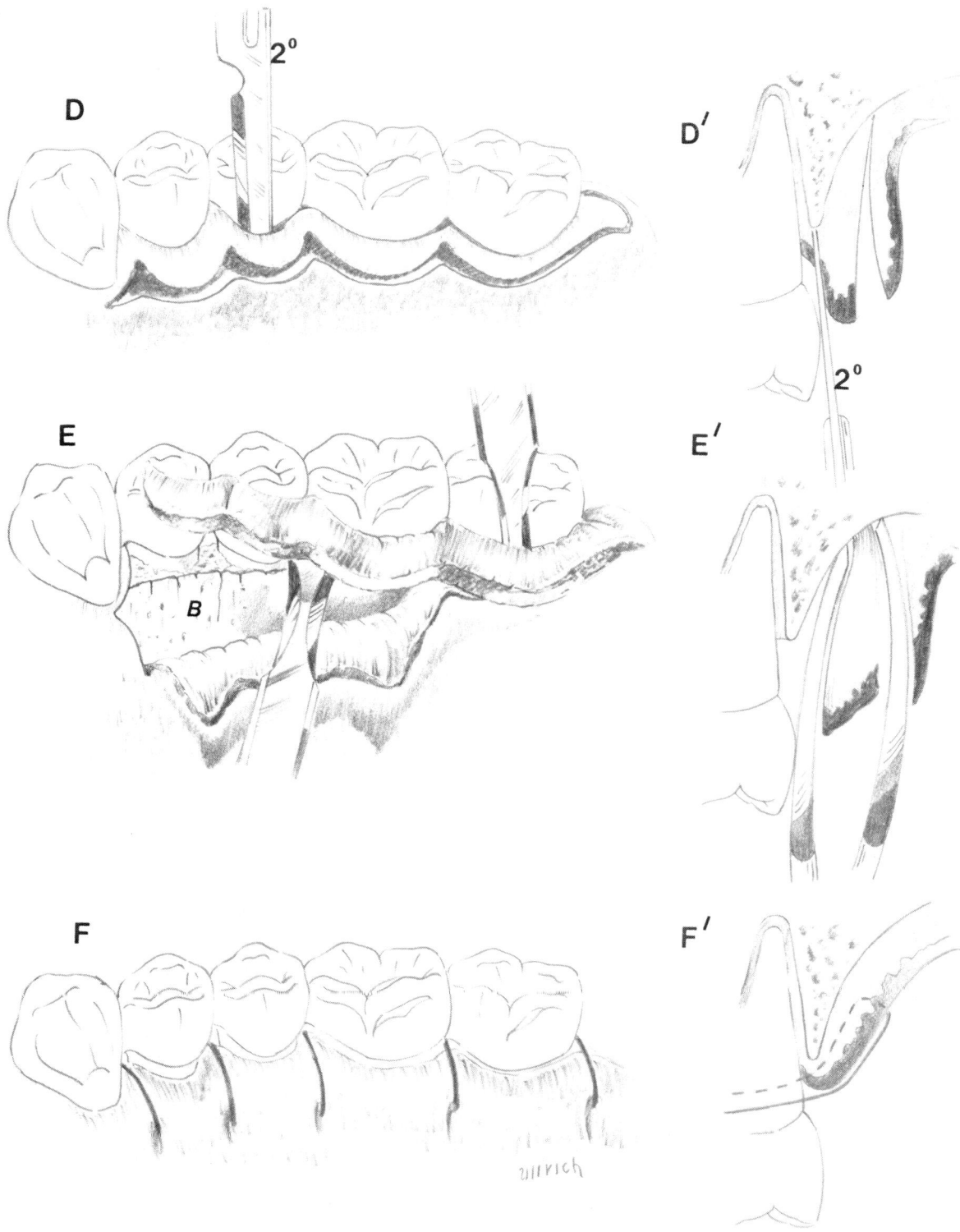

Fig. 6-5 (continued). **D,** A secondary, *sulcular* incision is now made to free the inner flap prior to removal. **D′,** The sulcular incision is made to the crest of bone. **E,E′,** Ochsenbein chisels are used to loosen and lift the inner flap for removal and bone exposure. **F,F′,** The thinned and shortened flap is positioned over the bone and sutured interproximally.

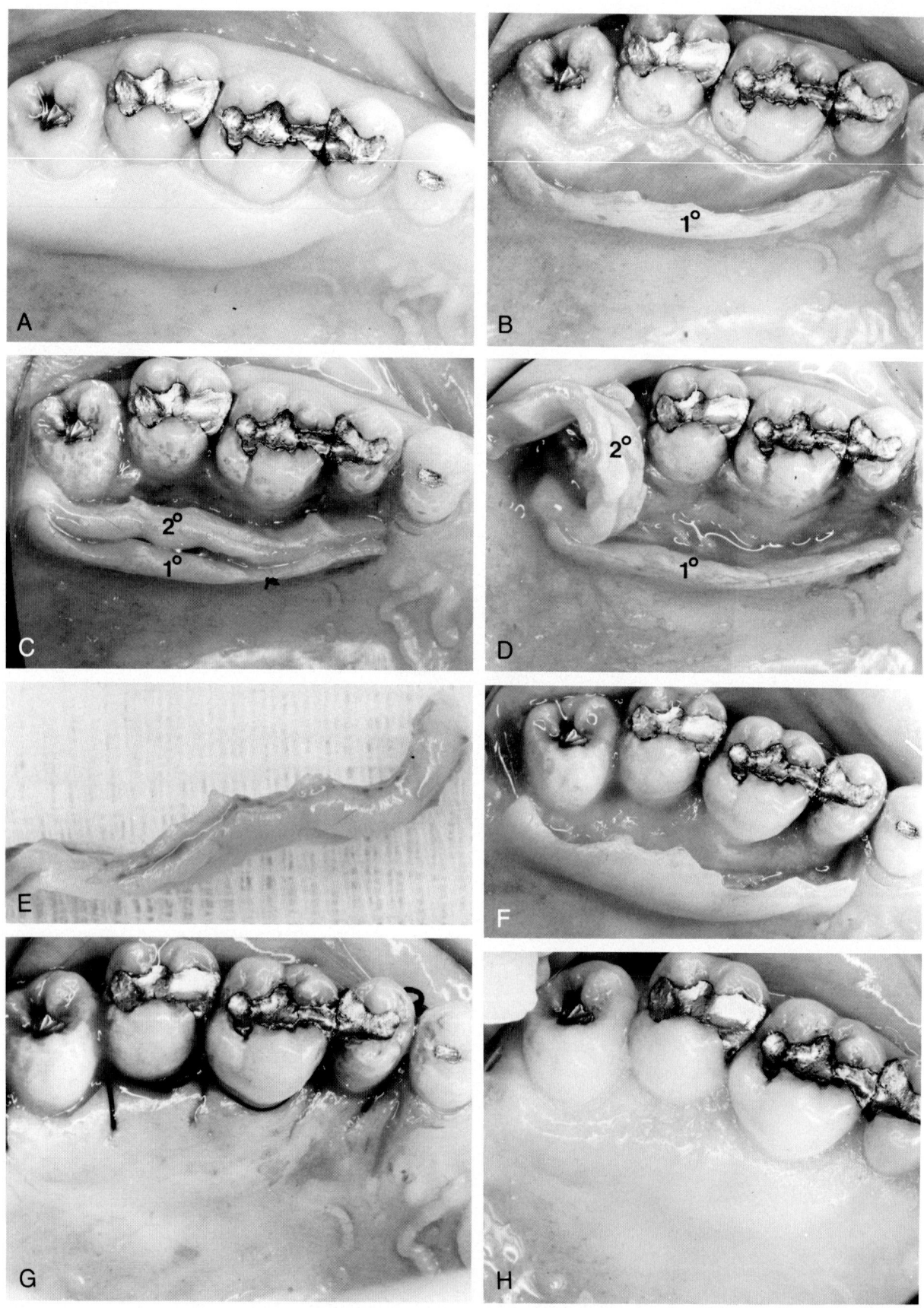

Fig. 6-6. Partial-Thickness Palatal Flap. **A,** Before, showing bulbous, enlarged tissue. **B,** Primary flap (1°) reflected. **C,** Secondary flap (2°) reflected. **D,** Removal of secondary inner flap. **E,** Secondary inner flap removed. **F,** Osseous contouring completed. **G,** Flap sutured. **H,** Seven months later. Note thin palatal contour with teeth fully exposed. Compare with A.

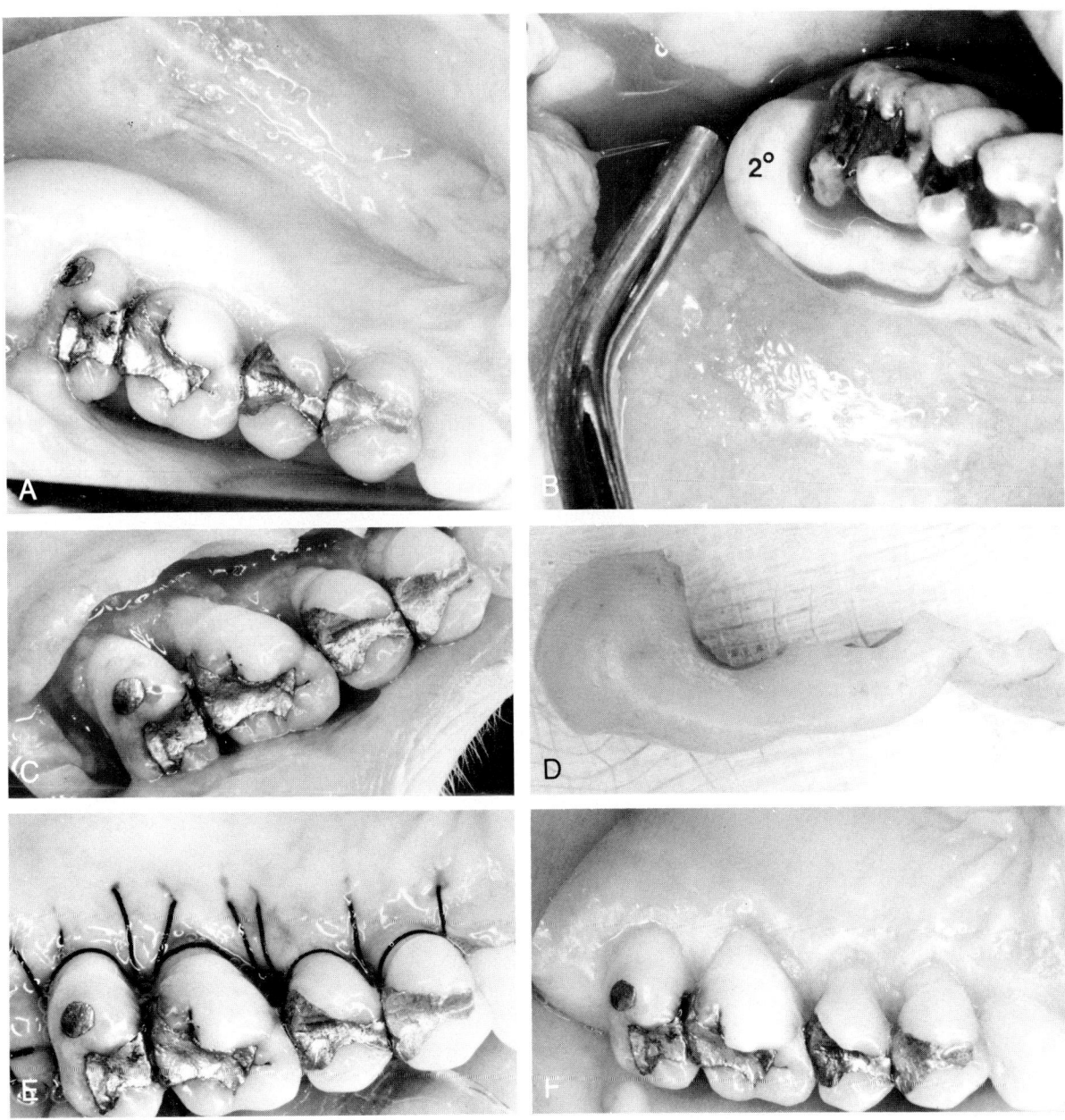

Fig. 6-7. Partial-Thickness Palatal Flap. **A,** Preoperative palatal view, showing severely enlarged bulbous tissue. **B,** Initial inverse beveled incision completed and secondary (2°) flap outlined. **C,** Secondary flap removed. Note extreme bulbousness of tissue. **D,** Flaps reflected and distal wedge removed. **E,** Flap sutured with primary closure. **F,** Eight months later; compare with A.

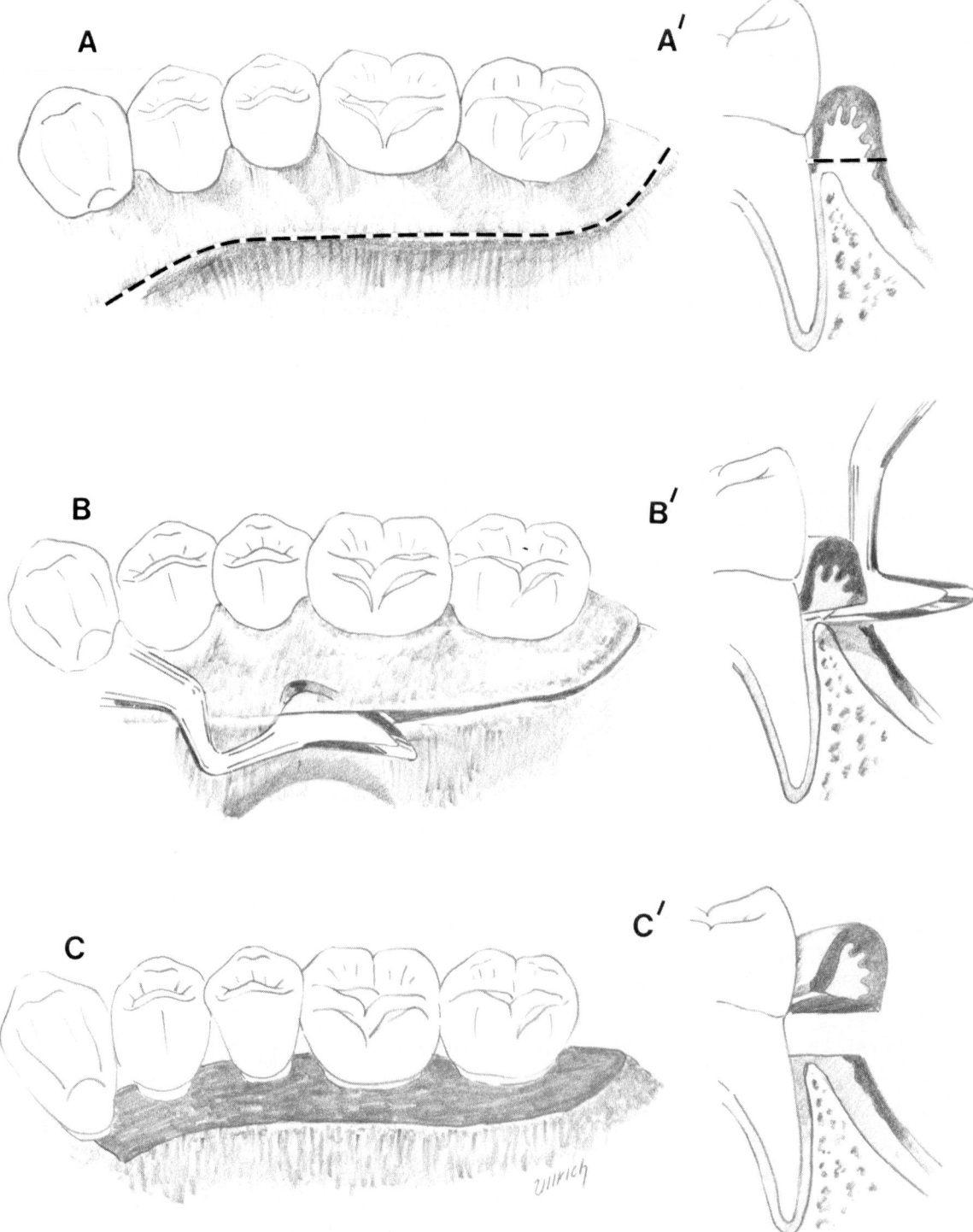

Fig. 6-8. Modified Partial-Thickness or Ledge-and-Wedge Palatal Flap. **A,** Outline of initial gingivectomy incision. **A',** Cross-sectional (CX) view showing a *non-beveled* initial gingivectomy incision above the bone. **B,B',** The initial gingivectomy incision is carried out using periodontal knives. **C,C',** Removal of the excised tissue and creation of a flat tissue ledge. Note that the tissue ledge allows the clinician to determine more easily the primary thinning incisions.

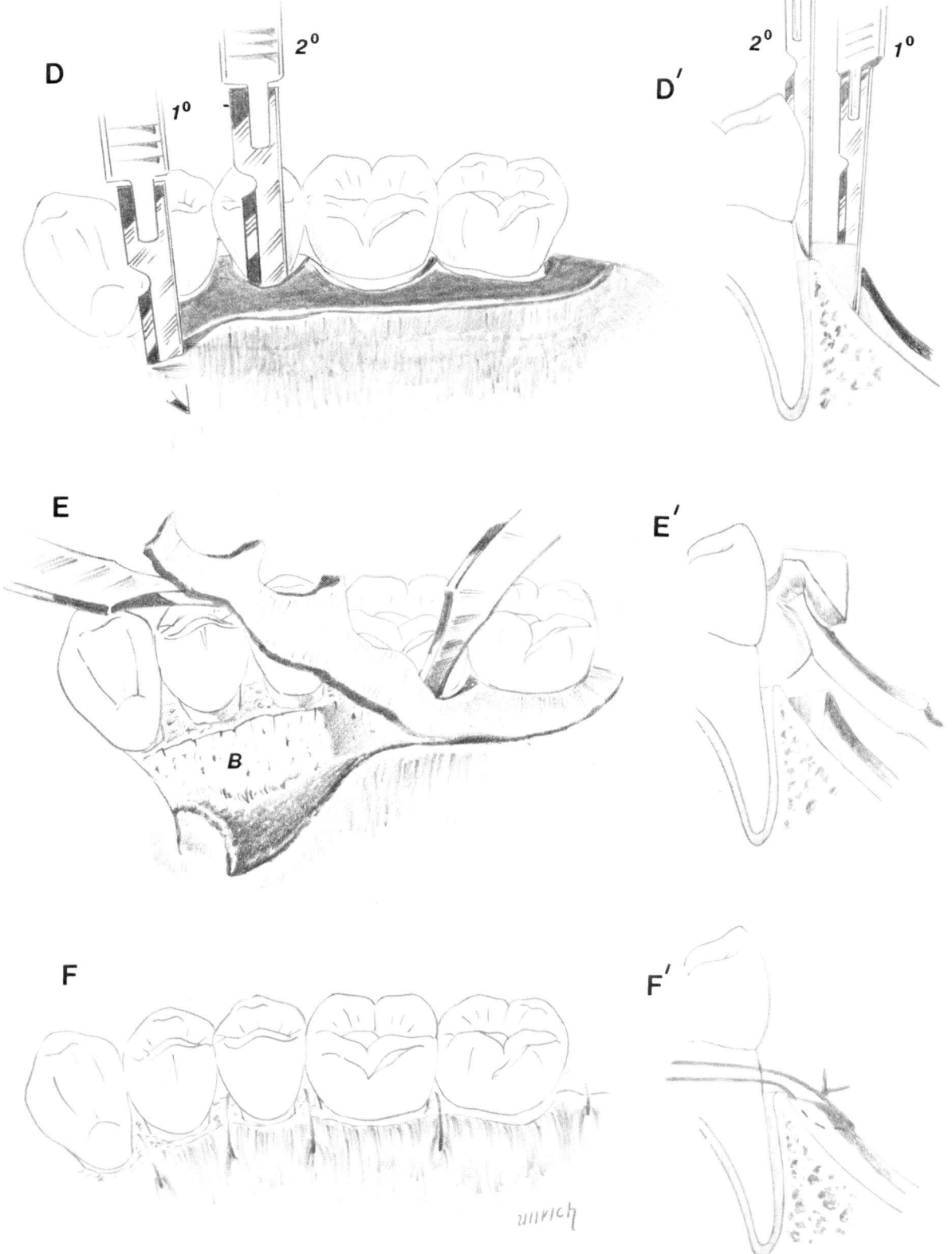

Fig. 6-8 (continued). D,D′, The primary and secondary incisions are completed. The primary incision is carried down to the bone, making sure the periosteum is severed at the base of the inner flap. The secondary incision is a sulcular incision made down to the crest of bone. **E,E′,** Ochsenbein chisels are used to remove the secondary inner flap and expose bone. **F,F′,** The flaps are sutured apically and the interproximal areas are permitted to granulate in by secondary intention.

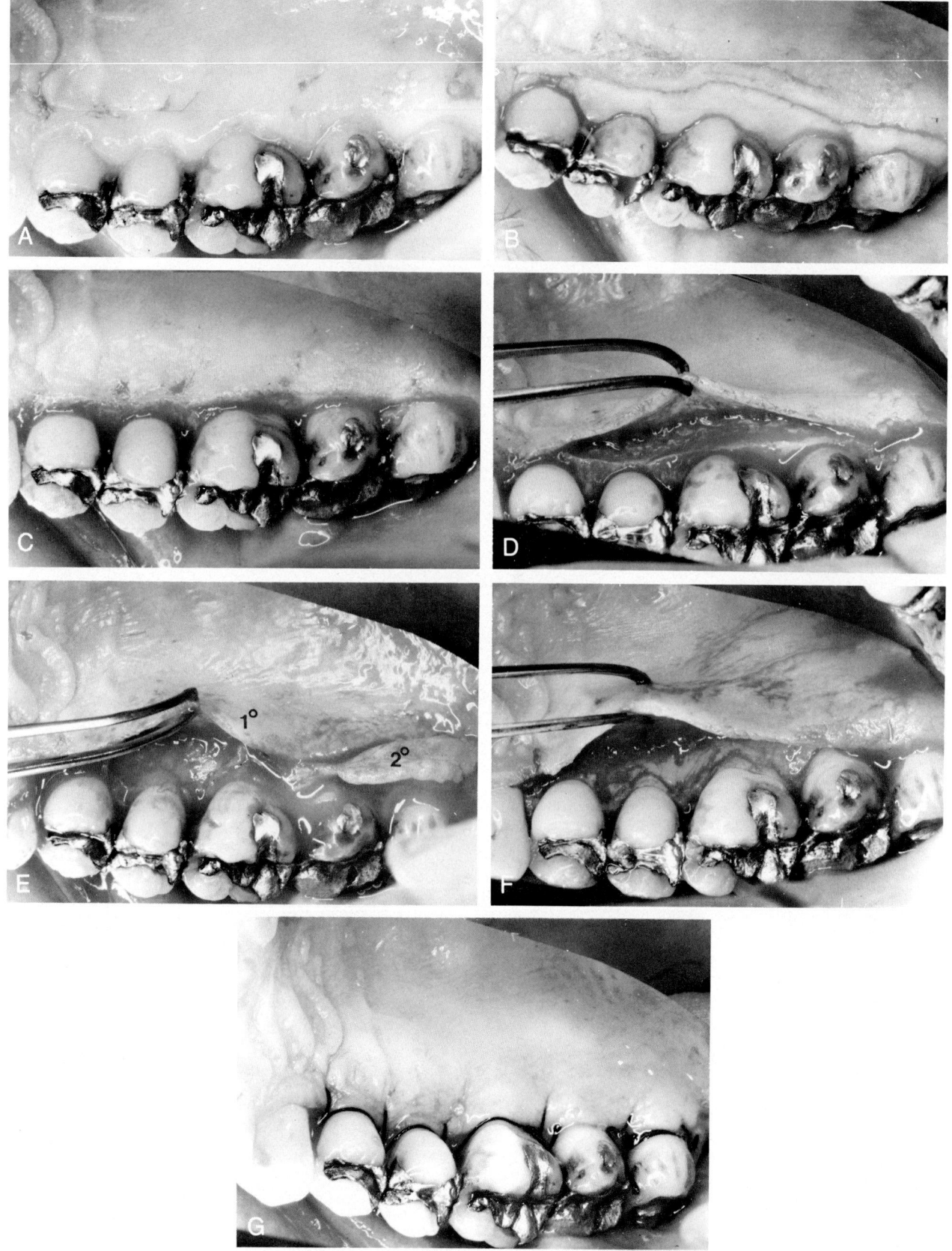

Fig. 6-9. Modified Partial Thickness Flap (Ledge-and-Wedge Technique). **A,** Before. **B,** Gingivectomy incision completed. **C,** Excised gingival tissue removed. **D,** Primary flap reflected. **E,** Secondary (2°) inner flap being removed. **F,** Secondary flap removed and osseous contouring completed. **G,** Flap sutured.

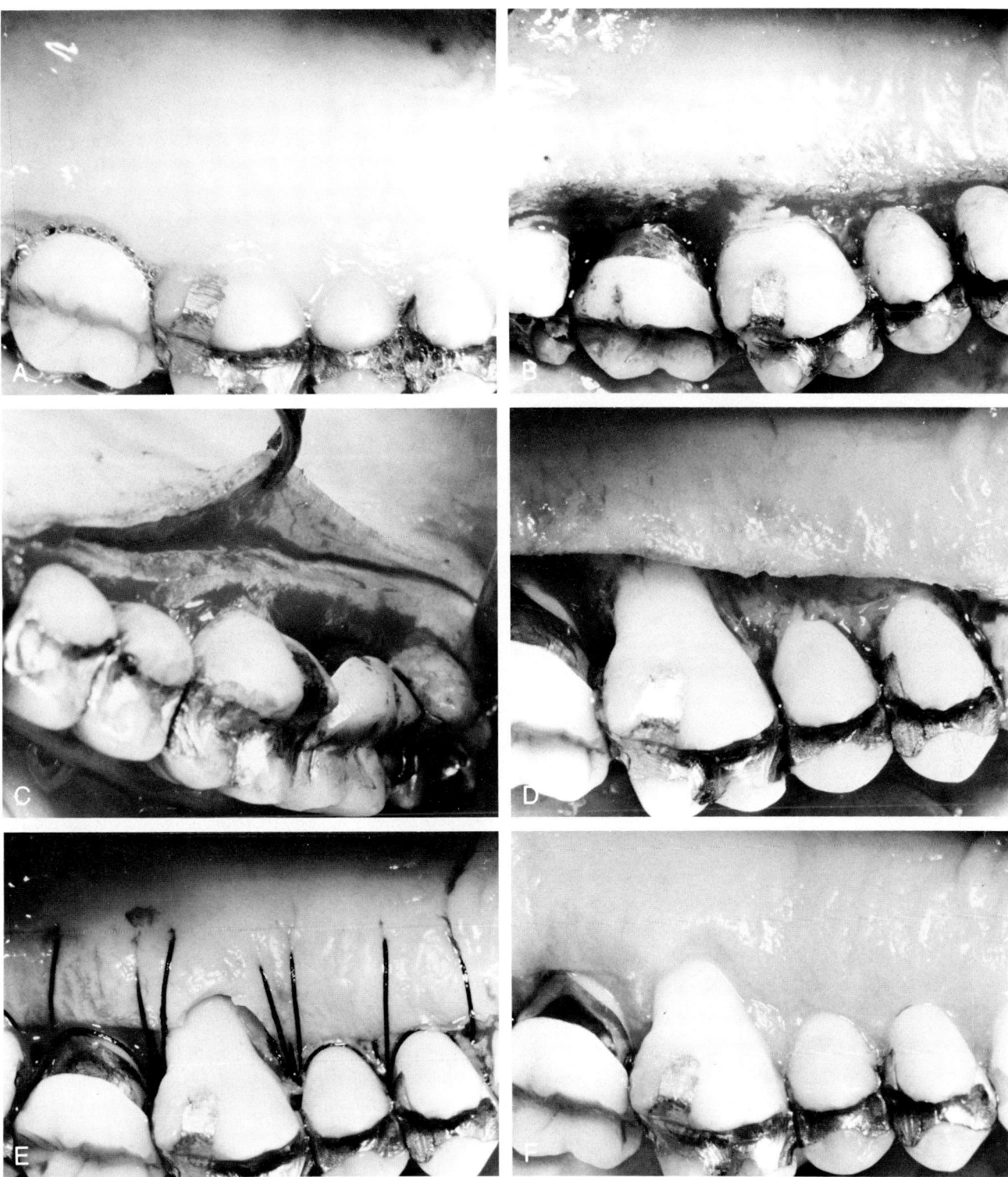

Fig. 6-10. Modified Partial-Thickness Palatal Flap. **A,** Before. **B,** Excised gingivectomy tissue. **C,** Primary partial-thickness flap reflected. **D,** Secondary inner flap removed. **E,** Palatal flap sutured. **F,** Five months later.

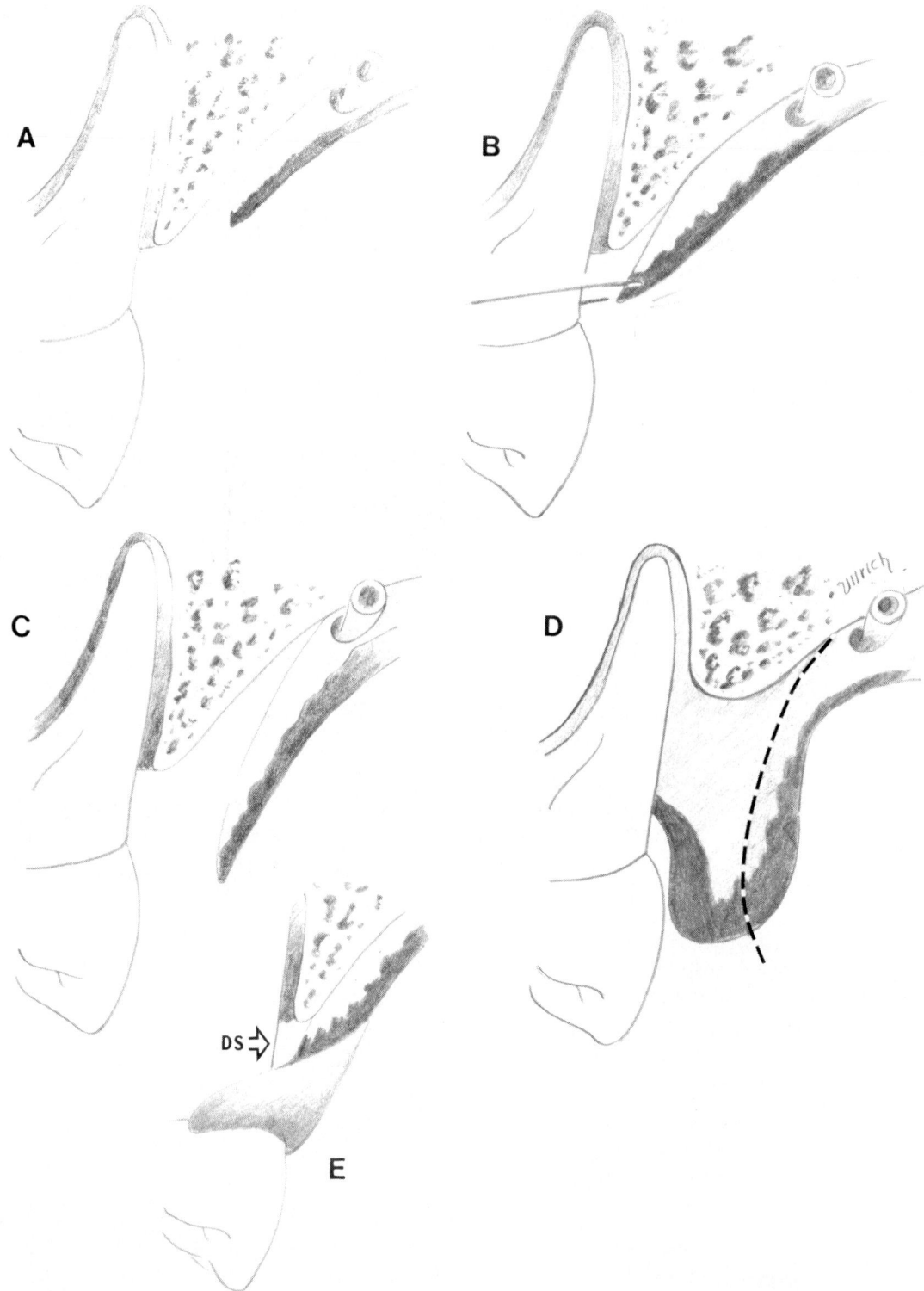

Fig. 6-11. Common Mistakes with Palatal Flaps. **A,** Flap is cut too short. **B,** Inadequate initial thinning of flap prevents proper placement. **C,** Initial thinning incision is too long, increasing chance of damage to palatal artery. **D,** Insufficient care in handling broad, shallow palates increases the chance of damaging the palatal artery. **E,** Inadequate flap design results in flap being placed too high onto teeth with resultant *dead-space* (DS) and pocket re-formation.

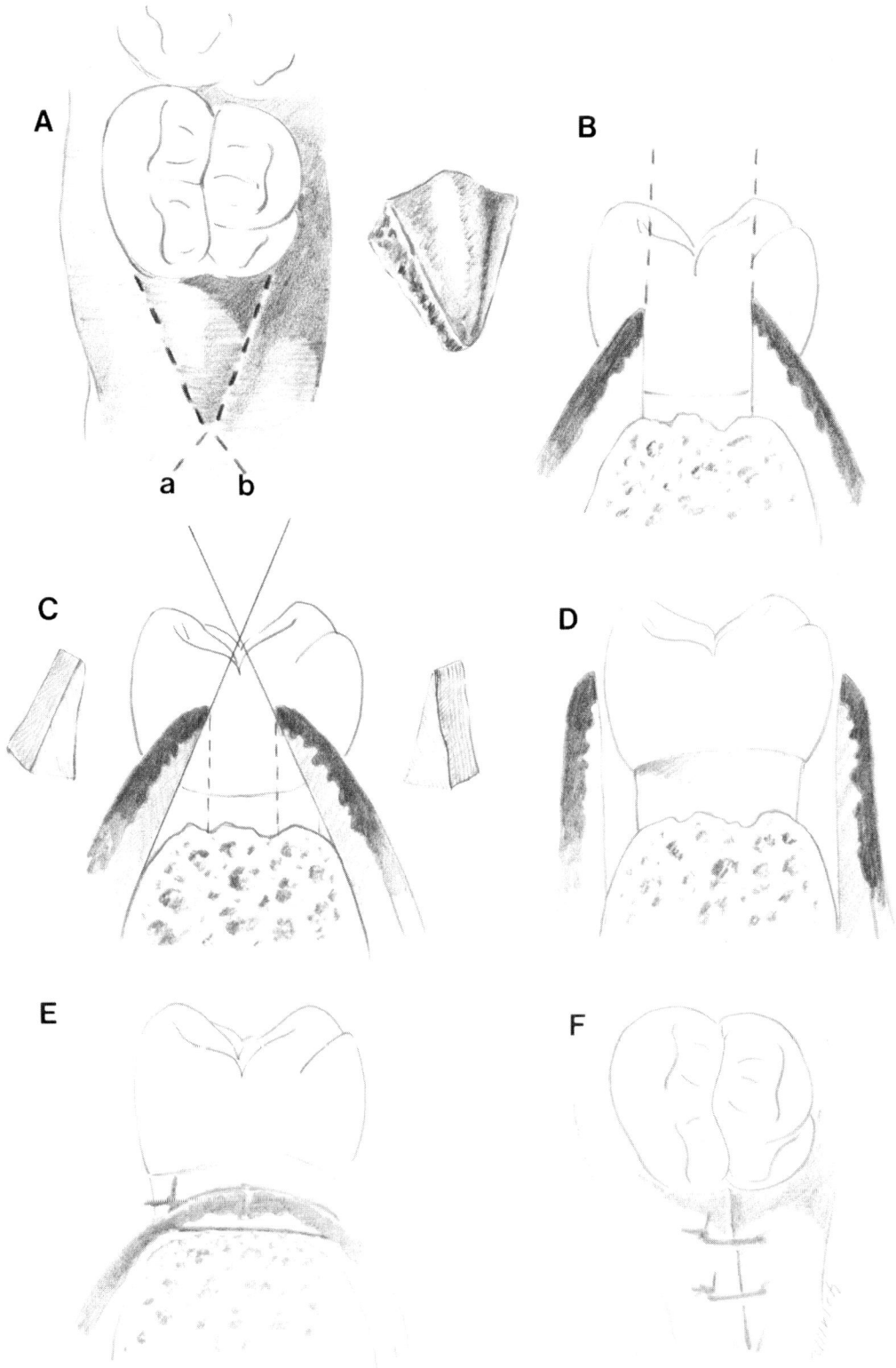

Fig. 6-12. Distal Wedge—Triangular Design. **A,** Outline of triangular incision distal to molar. Note outline of two small releasing incisions (a,b), which can be used if needed. **B,** Cross-sectional view showing wedge removal and thick tissue. **C,** *Undermining incisions* are used to thin the tissue. **D,** Reflection of flaps for osseous correction. **E,F,** Cross-sectional and occlusal views of sutured tissue.

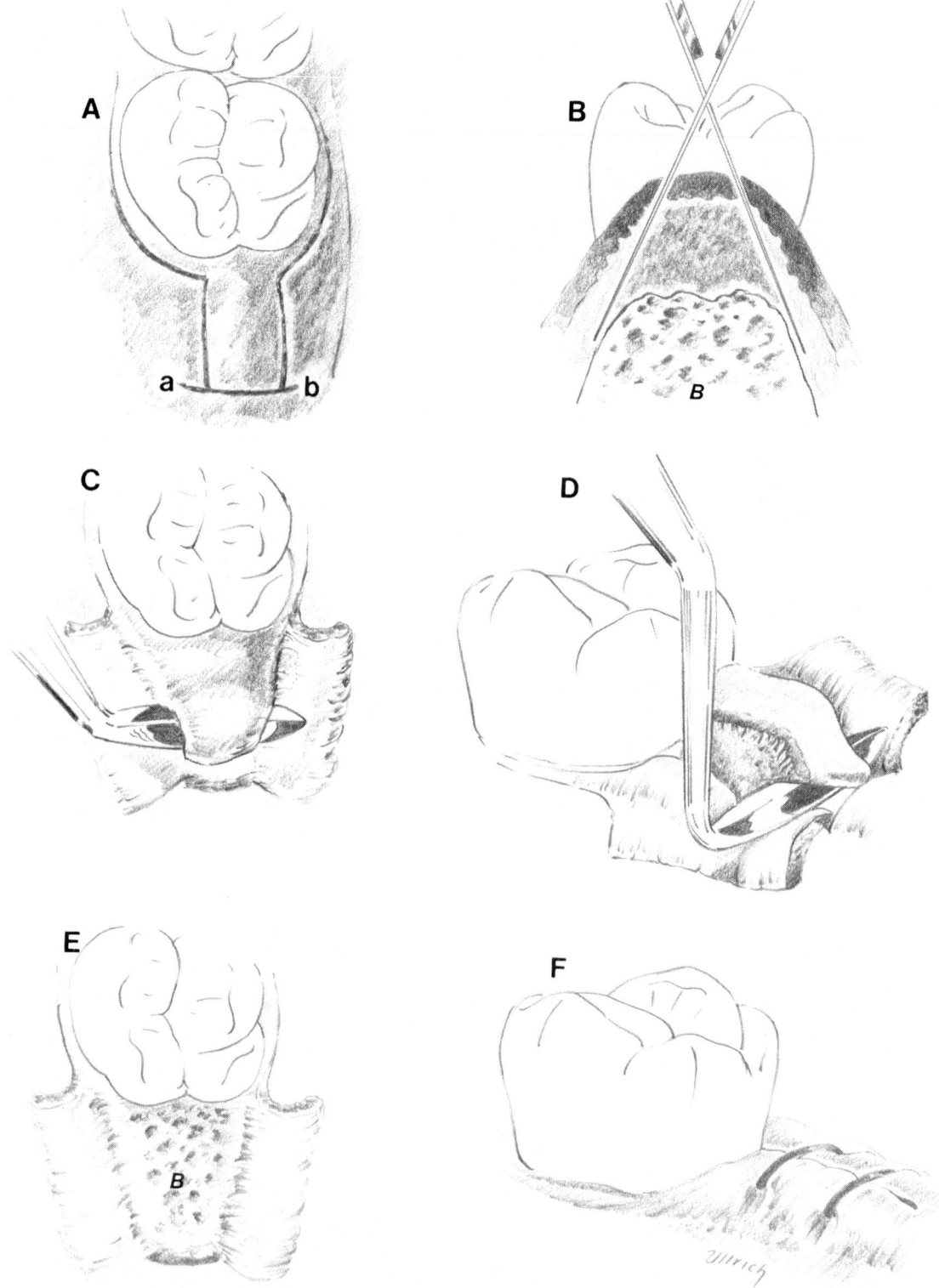

Fig. 6-13. Distal-Wedge—Square, Parallel, or H-Design. **A,** Occlusal view with incisions outlined. Note two parallel incisions over tuberosity joined by distal releasing incision (a,b). **B,** Cross-sectional view shows proper blade angulation in making initial incisions. **C,D,** Flaps reflected and tissue being removed from tuberosity, using a periodontal knife. **E,** Bone exposed for correction of osseous irregularities. **F,** Final suturing.

Palatal Flaps

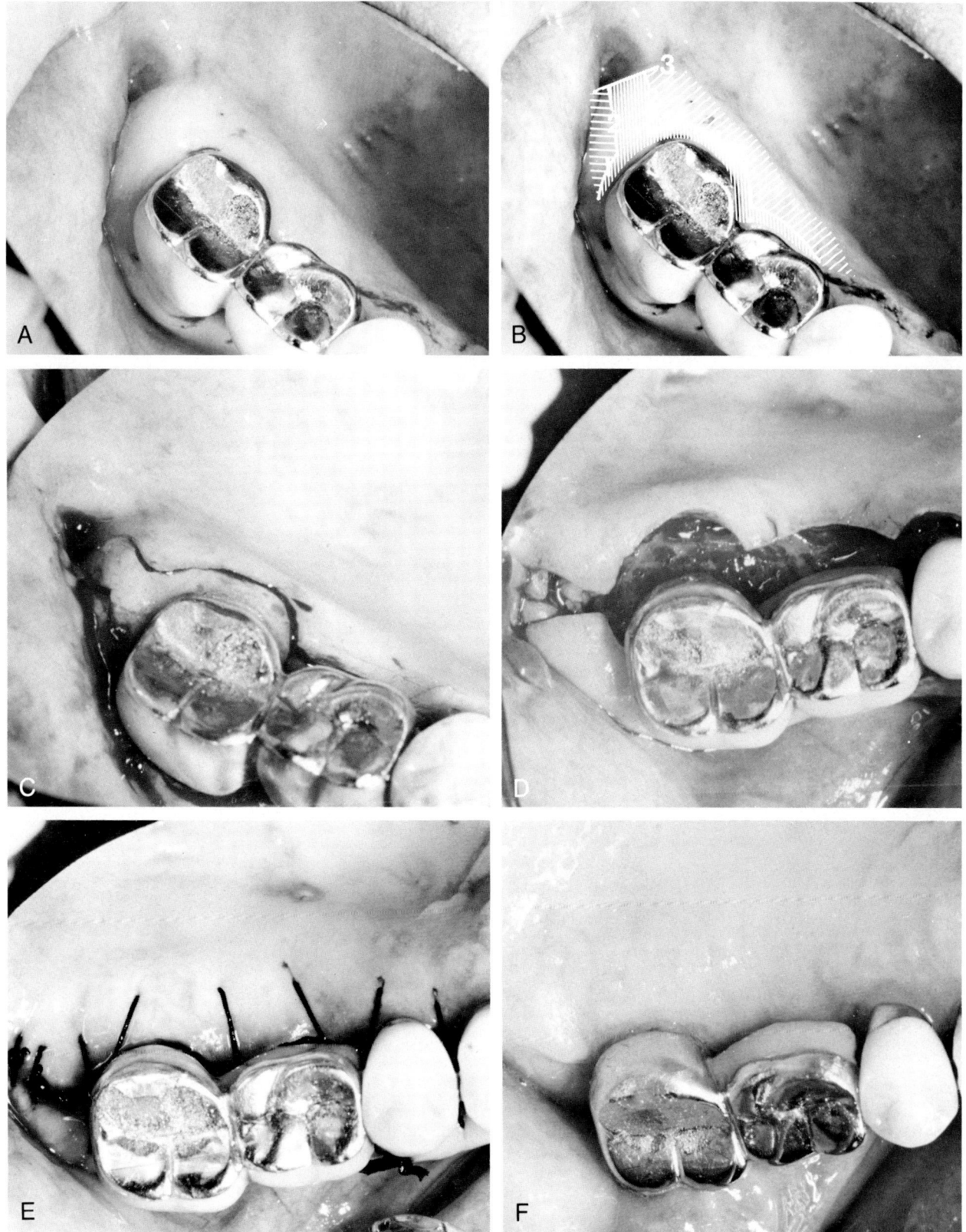

Fig. 6-14. Distal Wedge of Maxillary Tuberosity Area. **A,** Before. **B,** Outline of incisions: 1, scalloped, inverse beveled incision; 2, wedge-shaped parallel incisions; and 3, perpendicular incision at terminal ends of parallel incisions. **C,** Initial incision completed. **D,** Secondary flap removed and flap reflected. **E,** Flaps sutured. **F,** Case completed, 3 months later; compare with A.

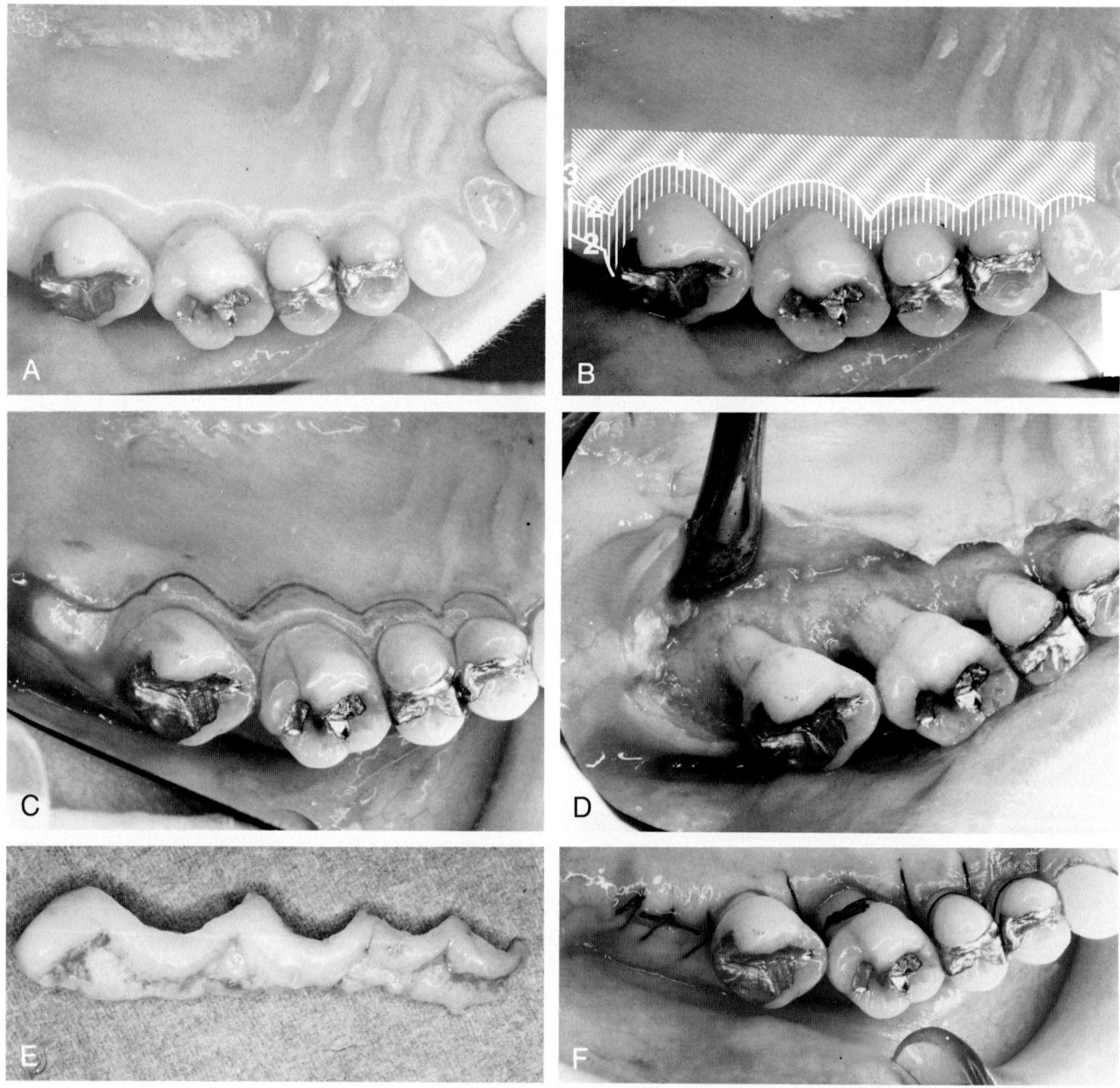

Fig. 6-15. Distal-Wedge and Partial-Thickness Palatal Flap Procedures Combined. **A,** Before. **B,** Incisions outlined: 1, scalloped partial-thickness primary incision; 2, parallel wedge incisions; and 3, perpendicular wedge incision. **C,** Initial incisions completed. **D,** Secondary flaps removed and flaps reflected. **E,** Wedge removed. **F,** Flaps sutured. Note primary closure of distal-wedge areas.

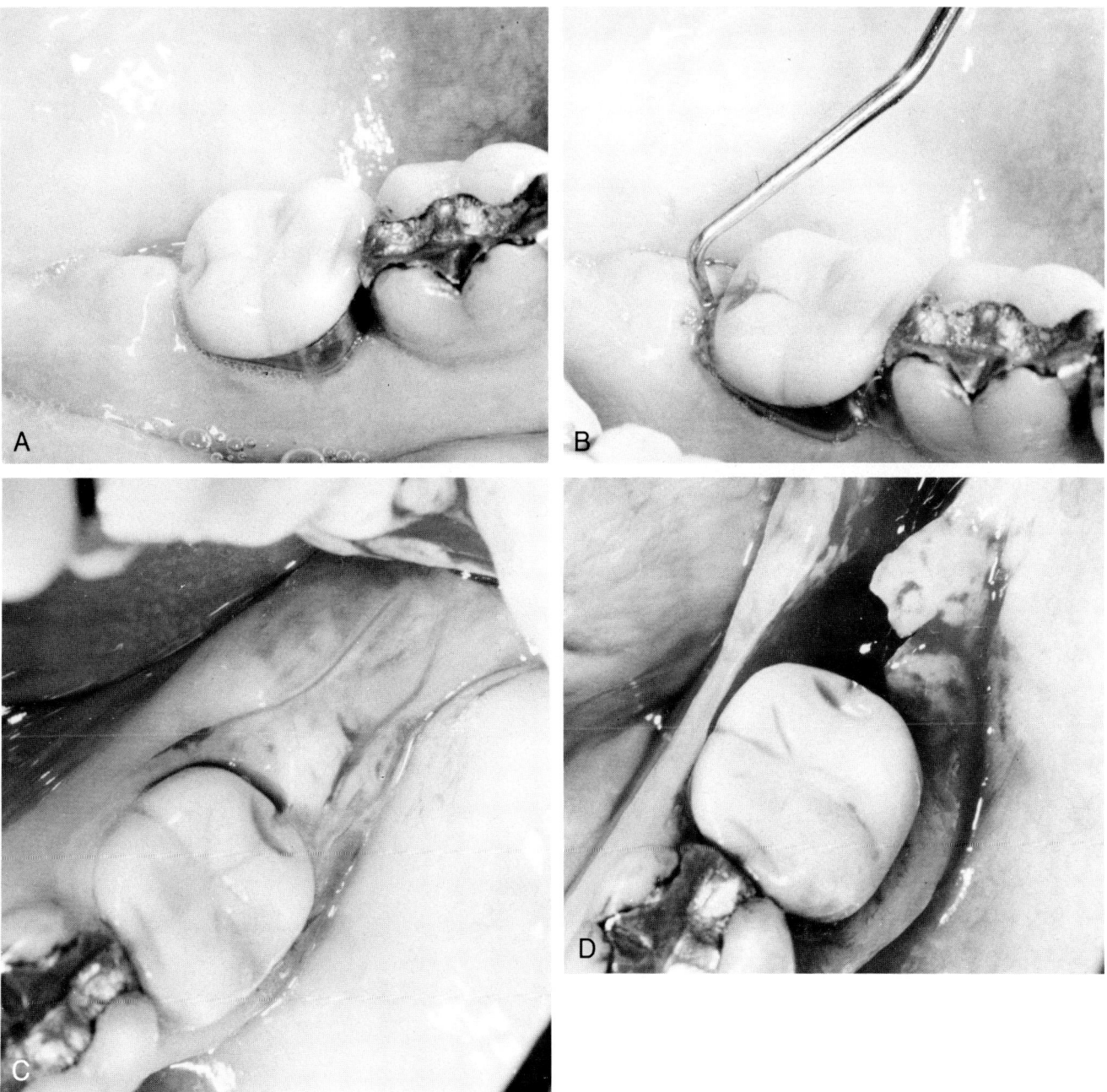

Fig. 6-16. Distal-Wedge of Retromolar Area of Mandible. **A,** Before. **B,** Probe showing 12-mm pocket. **C,** Parallel incisions made and joined distally later with perpendicular incision. **D,** Wedge removed.

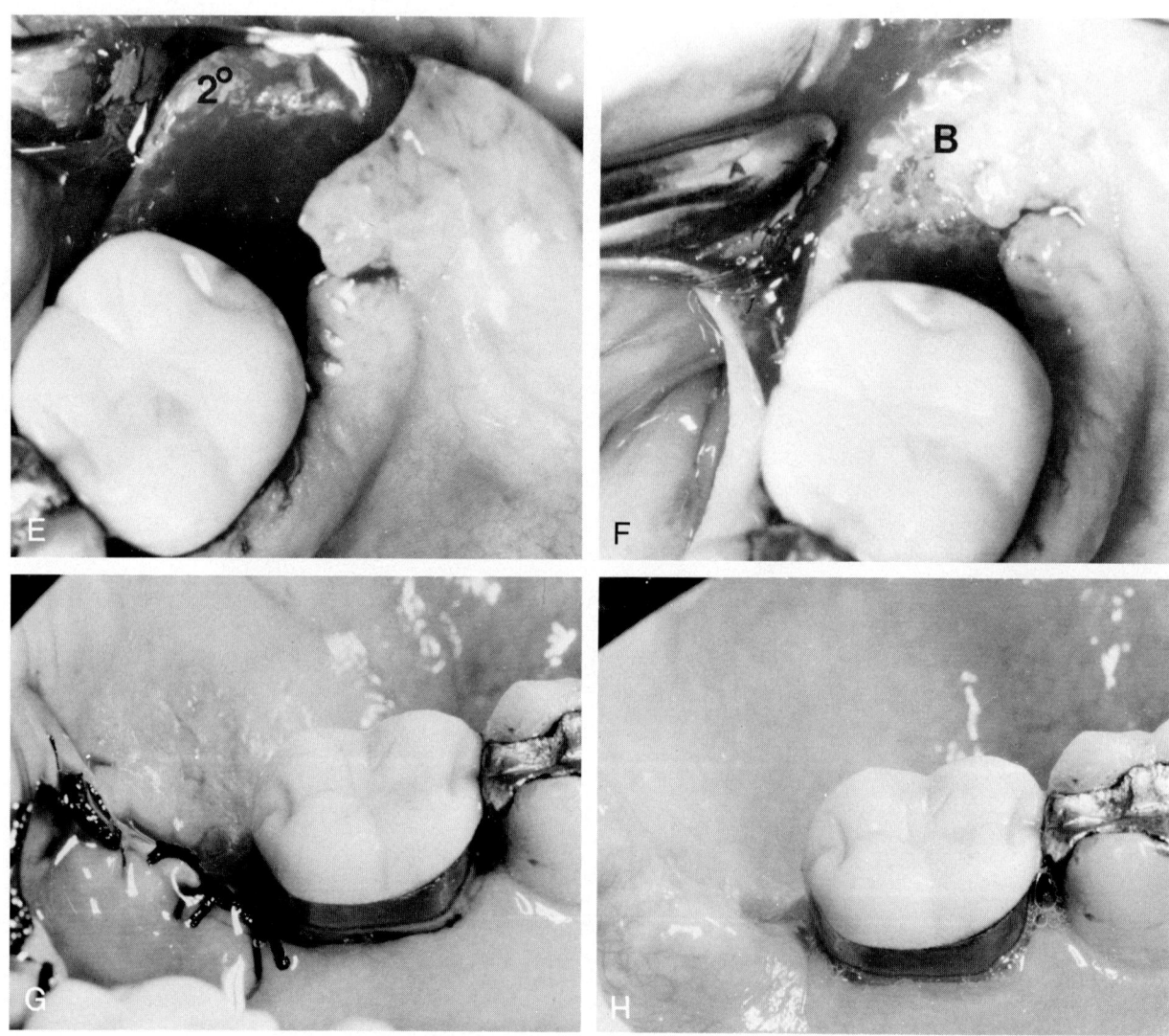

Fig. 6-16 (continued). **E,** Lingual flap thinned by secondary incision (2° flap). **F,** 2° flap removed and bone (B) exposed. **G,** Wedge sutured. **H,** Wedge healed, 3 months later.

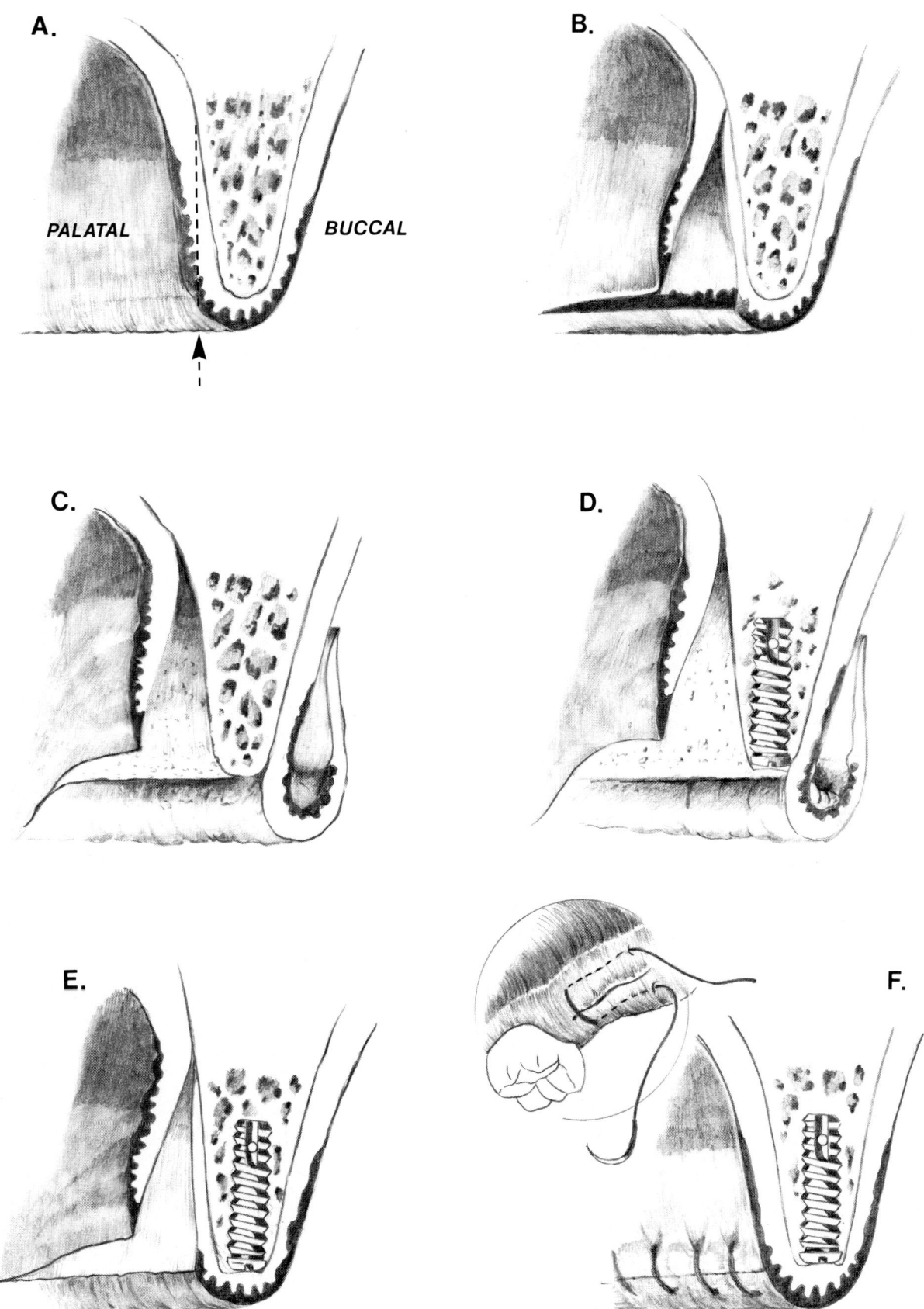

Fig. 6-17. Palatal Approach for Implant Placement. **A,** Cross section of maxillary alveolar ridge with incision outlined on palate. **B,** Partial-thickness palatal flap raised (see Fig. 6-5 for technique). **C,** Inner secondary flap reflected buccally, exposing osseous ridge. **D,** Implant placed. **E,** Secondary inner flap replaced. **F,** Primary and secondary flaps sutured with vertical or horizontal mattress sutures. Note that even if coronal aspects of incision were to open, apical overlap would maintain primary closure.

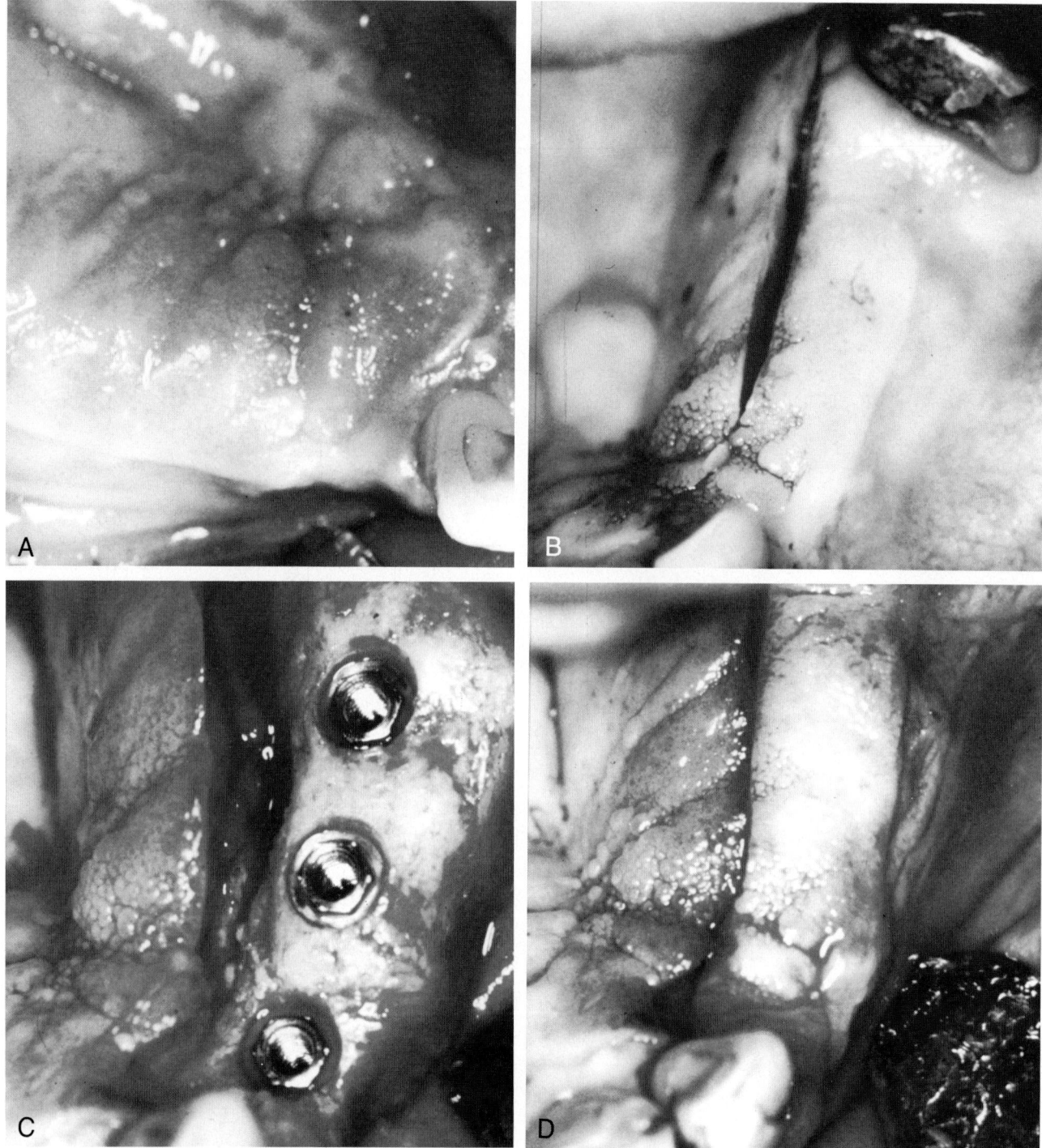

Fig. 6-18. Palatal Approach for Implant placement. **A,** Before surgery. **B,** Partial thickness palatal flap begun; initial incision. **C,** Implant placement completed. **D,** Flap reapproximated—note excellent primary closure.

Palatal Flaps

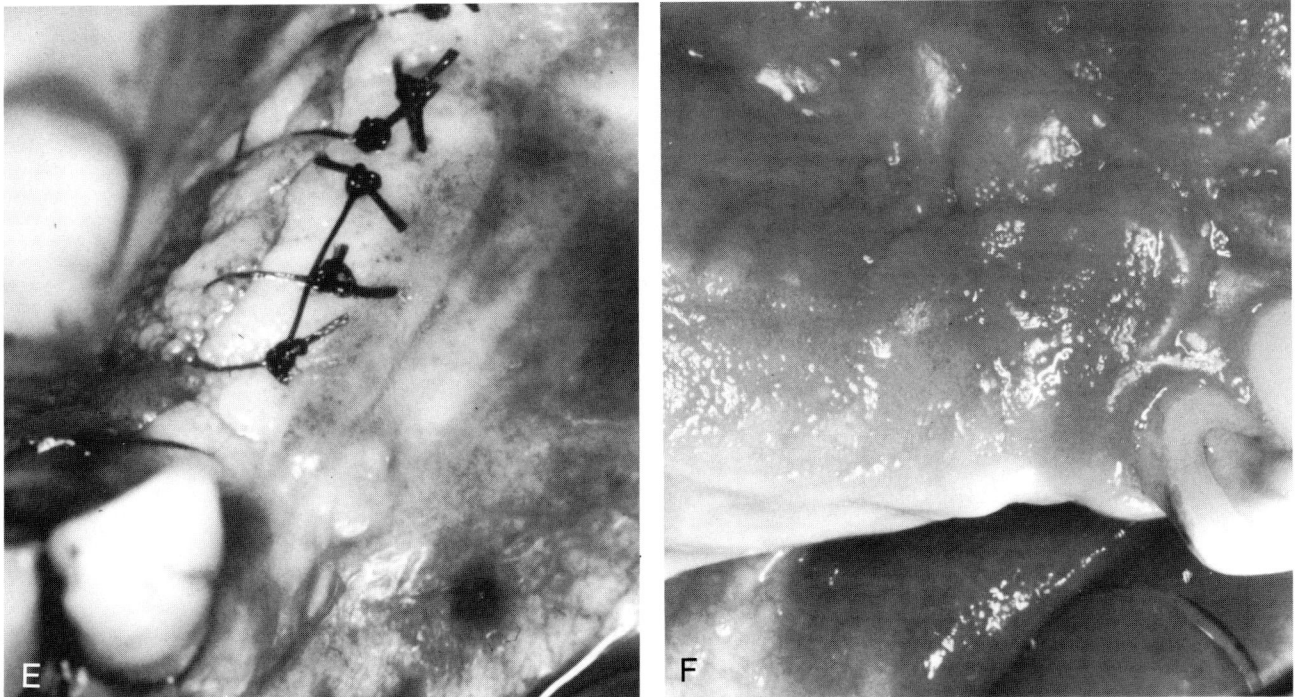

Fig. 6-18 (continued). **E,** Vertical mattress sutures for closure. **F,** Three months later.

7

COSMETIC TREATMENT OF MAXILLARY ANTERIOR POCKETING

MODIFIED SURGICAL APPROACH FOR MAXILLARY ANTERIOR ESTHETICS: THE CURTAIN PROCEDURE

One of the most distressing aspects of periodontal surgery is the unesthetic maxillary anterior results obtained after definitive surgical pocket elimination therapy. The elongation of the crowns with greater root exposure and increase in interproximal spacing results in a totally unacceptable *picket fence* appearance with varying degrees of speech difficulty.

In 1967, Frisch et al. developed a surgical technique that permitted conservation of the maxillary anterior esthetics. This modified surgical approach, or *curtain procedure*, which is somewhat similar to Kirkland's (1931, 1936) *semiflap technique* and *modified flap technique*, attempts to satisfy the esthetic and phonetic considerations of surgical procedures in this area.

This technique attempts to preserve all labial attached gingiva, even the labial third of the interproximal papillae. It was based on their finding that, even in the presence of interproximal disease, a healthy midlabial sulcus could exist with healthy labial tissue. Lie (1992) recently described the advantages and methodology of this procedure; he termed it the *modified resective (MR) technique*.

Advantages

1. Conservative
2. Esthetically acceptable
3. Technically simple and easy to do
4. Maintains phonetics, with normal speech

Disadvantages

1. Some labial shrinkage is unavoidable
2. Oral physiotherapy is more difficult because of tissue craters

Criteria for Treatment

Frisch et al. list several preoperative conditions, of which the most important is that the gingival tissue appears to be clinically healthy (firm, pink, and stippled) with a midlabial sulcus depth equal to or less than 4 mm, even when deep interproximal pockets are present.

This technique appears to satisfy all necessary criteria for treating the maxillary anterior teeth if esthetics are a problem. Long-term success is achieved by ease of access and maintainability of the area for oral hygiene. The round roots allow effective flossing, and palatal access to the longer roots is easy.

Procedure

1. Figure 7-1A displays the common finding of clinically healthy gingival tissue with significant underlying osseous destruction. This problem is further compounded by a high smile line.
2. Figure 7-1B shows the basic outline of the incision. The incisions are designed for maximum conservation of the facial gingiva and at least one-third of each of the labial papillae. Palatally, either a beveled gingivectomy or par-

tial-thickness palatal flap procedure can be performed.
3. The initial incisions are made with either a No. 11 or No. 15 scalpel blade. The blade is directed interproximally at right angles to the teeth from both the mesial and distal directions (Fig. 7-1C). This intersecting incision separates the labial one-third of the papilla, which combined with the labial tissue forms the **tissue curtain.** No further labial surgery is required.
4. Palatally, the objectives and need for osseous surgery determine whether a gingivectomy or flap procedure is used (Fig. 7-1D). Even though gingivectomy is faster and simpler, if the bony craters can be ramped palatally, plaque control will be facilitated.
5. Figure 7-1E and F shows the final suturing, which can be either interrupted or continuous.

In Figure 7-2 we see the same procedure except that a palatal flap was raised for treatment of underlying osseous depravities. In this technique the buccal two-thirds of the interproximal papillae is still retained to prevent shrinkage, and there is *no need* to release or reflect the papilla from the buccal surface.

The clinical examples that follow (Figs. 7-3 and 7-4) show the favorable results that can be achieved with this technique. Note carefully the minimal amount of labial recession even though significant recession occurs palatally.

PAPILLARY PRESERVATION TECHNIQUE

Takei et al. (1985, 1988, 1991) devised a surgical procedure to prevent partial or complete exfoliation of graft material by providing primary coverage of the entire interproximal defect. The authors acknowledge that it is a modification of a procedure originally described by Genon and Bender (1984) for esthetic treatment of the maxillary anteriors.

Indications

Embrasures wide enough to permit passage of the interproximal tissue.

Advantages

1. Esthetically pleasing
2. Primary coverage of implant material
3. Prevention of postoperational tissue craters

Disadvantages

1. Technically difficult
2. Time consuming

Contraindications

Narrow embrassures

Procedure

1. Buccally, interproximally, and palatally/lingually, the flaps are relieved with intrasulcular incisions, keeping the blade adjacent to the tooth.
2. Vertical incisions are made palatally/lingually adjacent to the papillae that are to be moved. The vertical incisions are extended far enough apically so that they will be *at least 3 mm apical to the margin of the interproximal bony defect and 5 mm from the gingival margin* (Fig. 7-5A,B).
3. The vertical incisions are joined by a horizontal incision, which can be made with a Kirkland knife (Fig. 7-5B).
4. For flap reflection, a curette or interproximal knife is used to free the interdental tissue from the underlying tissue. ***Note: The papilla must be completely mobile prior to reflection*** (Fig. 7-5C).
5. With a ***blunt*** instrument the papilla is carefully pushed through the embrasure, and excessive granulation is removed from the underside with a sharp scissors or curette. Overthinning is to be avoided (Fig. 7-5D).
6. Both flap and papilla are reflected off the bone with a periosteal elevator (Fig. 7-5E).
7. Once the defect area is debrided and filled, the flaps are repositioned and the papilla pushed back through the embrasure and sutured with either interrupted or horizontal mattress sutures (Fig. 7-5F).

The clinical procedure is seen in Figures 7-6 and 7-7.

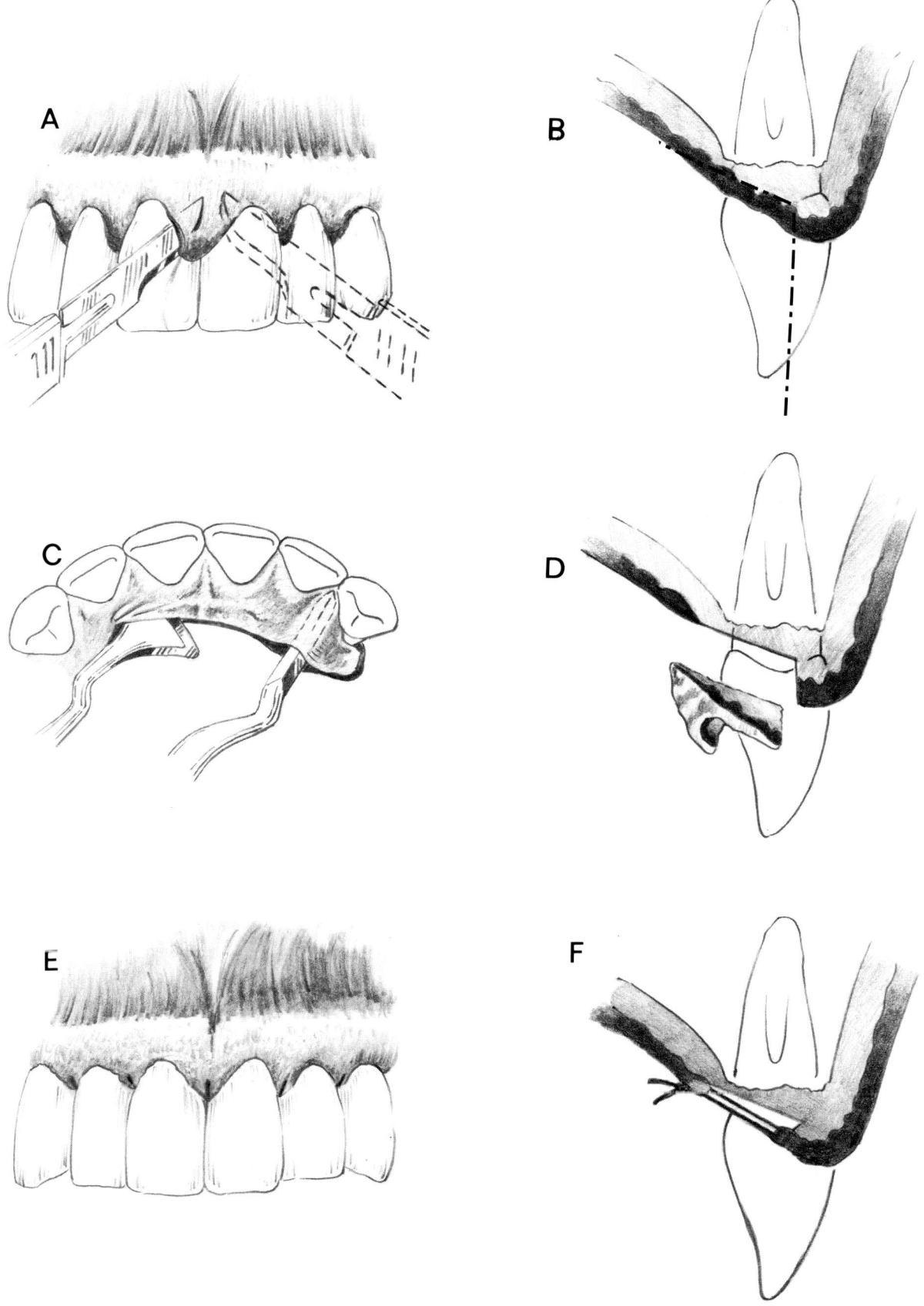

Fig. 7-1. Curtain Procedure. **A,B,** Before surgery. **C,D,** Palatal gingivectomy with side view showing removal of tissue. **E,F,** Buccal and side views showing suturing with no esthetic compromise. *Note:* If palatal bone exposure is shown in Figures 7-2 and 7-5.

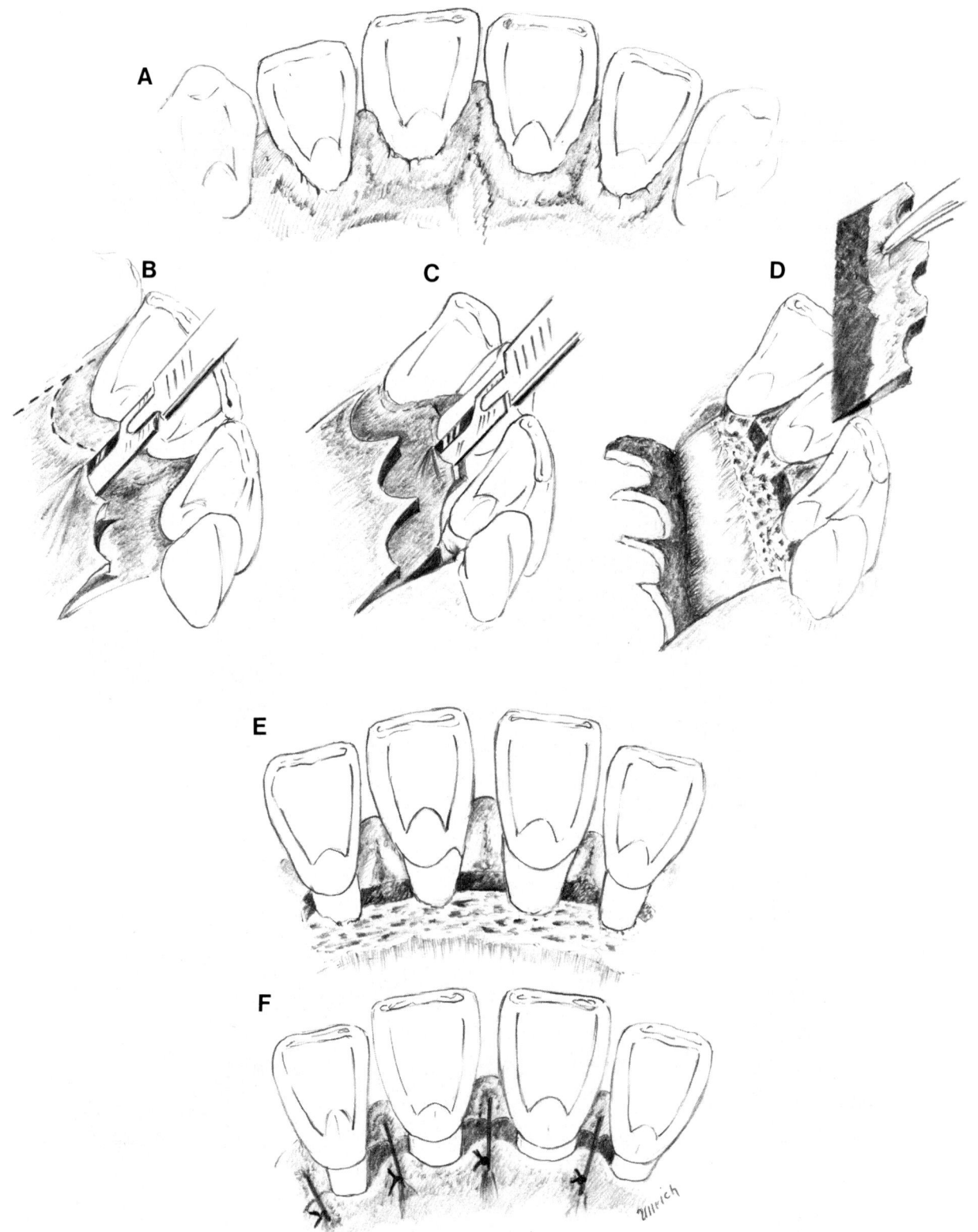

Fig. 7-2. Curtain Procedure Combined with Palatal Flap. **A,** Palatal view of anterior teeth with deep interproximal pockets. **B,** Scalloped palatal partial-thickness flap (see Chapter 6 for technique). **C,** Secondary inner flap is released with palatal sulcular incisions and extended interproximally from the palatal side only one-third of the distance interproximally. ***Note: No buccal release is required.*** **D,** The inner flap is reflected and removed. **E,** Scaling, root planing, and corrective osseous surgery are performed (inductive or receptive). **F,** Flaps are positioned and sutured.

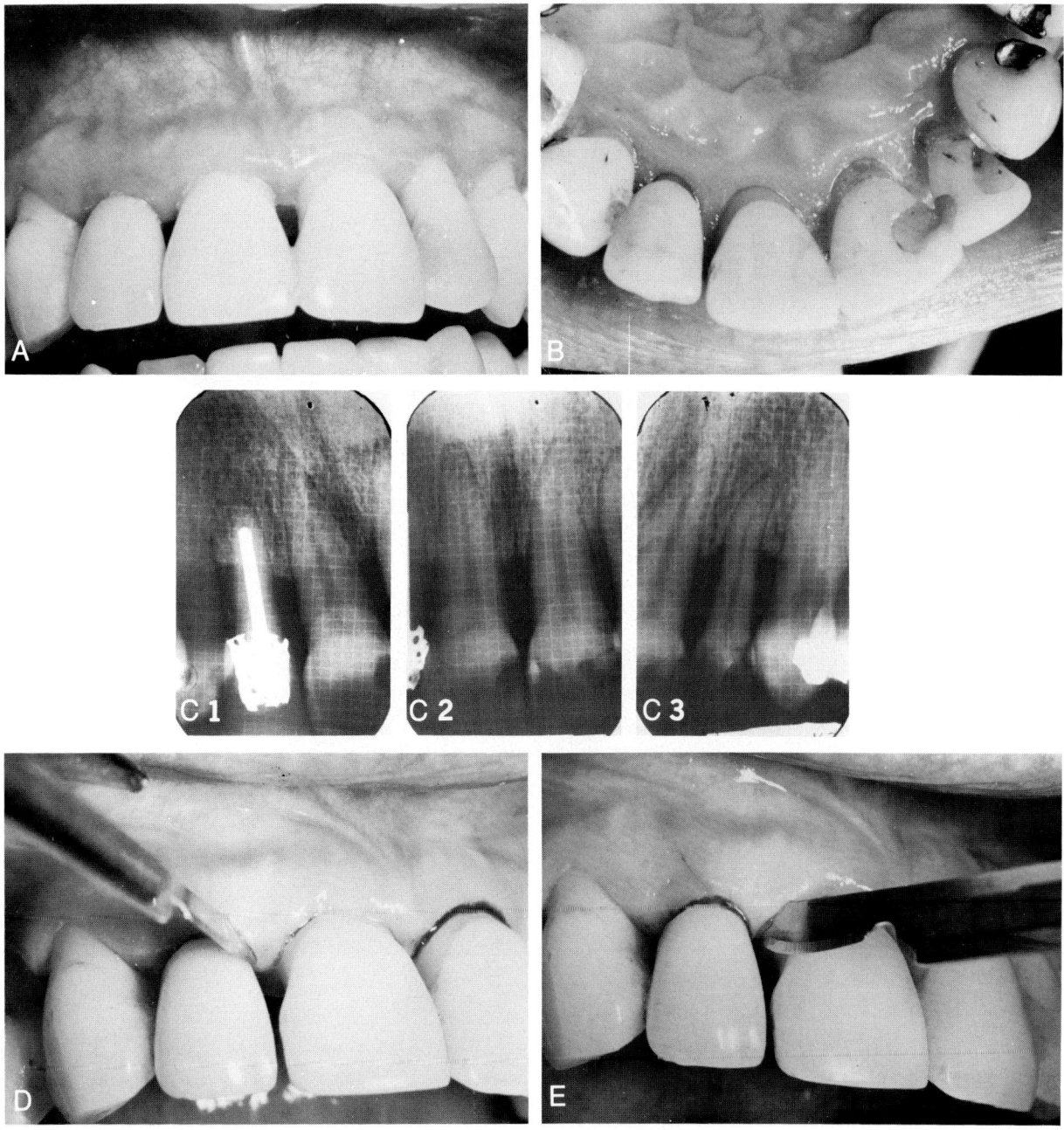

Fig. 7-3. Curtain Procedure. **A,B,** Before; buccal and palatal views. **C,** Preoperative x-ray studies show moderate bone loss. **D,E,** Sulcular interdental incisions maximize the buccal two-thirds of the papillae.

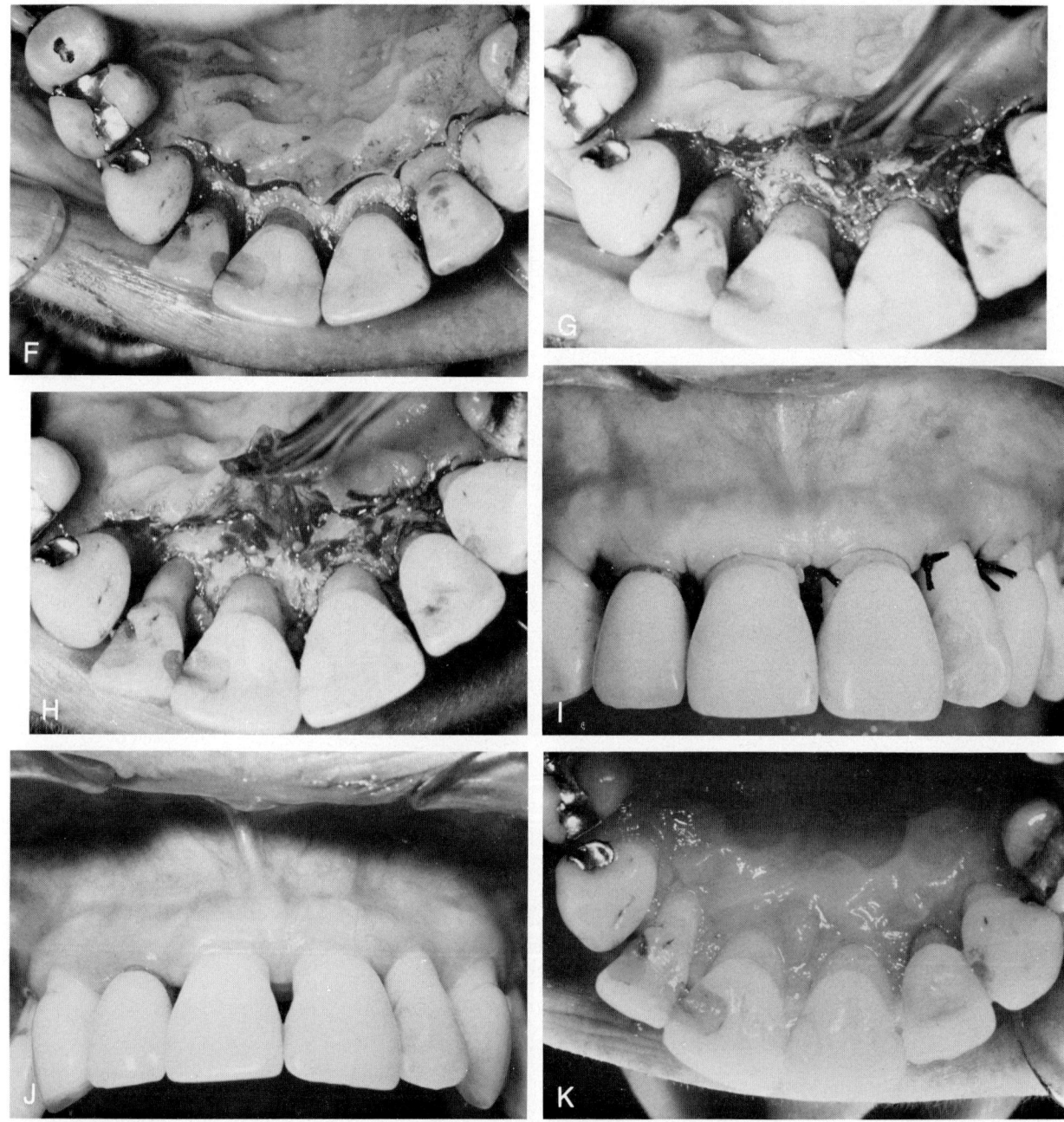

Fig. 7-3 (continued). **F,** Scalloped palatal incision for flap preparation. **G,** Flap reflected and secondary inner flap removed. **H,** Osseous surgery completed. **I,** Flaps sutured with interrupted sutures. **J, K,** After 4 months. Note minimal reduction of buccal tissue and esthetic result.

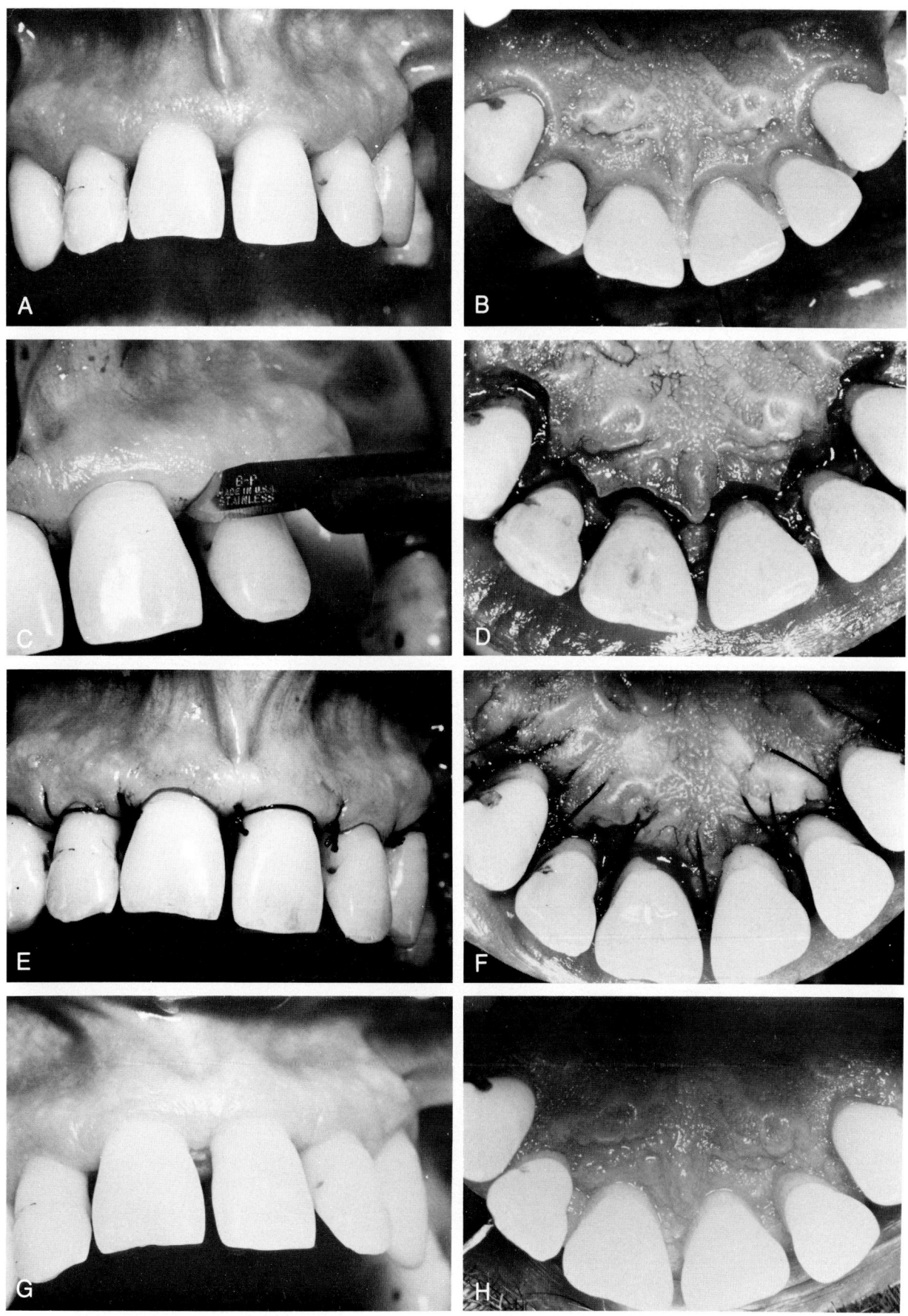

Fig. 7-4. Curtain Procedure. **A,B,** Before; buccal and palatal views. **C,** Sulcular interdental incisions maximizing the buccal two-thirds of the papillae. **D,** Palatal flap completed. **E,F,** Buccal and palatal flaps sutured. **G,H,** Completed case, 5 months later.

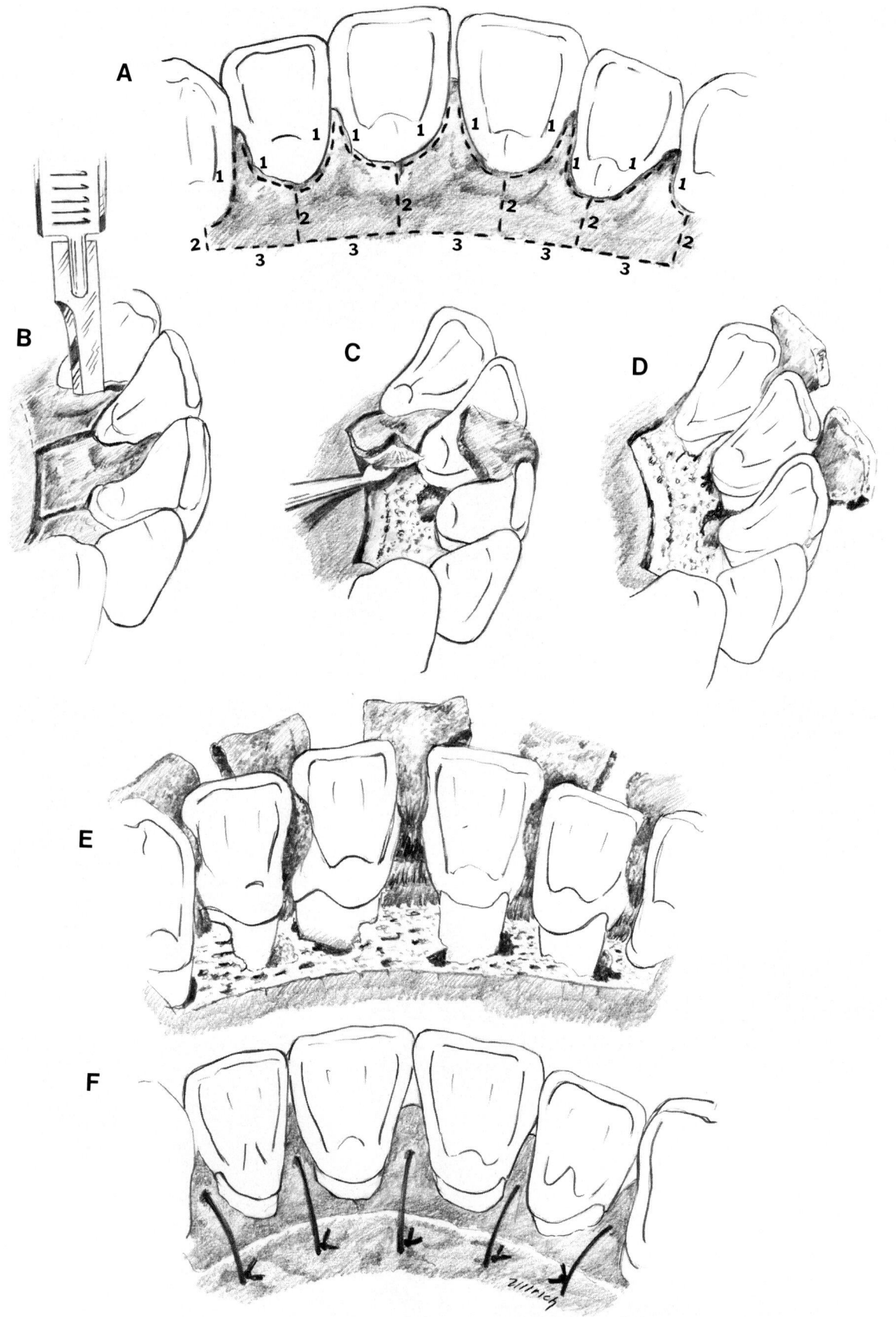

Fig. 7-5. Papillary Preservation Technique. **A,** Palatal view with incisions outlined. **B,** Completion of palatal incisions. **C,** A periosteal elevator is used to reflect individual papillary flabs. **D,** A blunt instrument used to push tissue buccally, exposing underlying osseous deformities and subgingival root deposits. **E,** Defects debrided and root scaled and root planed. **F,** Flaps sutured palatally. Suturing should avoid papillary compression, which may result in loss of interproximal tissue height.

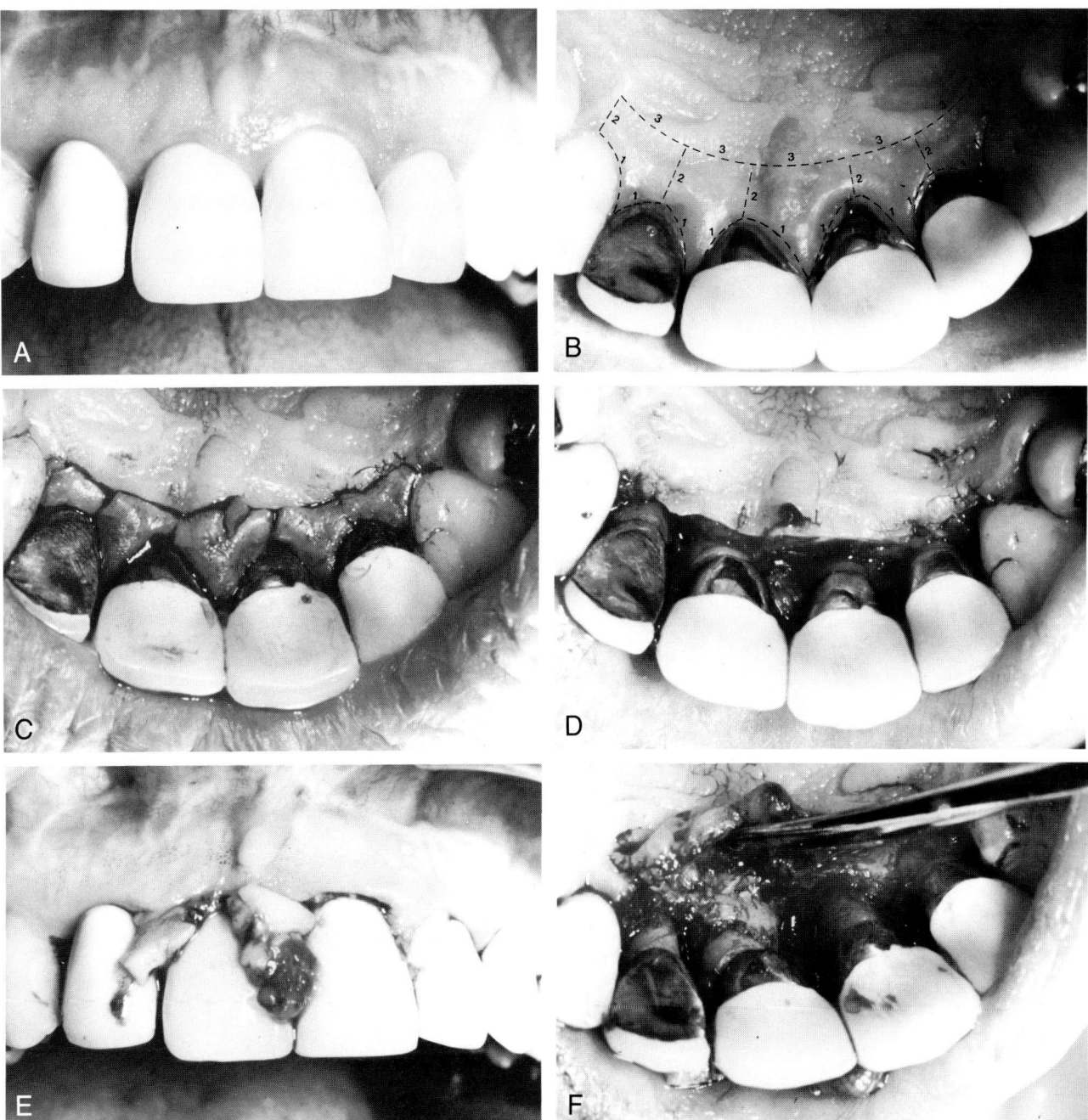

Fig. 7-6. Papillary Preservation Technique. **A,B,** Buccal and palatal views with incisions outlined before treatment. **C,** Initial horizontal and vertical incisions completed. Note vertical and horizontal incisions to facilitate flap elevation. **D,** Flap reflected buccally. **E,** Buccal view with papillary flaps reflected buccally. **F,** Palatal flap reflected prior to scaling.

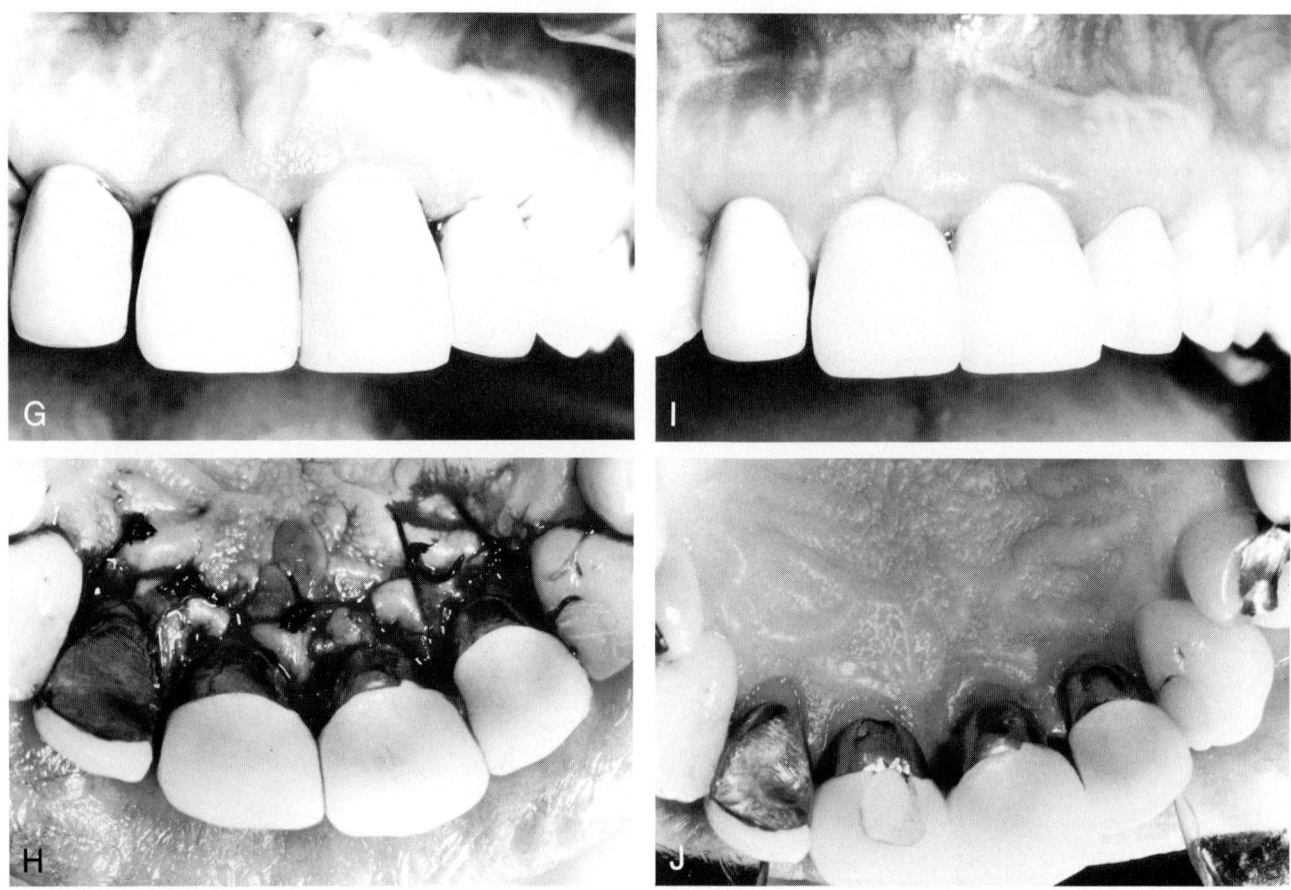

Fig. 7-6 (continued). G,H, Buccal and palatal views of flaps sutured. Note minimum conservation of interproximal tissue. Compare to A. **I,J,** Eight months later; buccal and palatal views. Note excellent cosmetics even though palate shows considerable recession. Compare to A and B.

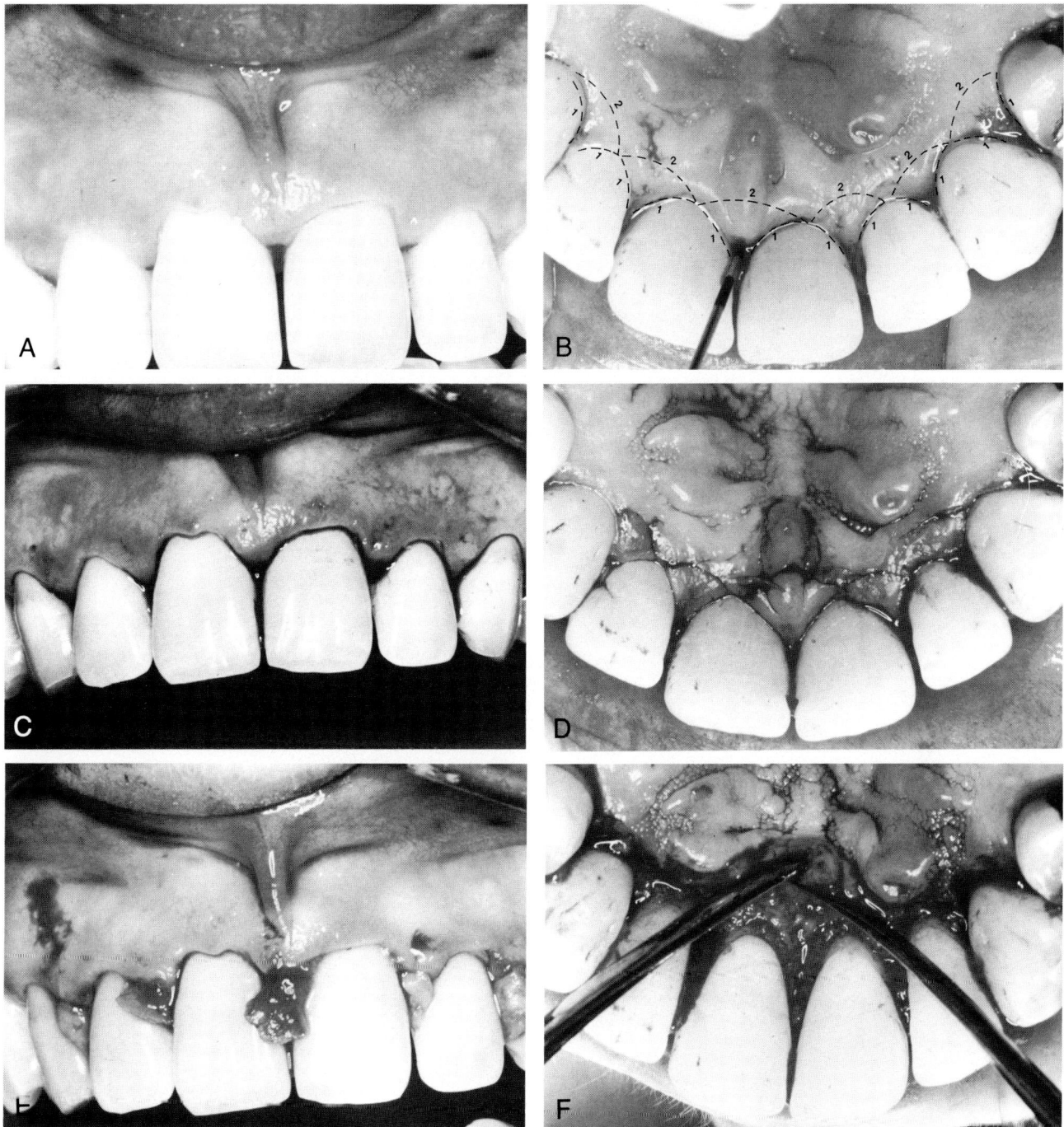

Fig. 7-7. Papillary Preservation Technique. **A,B,** Before treatment; buccal and palatal view with incisions outlined. **C,D,** Buccal and palatal views at time of initial incisions. Note primary gingivectomy incisions. **E,** Palatal papillary flap reflected buccally. **F,** Palatal flap reflected.

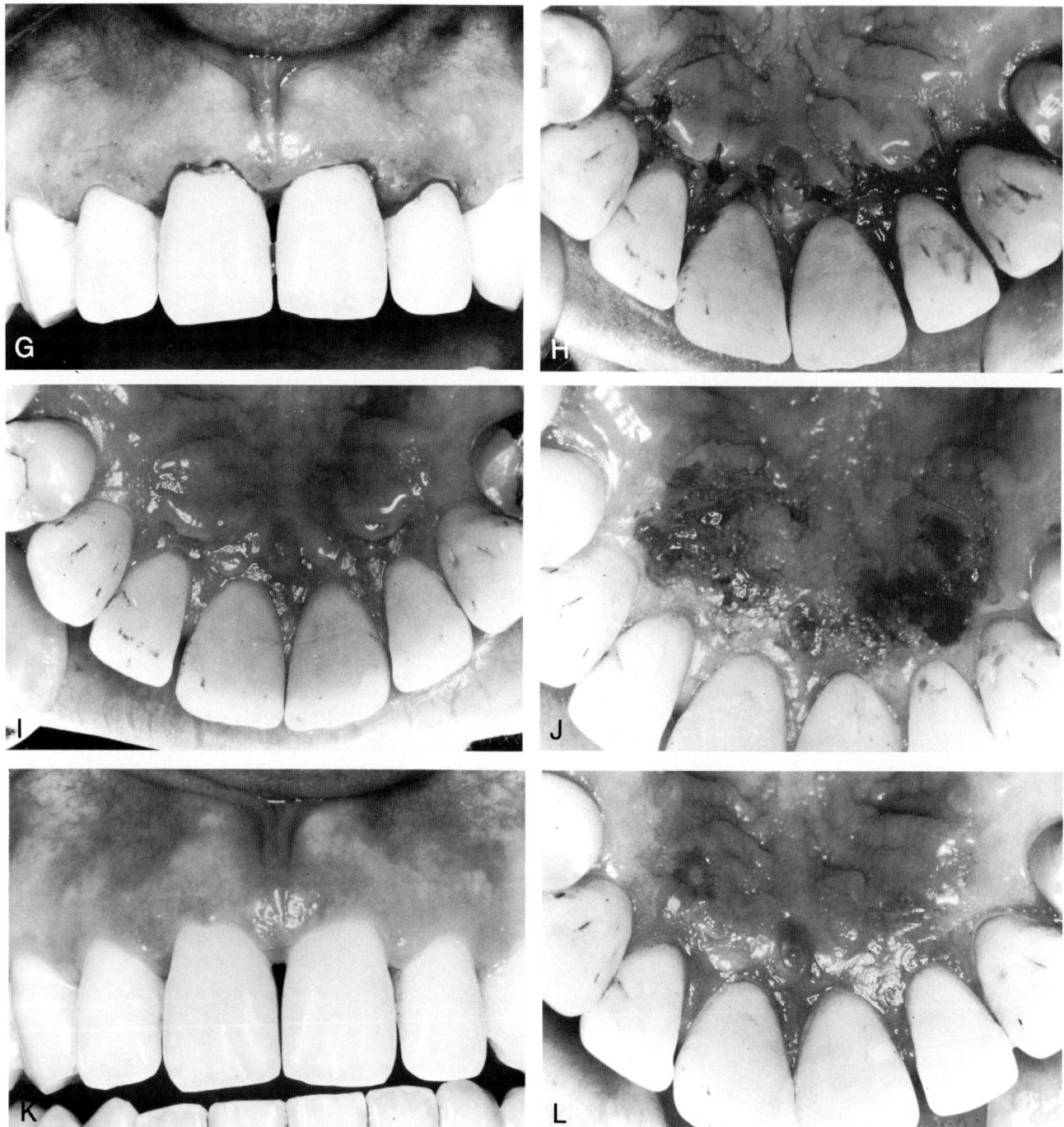

Fig. 7-7 (continued). **G,H,** Buccal and palatal views at time of suturing. **I,** Two months later; palatal view. Note uneven gingival margin. **J,** Gingivoplasty for tissue removal of uneven tissue. **K,** Three months later; excellent cosmetic result. **L,** One month after gingivoplasty.

8

BIOMECHANICAL ROOT PREPARATION

Periodontal disease, although multifactorial, has been shown to have bacteria, in the form of plaque, as its primary etiologic agent (Loe et al., 1965; Theilade et al., 1966). Bacteria initiate disease in many ways, one of which is by the production of endotoxin (Mergenhausen, et al., 1966; Simon, et al., 1970, 1971; Synderman, 1972). These endotoxins (complex lipopolysaccharides) have potent inflammatory agents as part of their cell walls and can be found in the cementum of teeth with untreated periodontal disease (Aleo, et al., 1974). This cementum-bound endotoxin has been shown to prevent the in vitro growth of fibroblasts (Aleo, et al., 1975; Fine et al., 1980) and to be cytotoxic (Hatfield and Bauhammers, 1971); and while it has been shown that in vitro mechanical removal of cementum is possible and does permit new growth of cells (Aleo, et al., 1975; Cogen, et al., 1983, 1984), it has also been shown that in vivo total removal of cementum is not possible (O'Leary and Kafrany, 1983; Borghetti, et al., 1987) and that trace amounts of endotoxin are left behind (Jones and O'Leary, 1978).

If the ultimate goal of periodontal therapy is restoration of lost support through complete regeneration or new attachment, then the root must be cleaned of the cementum-bound endotoxins, which are cytotoxic (Wirthlin, 1981) and which prevent regeneration or new attachment (Lopez, et al., 1980; Karring, et al., 1980). For this reason topical chemotherapeutic agents have been used for both detoxification and enhancement of new attachment in cosmetic gingival reconstruction (Miller, 1985B) and bone augmentation procedures (Yukna, 1980, 1990). *It is also an attempt to overcome the most significant limiting factor to new attachment, which is the rapid rate of epithelial proliferation down along the root* (Fig. 8-1).

Historically, the use of acids in lieu of scaling and root planing was first reported in the New York Dental Record in 1846 and later by Younger (1893, 1897) and Stewart (1899). These early clinicians sought to stimulate inductive activity on diseased root surfaces. Some of them reported attachment and bone induction to the demineralized root surfaces (Register, 1973).

CITRIC ACID

Register (1973, 1975, 1976), following in the footsteps of the early practitioners, based his rationale on present-day bone induction research (Urist, 1971; Yeomans and Urist, 1967; Bang et al., 1967; Dubuc, 1967), which demonstrated the formation of new bone or cementum on partially or totally acid demineralized allogenic bone or dentine matrix. He (Register and Burdick, 1975) showed that demineralization of the root surface produced cementogenesis and new attachment and that citric acid (CA) (pH 1.0) was the acid of choice with an optimal application time of 2 to 3 minutes. Sterratt et al. (1991) recently found the optimum pH to be 1.42, beyond which less demineralization took place.

Garrett (1978), using scanning electron microscopes (SEM) and transmission electron microscopes (TEM), demonstrated that CA, while having no effect on an unplaned root surface, did produce a 3- to 5-mm zone of demineralization on a planed root surface. He postulated that the failure was due to *hypermineralization* of the diseased root surface. Polson et al. (1984) further demonstrated by SEM that

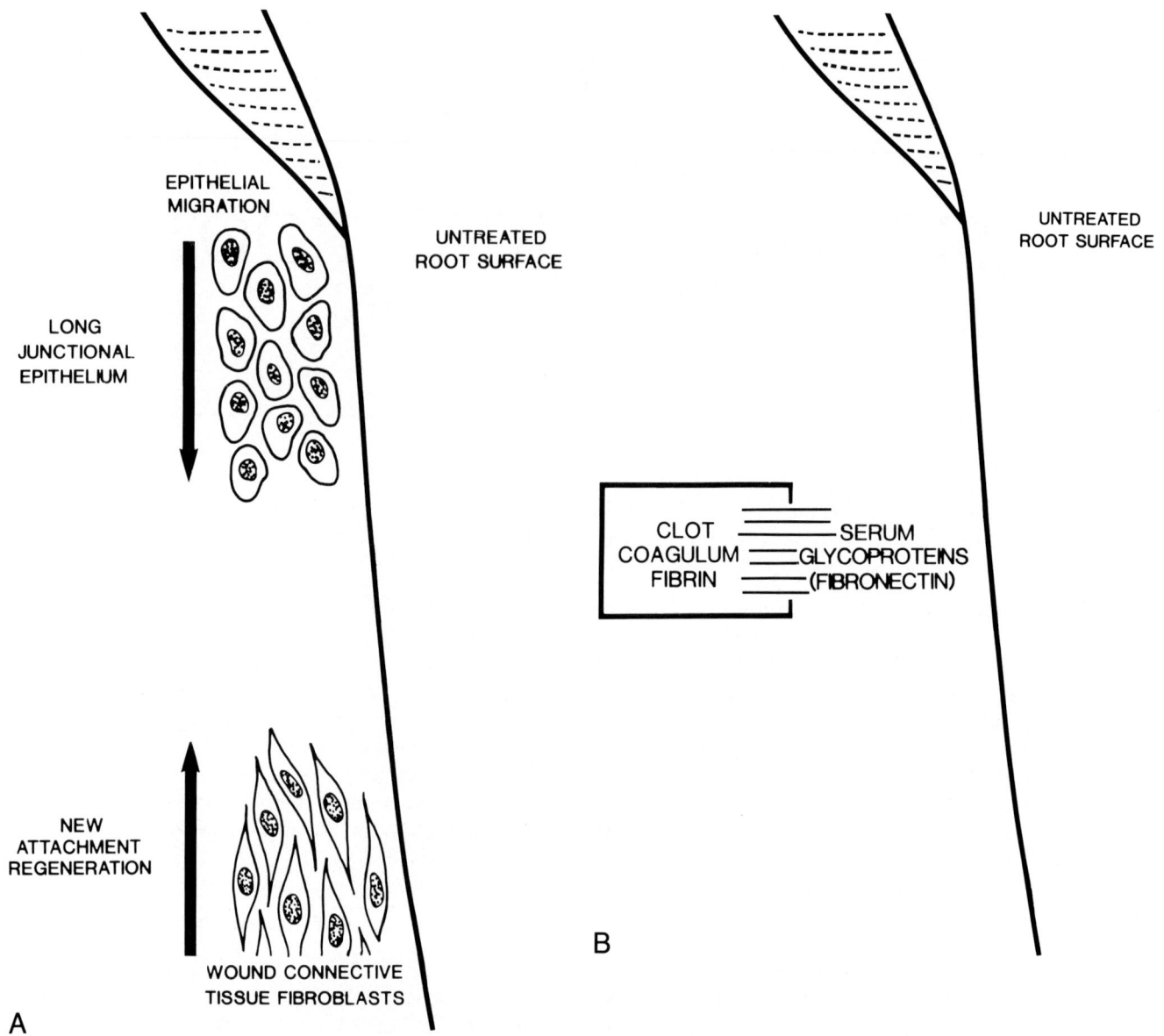

Fig. 8-1. Initial Healing—Cellular Response. **A,** Cellular phenotype determines nature of attachments. Epithelium-Long Junctional Epithelium; PDL-New attachment (Regeneration). **B,** Untreated root surface does not activate and/or maintain clot stability.

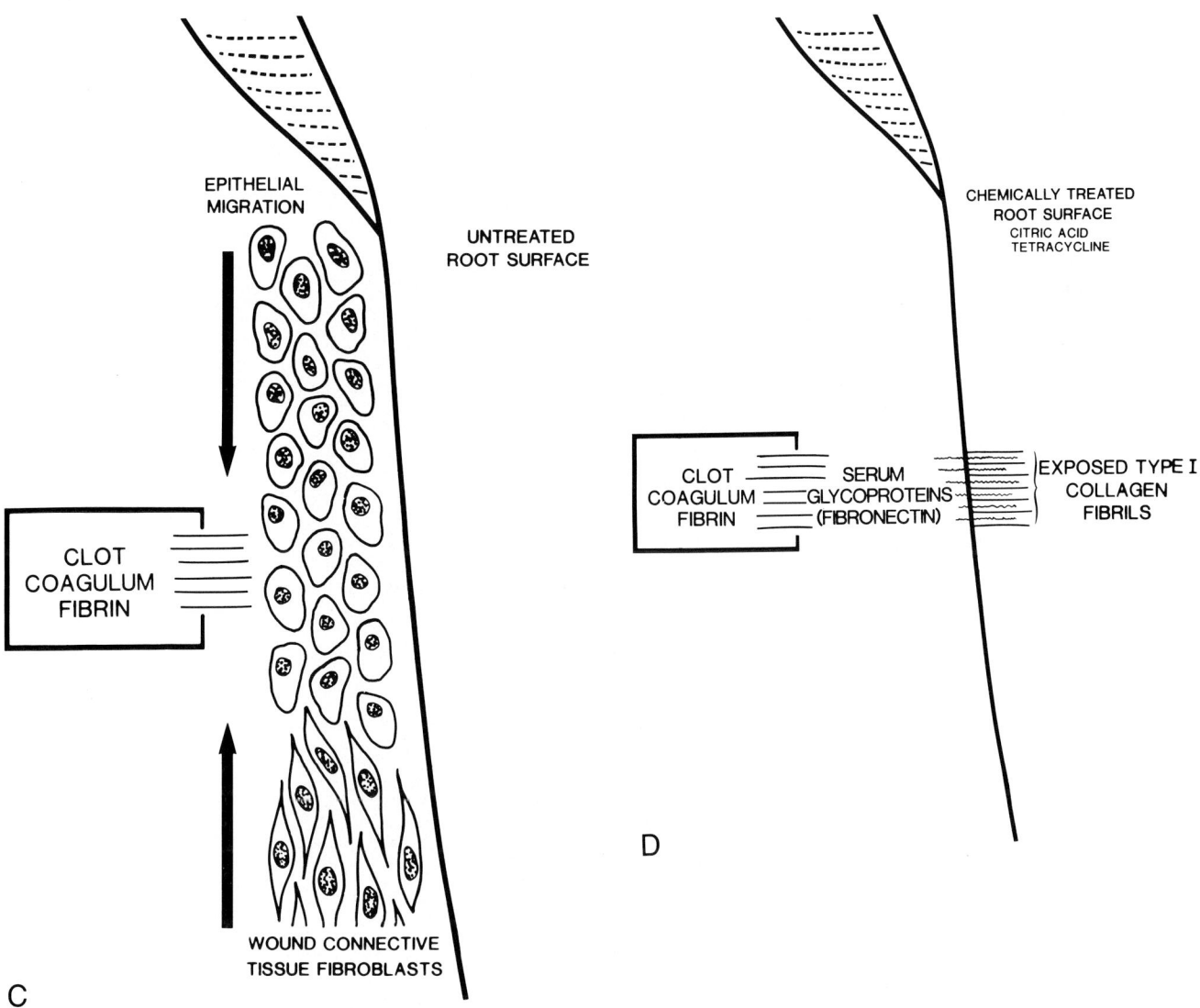

Fig. 8-1 (continued). C, Result is rapid epithelial proliferation and long junctional epithelium. **D,** Treated root surface promotes clot stability via fibrin linkage.

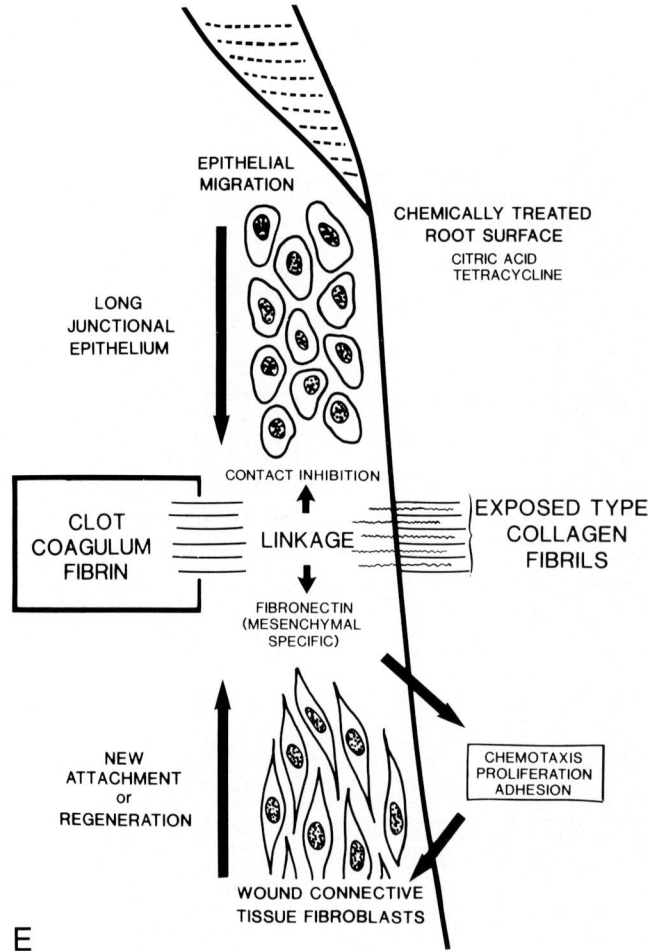

Fig. 8-1 (continued). E, The resulting cellular interactions as a result of root demineralization.

root planing alone produced a "smear layer" of residual debris, but when combined with CA application (pH 1.0; 2 to 3 minutes) the smear layer was removed, leaving a "mat-like" collagen surface with exposed dental tubules (Fig. 8-2). This demineralized *fiber* or *mat-like* surface was further shown in vitro to permit cells cultured from the periodontal ligament (PDL) and gingival fibroblasts to adhere better to the demineralized root surface (Boyko, et al., 1980). It was thought this was due to the exposed collagen rather than to the demineralized root surface (Leighton, 1982; Steinberg, 1987; Polson and Proye, 1982).

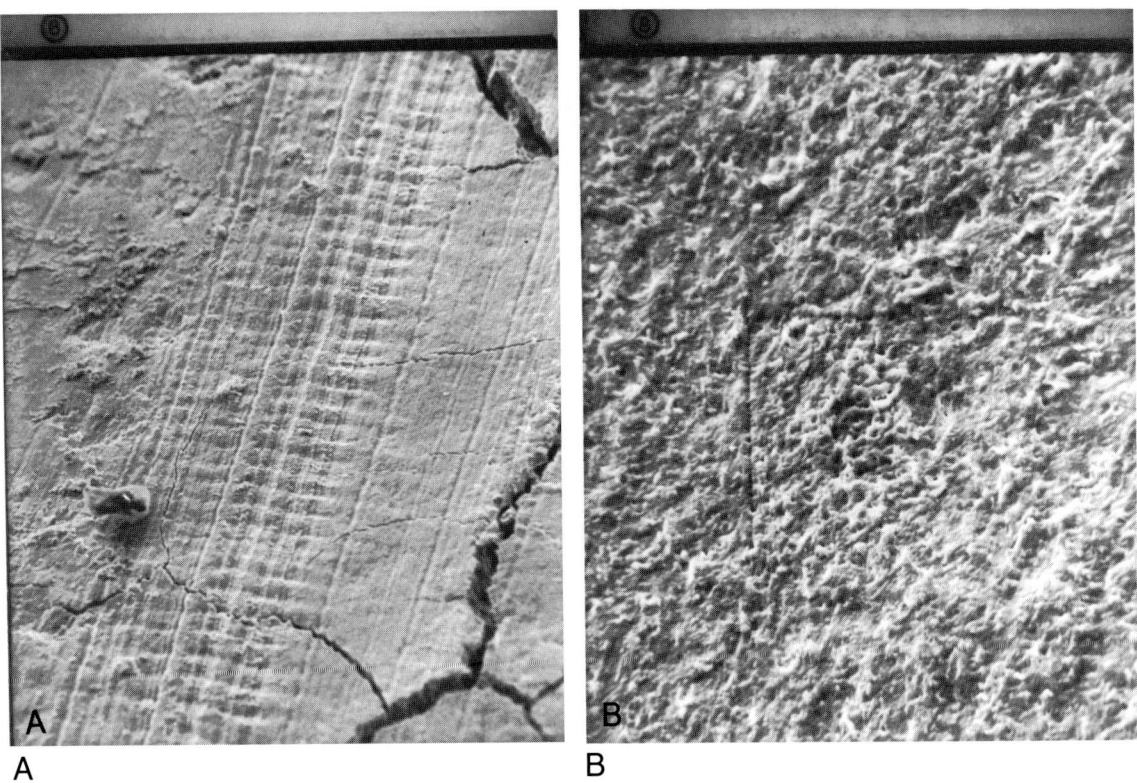

Fig. 8-2. Removal of Smear Layer. **A,** Scaled root surface showing smooth surface but closure of dentenal tubules (×1500). **B,** Scaled root surface after exposure to a saturated solution of citric acid (pH 1.0 for 3 minutes). The *smear layer* has been removed, the dentenal tubules have been exposed, and the fibrous matrix has been exposed (×1500). (Contributed by Knut A. Selvig, Bergen, Norway.)

Animal Studies

These early findings led to a series of animal studies. Through-and-through furcations were studied in dogs (Crigger et al., 1978; Nilveus et al., 1980; Nilveus and Egelberg, 1980; Ririe et al., 1980; Craig et al., 1980; Selvig et al., 1981, 1990), where high rates of bone regeneration and flap reattachment were seen with topical application of CA. It was concluded that the therapeutic use of CA was the critical factor irrespective of other factors (Fig. 8-3).

Reimplantation of teeth in primates was used to study the interrelationship between exposed root surface connective tissue fibers and reattachment (Polson and Proye, 1982, 1983; Proye and Polson, 1982; Polson and Caton, 1982). It was found that **"reattachment was dependent upon exposed healthy connective tissue root fibers"** and further that in cases where the fibers had been removed, either surgically or by disease, CA application prior to reimplantation permitted reattachment to occur. They concluded that "remnants of connective tissue fibers on the root resulted in reattachment whereas surgical denudation . . . resulted in epithelial migration."

The initial stages of clot formation and stabilization on CA-demineralized roots were found to be by a fibrin attachment via *"arcadelike"* formations (Steinberg, 1987). This fibrin–collagen linkage between the gingival fibers of the clot and the CA-demineralized root is mediated by a plasma fibronectin mechanism (Polson and Proye, 1982) (Fig. 8-4), which is an essential precursor to new attachment and is initiated by *platelet activation* (Steinberg, 1987). Platelet activation is dependent on root surface connective tissue and does not occur on surgically planed or diseased root surfaces resulting in clot instability (Polson and Proye, 1983; Wikesjo et al. 1991).

These findings may explain why human clinical studies using several different periodontal procedures (i.e., scaling and root planing, modified Widman flap, open-flap curettage, apically positioned flap) have shown healing only by a long junctioned epithelium.

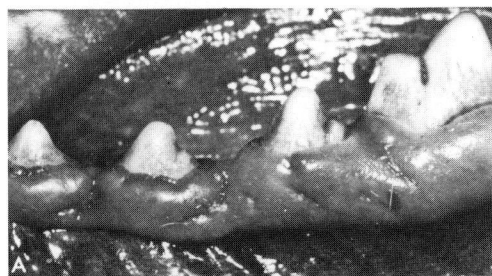
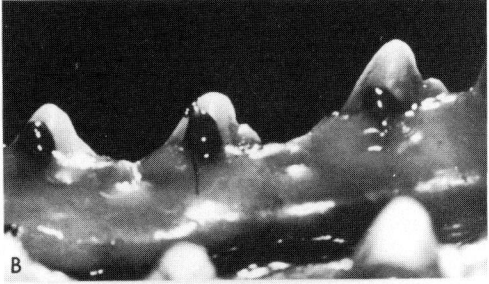
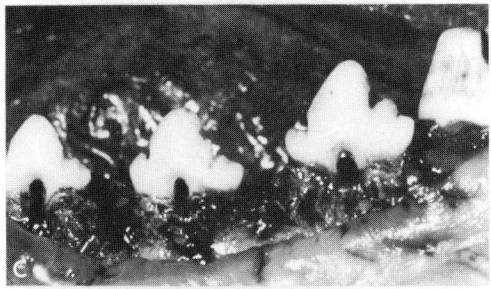
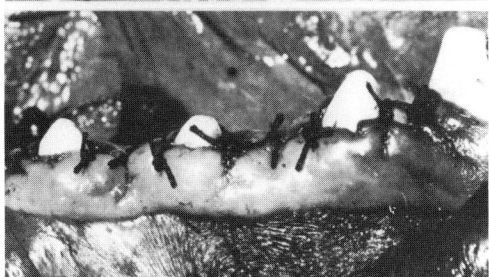
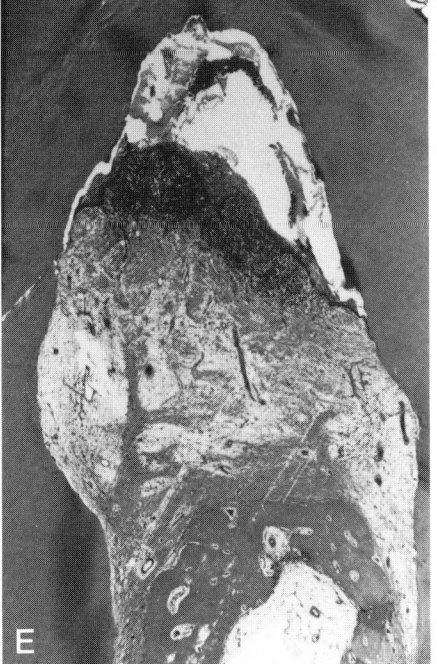
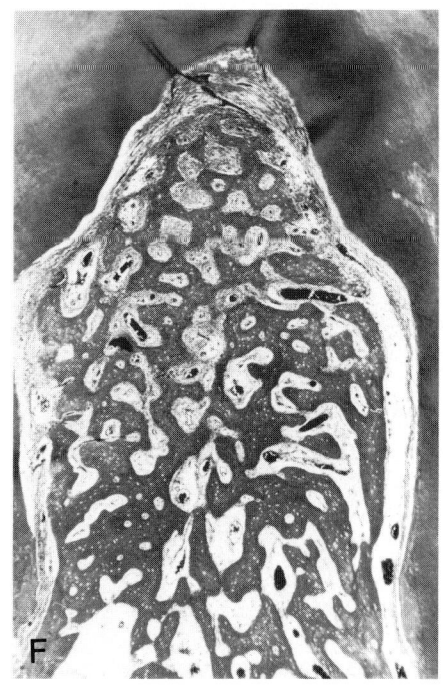

Fig. 8-3. Citric Acid and Coronally Positioned Flaps in Dogs. **A, B,** Before treatment. Buccal and lingual views of periodontally involved teeth. **C,** Flaps reflected, teeth scaled, and citric acid applied. **D,** Flaps coronally positioned. **E,** Photomicrograph ($\times 25$) of unhealed furcation defect of tooth treated with conventional flap surgery and mechanical debridement. **F,** Six weeks after furcation treated by mechanical debridement and citric acid application. (Contributed by Knut A. Selvig, Bergen, Norway.)

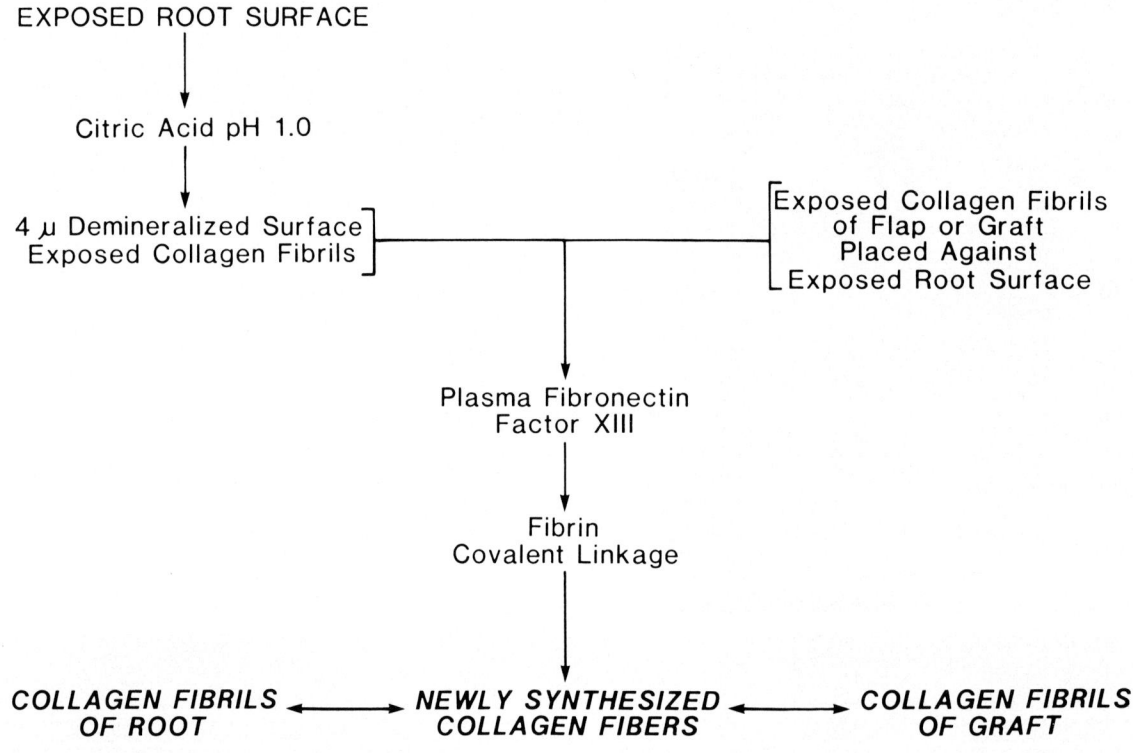

Fig. 8-4. Outline of Citric Acid Mechanism for Gaining Root Coverage. Note that the benefits of the use of citric acid in humans have not been substantiated.

Human Clinical Studies

Human clinical trials, although sparse, with studies showing both positive (Cole, 1980; Common and McFall, 1983; Frank, 1983; Stahl, 1985; Gantes et al., 1988A, 1988B; Stahl and Froum, 1991; Shiloah, 1980; Bogle et al., 1981, Hanes and Polson, 1989; Schallhorn and McClain, 1988; McClain and Schallhorn, 1993) and negative (Stahl and Froum, 1977; Marks and Mehta, 1986; Gottlow et al., 1986, Ibbott et al., 1985, Handelsman, 1991) results, have shown that there is a strong indication that when CA is combined with coronally positioned flaps a positive result can be achieved. A number of clinical studies (Gantes, et al., 1988, 1991) have shown that in CLII molar furcations (mandibular, buccal, and/or lingual; maxillary buccal) the combination of *CA-demineralization–coronal-flap* placement with or without demineralized freeze-dried bone allografts resulted in significant bone fill (66 to 70% fill of defect volume, 44 to 67% showing 100% bone fill). Stahl and Froum (1991) (Fig. 8-5), confirming the earlier work of Cole (1980), have shown an average gain in probing attachment of 4.5 mm in CA-demineralized coronally anchored sites (as opposed to the 1.7-mm gain for coronally anchored barrier membrane) with *histologic* evidence of new cementum with functionally inserted fiber in the calculus notch of all coronally anchored CA demineralized sites.

It can be concluded from the research that CA demineralization enhances new attachment or reattachment and regeneration by one or more of the following mechanisms:

1. Antibacterial effect (Daly, 1982)
2. Root detoxification (Aleo et al., 1975)
3. Exposure of root collagen and opening of dentinal tubules (Polson et al., 1984)
4. Removal of smear layer (Polson et al., 1984)
5. Initial clot stabilization (Wikesjo, 1991)
6. Demineralization prior to cementogenesis (Register, 1975, 1976)
7. Enhanced fibroblast growth and stability (Boyko et al., 1980)
8. Attachment by direct linkage (Stahl and Tarnow, 1985; Stahl, 1986) with or without cementogenesis (Levine and Stahl, 1972; Masileti, 1975)
9. No adverse effects to either the pulp (Hagner and Polson, 1986) or periodontal tissues (Polson and Haynes, 1986) have been reported.

TETRACYCLINE HCL

Tetracycline hydrochloride (TTC) has recently been used for acid root demineralization because it provides the same benefits as citric acid:

1. Antibacterial (Baker et al., 1983A)
2. Exposure of root collagen and opening of the dentinal tubules; removal of smear layer (Wikesjo et al., 1986)
3. Demineralization (Bjorvatn, 1983)
4. Detoxification of the root surface (Terranova et al., 1986)
5. Permits attachment by direct linkage with or without cementogenesis (Alger et al., 1990)

It also has a number of other advantages:

1. Anticollagenase activity (Golub et al., 1984)
2. Positive effects when placed in bone grafts (Papelarsi et al., 1991; Al-Ali et al., 1989)
3. Substantively antibacterial for 2 to 14 days (Baker, 1983B)
4. Enhances bone repair in extraction sockets (Hars and Massler, 1972)

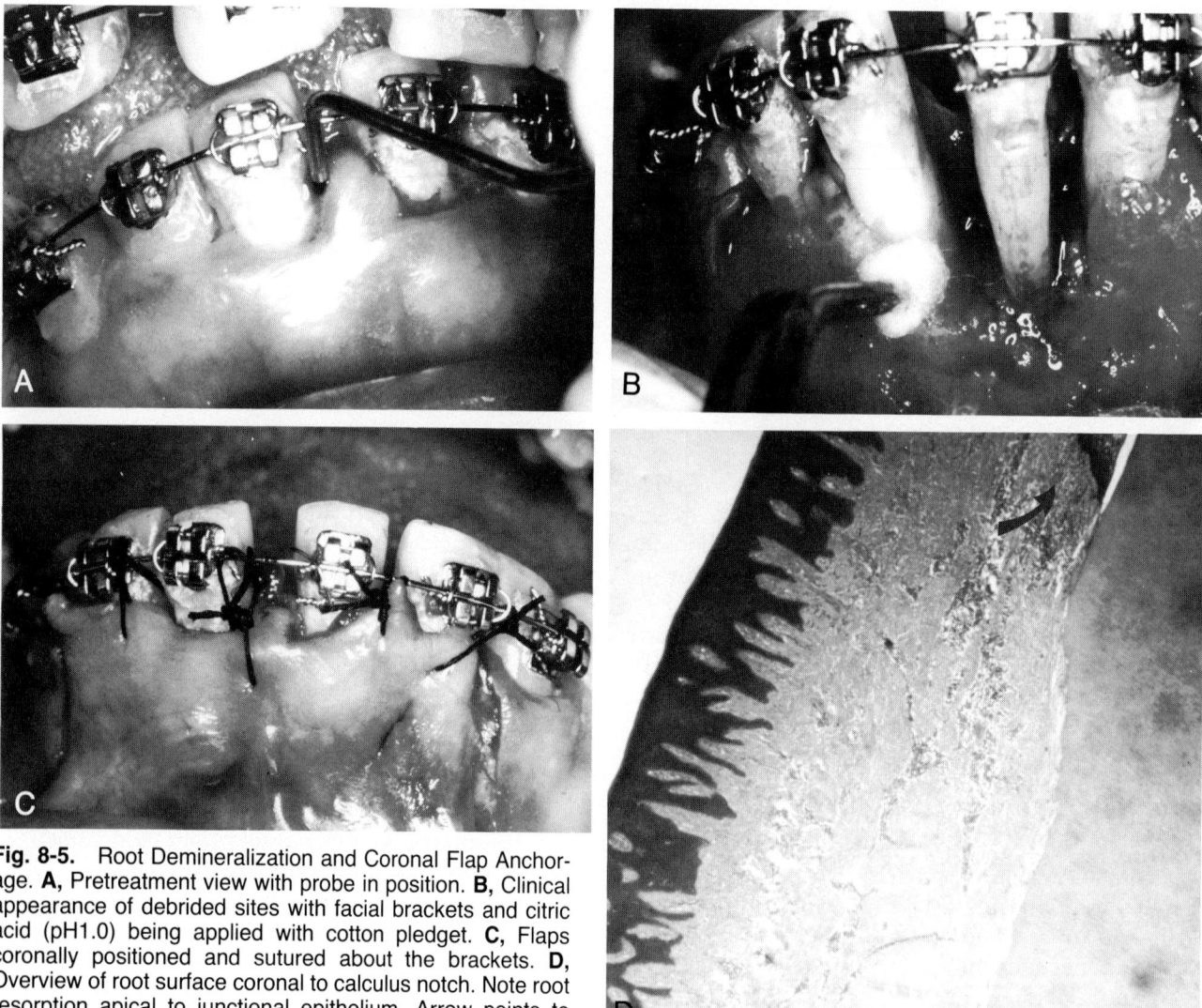

Fig. 8-5. Root Demineralization and Coronal Flap Anchorage. **A,** Pretreatment view with probe in position. **B,** Clinical appearance of debrided sites with facial brackets and citric acid (pH1.0) being applied with cotton pledget. **C,** Flaps coronally positioned and sutured about the brackets. **D,** Overview of root surface coronal to calculus notch. Note root resorption apical to junctional epithelium. Arrow points to apical position of JS.

5. Binds more fibronectin to demineralized surface (Terranova, 1986)

Unfortunately there appears to be a dosage dependent effect (>100mg/ml) on fibroblastic cell attachment and spreading (Somerman et al., 1988) about which they will not occur. Further, in comparative studies CA has been found not to be as effective in producing root demineralization, removal of the smear layer, or establishing new connective tissue attachment (Haynes et al., 1991). TTC may therefore require higher concentrations (>0.5%) and/or longer application times (>5 min). Finally, unlike for CA, no human histologic or clinical studies show the positive effects of TTC root demineralization.

FIBRONECTIN

Fibronectin (FN) is a high-molecular-weight glycoprotein (mol. wt. = 440,000) that is found in the extracellular tissue and is the main component that holds the clot together (Seelich and Redl, 1979; Baum and Wright, 1980). It promotes cell adhesion (Boyko et al., 1980; Kleinman et al., 1976) to both collagen (Ruoslahti et al., 1980) and scaled root surfaces (Terranova and Lundquist, 1981) and has a chemotactic effect on fibroblasts and mesenchymal cells (Kleinman et al., 1981, 1982; Mensing et al., 1983) (Figs. 8-6 and 8-7).

Periodontally, the application of FN to partially demineralized roots has been shown significantly to (1) enhance the effects of demineralization with regard to new attachment (Caffesse et al., 1987B), and (2) enhance cell proliferation from the PDL and supracrestal area (Caffesse et al., 1987B). The optimum concentration for use has been shown to be 0.38/ml saline (Smith et al., 1987). Finally, it has also been used as a substitute for sutures (Prato et al., 1987).

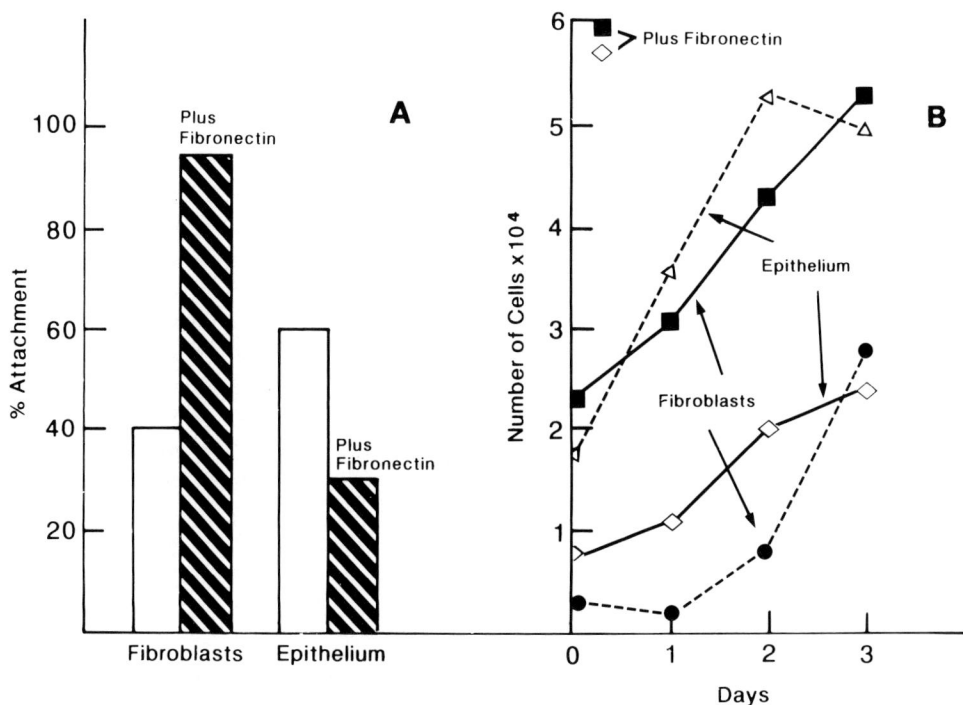

Fig. 8-6. **A,** Attachment of fibroblasts and epithelial cells on partially demineralized scaled root surfaces after incubation in Dulbecco's Modified Eagle's Media (DMEM) with and without the presence of fibronectin. Note that fibronectin potentiates fibroblasts while inhibiting epithelial cell. **B,** Growth curves for epithelial cells grown on scaled root surfaces (open triangles) and on partially demineralized and fibronectin-pretreated scaled root surfaces (open diamonds). Fibroblasts grown on scaled root surfaces (solid circles) and on scaled, partially demineralized, and fibronectin-pretreated (solid squares) root surfaces. (Drawn after Terranova, V.P., and Martin, G.F.: Molecular factors determining gingival tissue interaction with tooth structure. J. Periodontol. Res., 17:530, 1982.)

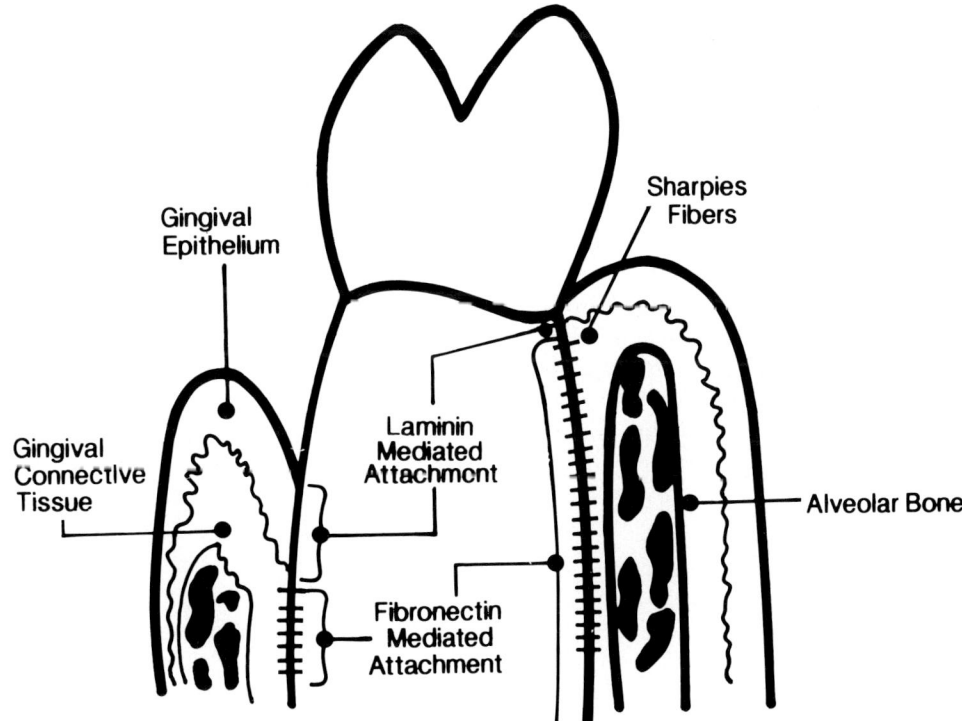

Fig. 8-7. Diagram of Tooth and Adjacent Supporting Structures in Health and Disease. The drawing depicts the laminin-mediated response (gingival epithelium and basement lamina) versus the fibronectin-mediated response (periodontal connective tissue adjacent to cementum and dentin). (Drawn after Terranova, V.P., and Martin, G.F.: Molecular factors determining gingival tissue interaction with tooth structure. J. Periodontol. Res., 17:530, 1982.)

The use of FN as a supplement to demineralization is therefore strongly supported by the following:
1. The initial stage after demineralization and prior to new attachment is fibrin formation and linkage (Polson and Proye, 1983)
2. It is the coronal growth of cells from the PDL that is responsible for new attachment (Karring et al., 1986) (fibronectin stimulates this growth from the PDL)
3. Favors the growth and attachment of fibroblasts over epithelial cells to the root surface (Terranova and Martin, 1982)
4. Speeds the linkage process by being chemoattractive for fibroblasts (Kleinman et al., 1981, 1982; Mensing et al., 1983; Ripamonti et al., 1986), acting as a tissue adhesive (Boyko et al., 1980; Mensing, et al., 1983; Ripamonti, et al., 1986), and stabilizing the clot between the exposed root surface collagen and new fibers within the tissue (Viljanto et al., 1981; Clark et al., 1982; Matras, 1988).

BIOCHEMICAL APPROACH TO PERIODONTAL REGENERATION

Early studies (Terranova and Martin, 1982) noted that epithelial cells and fibroblasts use the glycoproteins laminin (LM) (Terranova et al., 1980) and fibronectin (FN) (Klebe, 1974), respectively, to mediate their attachment to their collagenous and tooth substrates. Mineralized root surfaces favor the epithelial–LM combination, and demineralized surfaces favor the fibroblastic–FN combination. Terranova (Terranova and Martin, 1982) found an inverse relationship between epithelial cells and FN and fibroblasts and LM (Fig. 8-7) and that a *selective advantage* could be achieved by using FN on a demineralized root surface. He (Terranova, 1987) called this *"reciprocal utilization of biologic modifiers."*

The biochemical approach to periodontal regeneration uses acid demineralization (CA or TTC) and protein(s) activation [FN, LM, endothelial cell growth factor (ECGF), osteogenin, etc.]. ***The principle is that demineralization of the root surface will preferentially increase protein binding and promote fibroblastic attachment and at the same time epithelial exclusion (contact inhibition), while protein activation will enhance specific cell proliferation, chemotaxis, and enhanced cellular attachment.***

This theory has worked well in vitro and in the animal model, but no significant positive effects have been shown in humans. Pitaru (Pitaru et al., 1984) has noted that while FN is highly specific for fibroblasts, it also plays a role in epithelial wound healing (Pitaru et al., 1988) and partially restores epithelial cell migration on demineralized root surfaces. This blurring of protein functions may be the reason human results are not as yet forthcoming.

CONCLUSION

Citric acid root demineralization, although not yet fully supported by research on humans, does provide significant benefits that cannot be achieved by scaling and root planing alone. It assures root detoxification, removal of the smear layer, exposure of root collagen, antibacterial effects, and initial clot stabilization. Tetracycline HCL may further increase these advantages. Both CA and TTC provide a surface substrate for future use of protein modifiers.

Root demineralization (CA, TTC) (Miller, 1983, 1985; Allen and Miller, 1989) is recommended for use in cosmetic gingival reconstruction, prior to placement of bone implants (CA and TTC), infrabony defects, as an implant additive (TTC) (Schallhorn and McClain, 1988; McClain and Schallhorn, 1993) and as a primary treatment for CLII furcations (CA) with or without bone implants.

In the future periodontal regeneration will combine root detoxification with a combination of ***synthetic "biologic" protein modifiers*** *that will artificially stimulate tissue regeneration.*

9

COSMETIC ROOT COVERAGE: GINGIVAL AUGMENTATION

COSMETIC GINGIVAL RECONSTRUCTION

Gingival reconstruction is today not only possible but a routine part of periodontal practice. The ability to cover unsightly exposed and sensitive roots and crown margins, to reconstruct lost ridges and to enhance prosthetic reconstruction has undergone a rapid explosion.

This section deals exclusively with those procedures necessary for cosmetic and gingival enhancement:
1. Free gingival graft
2. Coronally positioned flap
3. Subepithelial connective tissue graft
4. Pedicle flap
5. Semilunar flap
6. Transpositional flap
7. Connective tissue pedicle graft

GRAFTING FOR ROOT COVERAGE

Historically, the free gingival autograft was not recommended for root coverage. Sullivan and Atkins (1968A,B) and later Hall (1984) advocated that it be used only for gingival augmentation or prophylactically to increase the width of the zone of attached keratinized gingiva. These views were not surprising when one considers that the only published study on the subject of root coverage reported only a 20% success rate (Mlinek, 1973). The major impediment to success was the large avascular area the graft had to bridge and the lack of predictability that resulted from it.

From 1972 to 1982 individual case reports of successful results were reported (Hawley and Staffilino, 1970; Livingston, 1975; Ward 1974), but it was not until Miller (1982, 1985B), modifying the basic grafting techniques, was able to demonstrate that successful root coverage was not only attainable but also predictable over denuded root surfaces even if they were of the Class II deep–wide variety. This was followed in rapid succession by others (Holbrook and Ochsenbein, 1983; Ibbott, et al., 1985; Bertrand and Dunlap, 1988; Borghetti and Gardella, 1990; Tolmie, 1991), all of whom were able to show that successful root coverage was not only attainable but also predictable.

CLASSIFICATION OF GINGIVAL RECESSION

Sullivan and Atkins (1968A) classified gingival recession into four categories: deep–wide, shallow–wide, deep–narrow, and shallow–narrow. Of these, they felt that the *deep–wide* gingival recession was the most difficult to treat and offered the least predictability for attaining root coverage. Miller (1985B) expanded this classification for gingival recession to take into account the nature and quality of gingival recession as well as its relationship to the adjacent interproximal tissue height.

Miller Classification

Class I   *Shallow–narrow* and *shallow–wide* gingival recession in which the marginal tissues have not receded beyond the mucogingival junction. There is no loss of interproximal soft tissue or bone. 100% root coverage is possible (Fig. 9-1A).

Class II **Deep–narrow** and **deep–wide** gingival recession in which the marginal tissues have receded beyond the mucogingival junction. There is no loss of interproximal soft tissue or bone. 100% root coverage is possible (Fig. 9-1B).

Class III **Class I or Class II gingival recession** combined with loss of interproximal bone such that the soft tissue is now apical to the cementoenamel interproximal junction but coronal to the marginal tissue. 100% root coverage is not possible (Fig. 9-1C).

Class IV **The loss of interproximal bone** and soft tissue is such that one or both of the adjacent interdental areas is level with the marginal gingiva. No root coverage is possible (Fig. 9-1D).

PROCEDURAL MODIFICATIONS

Preparation of the recipient and donor sites for the free soft-tissue graft for root coverage is shown in Figure 9-2. Certain modifications of principles or techniques that enhance success are needed when the recipient and donor sites are prepared.

1. Scaling and root planing are carried out to remove soft cementum, calculus, and plaque and to reduce the prominence of root convexities. Fine enamel finishing burs may be used to help flatten the root in the cervical third.
2. Citric acid (pH 10) is applied with a small cotton pledget and burnished in for 3 to 5 minutes (Miller 1982). This promotes root demineralization, detoxification of the root surface, opening of the dentinal tubules, and exposure of the connective tissue root fibers. This process has been shown to prevent apical migration of epithelium, to promote palate activation, to increase clot stability, and to enhance attachment by *linkage* (see Chapter 7).
3. The horizontal papillary incisions are made at right angles to the papilla *above* the level of the cementoenamel junction (CEJ) to create a butt joint. When **butt** joints cannot be achieved, all the epithelium over the papilla is removed to enhance bleeding and provide a connective tissue bed for graft contact (Fig. 9-2B).
4. The periosteal bed should be extended mesially, distally, and apically for about 4 to 6 mm on all sides of the denuded root to permit adequate graft extension (Fig. 9-2C).
5. Any epithelial remnants adjacent to the root should be removed.
6. A thick graft of 1.5 to 2.5 mm is preferred (Miller, 1982) (Fig. 9-2D,D'). Because of the size and thickness of the grafts required for root coverage, it is sometimes advantageous to fabricate a palatal stent for protection and comfort during healing (Fig. 9-6).
7. The graft should be of uniform thickness, with no beveled margins. All margins should be at right angles to the graft surface (Holbrook and Ochsenbein, 1983).
8. The graft, when placed at or slightly above the cementoenamel junction of the denuded root, should extend sufficiently to overlap the periosteal bed mesially, distally, and apically for 3 to 4 mm to ensure adequate plasmatic diffusion (Fig. 9-2D,D').
9. Tacking sutures are used for initial graft stabilization prior to suture modification (Fig. 9-2D,D').
10. The specialized suturing is now completed (Fig. 9-2E,E').
11. The final result is seen in Figure 9-2F.

The clinical procedures are depicted in Figures 9-3, 9-4, 9-5, and 9-6.

Suturing Modification for Root Coverage

Carvalho (1972) and Holbrook and Ochsenbein (1983) noted that when grafts are used for root coverage the underlying *anatomic osseous factors* must be taken into account: It is the teeth with the most prominent roots that generally exhibit the least amount of bone over them, the most dehiscences and fenestrations, the greatest gingival scalloping, the thinnest type of periodontium, the most esthetic form, and the most mucogingival problems. They point out that prominent, bulging roots produce deep interproximal valleys (Fig. 9-7), which require close adaptation of the grafts. These interradicular concavities necessitate graft stabilization to promote intimate graft contact and prevent dead space and hematoma formation.

Procedure

1. The first suture is a *horizontal "graft stretching" suture* (HS), which Sullivan and Atkins (1968A) noted was to counteract the primary contraction and open the blood vessels within the graft (Fig. 9-8A). The graft is usually stretched 2 to 3 mm.
2. The second suture is a *circumferential suture* (CS), which holds the graft against the denuded areas (Fig. 9-8B).
3. The third suture, the *interdental concavity suture* (ICS), prevents dead space formation in the interradicular concavities or depressions (Fig. 9-8C).

4. Figure 9-8D is a cross-sectional view, showing the *dead space* (DS) resulting when routine suturing techniques are used. Figure 9-8E is a cross section depicting the intimate contact between graft and underlying periosteal bed when proper suturing technique is employed.

This procedure is shown clinically in Figures 9-4 and 9-6.

Creeping Attachment

Goldman et al. (1964) and Matter (1976, 1980) noted a second mechanism of gaining root coverage by the phenomenon of *creeping attachment.* This occurred between 1 month and 1 year and was the result of the coronal migration of the newly grafted attached gingiva. The amount of anticipated coverage was totally unpredictable (see Fig. 9-9).

Coronally Positioned Flap

The coronally positioned flap has long been used as a means of gaining root coverage. This technique has met with varying degrees of success owing to minimal amounts of keratinized gingiva. It was not until 1965 when Harvey published the results of his combined technique, which used a first-stage free gingival graft to enhance the mucogingival complex and then coronally repositioned it in the second stage, that the technique received much attention. Bernimoulin (1975) graphically outlined the *combined procedure* as it is used in practice today. The combined procedure is used only when there is an inadequate zone of keratinized gingiva.

Allen and Miller (1989) used this procedure and were able to achieve 3.18-mm root coverage (97.8%) of shallow marginal recession. They used citric acid in combination with a partial-thickness pedicle flap that was coronally positioned.

Indications

1. Esthetic coverage of exposed roots
2. For tooth sensitivity owing to gingival recession

Requirements

The main prerequisite is an adequate zone of keratinized gingiva (≥ 3 mm).

Advantages

1. Treatment of multiple areas of root exposure
2. No need for involvement of adjacent teeth
3. High degree of success
4. Even if the procedure does not work, it does not increase the existing problem

Disadvantage

The main disadvantage is the need for two surgical procedures if the zone of keratinized gingiva is inadequate.

Procedure

Figures 9-10A and 9-10,1 display the common findings of a prominent cuspid with recession. The probable causes of the recession are the position of other teeth, prominent root convexity, orthodontic restoration, toothbrush abrasion, frenulum pull, or thin alveolar housing.

With the patient under anesthesia, the exposed root is scaled and root planed to remove softened cementum and reduce or eliminate prominent root convexities. Citric acid (pH 1.0) is burnished in with a moistened cotton pledget for 3 to 5 minutes.

A full-thickness flap is raised (Figs. 9-10B, 9-10,2) using two *parallel* vertical incisions to outline the surgical area. The incisions border the papillae that are to be moved coronally. A scalloped, inverse beveled incision is made, using a No. 15 scalpel blade to connect the two vertical incisions. *The scalloped incision is made at the gingival crest facially; but interproximally, care is taken to create new papillae that will fit their future locations.* The remaining portion of the papillae will undergo epithelial denudation with small ophthalmic scissors or tissue nippers.

The flap is positioned (Figs. 9-10C, 9-10,3) 1 mm coronal to the cementoenamel junction. To facilitate coronal movement, the base of the flap is undermined and separated from the periosteum with scissors.

The flap is sutured coronally with a sling-type papillary suture around the neck of the tooth. This positions and stabilizes the flap coronally. Interrupted sutures are used laterally. Figure 9-10,4 shows the completed case. See also Figure 9-11.

SUBEPITHELIAL CONNECTIVE TISSUE GRAFT

This procedure is the single most effective way to achieve predictable root coverage with a high degree of cosmetic enhancement.

History

Historically, the underlying gingival connective tissue has been shown to be a viable source of cells for repopulating the epithelium (Karring, et al., 1971) and a somewhat predictable source for increasing the zone of keratinized gingiva (Edel, 1974; Becker and Becker, 1986).

Langer and Langer (1985) published an article that introduced and outlined the indications and proce-

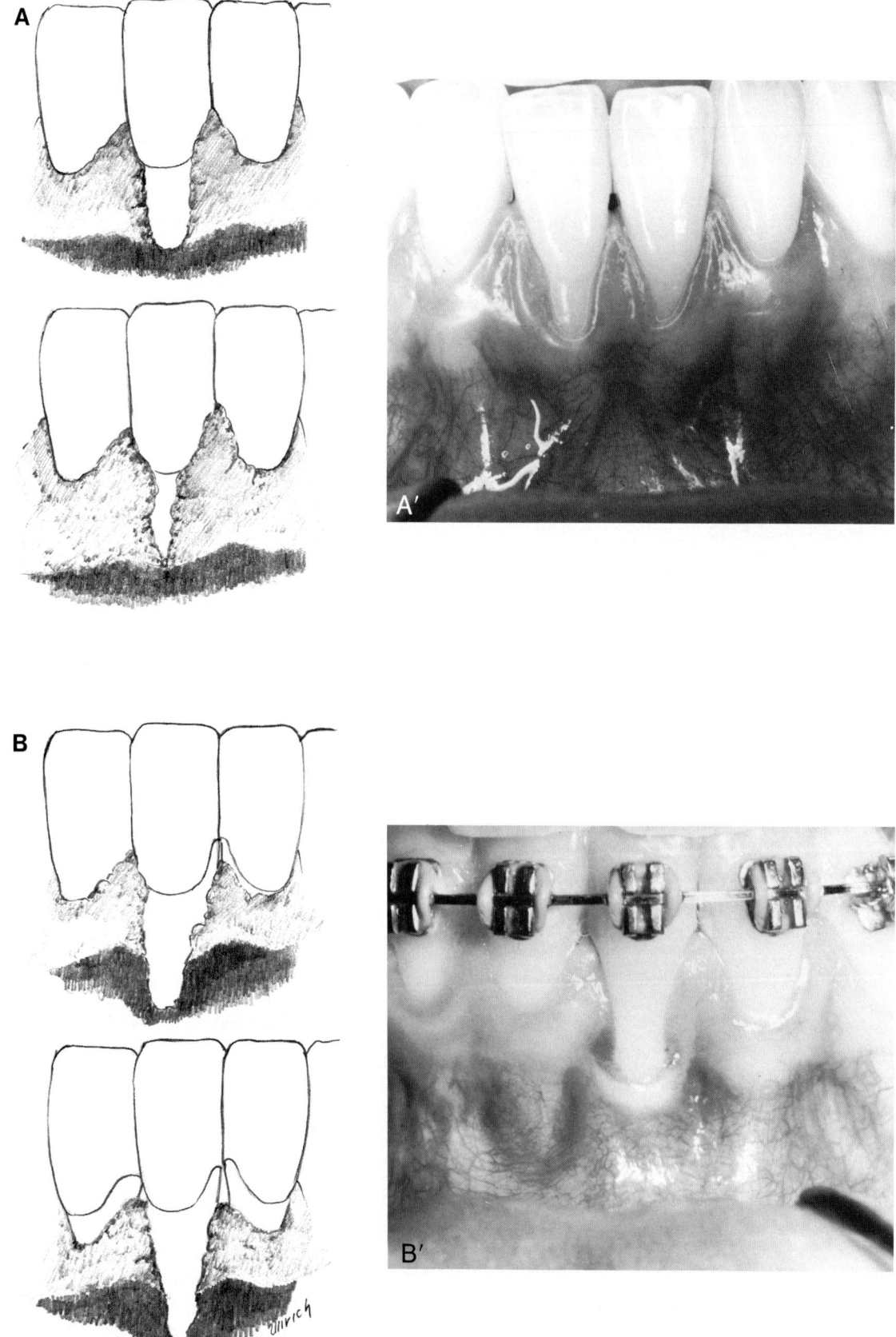

Fig. 9-1. Classification of Gingival Recession. **A,A′**, Class I. **B,B′**, Class II.

Cosmetic Root Coverage: Gingival Augmentation

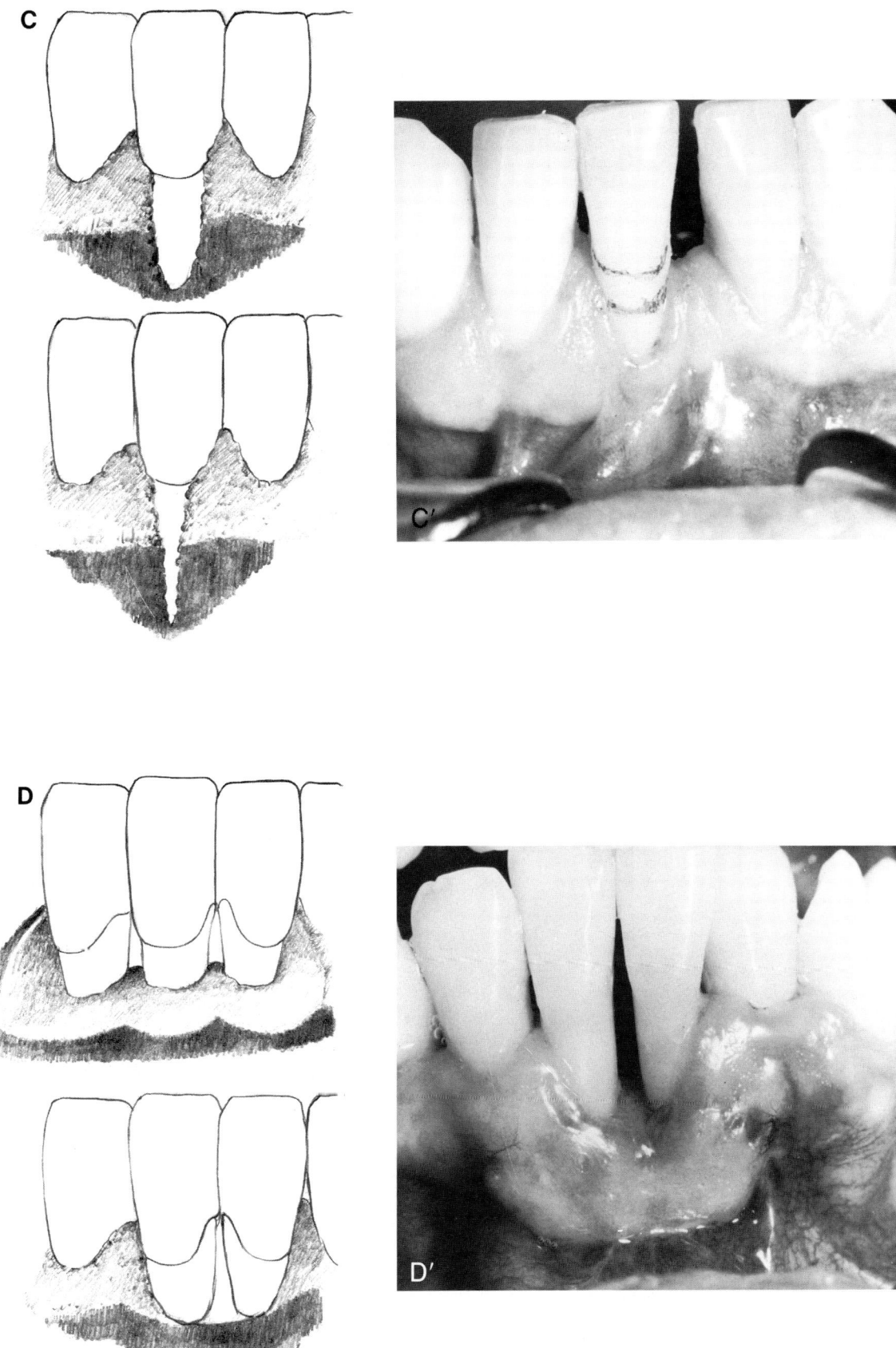

Fig. 9-1 (continued). C,C′, Class III. D,D′, Class IV.

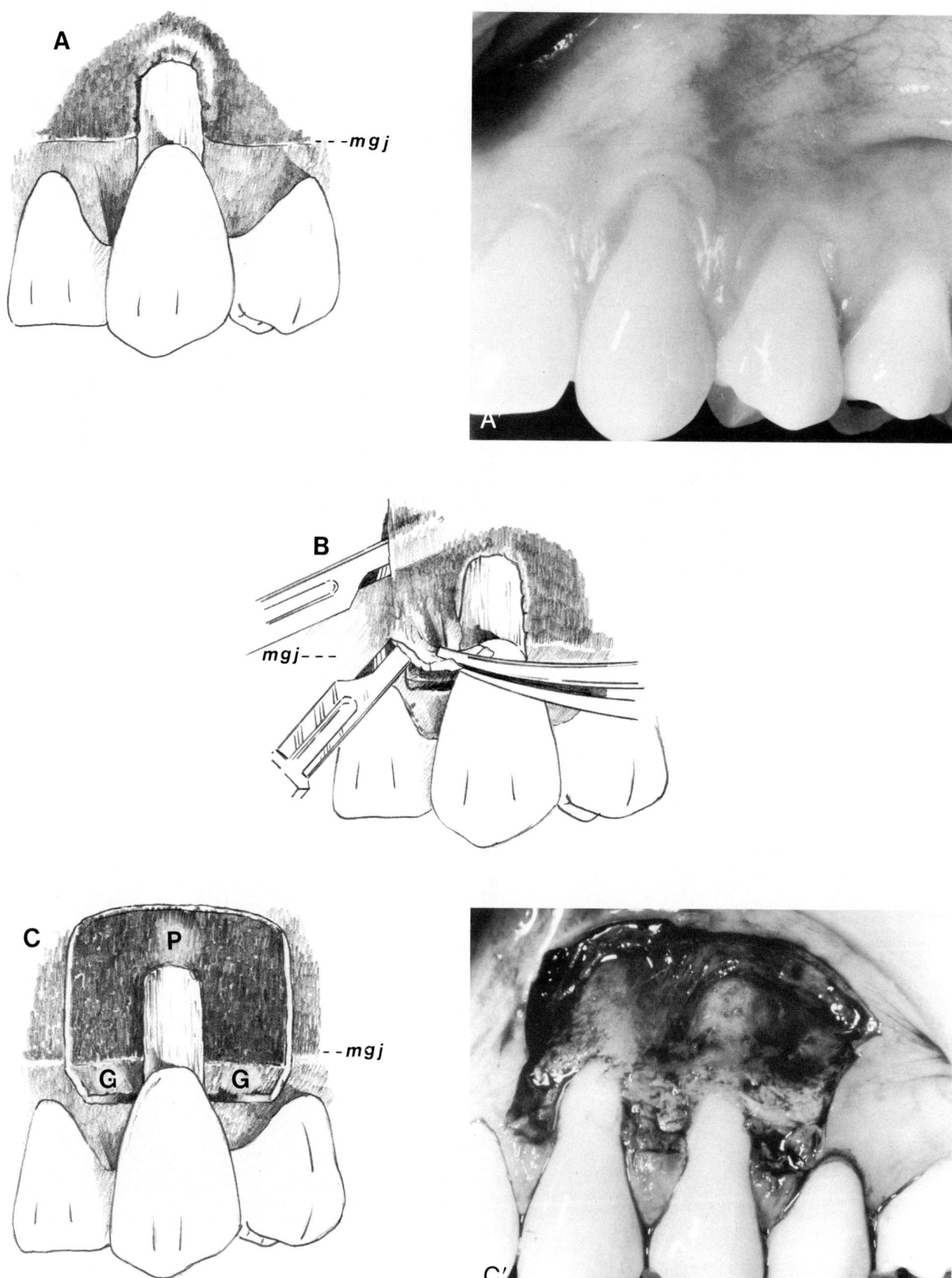

Fig. 9-2. Free Soft-Tissue Graft for Root Coverage. **A,A′,** Before surgery; note clinical gingiva recession of cuspid and bicuspid. **B,** Periosteal bed prepared by sharp dissection. **C,C′,** Periosteal bed augmentation completed.

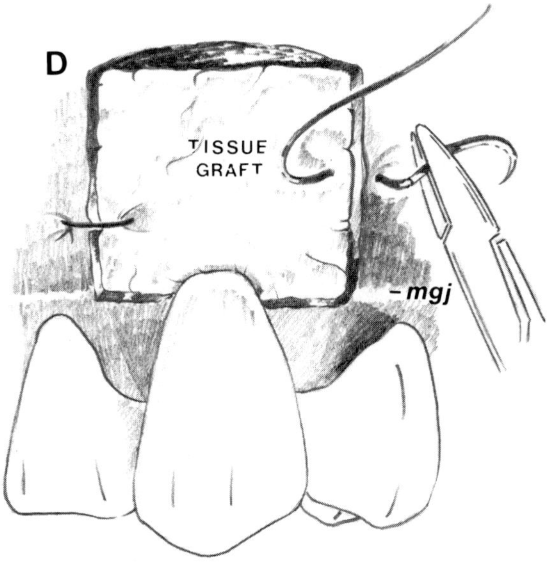

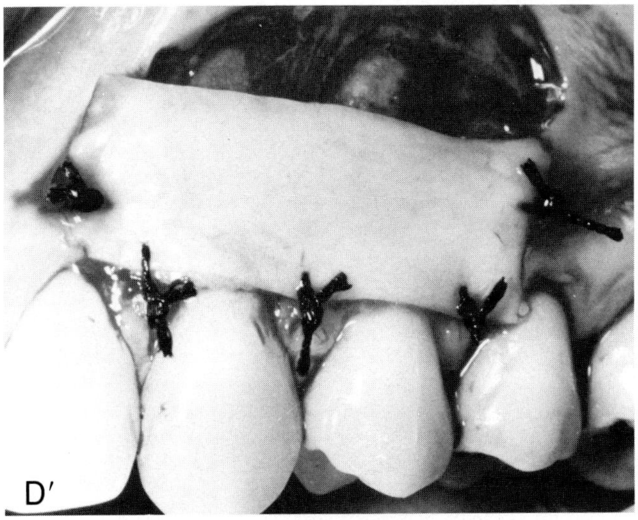

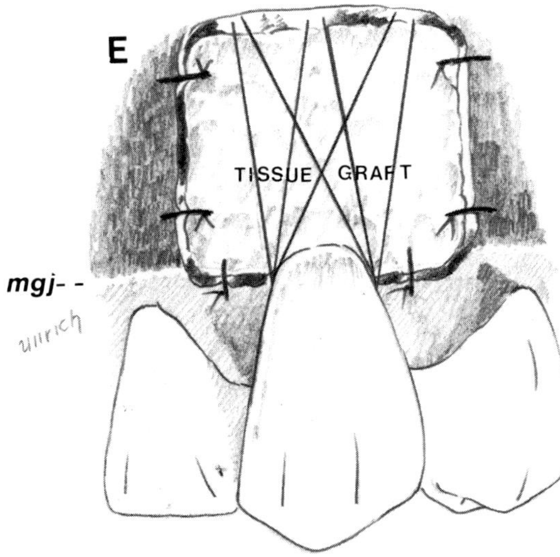

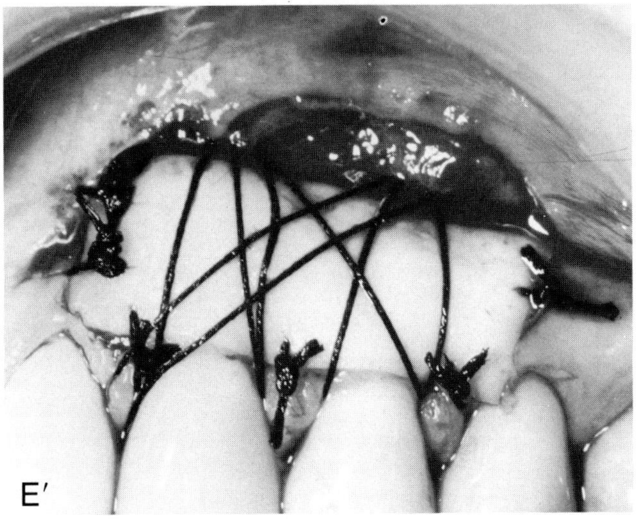

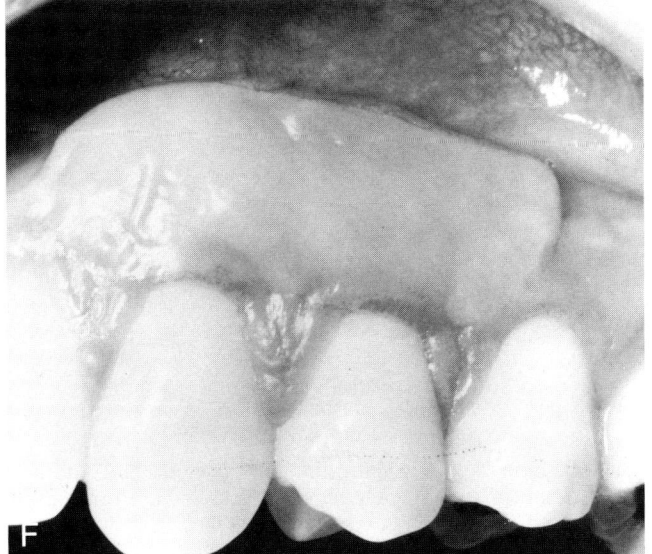

Figure 9-2 (continued). D,D', Graft is first tacked in position by interrupted sutures. **E,E'**, Modified suturing technique for improved graft stability. **F**, Eight months later.

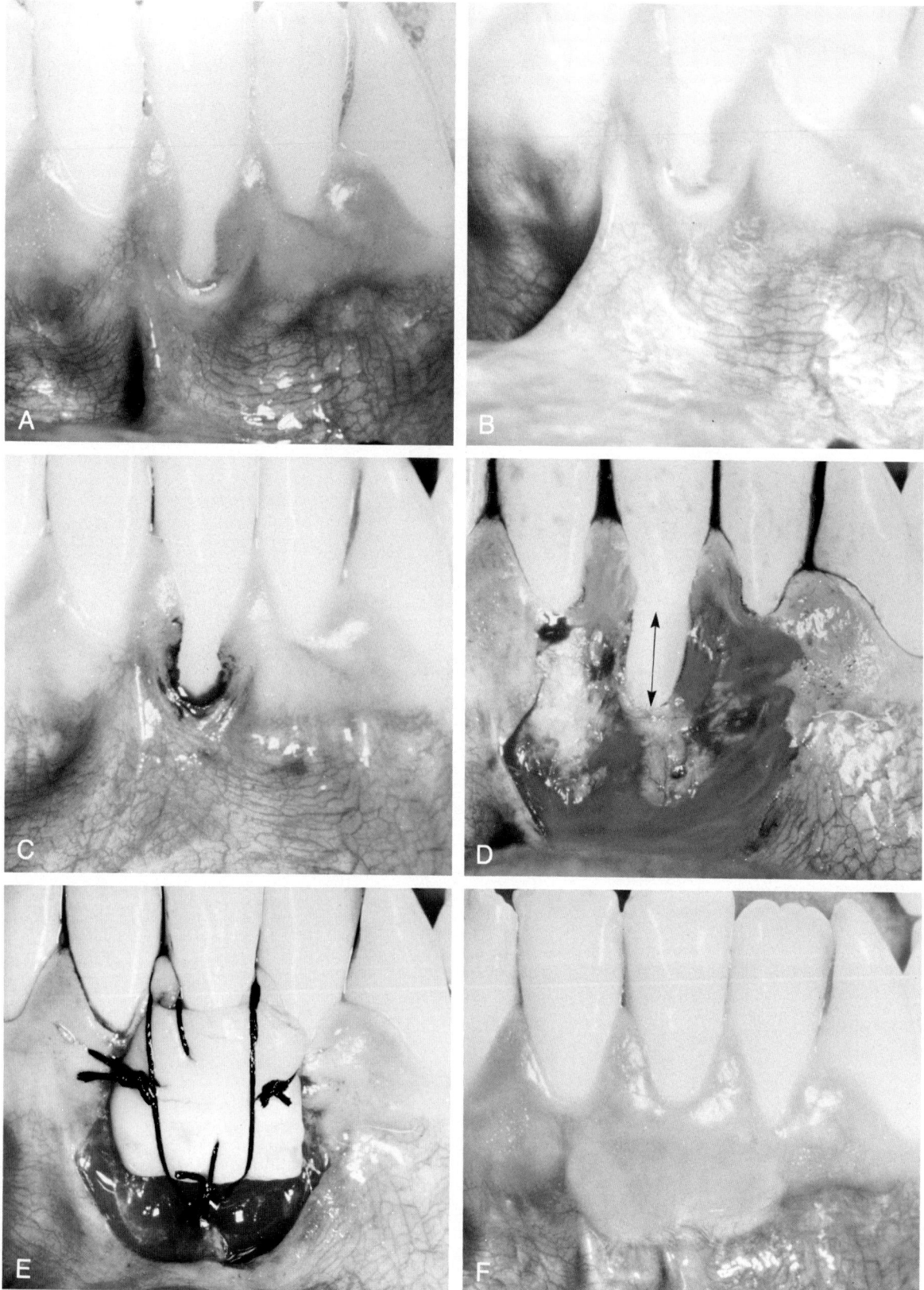

Fig. 9-3. Free Soft-Tissue Autograft for Root Coverage. **A,** Before. **B,** Side view showing prominent frenum. **C,** Citric acid applied. **D,** Periosteal bed prepared; note adequate extension mesially, distally, and apically. **E,** Full-thickness graft placed. **F,** Seven months later; total coverage achieved.

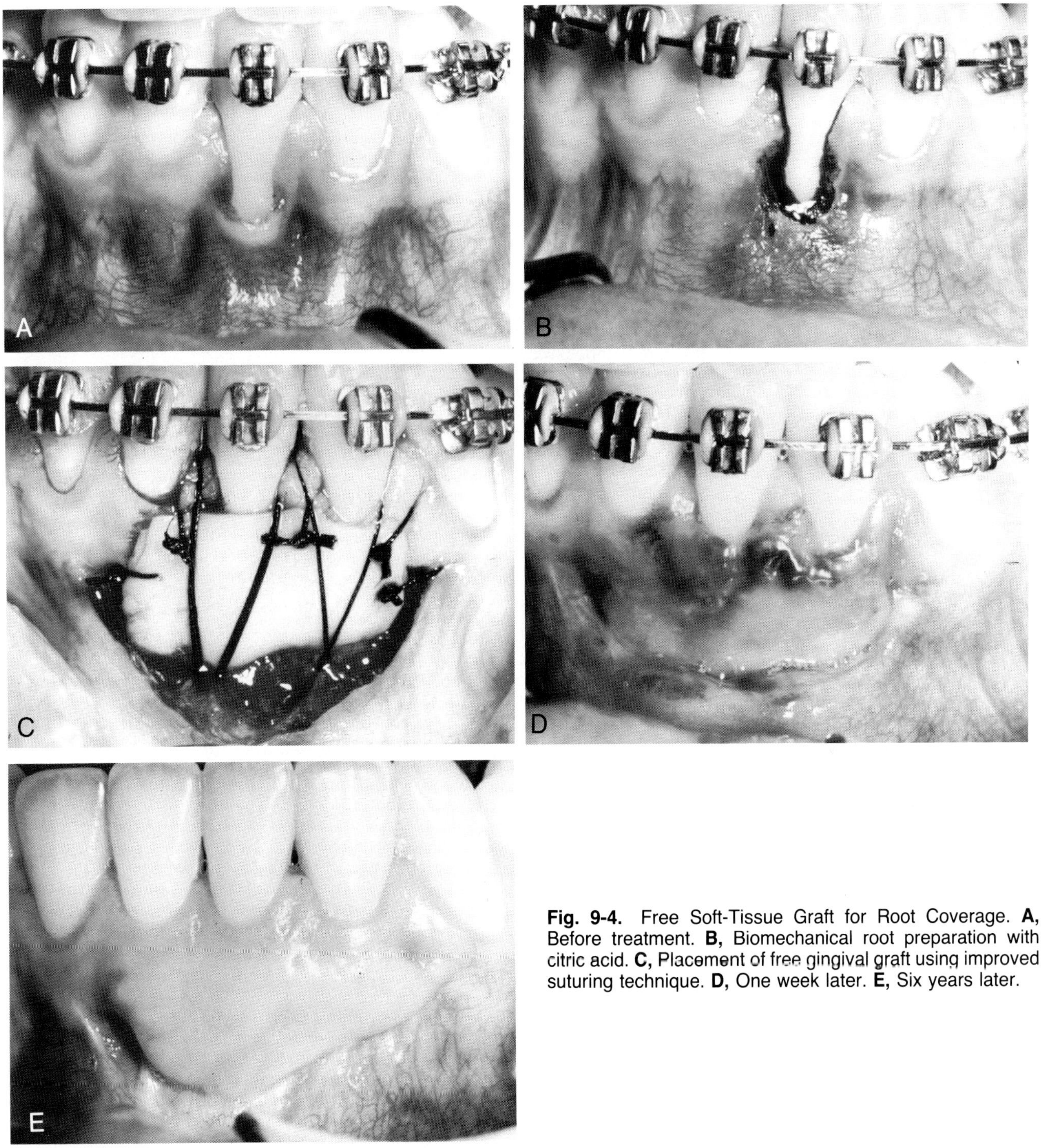

Cosmetic Root Coverage: Gingival Augmentation

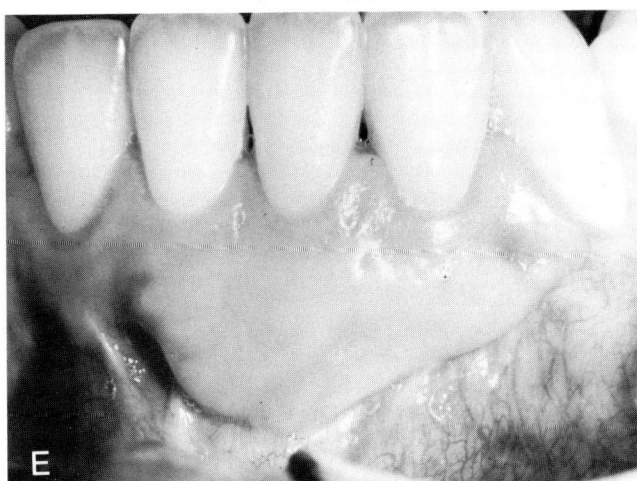

Fig. 9-4. Free Soft-Tissue Graft for Root Coverage. **A,** Before treatment. **B,** Biomechanical root preparation with citric acid. **C,** Placement of free gingival graft using improved suturing technique. **D,** One week later. **E,** Six years later.

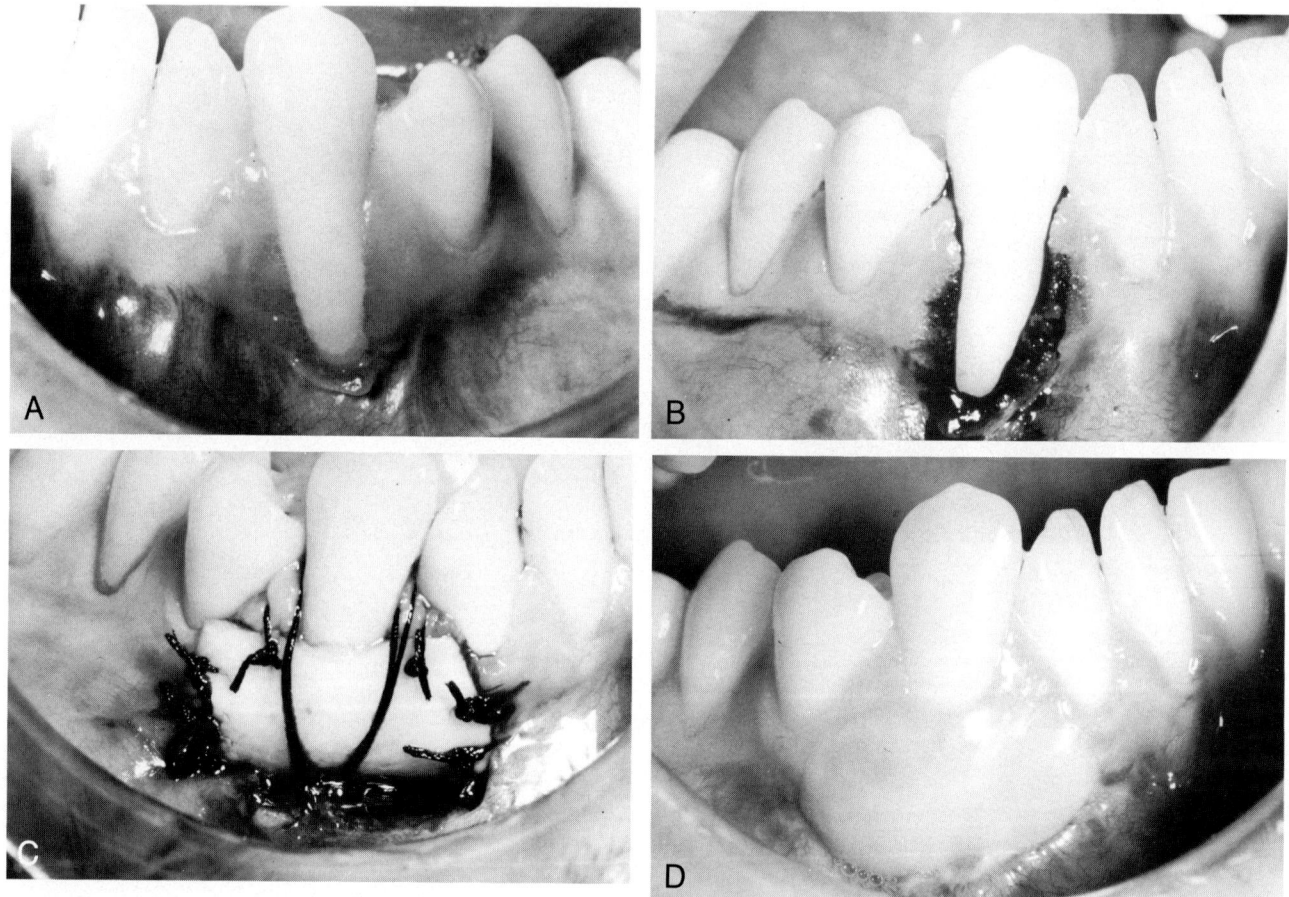

Fig. 9-5. Free Soft-Tissue Graft for Root Coverage. **A,** Before treatment. **B,** Biomechanical root preparation with citric acid. **C,** Graft placement over large Class II deep wide recession and sutured. **D,** One year later, note complete root coverage.

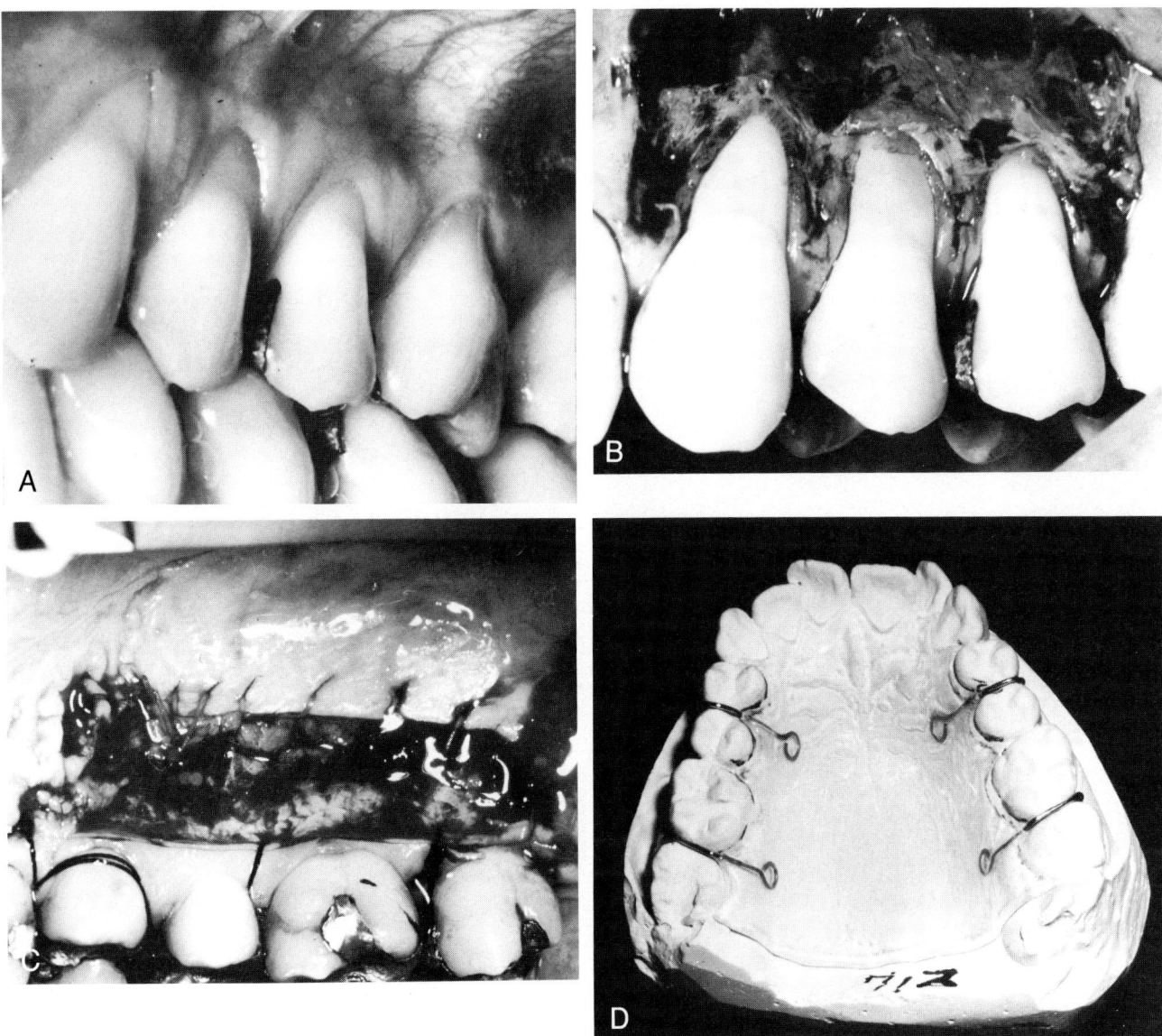

Fig. 9-6. Free Soft-Tissue Graft for Root Coverage. **A,** Before treatment showing multiple areas of recession. **B,** Mucosal flap reflected, showing significant Class II deep–wide gingival recession. **C,** Deep–wide gingival graft removed from palate. Palate sutured with chromic gut sutures for hemostasis. **D, E,** Palatal stent that was fabricated to protect palate.

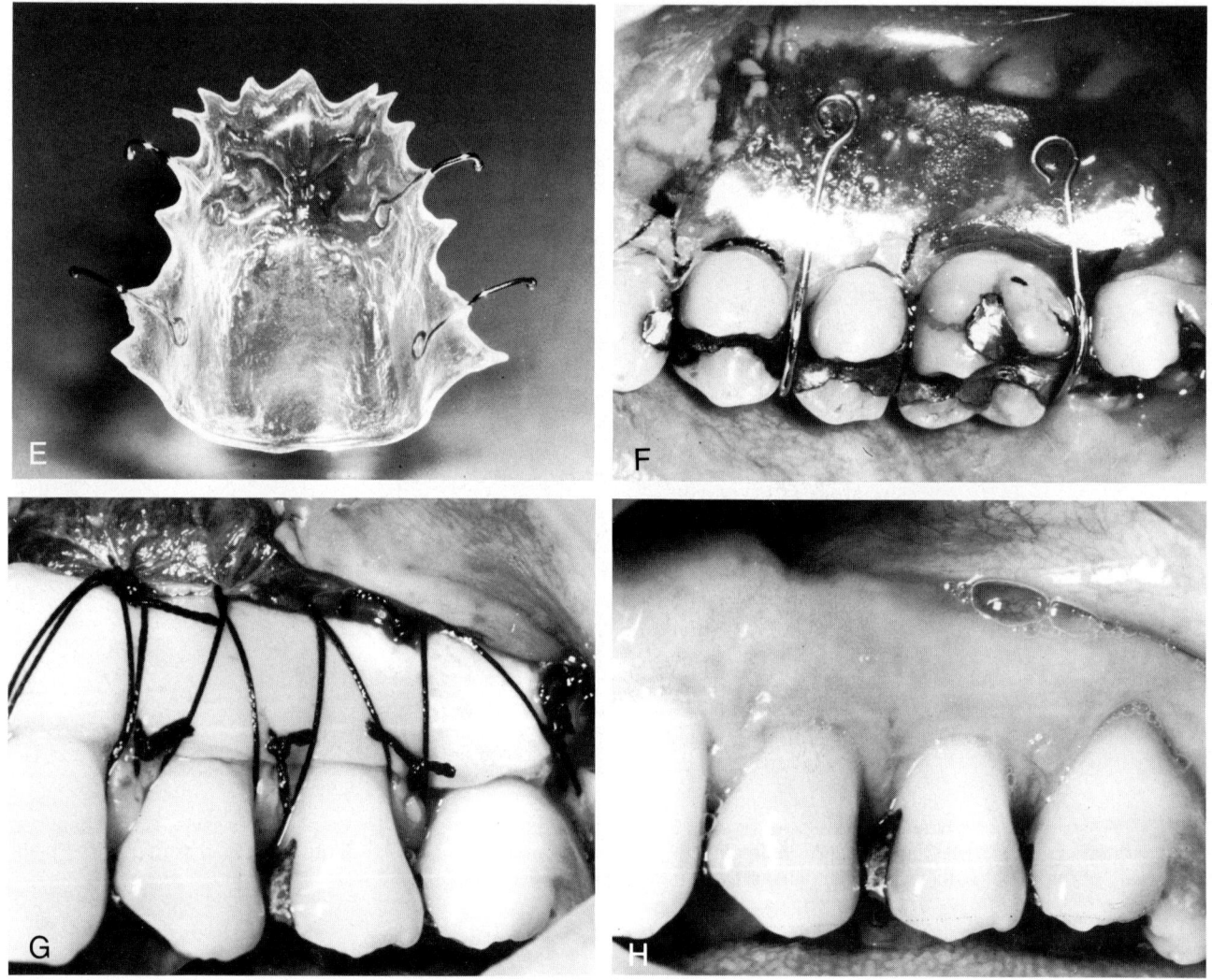

Fig. 9-6 (continued). **F,** Stent positioned on palate. **G,** Free gingival graft positioned and sutured. **H,** Two years later; note excellent result and complete root coverage. Compare with A and B.

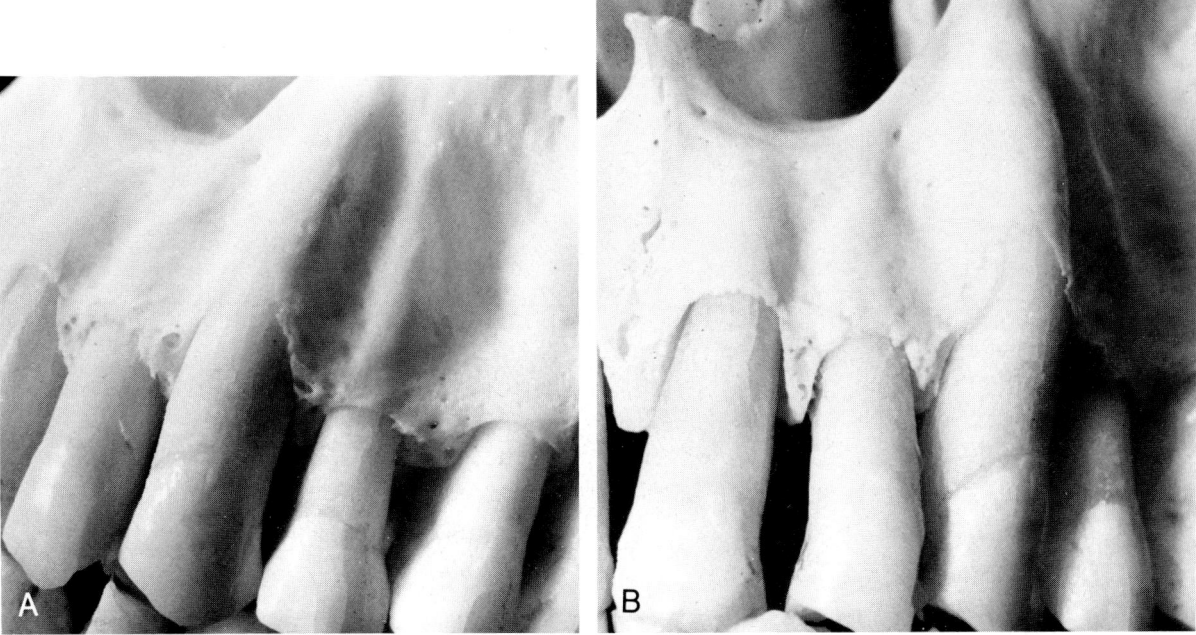

Fig. 9-7. Dry Skull Representation of Prominent Root with Deep Interproximal Concavities. **A,** Side view. **B,** Facial view. Note cuspid prominence.

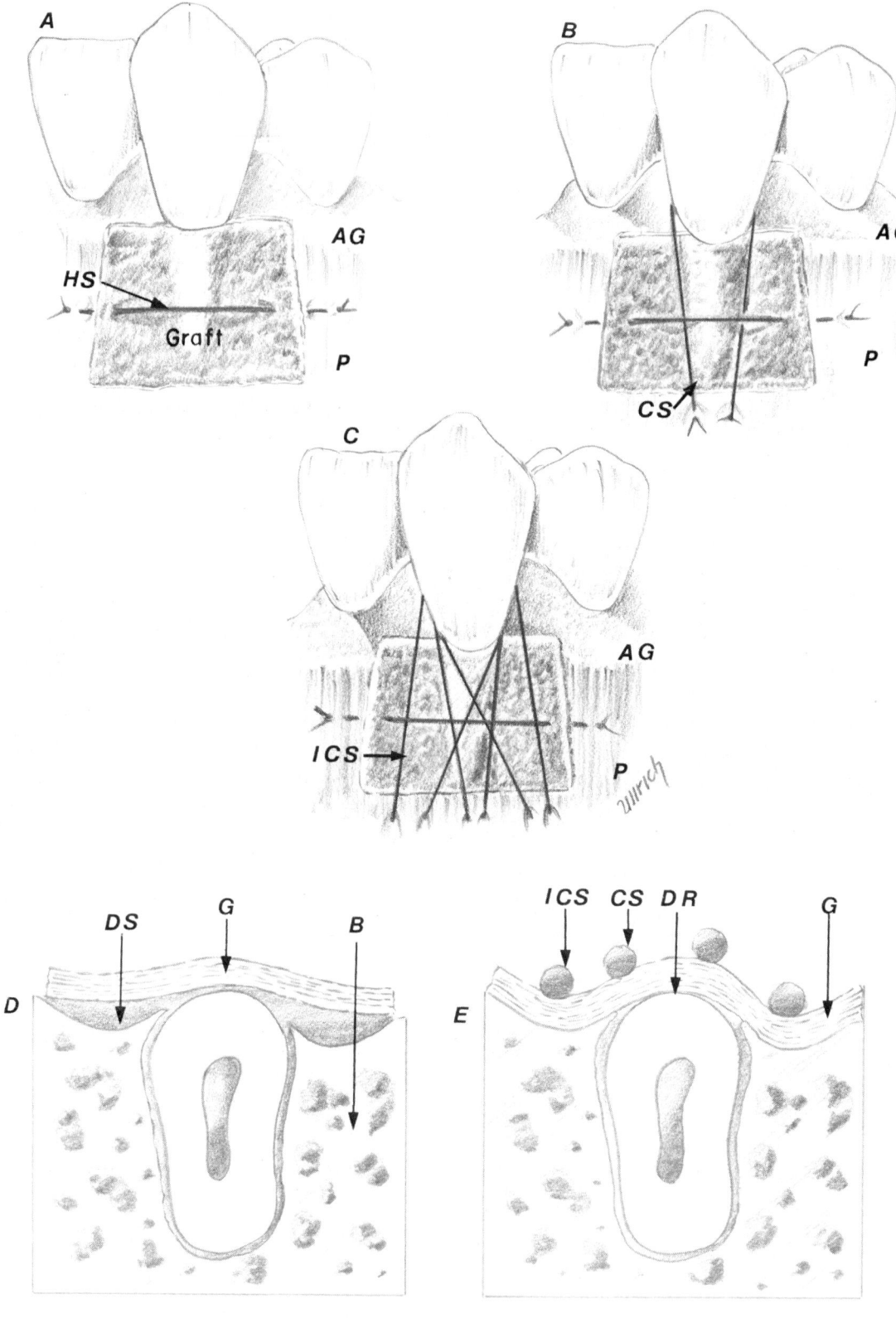

Fig. 9-8. Suturing Modification for Root Coverage (Holbrook and Ochsenbein Technique). **A,** Graft placement with initial horizontal stretching (HS) suture. **B,** Circumferential suture (CS) placed. **C,** Interdental concavity sutures (ICS) are now placed. **D,** Graft–periosteum relationship with normal suturing; note dead space (DS) between graft and concavity. **E,** Intimate graft–periosteum contact using suturing modification.

Cosmetic Root Coverage: Gingival Augmentation

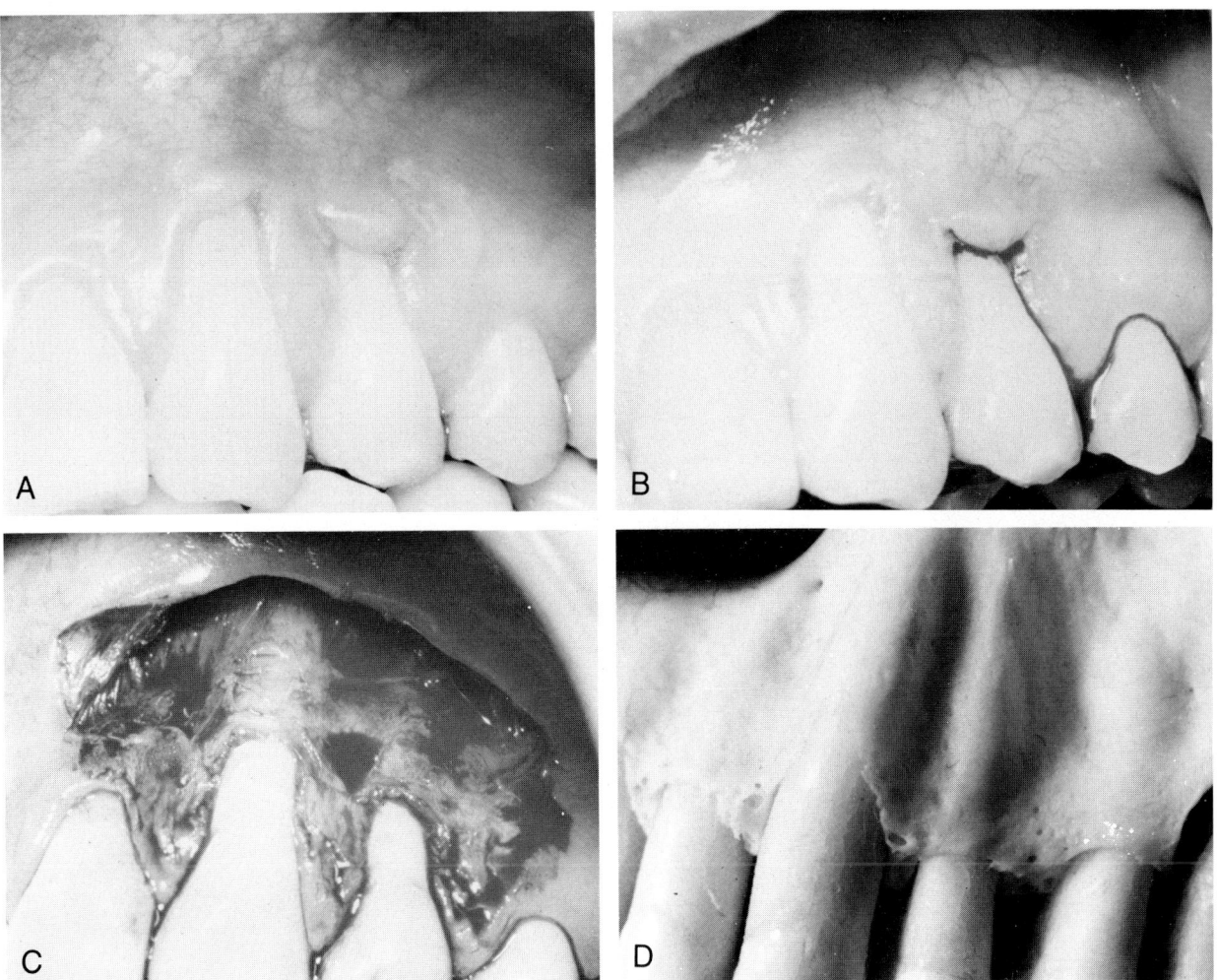

Fig. 9-9. Free Soft-Tissue Autograft with *Creeping Attachment.* **A,** Before. **B,** Citric acid applied. **C,** Mucosal flap reflected, showing prominent roots. **D,** Skull specimen showing prominent roots with depressions, similar to clinical situation.

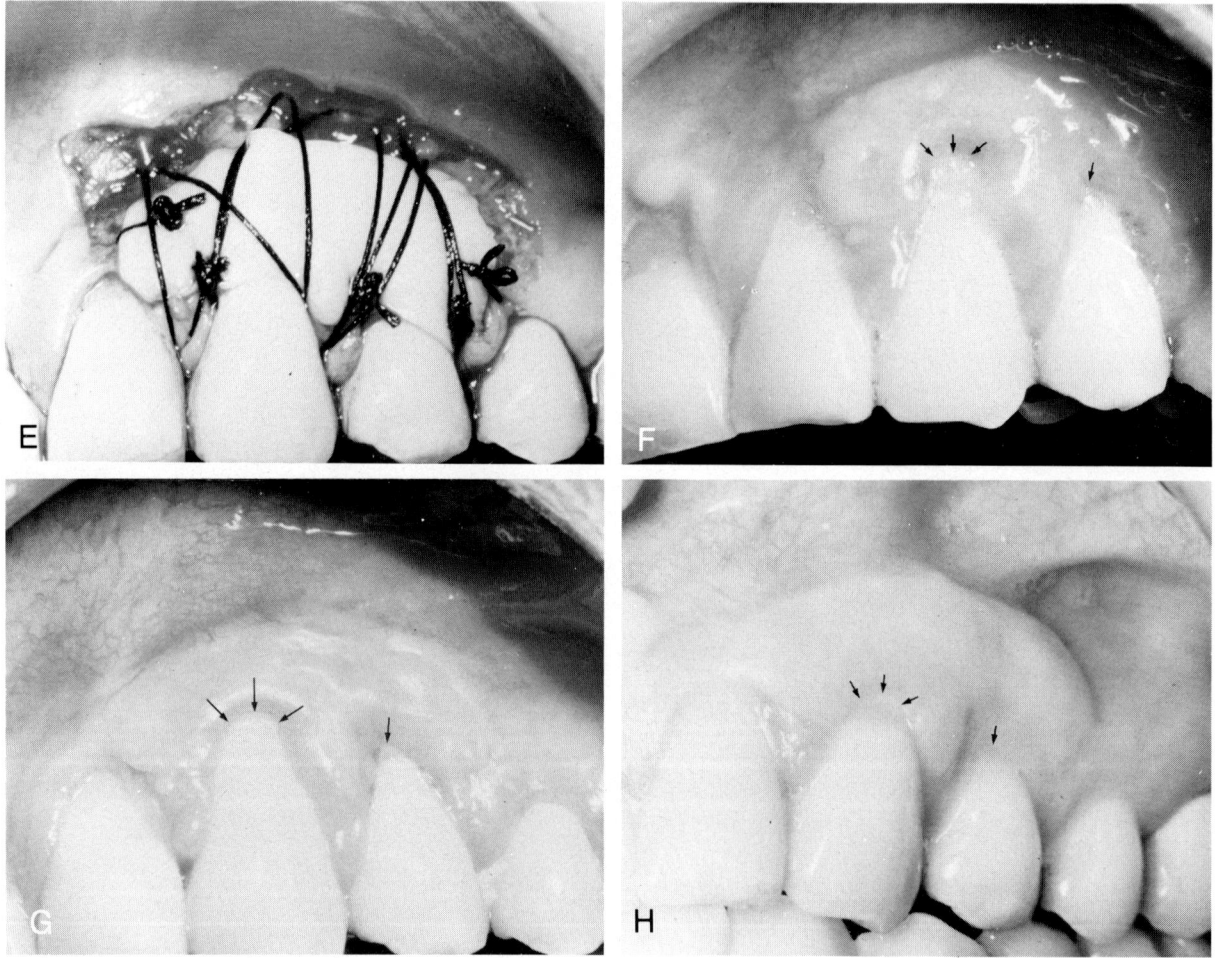

Fig. 9-9 (continued). **E,** Graft sutured in position, using Holbrook and Ochsenbein suturing modification. **F,** Three weeks later; arrows indicate extent of root coverage. **G,** Ten weeks later; arrows indicate coronal migration of tissue. **H,** Six months later; coronal migration of creeping attachment complete. Compare with A and F.

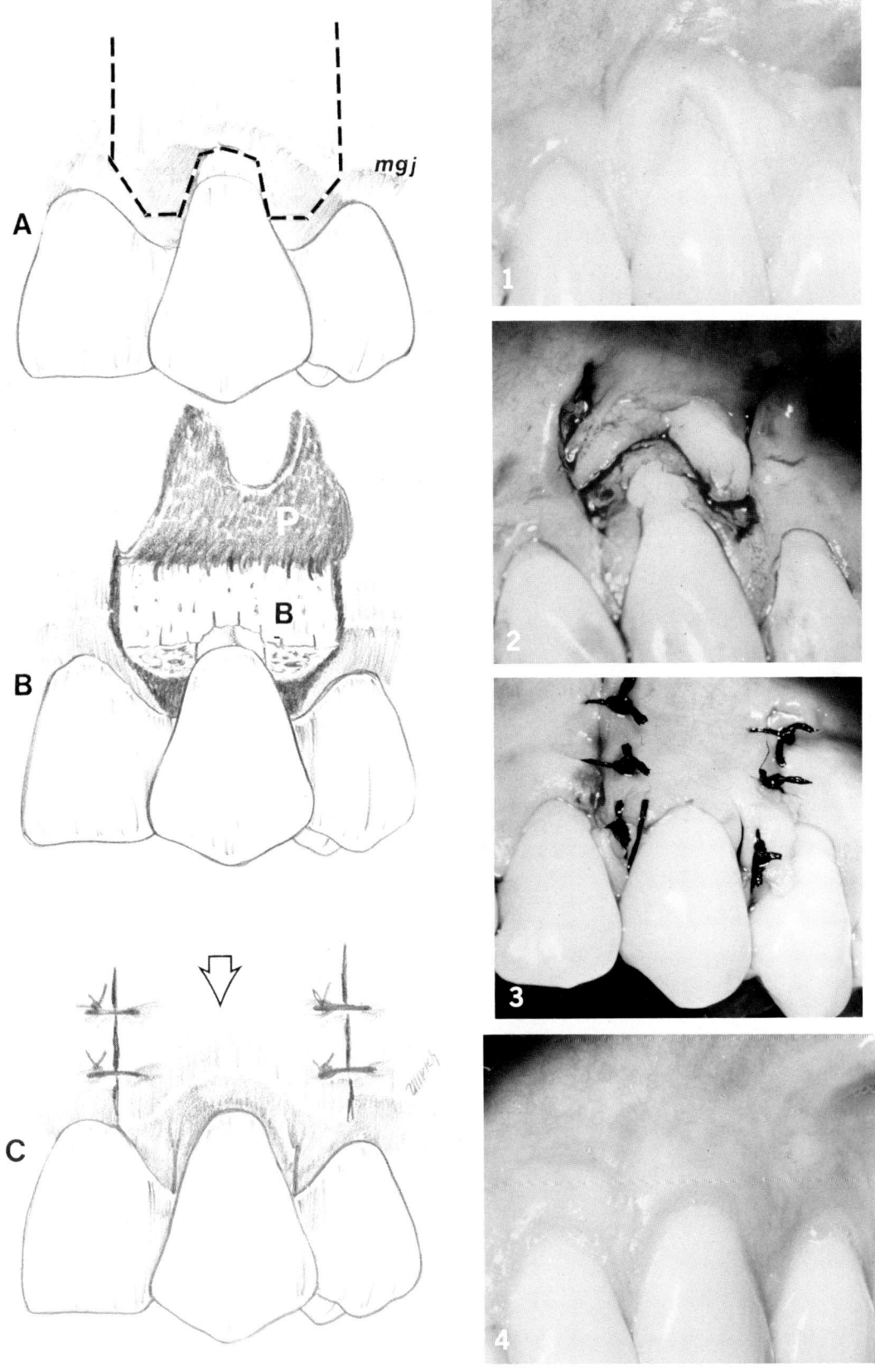

Fig. 9-10. Coronally Positioned Pedicle Flap. Diagrammatic View: **A,** Incisions outlined preoperatively. Note that incisions do not go to the tips of the papillae. **B,** A full-thickness flap is reflected, exposing the underlying bone (B). The epithelium overlying the remaining portion of the papillae is removed. **C,** The flap is sutured coronally for root coverage. Clinical View: **1,** Before. **2,** Full-thickness flap reflected. **3,** Epithelium over remaining papillae removed and flap sutured coronally. **4,** Two years later; compare with 1.

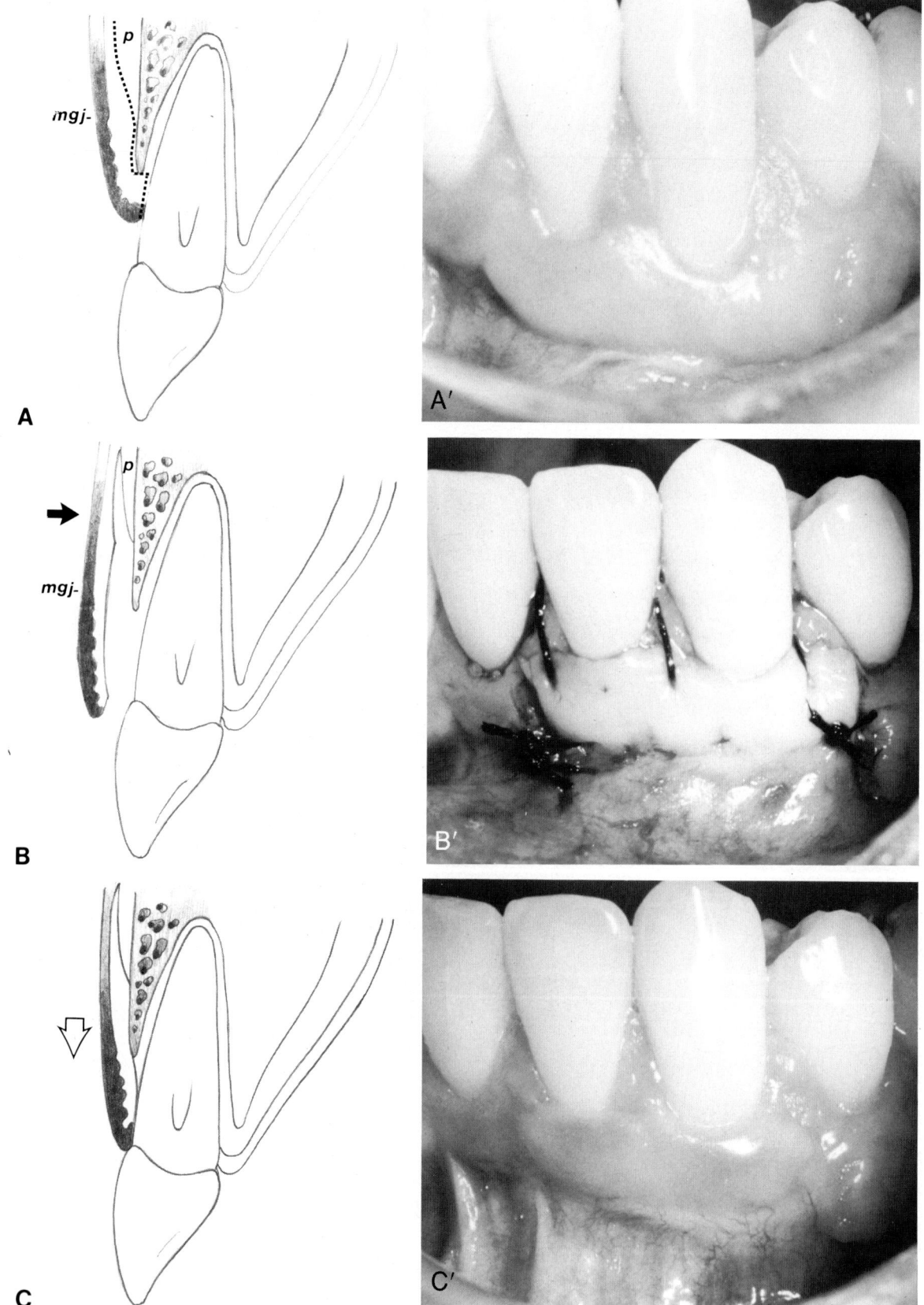

Fig. 9-11. Coronally Positioned Flap. **A, A′,** Before treatment. Incisions are outlined to show sulcular incisions, partial or full thickness over bone, and apical release to permit coronal movement of flap. **B,** Flap reflected. **B′, C,** Coronal positioning of flap to CEJ. **C′,** Completed clinical case.

dures necessary for achieving success with the subepithelial connective tissue graft. Nelson (1987) modified the procedure somewhat to further enhance clinical predictability (≧90%).

The technique gains its clinical predictability by use of a *bilaminar flap* (Nelson 1987, Harris 1992) design to assure graft vascularity and a high degree of gingival cosmetics from the secondary-intention healing of the connective tissue graft. This seems to avoid the *"tire patch"* look often associated with free gingival grafts. Jahnke et al. (1993), in comparing free gingival grafts (FGG) to subepithelial connective tissue grafts (CTG), found the CTG to be significantly ($p<0.03$) more effective than the FGG.

Indications

1. Esthetics
2. Predictability
3. One-step procedure
4. Minimum palatal trauma
5. Can treat multiple teeth
6. Increased graft vascularity

Disadvantages

1. High degree of technical skill required
2. Complicated suturing

Contraindications

1. Broad, shallow palates where contact with the palatal artery may be anticipated.
2. Excessively glandular or fatty palatal submucosa.

Procedure

The procedure is basically a combination of a partial-thickness coronally positioned flap and a free connective tissue graft.

Recipient Site

1. The root surface is scaled and root planed to flatten prominent convexities and to remove any softened root structure, endotoxins, and composite restorations. Enamel finishing burs may be used to help flatten the root convexity in the central portion of the root or after removal of composite restorations.
2. Optional use of chemical root modifiers: citric acid (pH 1.0 for 3 to 5 minutes) or tetracycline (3 to 5 minutes).
3. A No. 15 scalpel is used to outline the surgical site, making sure to raise a partial thickness flap (no incisions are made down to bone). The scalloped papillary incisions must be made above the CEJ to assume total root coverage and so that an adequate bleeding surface is prepared (Fig. 9-12A,B).
4. Two vertical incisions are extended adequately into the mucosal tissues to permit coronal positioning of the flap. The partial-thickness flap is raised by sharp dissection (Fig. 9-12C).
5. Apically the undersurface of the flap is released from the underlying periosteum via a horizontal incision. This will permit coronal positioning of the flap (Fig. 9-12D).

Donor Site

Unlike the free gingival graft, the connective tissue graft is taken internally and *is not* limited by rugae.

1. A straight, horizontal incision is begun approximately 5 to 6 mm from the free gingival margin with a No. 15 scalpel blade. The incision is begun in the molar areas and extended anteriorly. The blade is used to undermine a partial-thickness palatal flap (Fig. 9-13A,A'). *Note:* The length and width of the partial-thickness palatal flap will vary with the size of exposed root to be covered. *It is also important to note that if additional graft length is required the incisions may be carried anteriorly into the rugae area since the connective tissue graft is not adversely affected by the rugae.*
2. A second, more coronally positioned parallel incision is now made approximately 3 mm from the gingival margin with a No. 15 blade. It is continued apically to the same level as the first incision. The blade may have to be angled toward the bone to ensure adequate graft thickness (Fig. 9-13B,B'). *Note:* This second incision will produce a connective tissue wedge with a 2- to 3-mm-wide epithelial border and is 1.5 to 2 mm in thickness.
3. Vertical incisions (optional) are used for graft release mesially and distally. They are made from the outer epithelial surface down through the submucosa. This will free the terminal ends of the graft (Fig. 9-13C,C').
4. To completely free the graft, a horizontal incision is made at its most apical border (Fig. 9-13D,D').
5. Upon removal the graft is placed on a saline moistened gauze sponge (Fig. 9-13E,E').
6. The palate is now sutured with a combination of horizontal mattress sutures or continuous basting sutures. Immediate suturing will promote hemostasis and prevent excessive clot formation (Fig. 9-13F,F').

The clinical procedure of donor site management is depicted in Figure 9-14.

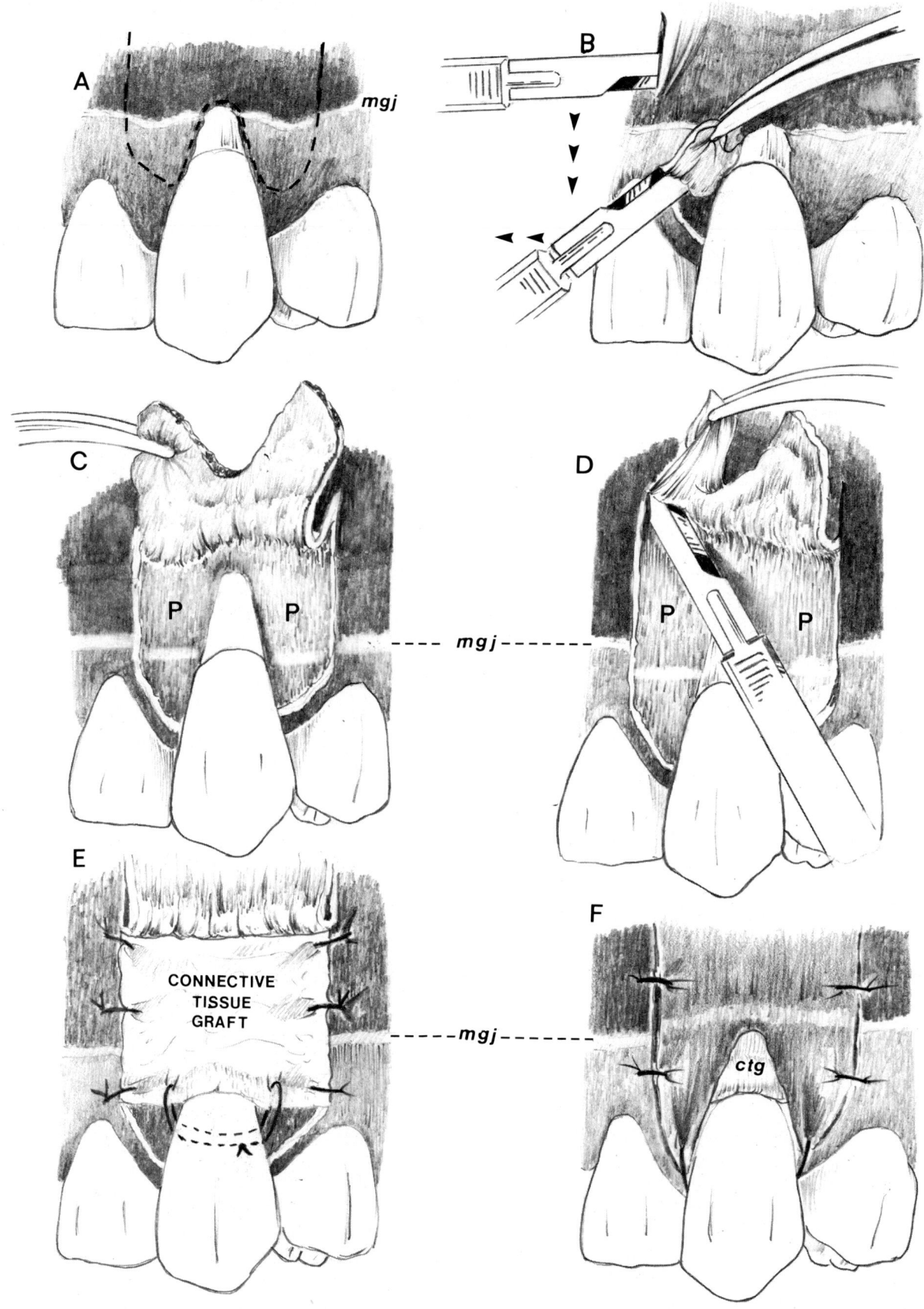

Fig. 9-12. Subepithelial Connective Tissue Graft: Recipient Site. **A,** Before treatment with incisions outlined. **B,** Partial-thickness pedicle flap reflected by sharp dissection. **C,** Partial-thickness pedicle flap is reflected. **D,** Apical border of pedicle flap is released to permit coronal repositioning. **E,** Connective tissue graft positioned and sutured with epithelium positioned onto the enamel. **F,** Flap coronally positioned and sutured.

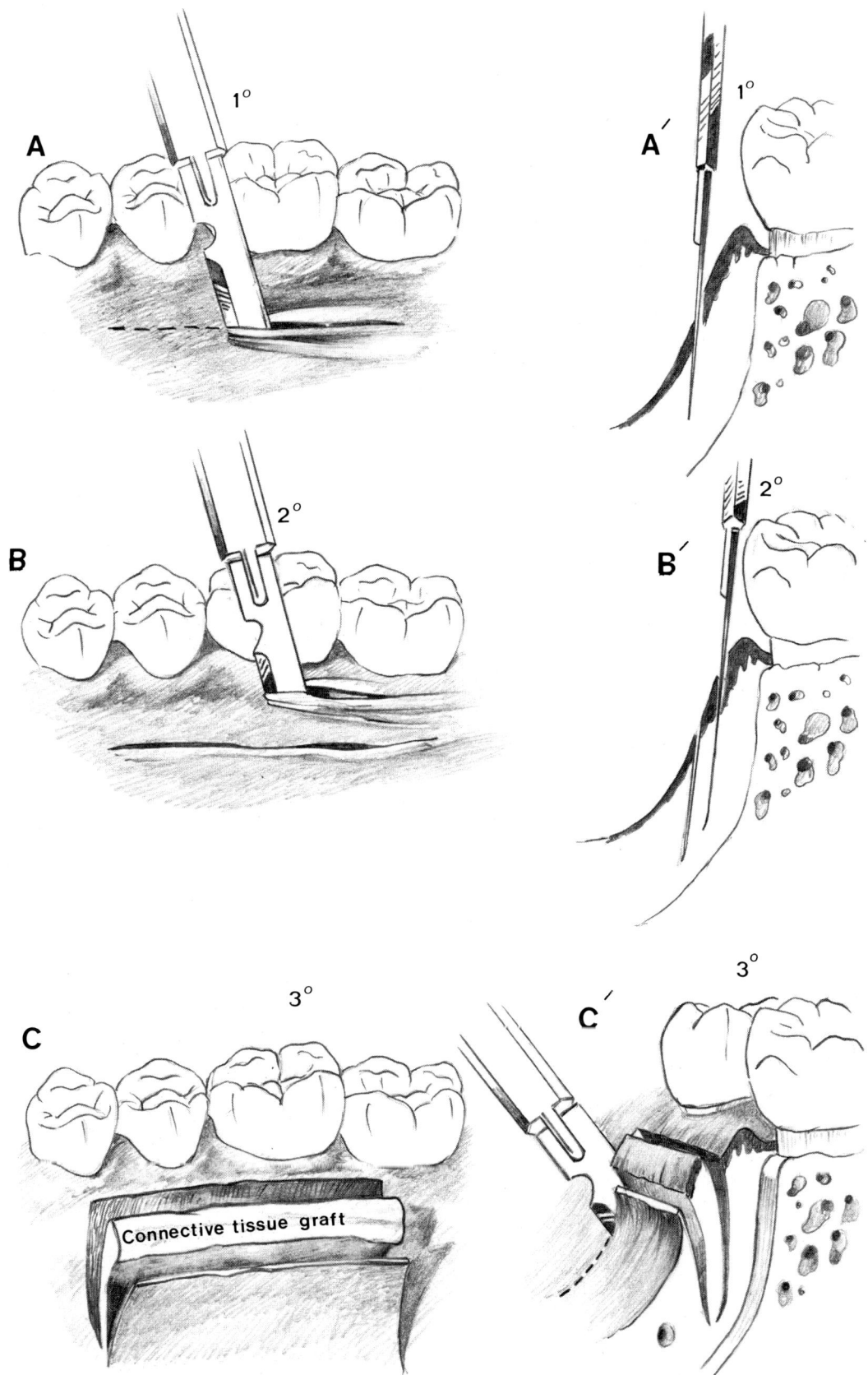

Fig. 9-13. Subepithelial Connective Tissue Graft: Donor Site (Palatal and Cross-Sectional Views). **A,A′,** Primary horizontal partial-thickness incision begun 5 to 7 mm from free gingival margin. **B,B′,** Secondary horizontal incision made 2 to 3 mm from gingival margin. Incisions are directed apically to provide a connective tissue graft 1.5 to 2 mm in thickness and a length sufficient to cover the exposed root surface to be covered. **C,C′,** Optional vertical incisions are made at the terminal ends of the graft.

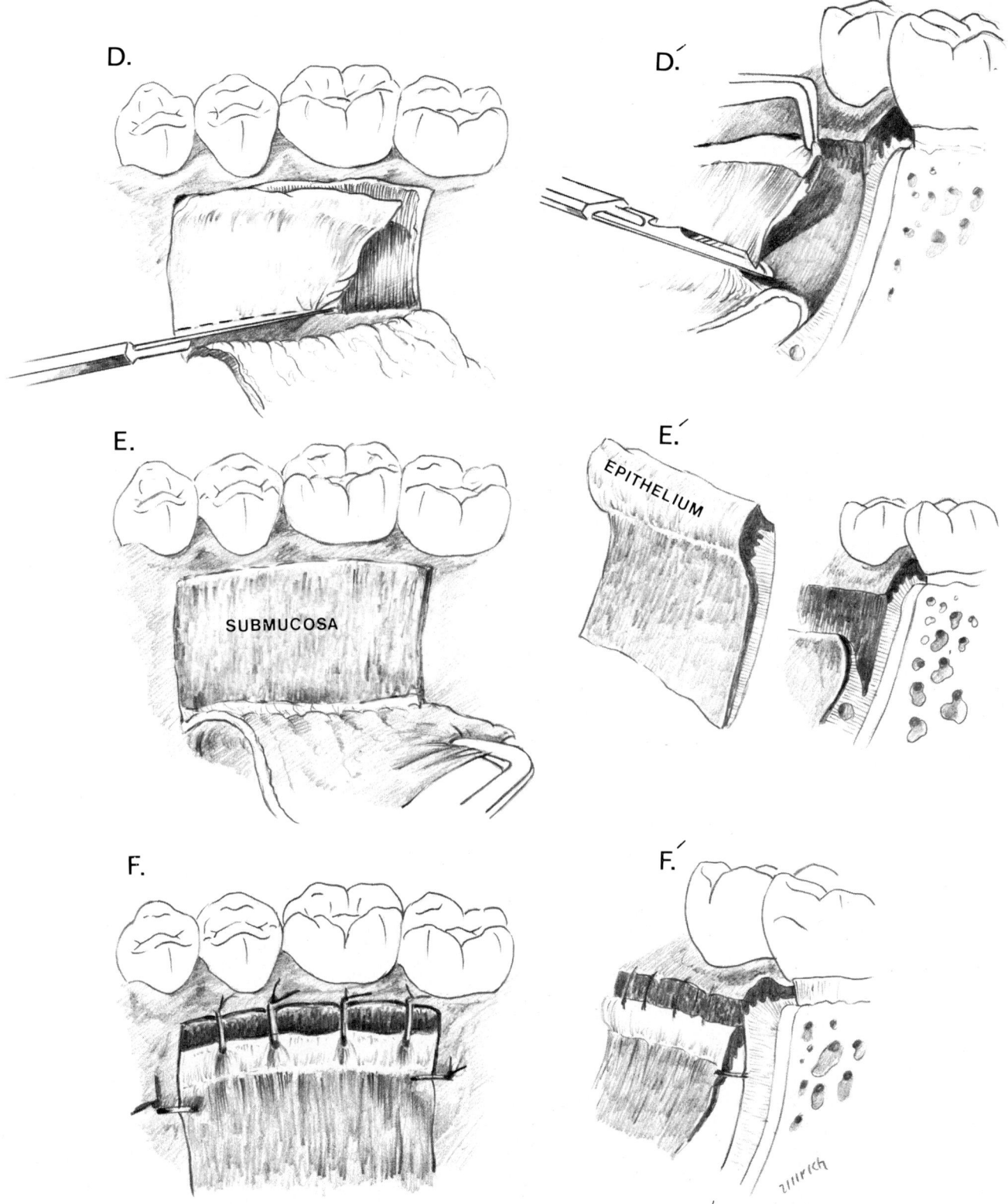

Fig. 9-13 (continued). **D,D′,** The primary flap is reflected. With the graft held in a tissue forceps, it is released apically with a sharp horizontal incision. **E,E′,** The subepithelial graft is removed and the underlying submucosa exposed. **F,F′,** Primary flap sutured with almost complete coverage obtained. Suturing can be interrupted, continuous, or suspensory.

Cosmetic Root Coverage: Gingival Augmentation

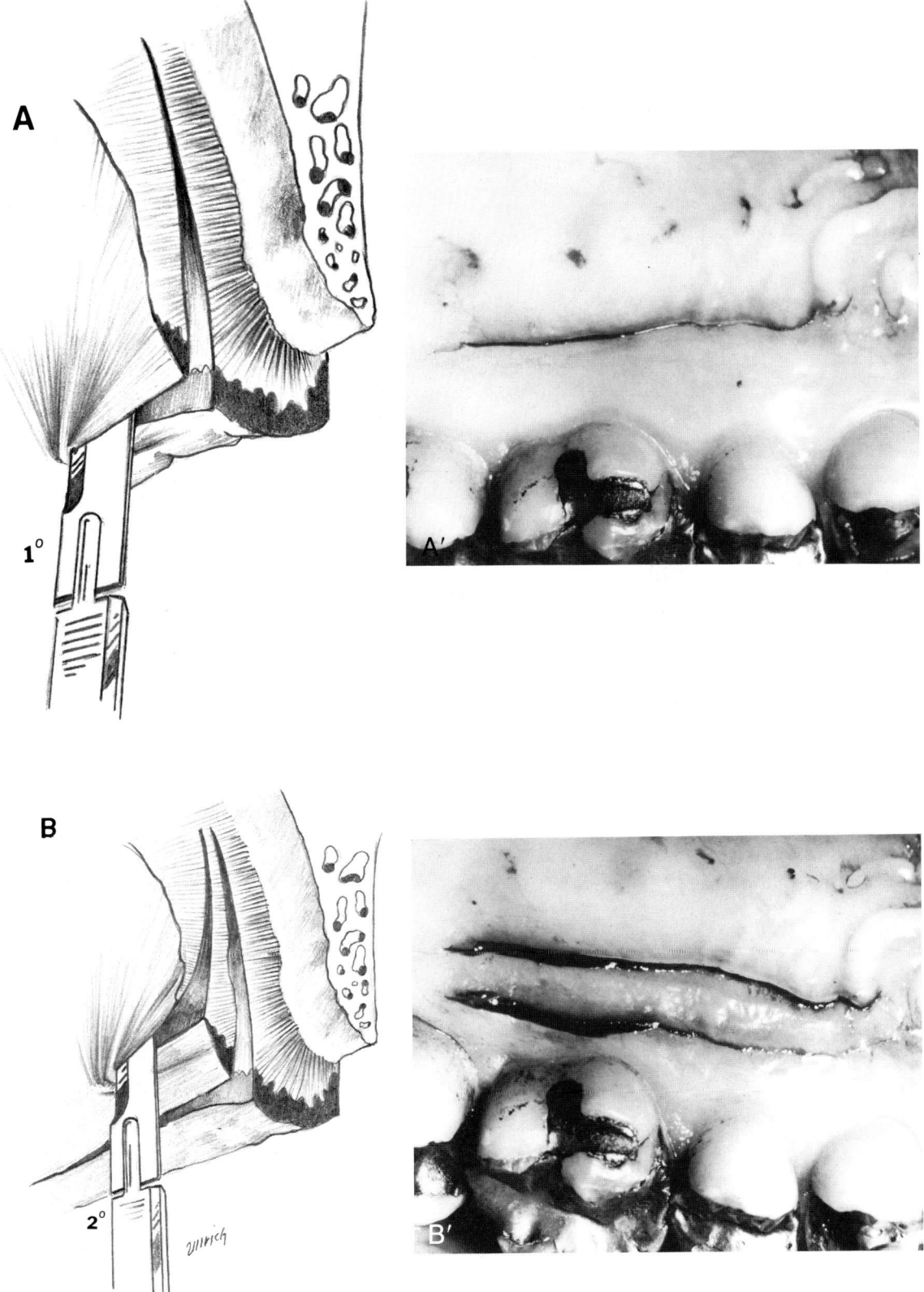

Fig. 9-14. Subepithelial Connective Tissue Graft Donor Site. **A,A′,** 1° horizontal incision being made. **B,B′,** 2° horizontal incision being made.

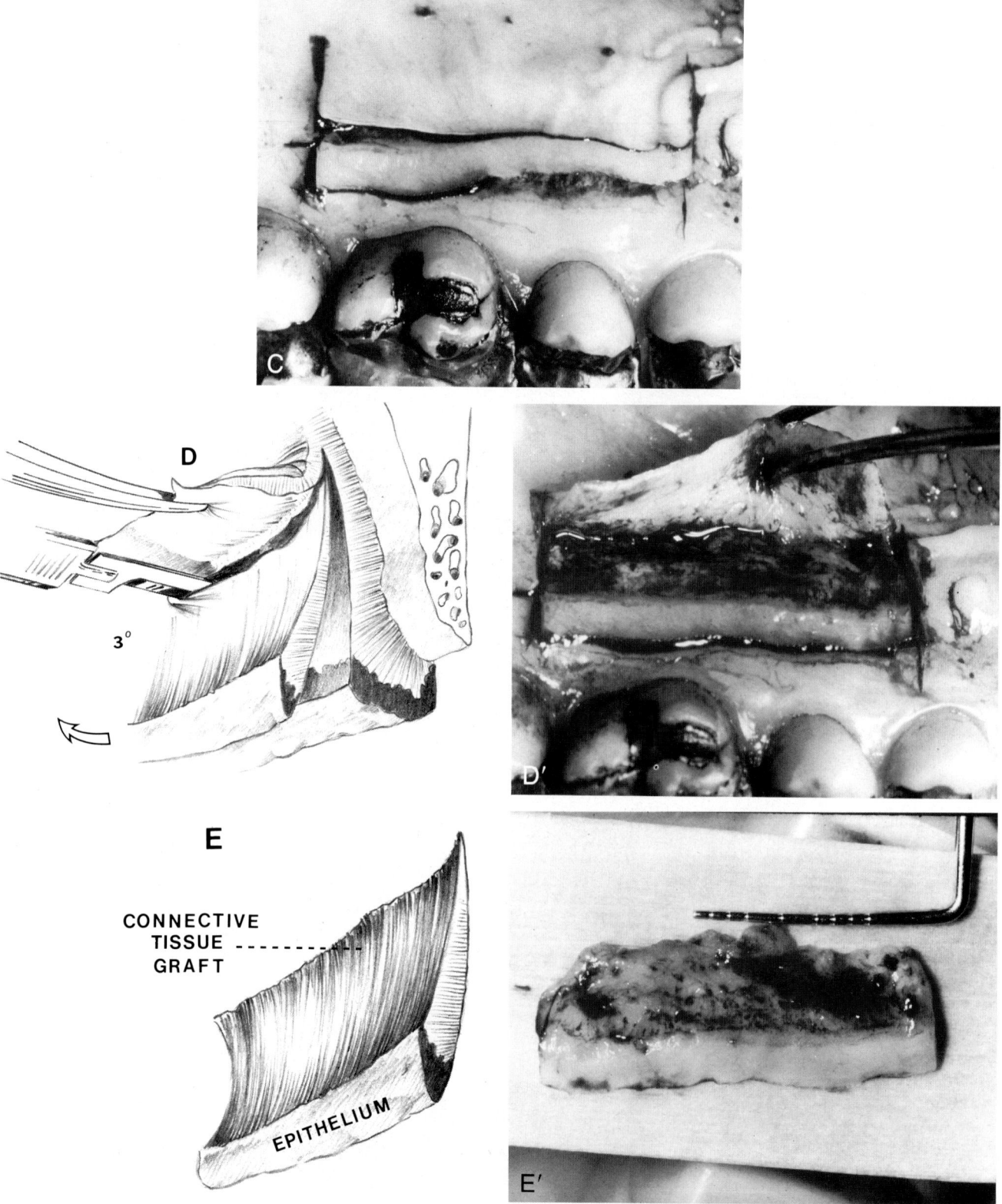

Fig. 9-14 (continued). C, Vertical incisions outline the graft. **D,D',** Apical horizontal incision is now made for graft release. **E,E',** Connective tissue graft is freed.

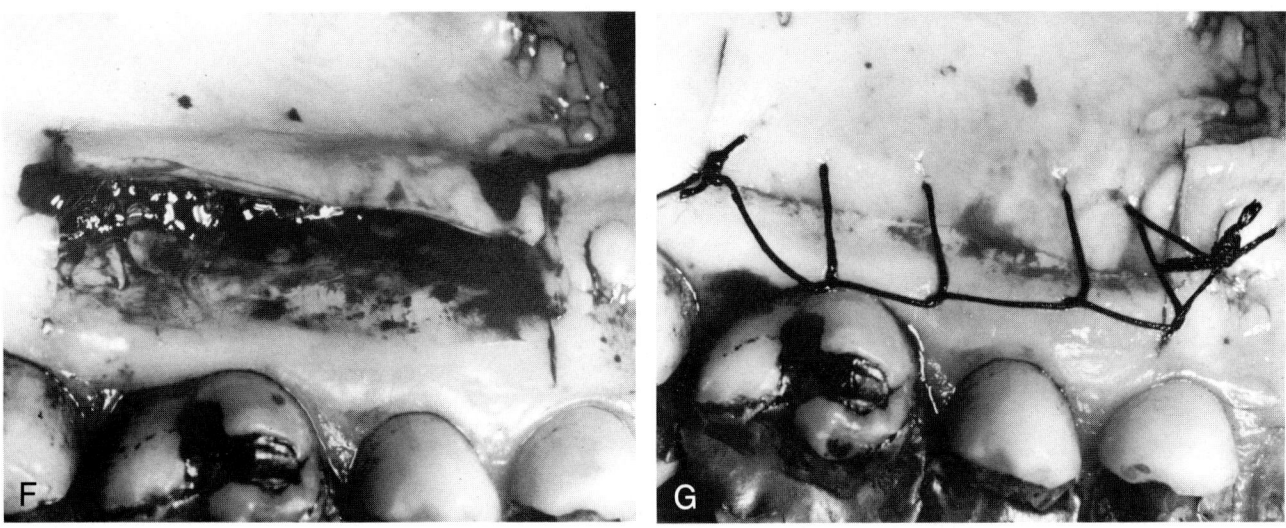

Fig. 9-14 (continued). **F,** Submucosa after graft removal. **G,** Palatal primary flap sutured with horizontal basting suture.

Graft Placement

1. The graft is trimmed to size with a sharp scissors or No. 15 blade. *There is no need for complete removal of glandular or fatty tissue.*
2. The graft is placed so that the epithelial border is positioned *above the CEJ and onto the enamel.* This will assure greater root coverage, predictability, and enhanced esthetics (Fig. 9-12E).
3. Intimate graft–root contact is achieved by stabilizing the graft first laterally with interrupted sutures and second by using a continuous sling suture about the necks of the teeth for cervical positioning and stabilization. To avoid problems of retrieval, chromic gut sutures are recommended for graft positioning and stabilization (Fig. 9-12E). *Note:* This suturing technique will inhibit graft mobility, prevent underlying clot formation, and promote initial graft viability.
4. The primary flap is now coronally positioned and sutured with 4-0 silk (P-3 needle) to cover as much of the graft as possible. The flap is positioned laterally with interrupted sutures and coronally with a suspensary sling suture (Fig. 9-12F).

It is important to note that 6 to 10 weeks after surgery a gingivoplasty is often required for establishing final gingival contours and for reduction of tissue bulk.

Common Reasons For Failure

According to Langer and Langer (1992), common reasons for failure of this procedure are

1. Recipient bed is too small to provide an adequate blood supply.
2. Flap perforation(s).
3. Inadequate graft size.
4. Inadequate coronal positioning of flap.
5. Too thick a connective tissue graft.
6. Poor root preparation.
7. Poor papillary bed preparation.

The clinical procedure is depicted in Figures 9-15, 9-16, 9-17, and 9-18.

SUBPEDICLE CONNECTIVE TISSUE GRAFT

Nelson (1987) modified Langer and Langer's (1985) original technique by using a pedicle flap to cover the connective tissue graft. He called this a *subpedicle bilaminar graft.* He was able to achieve an average of 88% root coverage in a group of advanced cases having recession of 7 to 10 mm. Harris (1992) achieved 97.4% root coverage with the combination of double pedicle flap over a connective tissue graft.

Advantages

1. Predictable root coverage
2. Ability to increase the width of keratinized gingiva

Disadvantages

The main disadvantage is the difficulty in handling, positioning, and suturing small pedicle flaps.

Procedure

In Figures 9-19 and 9-21 we see the procedures depicted.
1. The root surface is scaled and root planed to reduce and remove prominent cervical convexities. Finishing burs and biochemical root modifiers are optional.
2. A No. 15 scalpel is used to outline the surgical site, and a partial thickness flap is chased by sharp dissection (Figs. 9-19B and 9-21B). As always, the sharp dissection is begun at the mucogingival junction and carried coronally.
3. The flaps are reflected (Figs. 19-19C and 19-21C), and the connective tissue graft is obtained and sutured as previously described (Figs. 19-19D and 19-21D).
4. The pedicles are either singularly, as in a rotated pedicle flap (Fig. 9-21E), or dually, in a double papilla pedicle flap, sutured in place with 4-0 or 5-0 silk using a P-3 needle (Figs. 9-19F and 9-20F).

The clinical procedure is depicted in Figs. 9-20 and 9-22.

SEMILUNAR FLAP

The semilunar flap, a modification of the coronally positioned flap, was originated by Tarnow (1986). It is designed primarily for attaining esthetic root coverage where only 2 to 3 mm of root coverage is required.

Indications

Areas where gingival recession is only 2 to 3 mm.

Advantages

1. No vestibular shortening as occurs with the coronally positioned flap
2. No esthetic compromise of interproximal papillae
3. No need for sutures

Cosmetic Root Coverage: Gingival Augmentation

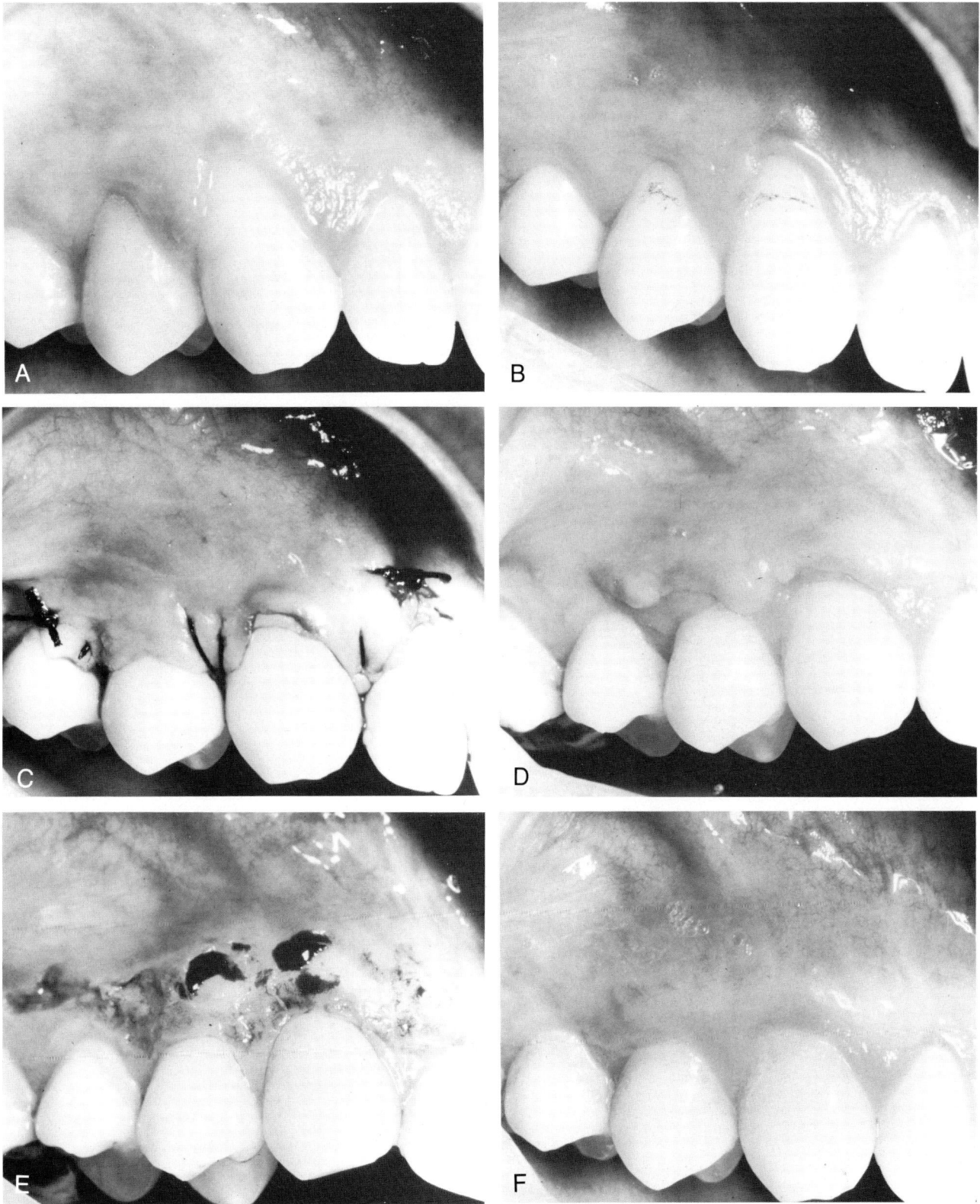

Fig. 9-15. Subepithelial Connective Tissue Graft. **A,B,** Before treatment. Pencil outlines CEJ. **C,** Connective tissue graft secured and covered by coronally positioned flap. **D,** Eight weeks later, tissue shows uneven gingival margin. **E,** Gingivoplasty 8 weeks later. **F,** Four months later with complete esthetic coverage.

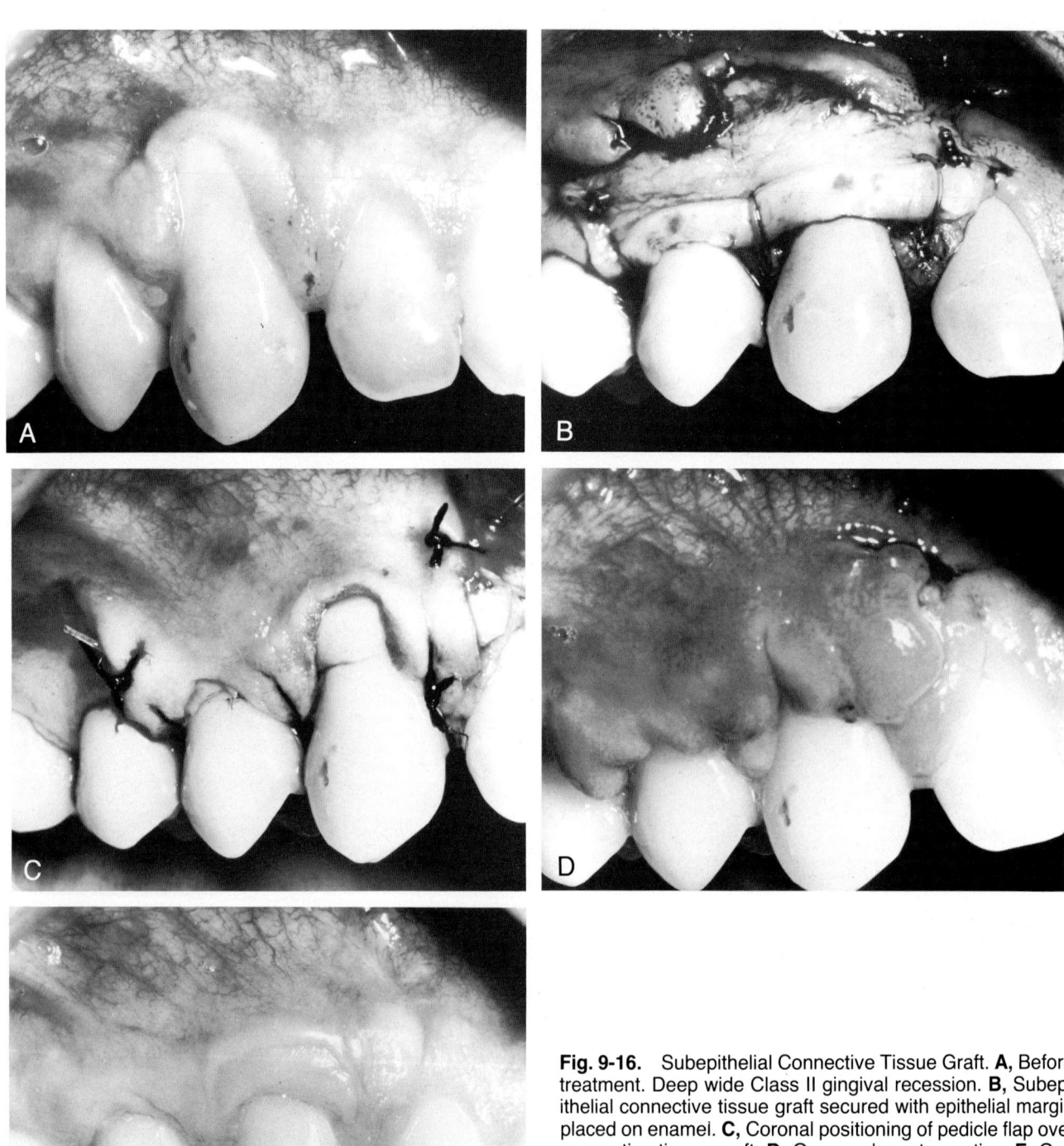

Fig. 9-16. Subepithelial Connective Tissue Graft. **A,** Before treatment. Deep wide Class II gingival recession. **B,** Subepithelial connective tissue graft secured with epithelial margin placed on enamel. **C,** Coronal positioning of pedicle flap over connective tissue graft. **D,** One week postoperative. **E,** One year later. Note excellent result with no gingivoplasty.

Cosmetic Root Coverage: Gingival Augmentation

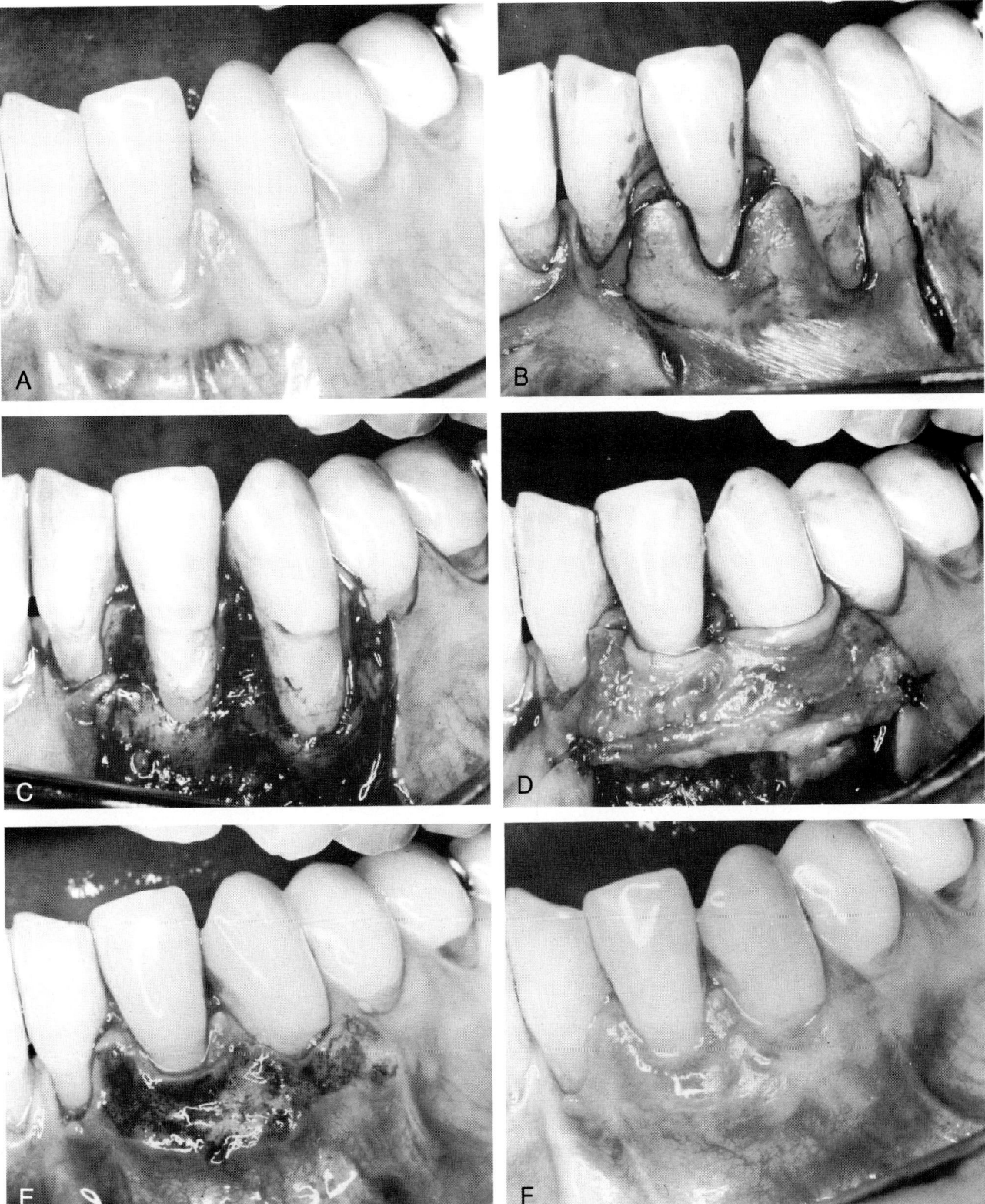

Fig. 9-17. Subepithelial Connective Tissue Graft. **A,** Flaps reflected. **B,** Partial-thickness pedicle flap outlined prior to reflection. **C,** Flap reflected and recession exposed. **D,** Connective tissue graft positioned and sutured. **E,** Gingivoplasty for enlarged, uneven gingival margin 6 to 8 weeks later. **F,** Final healing 1 month after gingivoplasty. Compare to A and C.

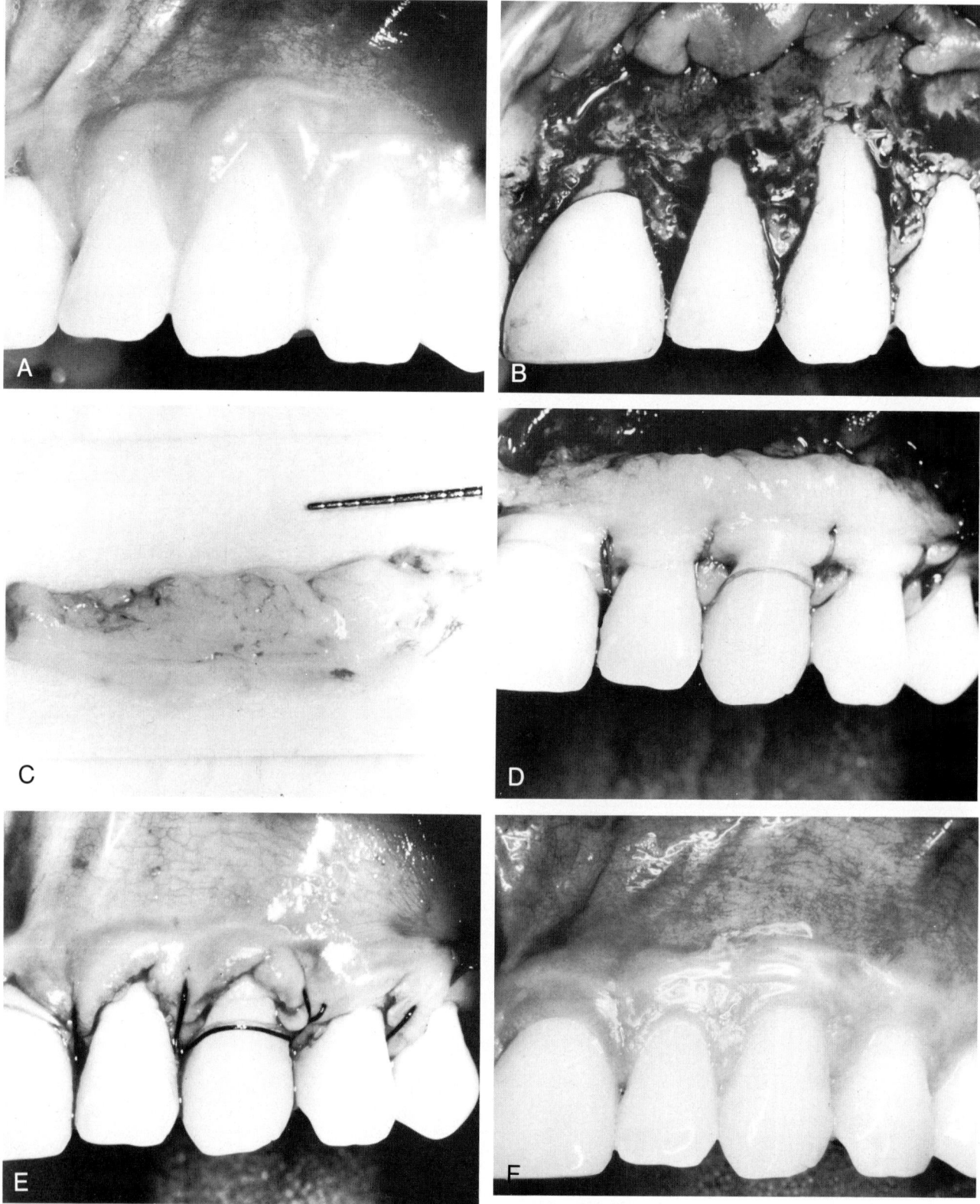

Fig. 9-18. Subepithelial Connective Tissue Graft. **A,** Before treatment; note multiple areas of recession. **B,** Partial-thickness flap reflected and recession exposed. **C,** Large connective tissue graft obtained. **D,** Connective tissue graft sutured with chromic gut sutures. **E,** Pedicle flap positioned and sutured coronally over graft. **F,** Six months later; note excellent result.

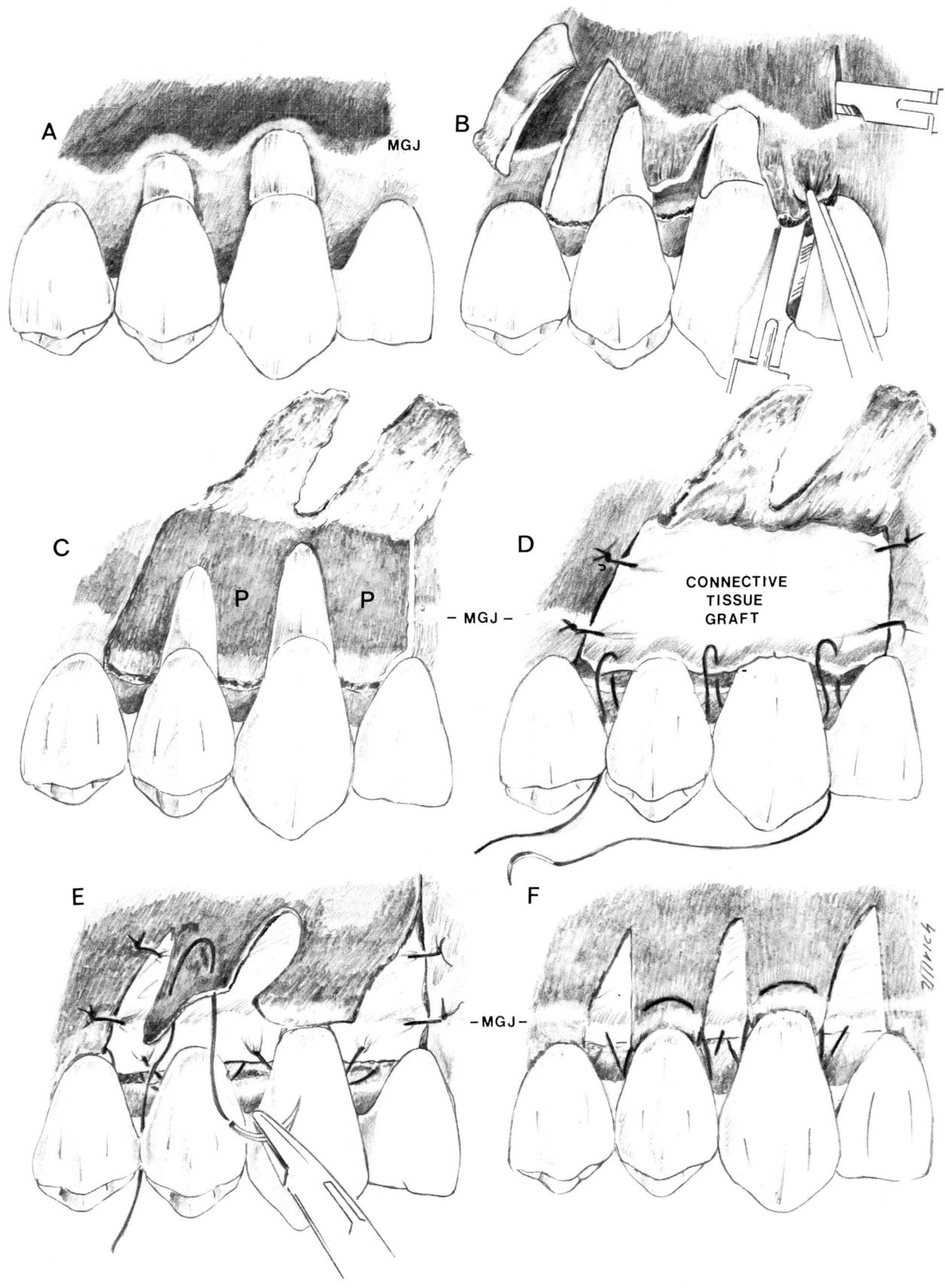

Fig. 9-19. Subepithelial Connective Tissue Graft: Modified Technique. **A,** Before surgery with incisions outlined. **B,** Sharp dissection of partial-thickness pedicle flap. **C,** Periosteal bed prepared. **D,** Connective tissue graft sutured. **E,** Pedicle flaps being sutured over radicular surface. **F,** Final suturing with pedicles covering facial aspect of graft.

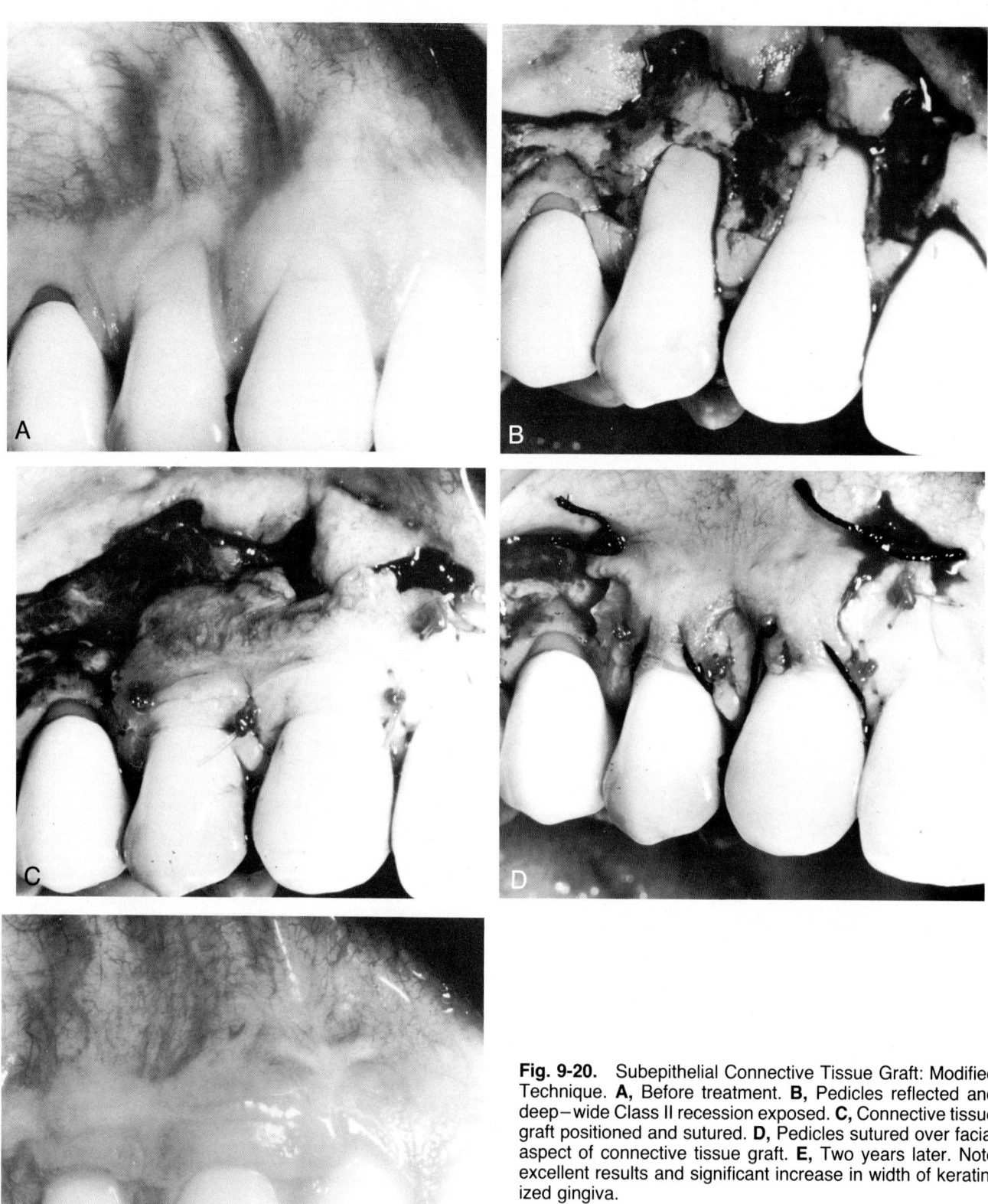

Fig. 9-20. Subepithelial Connective Tissue Graft: Modified Technique. **A,** Before treatment. **B,** Pedicles reflected and deep-wide Class II recession exposed. **C,** Connective tissue graft positioned and sutured. **D,** Pedicles sutured over facial aspect of connective tissue graft. **E,** Two years later. Note excellent results and significant increase in width of keratinized gingiva.

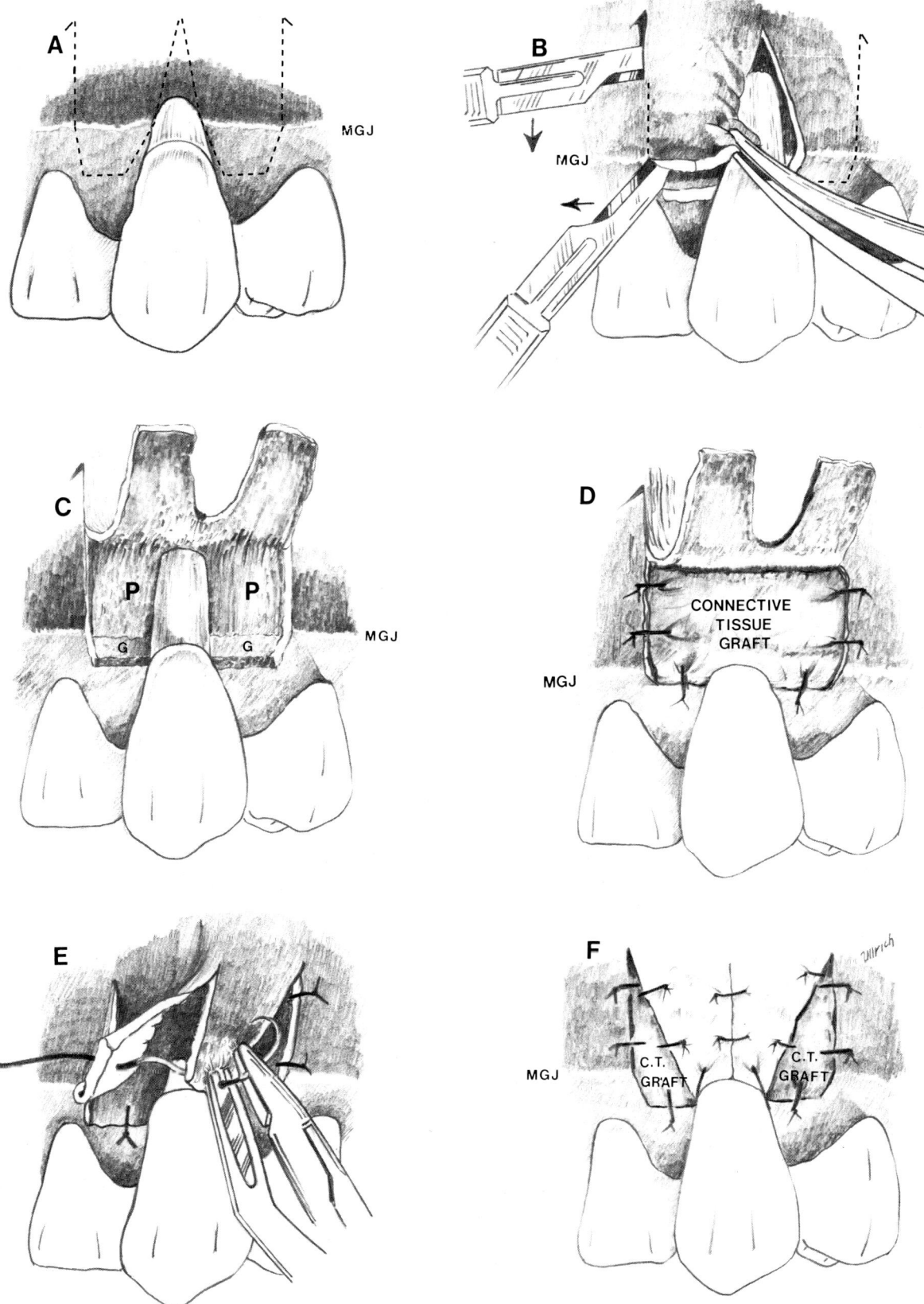

Fig. 9-21. Subepithelial Connective Tissue Graft: Modified Technique. **A,** Double papilla incisions outlined (see Double Papilla Flap in Chapter 5 for technique). **B,** Partial-thickness flap completed by sharp dissection. **C,** Periosteal bed prepared. **D,** Connective tissue graft sutured. **E,** Double-papilla flaps being sutured over the graft. **F,** Suturing completed. Radicular surface of graft covered by tissue.

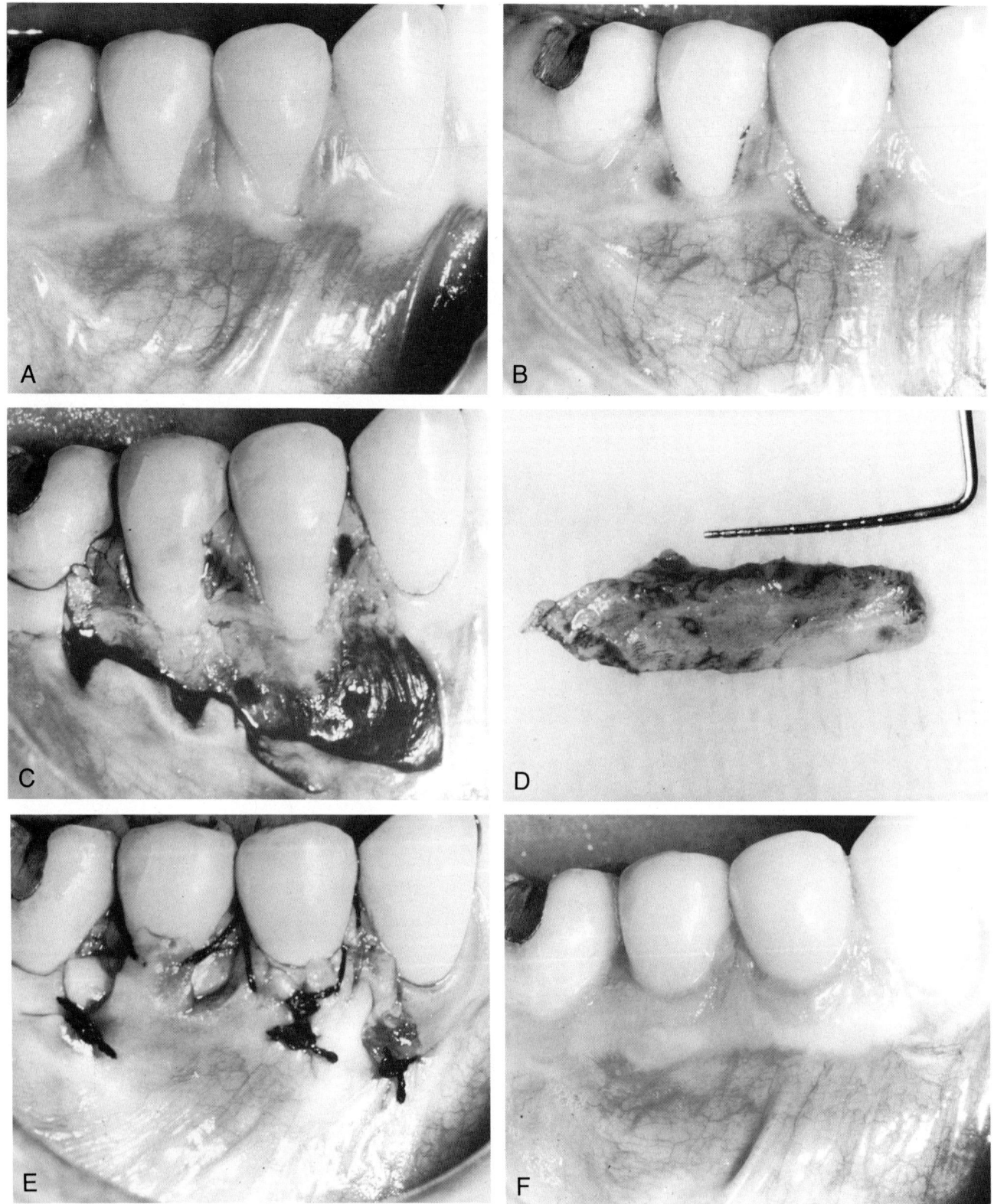

Fig. 9-22. Subepithelial Connective Tissue Graft: Modified Technique. **A,** Before treatment. **B,** Biomechanical root preparation with citric acid. **C,** Partial thickness flap reflected. **D,** Subepithelial connective tissue graft. **E,** Pedicles sutured over buccal radicular surface of teeth. **F,** Three years later. Complete root coverage with increased zone of keratinized gingiva.

Cosmetic Root Coverage: Gingival Augmentation

Disadvantages

1. Inability to treat large areas of gingival recession
2. The need for a free gingival graft if there is an underlying dehiscence or fenestration

Requirements

1. Lack of tissue inflammation
2. Minimal pocket depth labially

Procedure

1. The exposed root surface is root planed and biochemically modified (optional).
2. The incisions are outlined in Figure 9-23A and B. This is a partial-thickness procedure.
3. A No. 15 scalpel blade is used to outline a semilunar incision that follows the curvature of the gingival margin (Fig. 9-23C). The incision is not made down to bone.
4. The midfacial part of the incision should be high enough to ensure that after flap is coronally positioned the apical portion of the flap will still rest on bone (Fig. 9-23B). *Note:* If there is not enough keratinized gingiva the semilunar incision is made in the mucosal tissue (Fig. 9-23C).
5. The incision is extended into the papillae on each side, making sure that at least 2 mm of lateral tissue is left to ensure an adequate blood supply (Fig. 9-23D).
6. A partial-thickness flap is raised from the initial sulcular incision to the semilunar incision (Fig. 9-23E).
7. The midfacial tissue is positioned coronally to the CEJ. Pressure is applied for 5 minutes. The area is packed, and the patient is placed on a soft diet for 10 days with careful brushing (Fig. 9-23E).

The clinical procedure is depicted in Figures 9-24 and 9-25.

TRANSPOSITIONAL FLAP

This technique, as outlined by Bahat et al. (1990), appears to be a modification of the laterally positioned papillary flap as originally described by Pennel (1965), Hattler (1967), Garber, and Rosenberg (1984).

Advantages

1. Simple
2. Predictable for narrow areas of root exposure
3. Versatile
4. Avoids recession at donor site

Disadvantages

1. Cannot treat multiple teeth
2. Limited primarily to narrow areas of recession
3. Requires a wide papilla

Procedure

1. A No. 15 scalpel blade is used to outline two partial-thickness flaps (primary or donor; secondary or recipient). *The primary, or donor, flap is partial thickness to the mucogingival line and full thickness apical to it.* (Fig. 9-26A,B).
2. The outlined incisions of the primary flap follow obliquely along the exposed root surface, resulting in a pedicle flap with a wider base. These incisions are extended apically enough to ensure freedom of movement and permit a thick base (1.5 to 2 mm) with adequate vascularity (Fig. 9-26B).
3. The recipient periosteal bed is prepared by raising and disregarding the secondary flap using sharp dissection with a No. 15 blade (Fig. 9-26C).
4. Sharp dissection beginning below the mucogingival junction and moving the blade in an apicocoronal direction is used to raise the partial-thickness primary flap (Fig. 9-26C).
5. The pedicle is freed and released apically to assure freedom of movement (Fig. 9-26D).
6. The flap edge is sutured to the adjacent interproximal papilla at least 2 mm anterior to the defect. This is to avoid possible cleft formation (Fig. 9-26E).
7. The flap is now secured about the neck of the tooth by suturing the midflap portion to the remaining exposed papilla. Lateral sutures are for stabilization and approximation of the flap to the adjacent tissues (Fig. 9-26F).
8. Pressure is applied for 10 minutes for initial clot stability.

The clinical procedure is depicted in Figures 9-27 and 9-28.

CONNECTIVE TISSUE PEDICLE GRAFT

Carvalho et al. (1982) published a report on a modification in which the periosteum from the periosteal bed is used as a single or double pedicle flap for enhancing root coverage. The theory is that the pedicle increases the chance for graft survival over the denuded root by increasing the plasmatic circulation in the avascular area.

Procedure

The periosteal bed at the recipient site is prepared by sharp dissection in the usual way; epithelial denudation is completed (Fig. 9-29A).

The connective tissue pedicle flap is obtained by making an oblique incision on one or both sides of the tooth (Fig. 9-29B). The size of the pedicle varies with the size of the denuded root surface.

The pedicle(s) is raised by blunt dissection and held with Corn suture pliers as a 5-0 silk suture is passed through it (Fig. 9-29C).

Figures 9-29D and E show the suturing used when one or two pedicles are employed. Figure 9-29F represents graft placement and suturing.

This procedure is depicted clinically in Figure 9-30.

GUIDED TISSUE REGENERATION AND GINGIVAL RECESSION

Cortellini et al. (1991), Tinti et al. (1992), McGuire (1992), and Prato et al. (1992) recently advocated the use of guided tissue regeneration for correction of gingival recession. Although successful results are achievable, they do not surpass those of the free gingival graft or the subepithelial connective tissue graft. The procedure is more complex, in that it requires the need for a second surgical procedure. For that reason, it is not advocated for routine use unless bone regeneration is desired.

Cosmetic Root Coverage: Gingival Augmentation

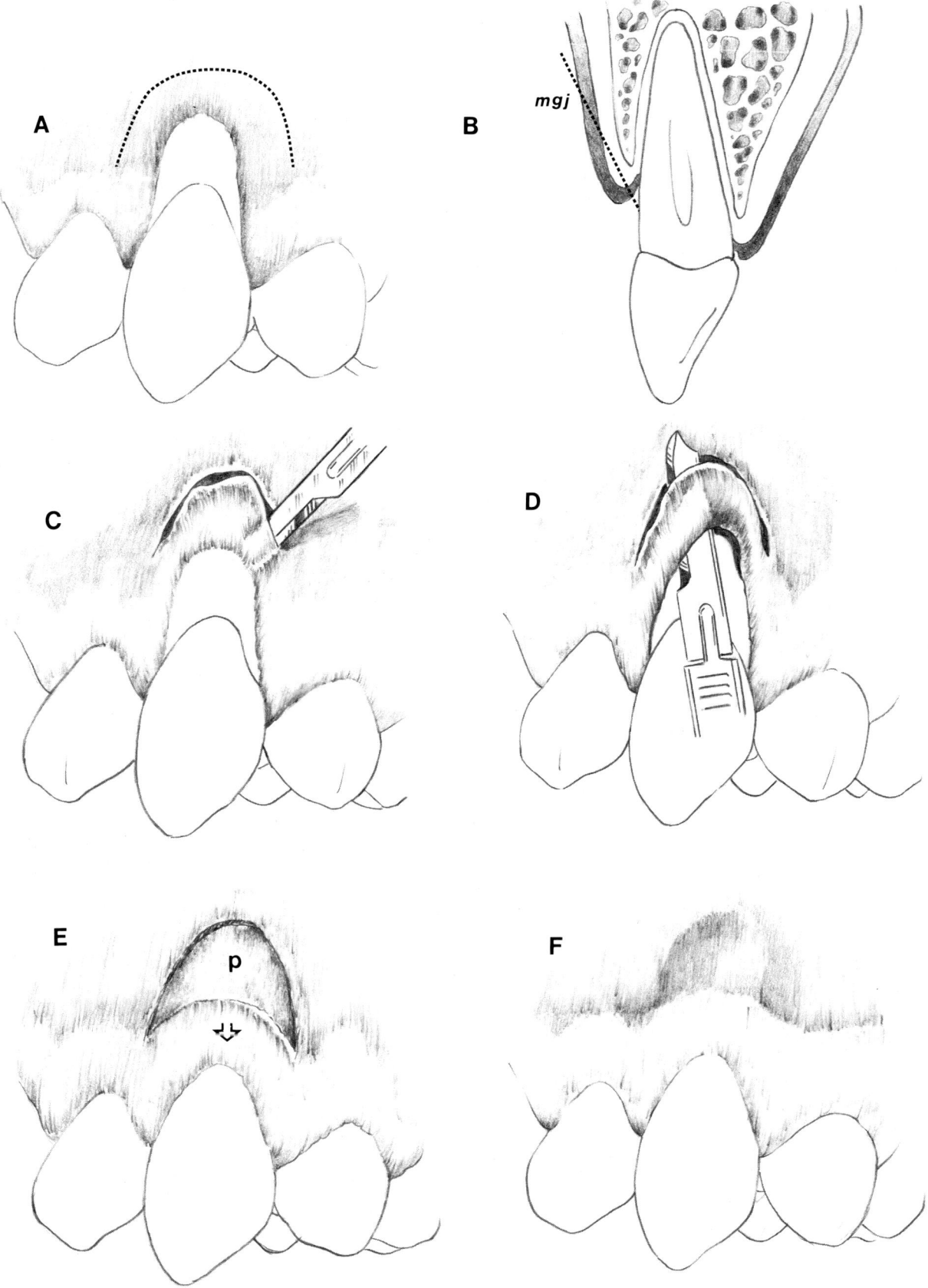

Fig. 9-23. Semilunar Flap. **A,** Before treatment. Incisions outlined buccally. **B,** Side view showing that incision is extended far enough apically. **C,** Semilunar incision is made by sharp dissection but not down to bone. **D,** The partial-thickness flap is via the sulcus. **E,** The semilunar flap is now moved coronally. **F,** Completed case.

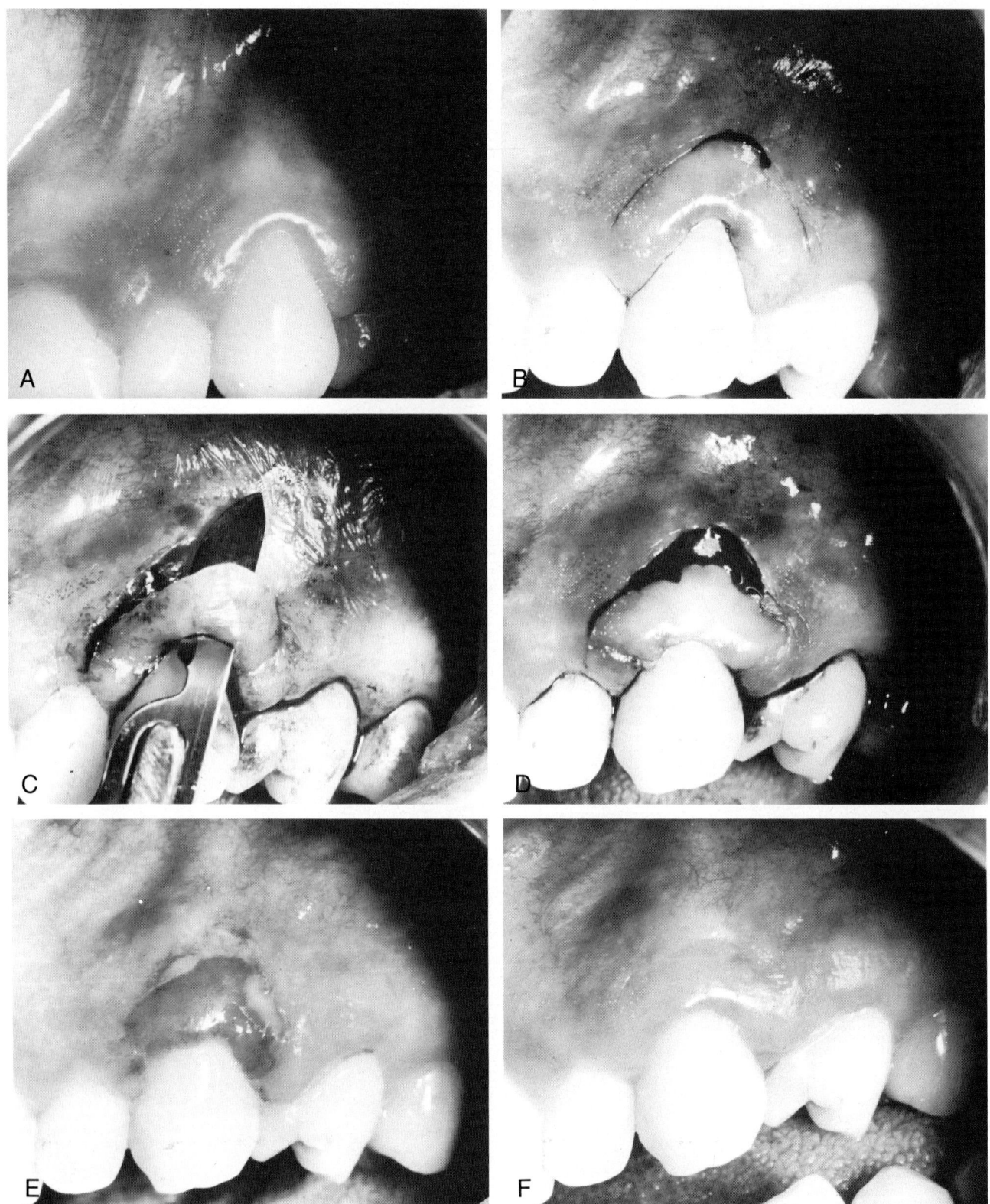

Fig. 9-24. Semilunar Flap. **A,** Before treatment. **B,** Partial-thickness semilunar incision. **C,** Semilunar flap raised by partial dissection. **D,** Flap moved coronally and stabilized in position by pressure. **E,** One week later. **F,** Three months later. Complete root coverage.

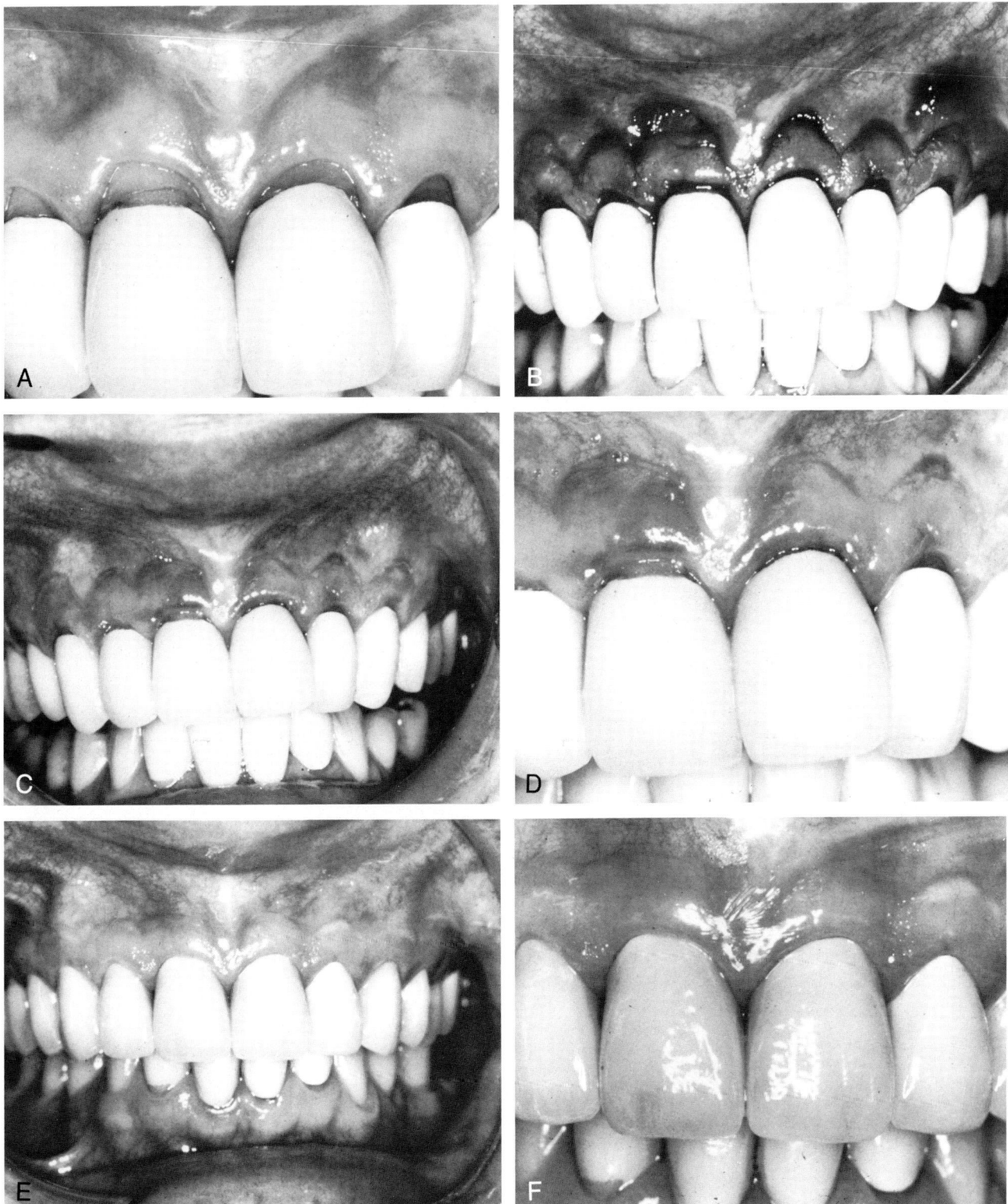

Fig. 9-25. Semilunar Flap: Multiple Teeth. **A,** Before treatment. **B,** Multiple semilunar flaps outlined and positioned coronally. **C,D,** One week later. **E,F,** One year later, after completion of prosthetics. Note excellent result. (Contributed by Dr. Dennis Tarnow, New York, New York).

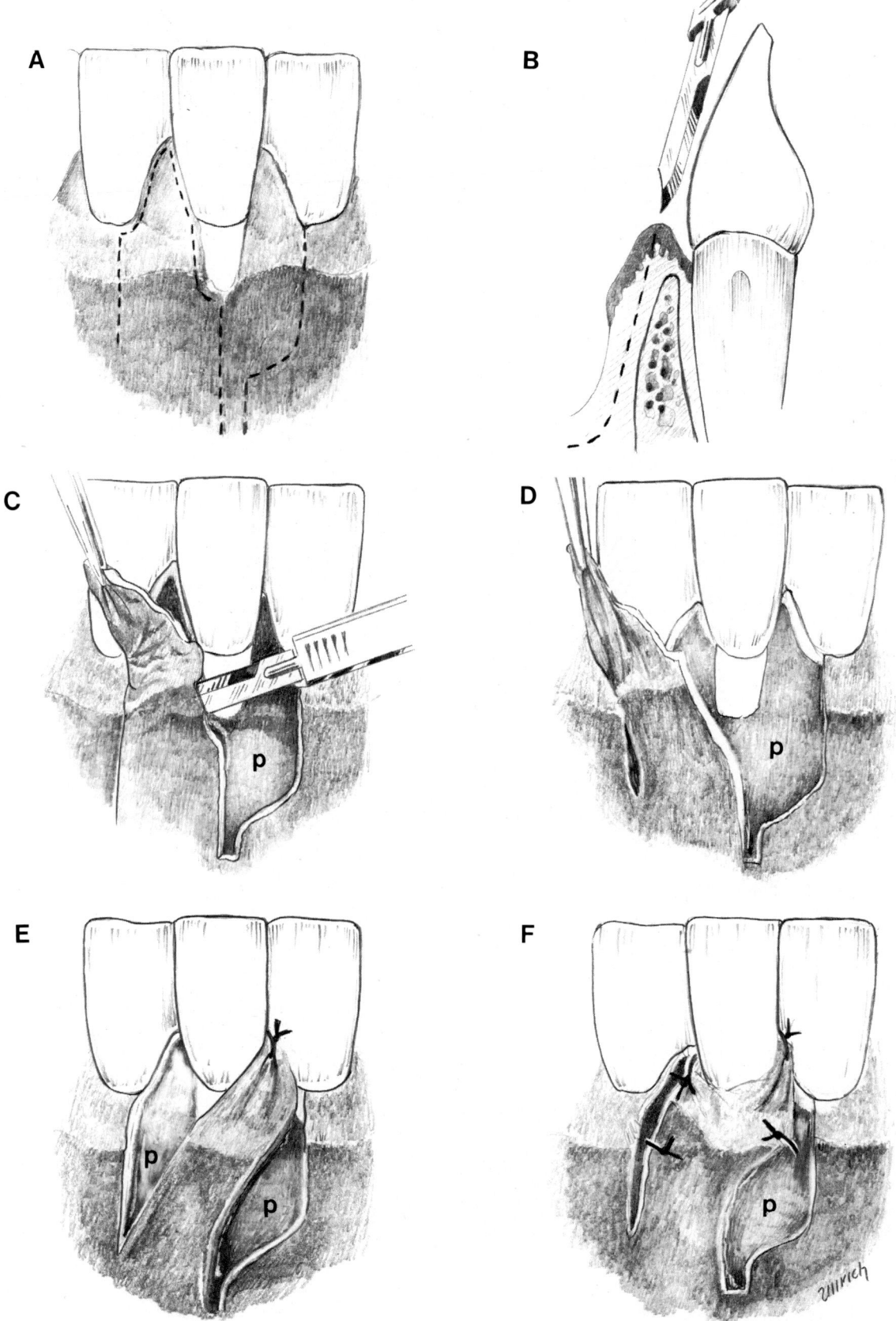

Fig. 9-26. The Transpositional Papillary Flap. **A,** Before surgery; incisions are outlined. **B,** Side view showing a partial-thickness flap design. **C,** The recipient site has been prepared, and the donor pedicle is prepared by sharp dissection. **D,** The pedicle flap is released apically. **E,** The initial suture positions the papilla at the CEJ to the underlying recipient bed. **F,** The papilla is now anchored mesially, distally, and apically.

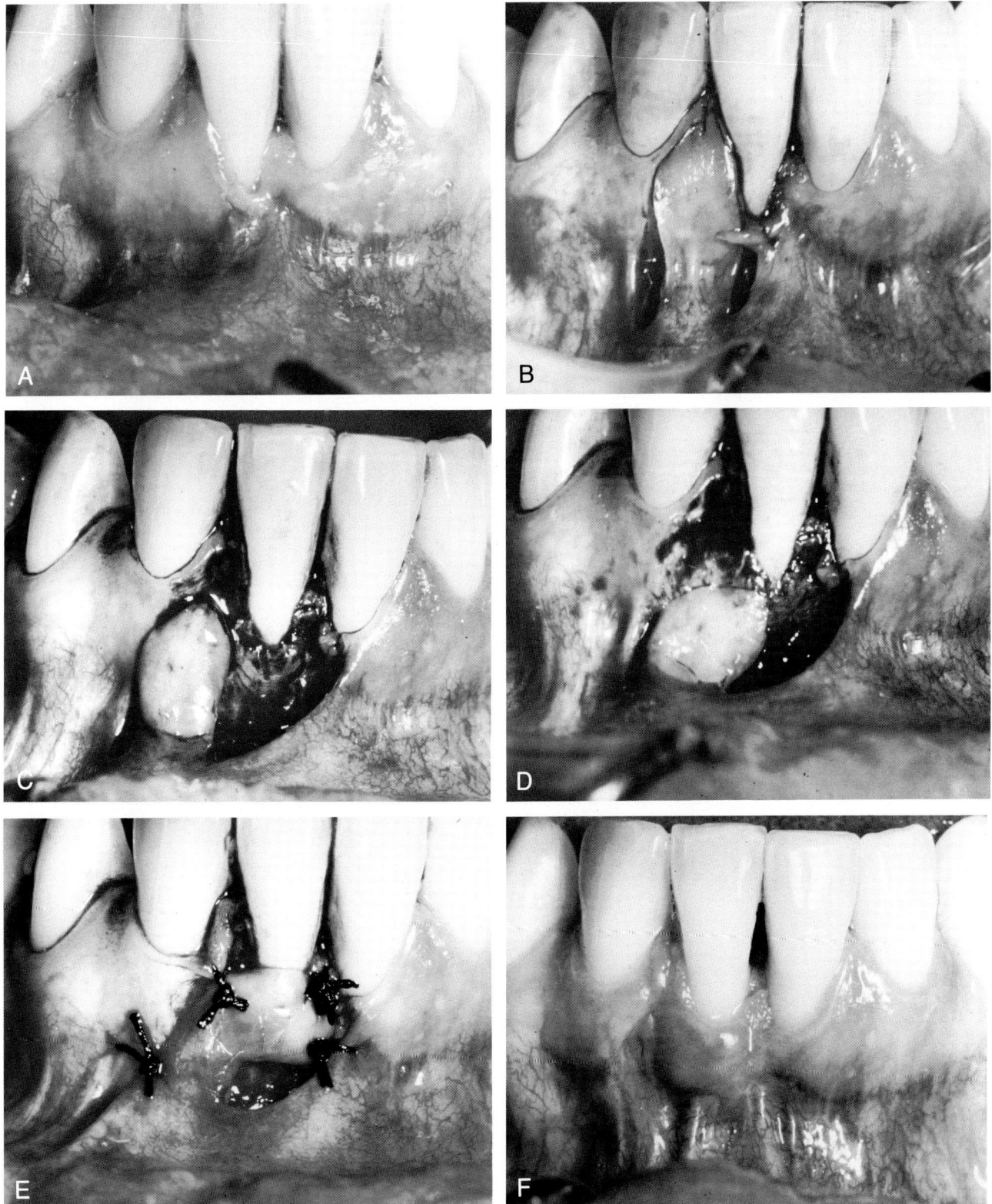

Fig. 9-27. Transpositional Rotated Pedicle Flap. **A,** Before treatment. **B,** Partial-thickness pedicle flap outlined. **C,** Partial-thickness recipient bed prepared. **D,** Pedicle flap released and removed apically. **E,** Pedicle rotated and sutured over denuded root surface. **F,** Five months later.

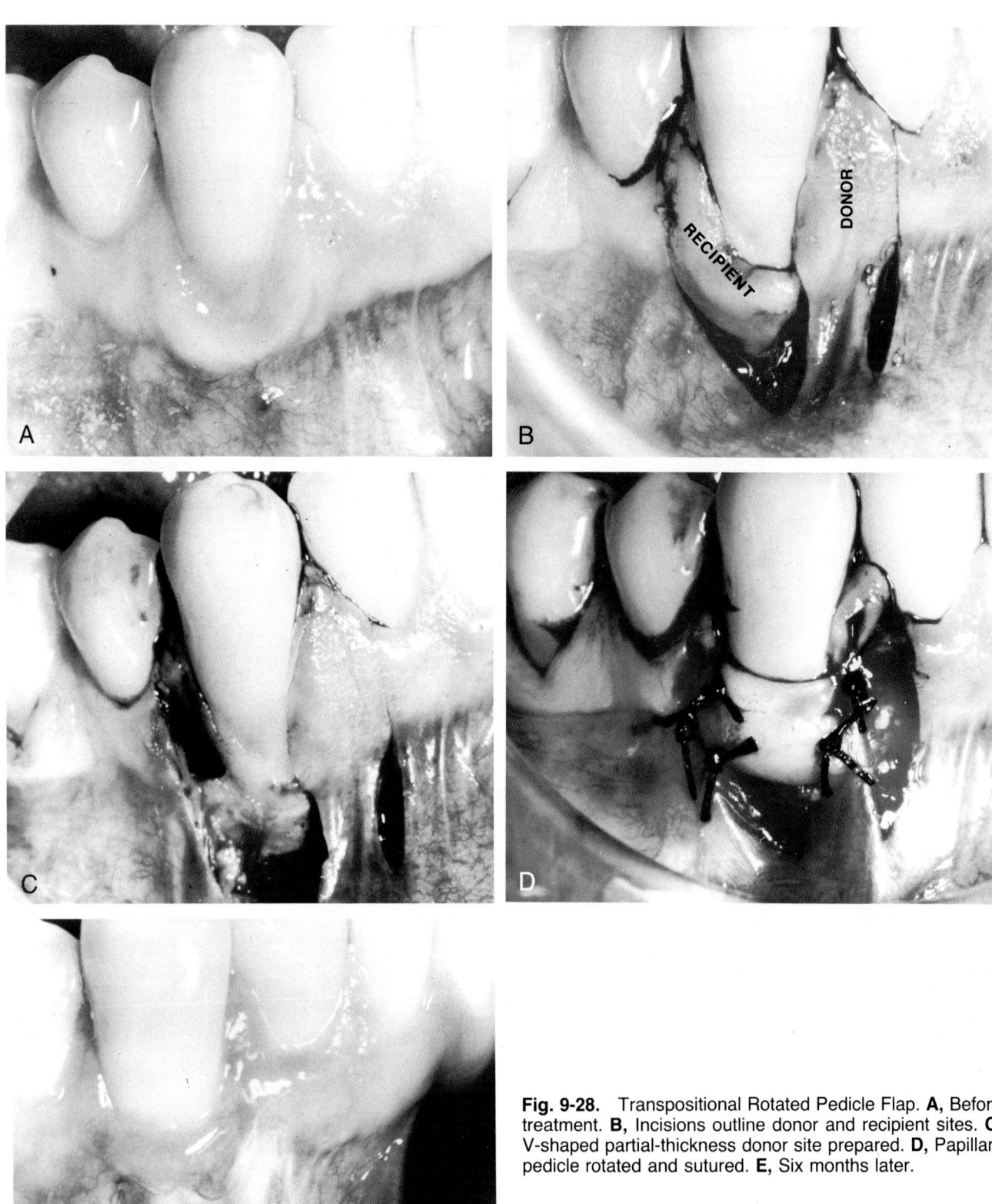

Fig. 9-28. Transpositional Rotated Pedicle Flap. **A,** Before treatment. **B,** Incisions outline donor and recipient sites. **C,** V-shaped partial-thickness donor site prepared. **D,** Papillary pedicle rotated and sutured. **E,** Six months later.

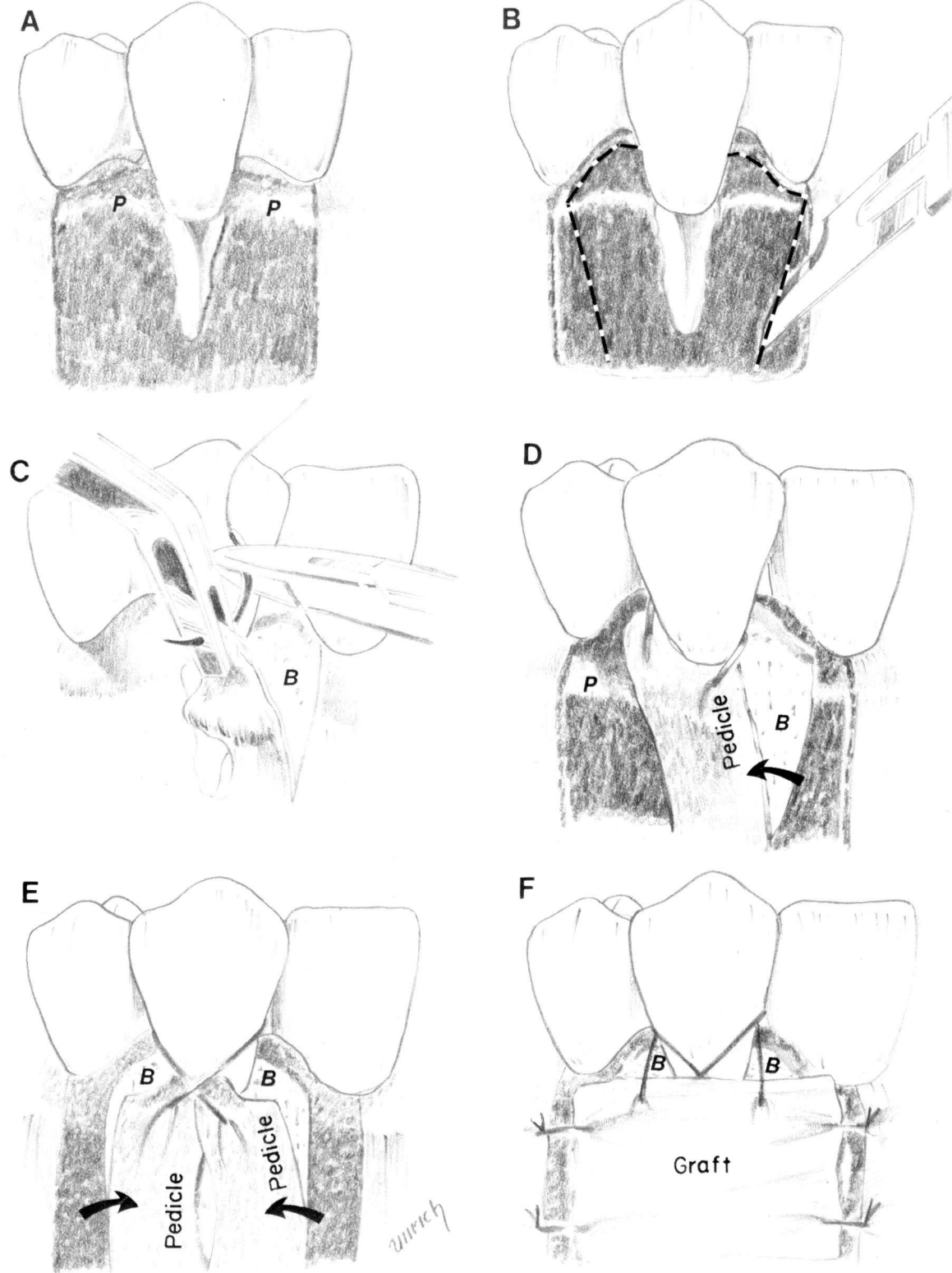

Fig. 9-29. Periosteal Pedicle for Root Coverage (Carvalho Technique). **A,** Facial view of prepared periosteal bed (P) with exposed root. **B,** Dotted lines outline design of periosteal pedicle flaps (PPF). **C,** Pedicle raised, underlying bone exposed (B), and suturing begun. **D,** Single pedicle sutured in place. **E,** Use of two pedicles if area is large. **F,** Graft positioned and sutured over exposed root and PPF.

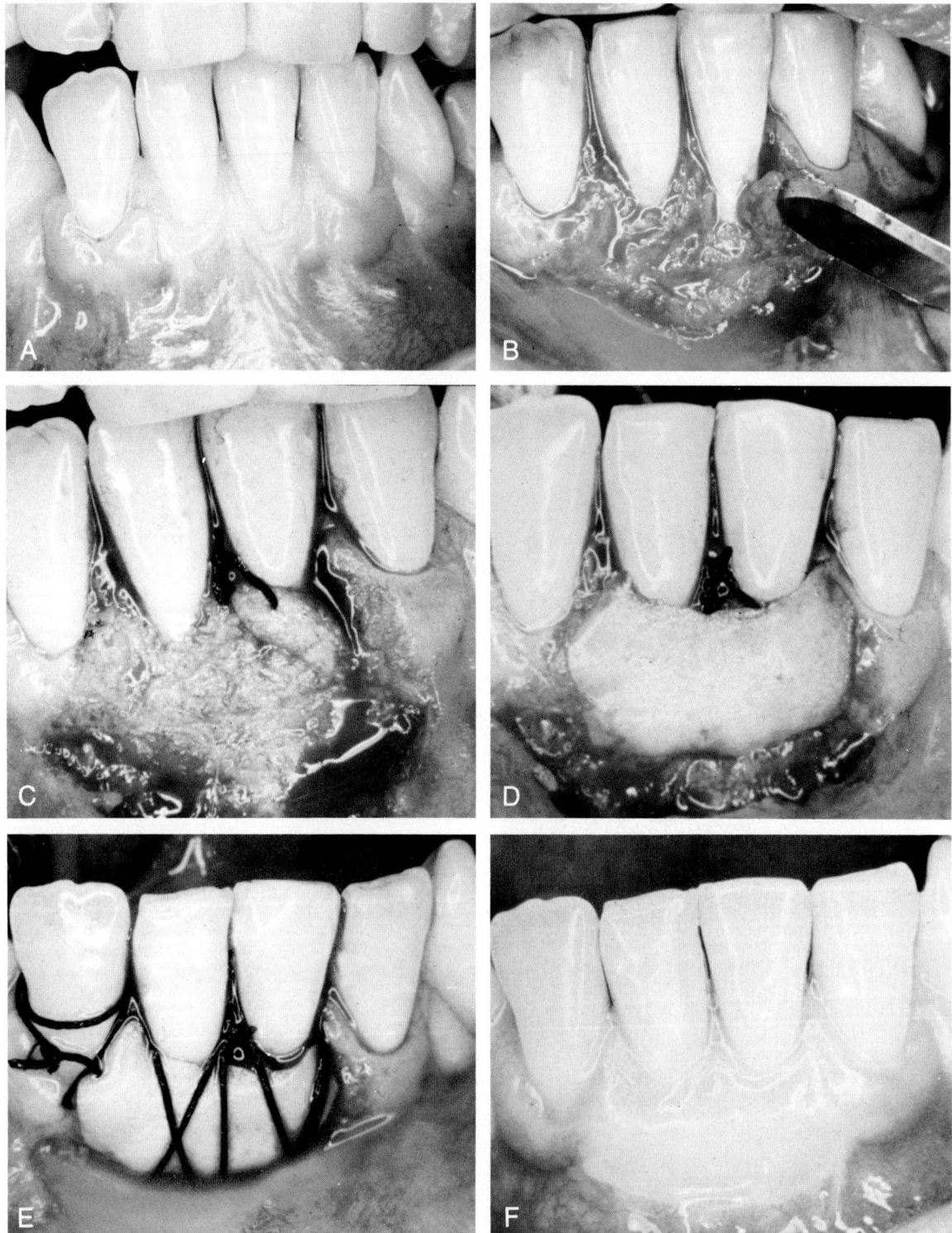

Fig. 9-30. Free Soft-Tissue Autograft with Periosteal Pedicle Flap for Root Coverage. **A,** Before; note recession on teeth on lower centrals. **B,** Periosteal pedicle flap reflected. **C,** Periosteal pedicle flap sutured. **D,** Graft placed. **E,** Graft sutured. **F,** One year later; note root coverage and increased zone of attached gingiva. (From Carvalho, J.C., Putiglioni, F.E., and Kon, S.: Combination of a connective tissue pedicle flap with a free gingival graft to cover localized gingival recession. Int. J. Periodont. Rest. Dent., *4*:27, 1982.)

10

RIDGE AUGMENTATION

Excessive bone resorption is commonly found when teeth are extracted. This is a problem anteriorly, since it will result in an unesthetic long pontic on a narrow, hollowed-out ridge. Special techniques have been developed to treat problems of vertical and horizontal ridge resorption.

CLASSIFICATION OF RIDGE DEFECTS

Seibert (1983) classified the various types of ridge loss into three classes:

Class I: Buccolingual loss of tissue with normal ridge height in the apicocoronal dimension (Fig. 10-1).

Class II: Apicocoronal loss of tissue with normal ridge width in a buccolingual dimension (Fig. 10-2).

Class III: Combination buccolingual and apicocoronal loss of tissue resulting in loss of normal height and width (Fig. 10-3).

FULL-THICKNESS SOFT-TISSUE GRAFTS

Meltzer (1979) published the first clinical report on using a soft-tissue graft solely to correct an esthetic anterior *vertical* ridge defect. Seibert (1983A,B) published a series of classic articles that detail the technique and its application. Figures 10-4 and 10-5 show the clinical application of the technique. Note in Figure 10-5G, after the epithelial denudation is complete, vertical slices are made to enhance the bleeding surface. This is to permit adequate diffusing of the full-thickness graft. The tuberosity or dentulous ridge is the best source for donor tissue. The procedure is limited by the availability of thick graftable tissue.

POUCH PROCEDURE

Garber and Rosenberg (1981) developed a technique for treating ridges that had a *horizontal* loss of dimension. Using a connective-tissue graft from the tuberosity for subepithelial placement, the procedure provides both stabilization of the graft and ridge enhancement. This technique was a refinement and an advancement of those devised by Langer (1980) and by Abrams (1980).

Figure 10-6A shows an occlusal view of the initial horizontal incision made at the crest of the ridge. A partial-thickness incision is made with a No. 15 scalpel blade and extended apically and laterally over the deformity (Fig. 10-6B). Blunt dissection may be used to extend the pouch.

The connective-tissue graft is sutured, using 4-0 or 5-0 silk or gut. The suture is passed first through the base of the pouch (Fig. 10-6C). This provides apical stabilization of the graft. Figure 10-6D shows the addition of a second middle suture and closure of the initial horizontal incision. Figure 10-6E is an occlusal view of the graft sutured, showing the correction of the deformity. Figure 10-6F is a cross-sectional view of the graft stabilized in position.

This procedure is shown clinically in Figure 10-7 and 10-8.

RIDGE AUGMENTATION—IMPROVED TECHNIQUE

In 1985, Allen et al. outlined an improved surgical technique for localized ridge augmentation that was similar to that previously described by Kaldahl et al. (1982) except that the graft material was an hydroxyapatite implant.

The use of an hydroxyapatite implant permitted an unlimited donor source, with greater predictability of results. The use of a partial-thickness palatal flap prevents separation and opening of the pouch.

Procedure

In Figures 10-9A and B, the flap is outlined. Two partial-thickness vertical parallel incisions are joined by a horizontal incision. The incisions are begun 6 to 12 mm palatal to the crest of the ridge. Care is taken to avoid the sulci of the adjacent teeth. The partial-thickness flap will extend to the crest of the ridge.

A partial-thickness flap is raised, using sharp dissection to the crest of the ridge (Fig. 10-9C).

At the crest of the ridge, a full-thickness pouch is reflected off the bone and extended far enough apically for correction of the ridge deformity (Fig. 10-9C,D). The pouch is now filled with any of the hydroxyapatite materials (Perigraf, Alveograf, or Calcitite) as seen in Figure 10-9E and F.

The pouch is closed and the flap is sutured. Even if the flap is not totally approximated palatally, it will still not open because of the adequate overlap of the tissue palatally (Fig. 10-9G).

This procedure is shown clinically in Figures 10-10 and 10-11.

SUBEPITHELIAL CONNECTIVE TISSUE GRAFT FOR RIDGE AUGMENTATION

Langer and Calagna (1980, 1982) designed a procedure for ridge augmentation that uses a combination of a partial-thickness flap (buccally and palatally) and a connective tissue graft.

Advantages

1. Versatility
2. Primary closure
3. Good vascularity
4. May be combined with adjacent root coverage procedures
5. Reduced trauma

Disadvantages

1. Technically difficult
2. Possible need for secondary mucogingival surgery due to altered coronal position of the mucogingival junction

Indications

For correction of all types of ridge deformities.

Procedure

1. With a No. 15 scalpel blade, a partial-thickness flap is begun at the crest, or palatal to crest of the edentulous ridge (only if flap overlap is desired) (Fig. 10-12A).
2. The incisions are carried mesially and distally to the terminal ends of the edentulous ridge (Fig. 10-12B).
3. Vertical incisions are now made bucally and palatally. Buccally, they are carried far enough apically beyond the mucogingival junction to permit freedom of movement. Palatally, the flap is reflected just far enough to permit placement of the graft (Fig. 10-12A).
4. A horizontal apical releasing incision of the buccal flap may be necessary for greater flap mobility and coronal positioning (Fig. 10-12C).
5. The connective tissue grafts (see subepithelial connective tissue graft for root coverage), without the epithelial borders, are sutured in place using chromic gut sutures. One or more pieces may be used, depending upon the defect (Fig. 10-12D,D').
6. The buccal flap is coronally positioned and sutured at the crest of the ridge or overlapped palatally. The flap is also sutured laterally for enhanced stability (Fig. 10-12E).

The clinical procedure is depicted in Figures 10-13, 10-14, and 10-15.

SOCKET PRESERVATION (RIDGE AUGMENTATION)

This technique is designed to prevent ridge collapse anteriorly and is carried out at the time of extraction. It was described by Greenstein (1985).

Indications

1. Ridge preservation and enhancement for increased anterior esthetics
2. Ridge maintenance for future implant placement

Advantages

1. Simple
2. Effective
3. Minimizes postoperative pain
4. Will prevent future need for secondary surgical procedures for ridge augmentation.

Procedure

1. The individual teeth are extracted (Fig. 10-16B).
2. All granulation is removed from the sockets (Fig. 10-16B).
3. The undersurfaces of the flaps are thinned by sharp dissection, and all granulation tissue is removed.
4. The flaps are reflected for only a short distance off the bone.
5. The sockets are now filled with any of the bone augmentation materials, DFDBA, hydroxyapatite, or HTR, depending on operator preference. *Note: If future implant placement is a consideration, it is the author's recommendation the DFDBA be used (Fig. 10-16C).*
6. A biologic bandage (connective tissue, collagen, facia-laria, etc.) is now placed to cover the sockets, help augment the ridge and prevent loss of implant material (Fig. 10-16D). *Note: If implants are to be placed, a guided tissue augmentation material (GTAM) membrane is recommended for implant coverage.*
7. The flaps are sutured to secure implant and bandage (Fig. 10-16E,F).

The clinical procedure is depicted in Figure 10-17.

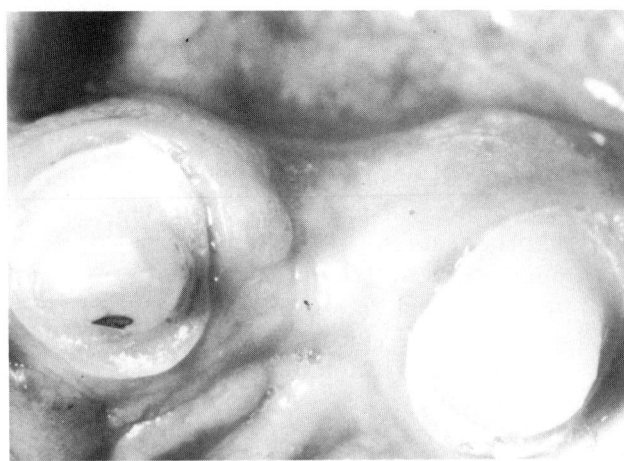

Fig. 10-1. Class I Ridge Loss.

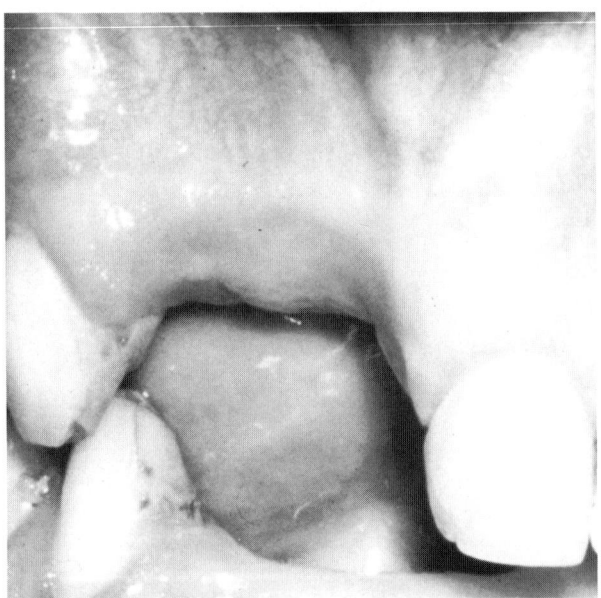

Fig. 10-2. Class II Ridge Loss.

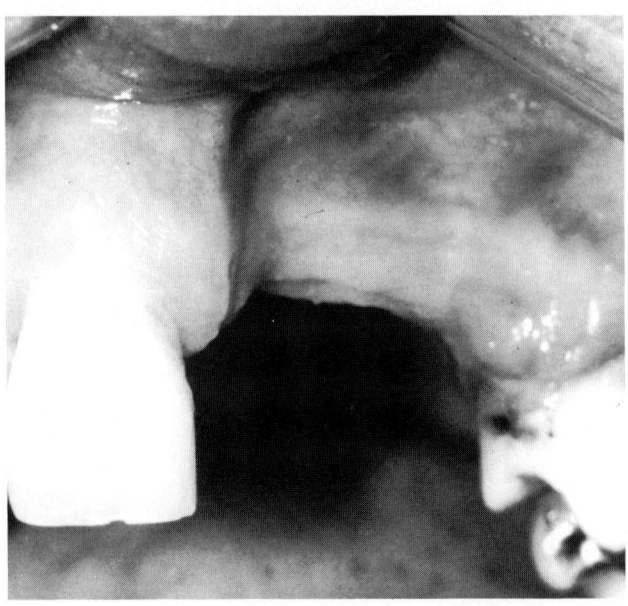

Fig. 10-3. Class III Ridge Loss.

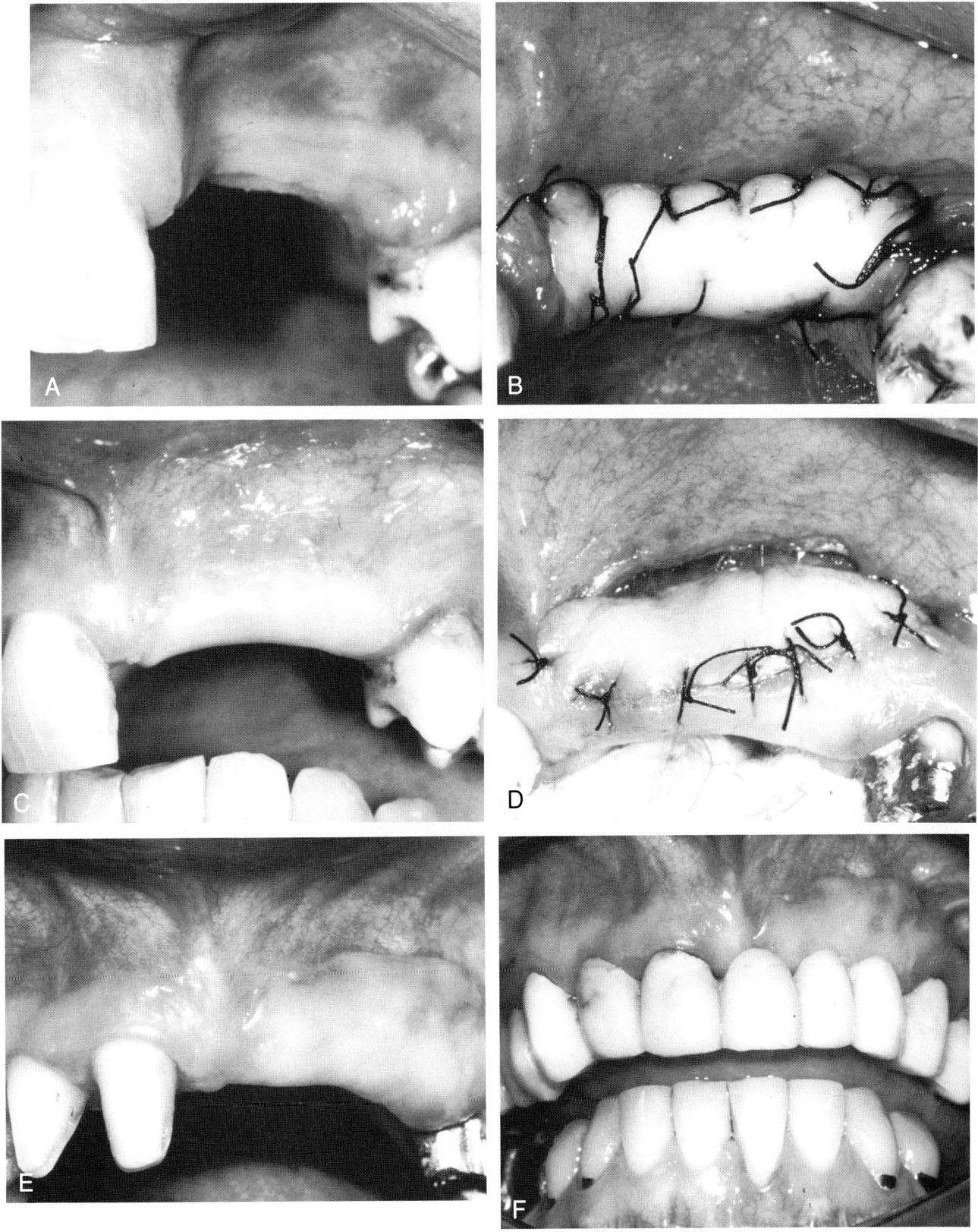

Fig. 10-4. Free Gingival Onlay Graft for Correction of *Class III Ridge Defect.* **A,** Pretreatment view of an extensive *Class III ridge defect.* The patient has used a removable prosthesis for many years and wished to have a fixed prosthesis made. **B,** First stage of soft-tissue reconstruction. A large, thick onlay graft was sutured into position. **C,** Two months postsurgery. The onlay graft produced gain in ridge height. A second procedure was performed to augment the ridge further in buccolingual dimension. **D,** A veneer type of free graft was used to gain augmentation in a buccolingual direction. **E,** Appearance of the reconstructed ridge 2 months after the final grafting procedure. Compare the contour of the healed augmented ridge with that shown in Figure 10-4A. **F,** Provisional prosthesis in place. (Contributed by Dr. Jay Seibert, Philadelphia, PA.)

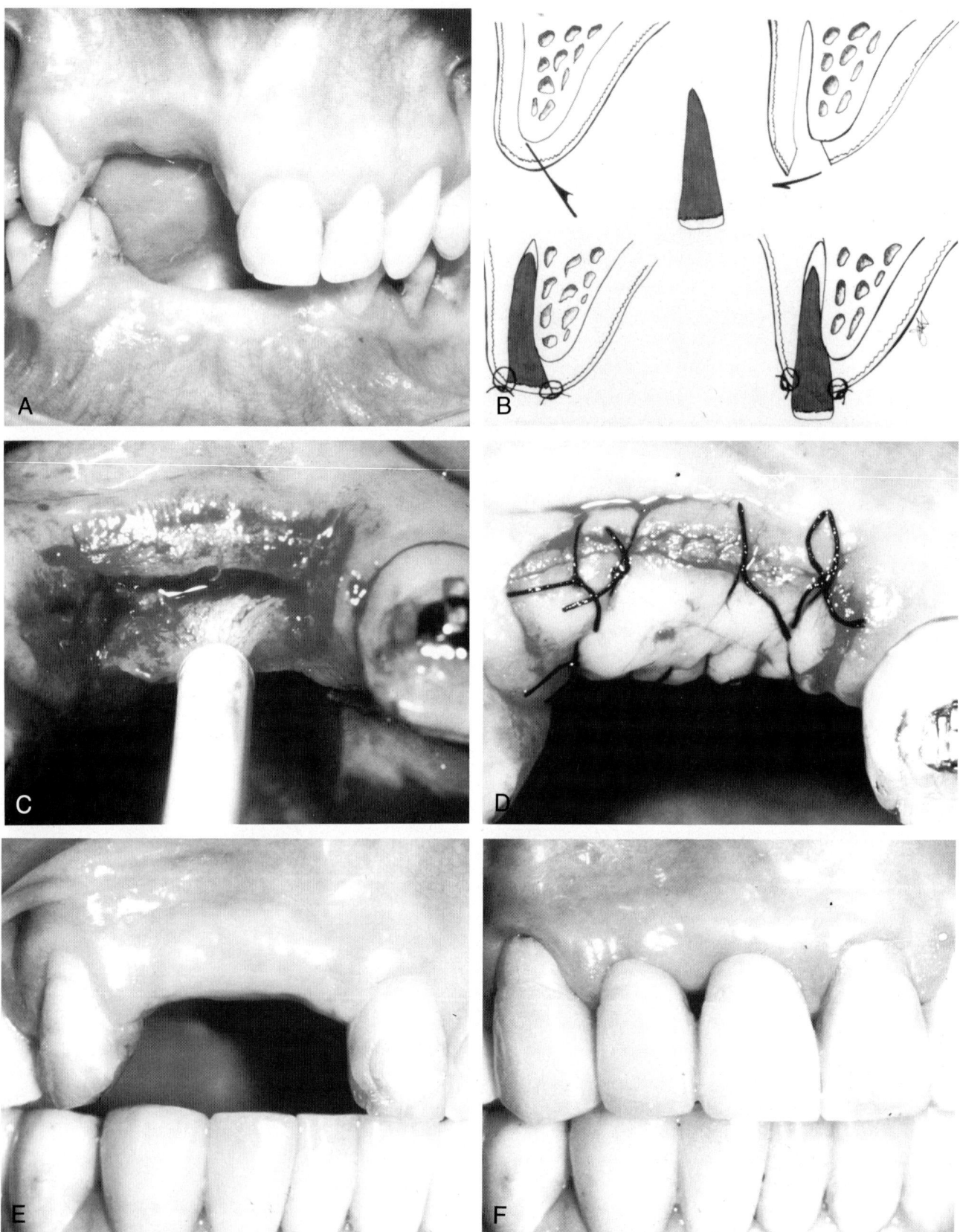

Fig. 10-5. *Wedge Procedure* in Conjunction with Second-Stage Onlay Graft for Correction of Class III Ridge Defect. **A,** Pretreatment view. The patient had a large Class III ridge defect. **B,** Sequence of steps in the wedge procedure. A wedge-shaped section of connective tissue with its epithelium was removed from the palate and was inserted between the elevated pouch-like flap and the ridge. **C,** The pouch was prepared to receive the wedge (inlay-onlay) graft. **D,** The graft was sutured into position. **E, F,** Two months post surgery. Note the amount of ridge height that was obtained. A second-stage procedure was performed to gain more ridge height and to fill in the "dark triangles" between the teeth.

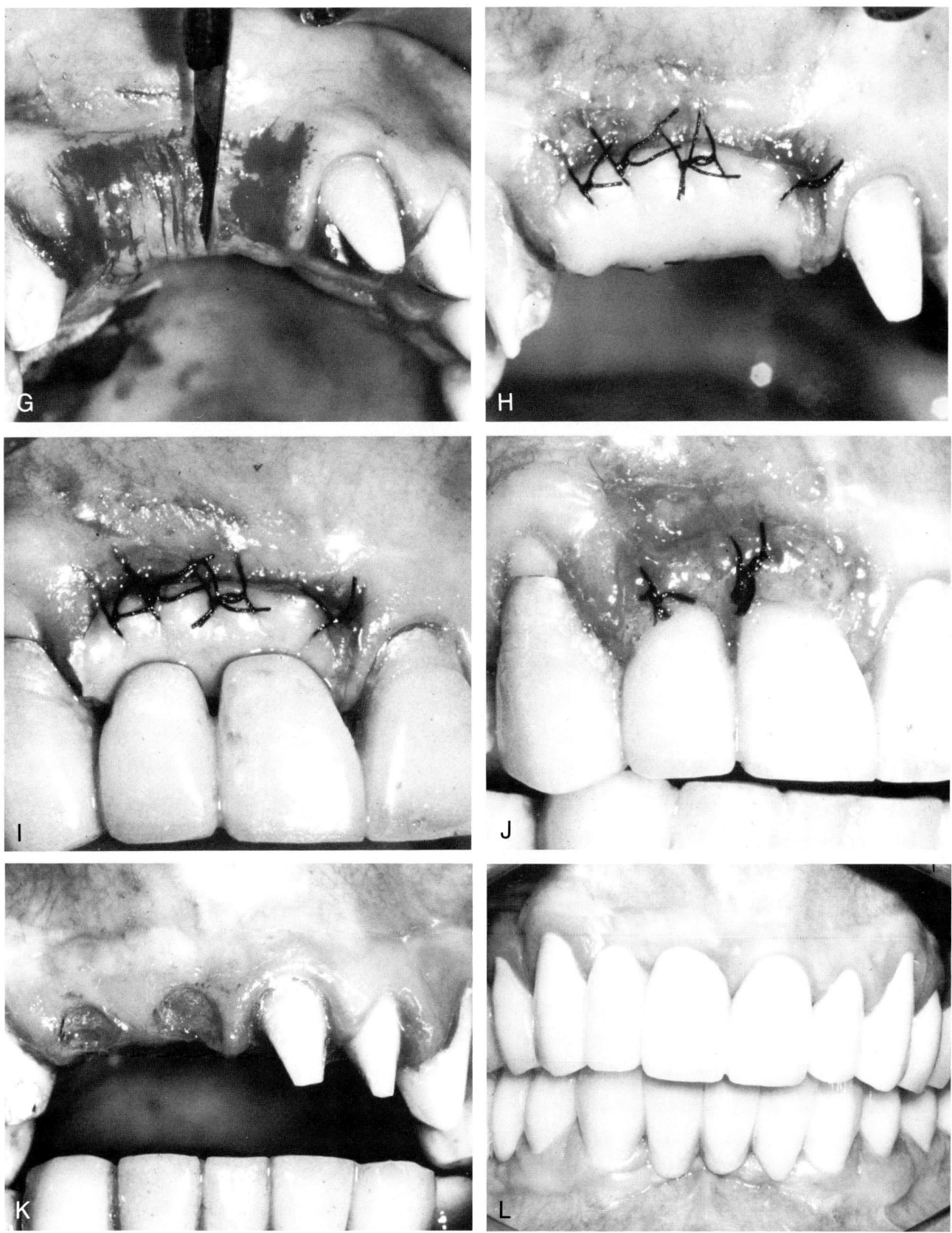

Fig. 10-5 (continued). **G,** Two months after the first surgical procedure, the ridge was de-epithelialized and cuts were made into the connective tissue prior to placing the second-stage onlay graft into position. **H,** The onlay graft was sutured into position. **I,** The pontics were adjusted and brought into light contact with the graft. **J,** Marked swelling occurred within the graft 14 days postsurgery. **K,** Two months following the second surgical procedure, a gingivoplasty was performed to deepen the pontic sites for the ovate pontics. **L,** Post-treatment view 1 year after the final surgical procedure. (Contributed by Dr. Jay Seibert, Philadelphia, PA.)

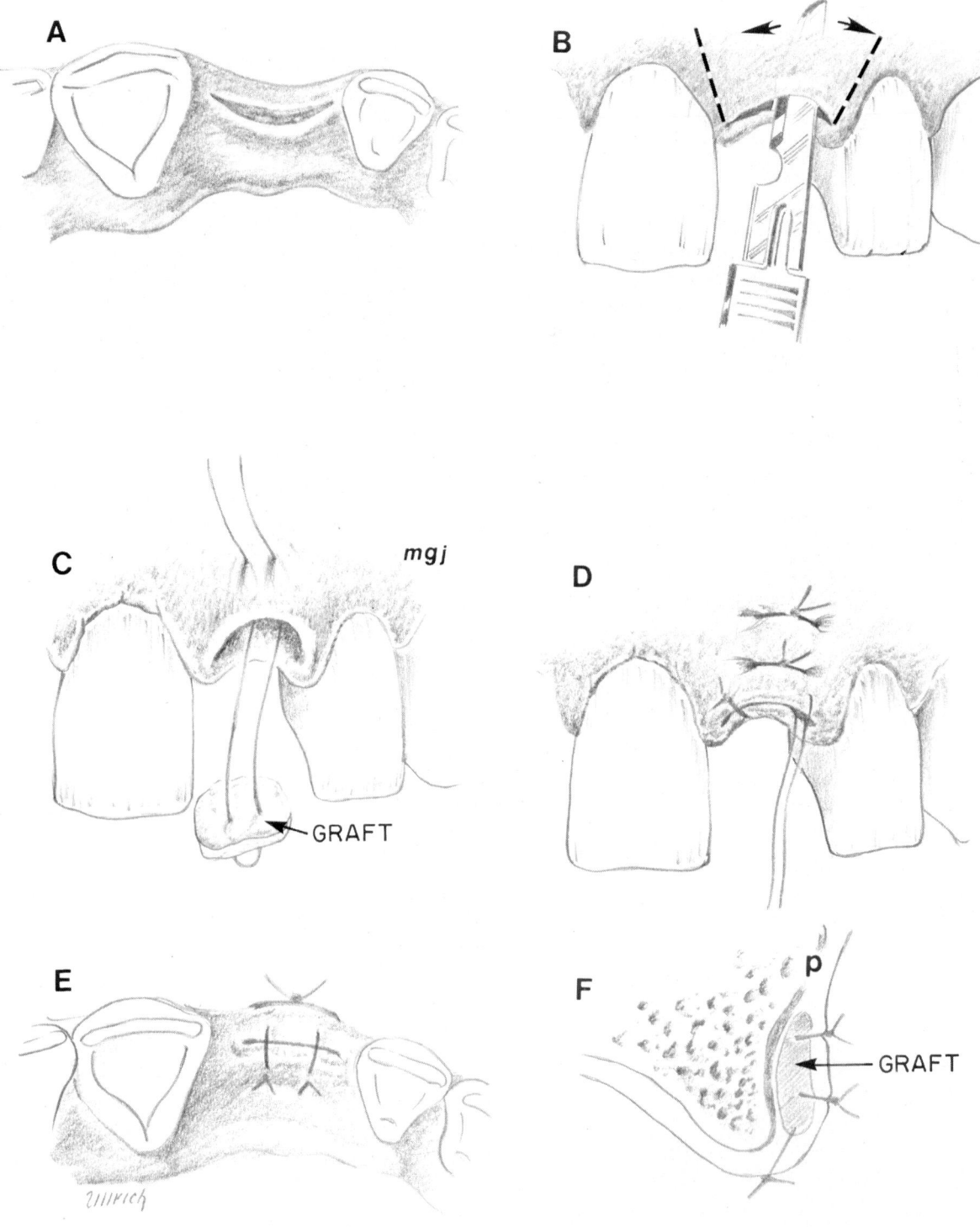

Fig. 10-6. Pouch Procedure. **A,** Deformed ridge as a result of a buccolingual loss in dimension. Initial incision placed over crest of ridge. **B,** Pouch created by extension of crestal incision apically. Dotted lines represent extension mesiodistally. **C,** Connective tissue flap being sutured. **D,** Flap closure. **E,** Occlusal view showing ridge enhancement. **F,** Cross-sectional view of tissue–graft relationships.

Ridge Augmentation

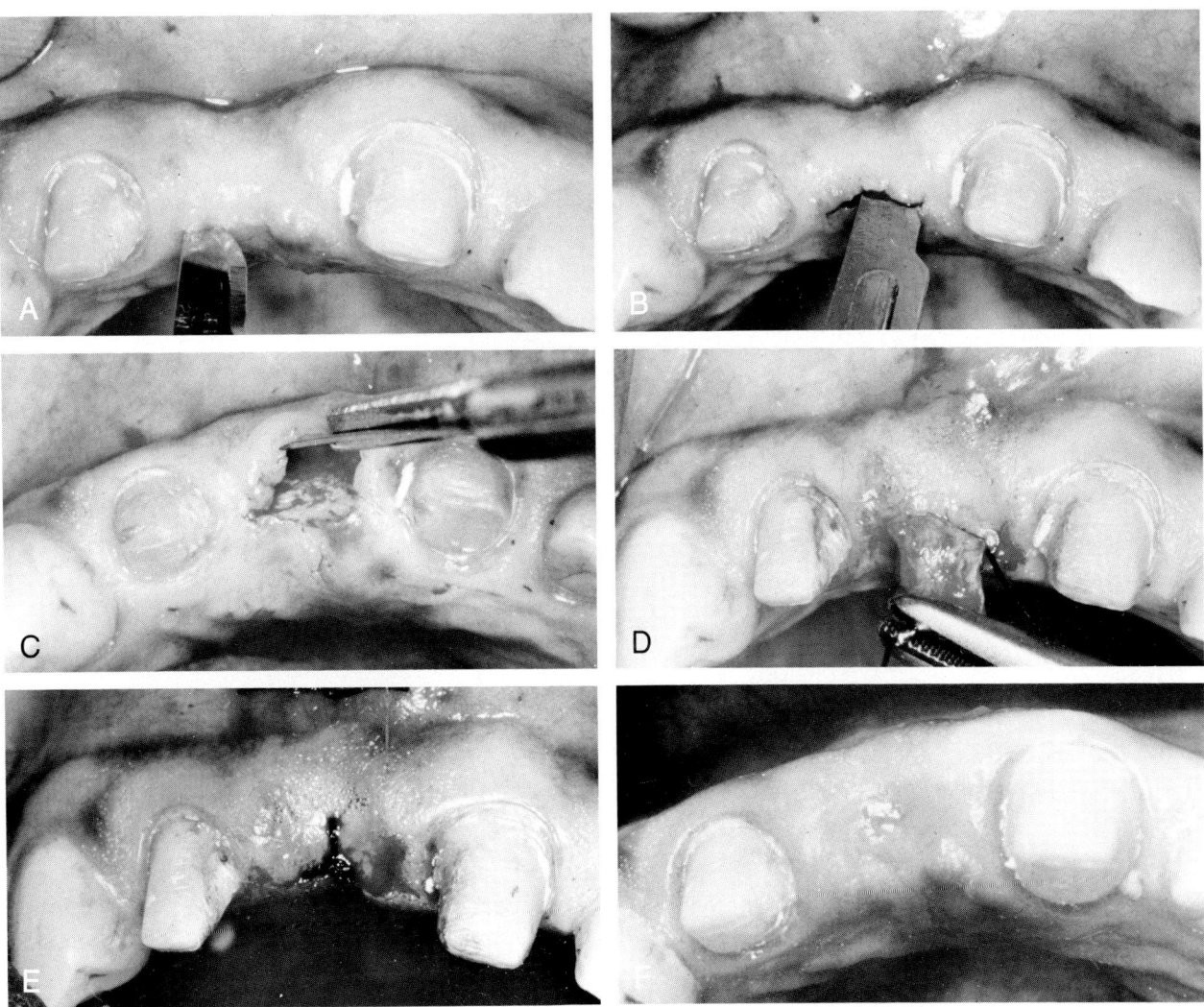

Fig. 10-7. Pouch Procedure for Ridge Augmentation. **A,** Before, as incision is to begin. Note horizontal loss of ridge dimension. **B,** Horizontal ridge incision begun. **C,** Pouch formed. **D,** Connective tissue graft being placed and sutured. **E,** Graft placed and pouch sutured. **F,** Three months later. Note restoration of ridge. (From Garber, D. and Rosenberg, E.: The edentulous ridge in fixed prosthodontics. Compend. Cont. Ed. Gen. Dent., 2:212, 1981.)

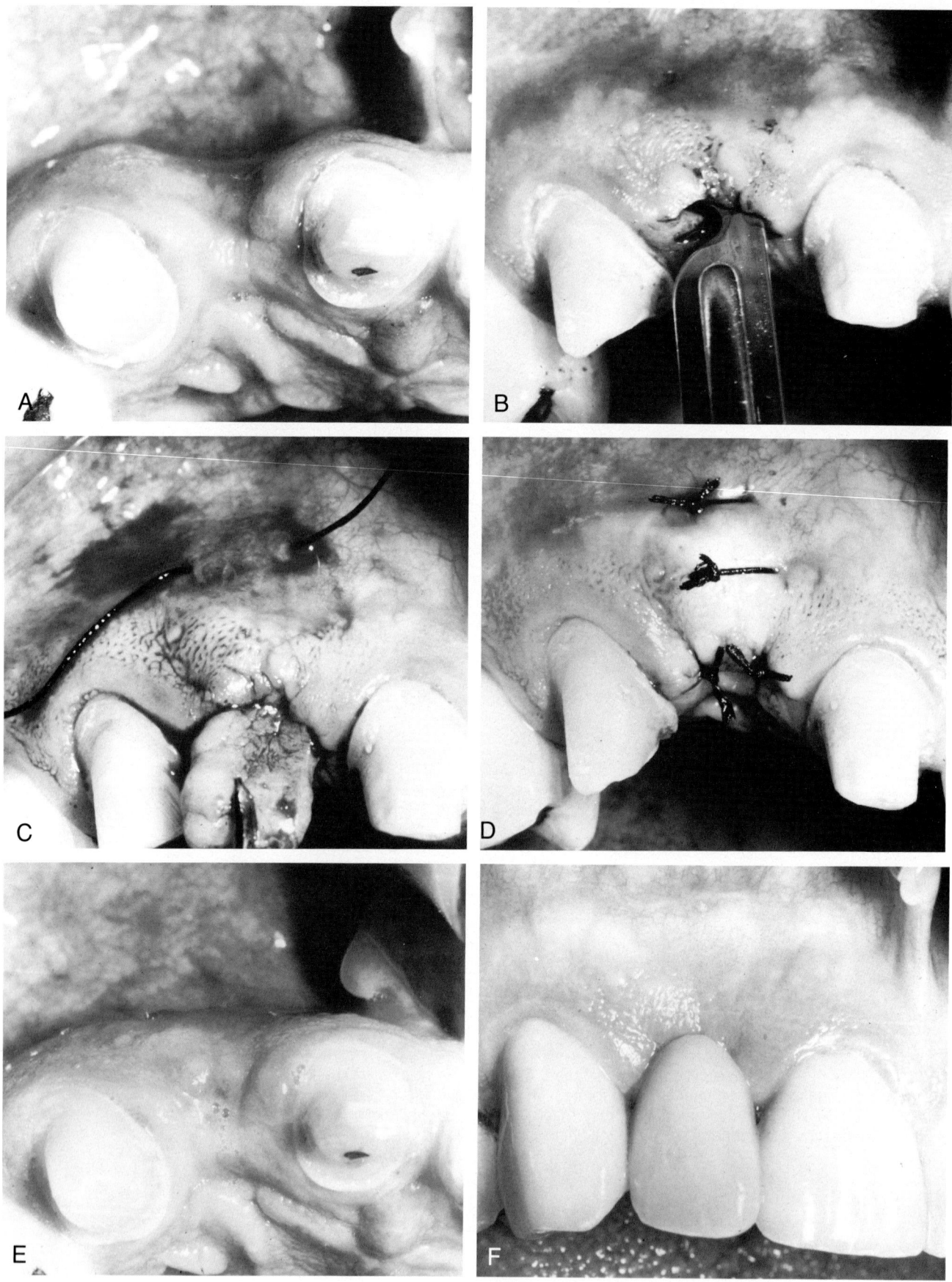

Fig. 10-8. Pouch Procedure. **A,** Before treatment; Class I ridge deformity. **B,** Horizontal ridge incision is made. **C,** Connective tissue graft being placed and sutured. **D,** Graft placed and sutured. **E,** Two months later. Note correction of buccal deformity. **F,** Final prosthetics.

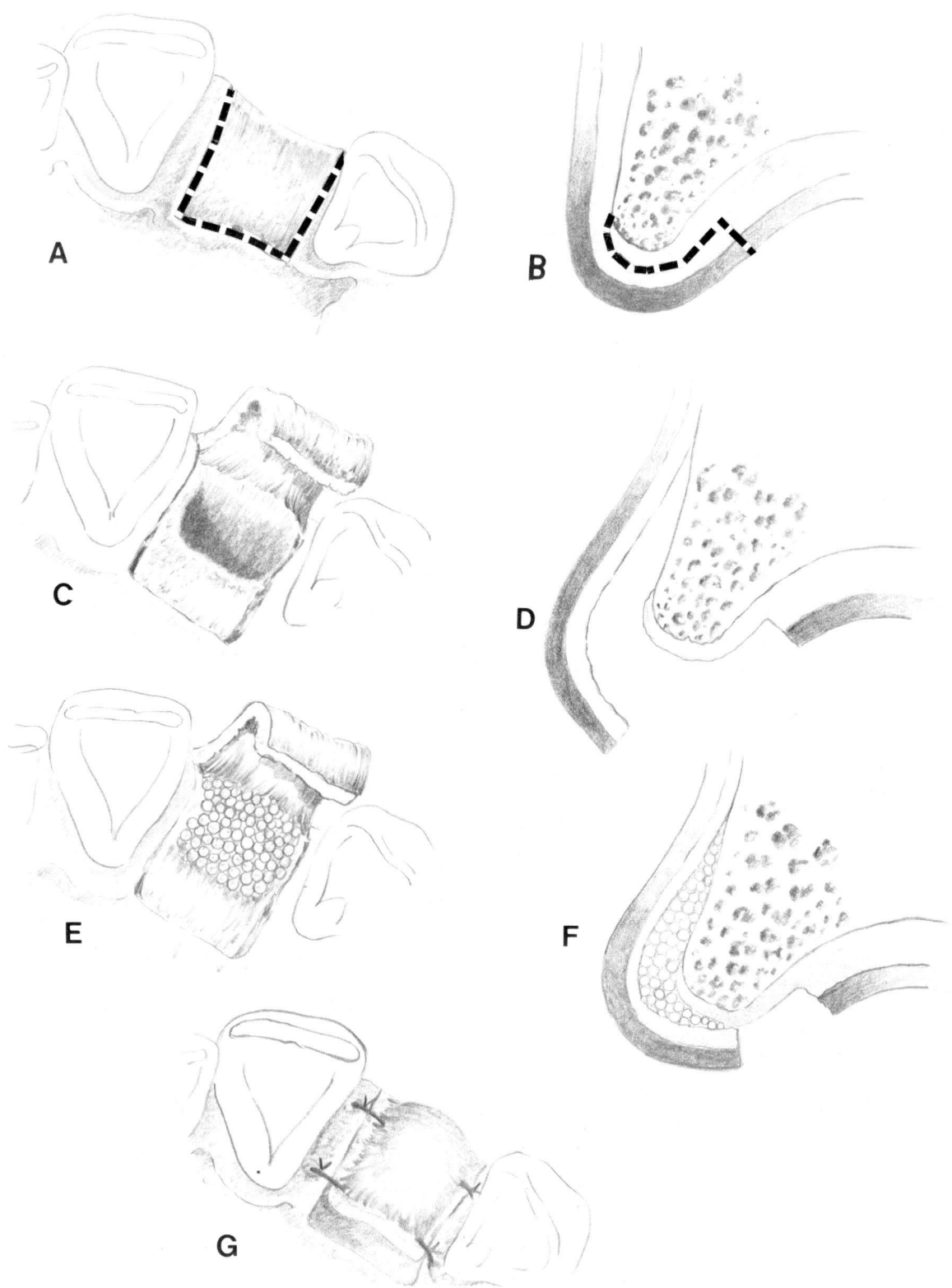

Fig. 10-9. Ridge Augmentation: Improved Technique. **A,** Palatal view, with initial incisions outlined. **B,** Cross-sectional view showing partial-thickness design of flap to crest of ridge. **C,** Flap reflected and pouch formed. **D,** Cross-sectional view of partial-full-thickness pouch design. **E,** Hydroxyapatite placed in pouch. **F,** Cross-sectional view of filled pouch. **G,** Pouch sutured closed.

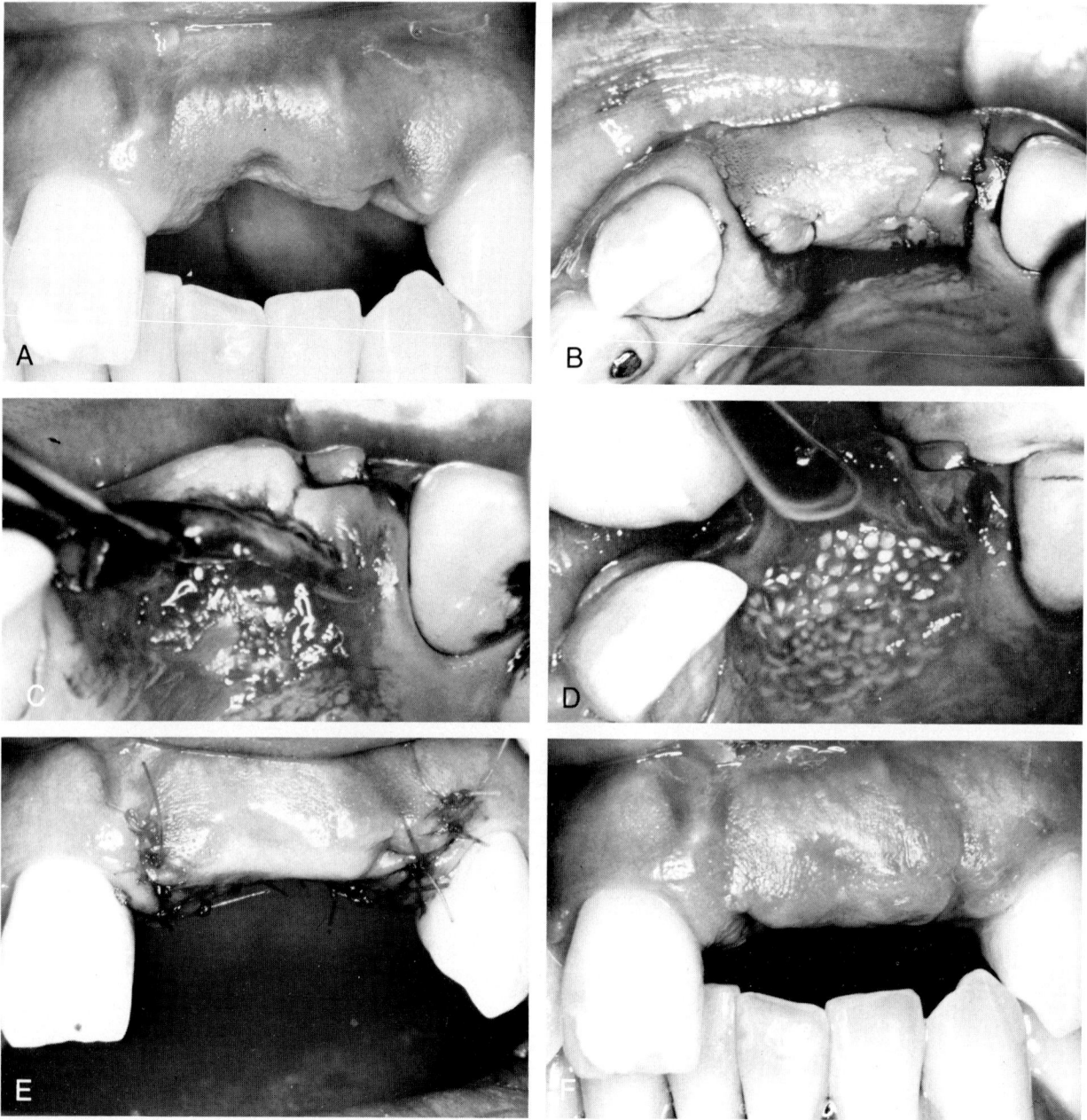

Fig. 10-10. Ridge Augmentation: Improved Technique. **A,** Before; note vertical ridge deformity. **B,** Initial incisions outlining palatal pedicle flap. **C,** Pedicle flap reflected and full-thickness pouch created. **D,** Hydroxyapatite implant material inserted. **E,** Flap sutured. **F,** Four weeks later. (From Allen, P.E., et al.: Improved technique for localized ridge augmentation—A report of 21 cases. J. Periodontol., 56:187, 1985.)

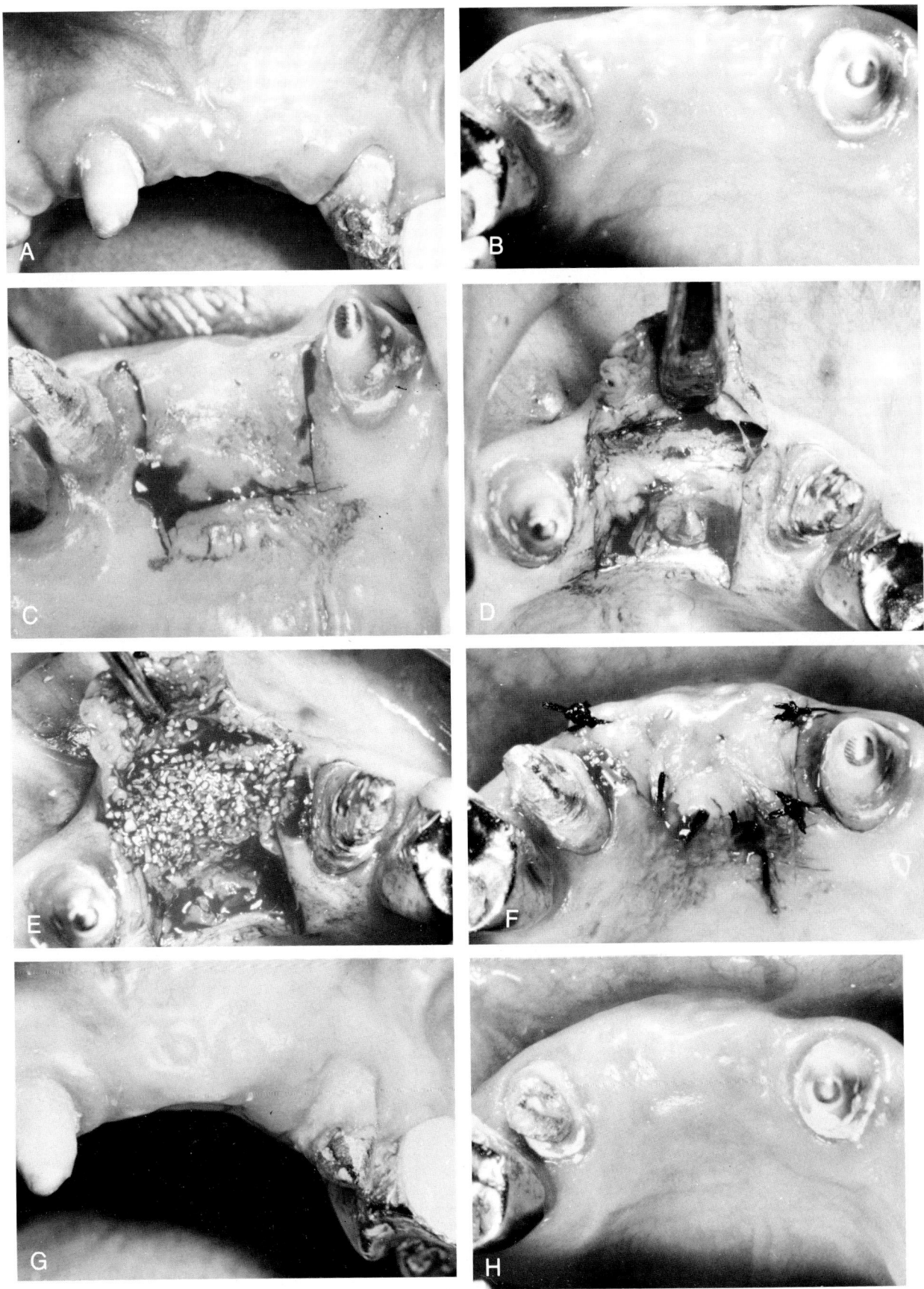

Fig. 10-11. Ridge Augmentation: Improved Technique. **A, B,** Before, buccal and occlusal views, respectively, showing some loss of vertical and horizontal height. **C,** Palatal incisions outlined; note that they begin 10 to 15 mm palatal to ridge and avoid the sulcus areas. **D,** Partial-thickness palatal flap and full-thickness pouch reflected. **E,** Hydroxyapatite graft placed. **F,** Flap sutured. **G, H,** Buccal and occlusal views 2 months later, with increased vertical and horizontal dimensions.

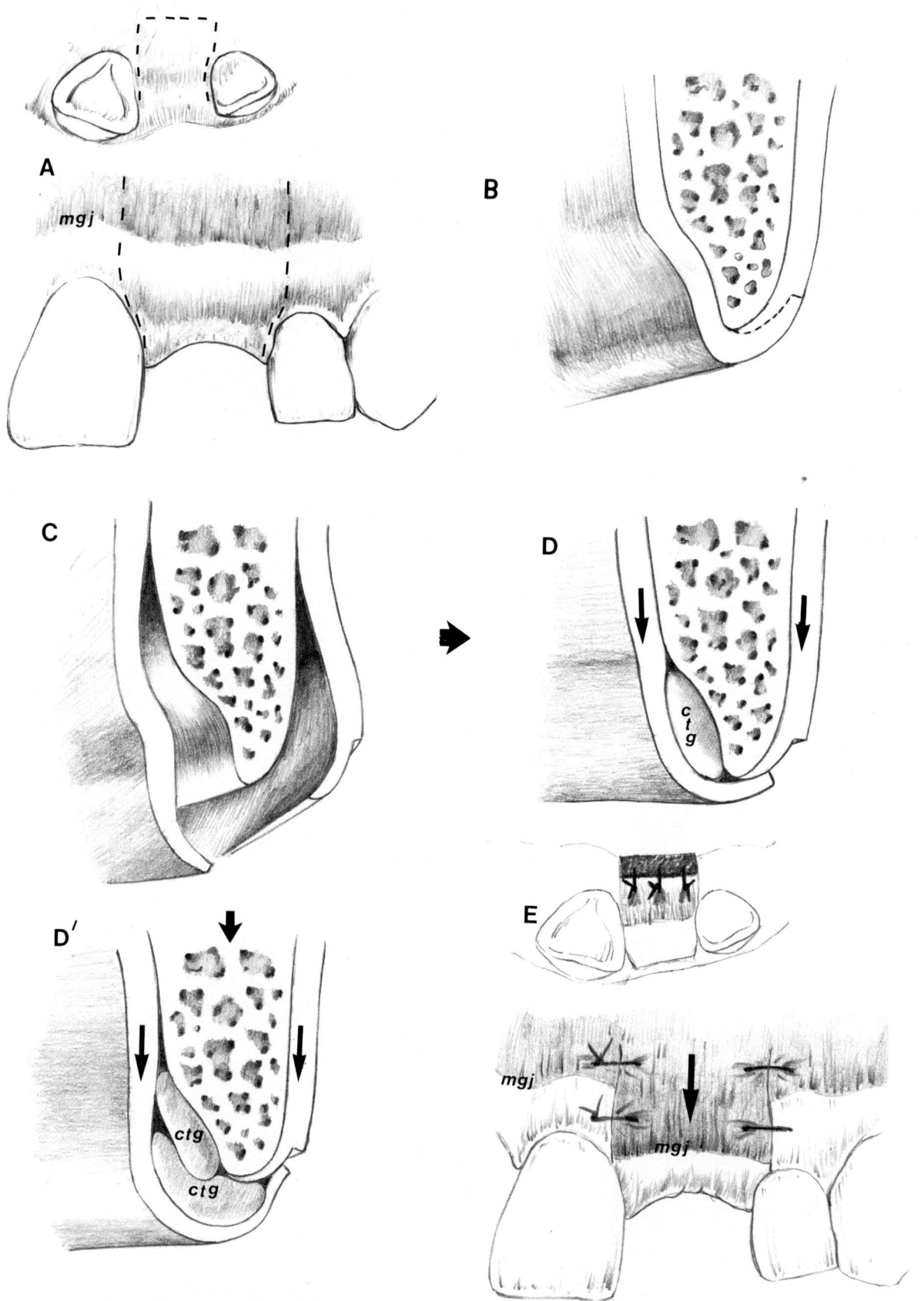

Fig. 10-12. Subepithelial Connective Tissue Graft for Root Coverage. **A,** Incisions outlined buccally. **B,** Palatal partial-thickness flap raised to assure overlap. **C,** Partial-thickness flaps reflected. **D,** Single connective tissue graft placed. **D',** Alternatively, multiple connective tissue grafts placed. Arrows indicate coronal placement of flaps. **E,** Final suturing. Note coronal movement of mucogingival function.

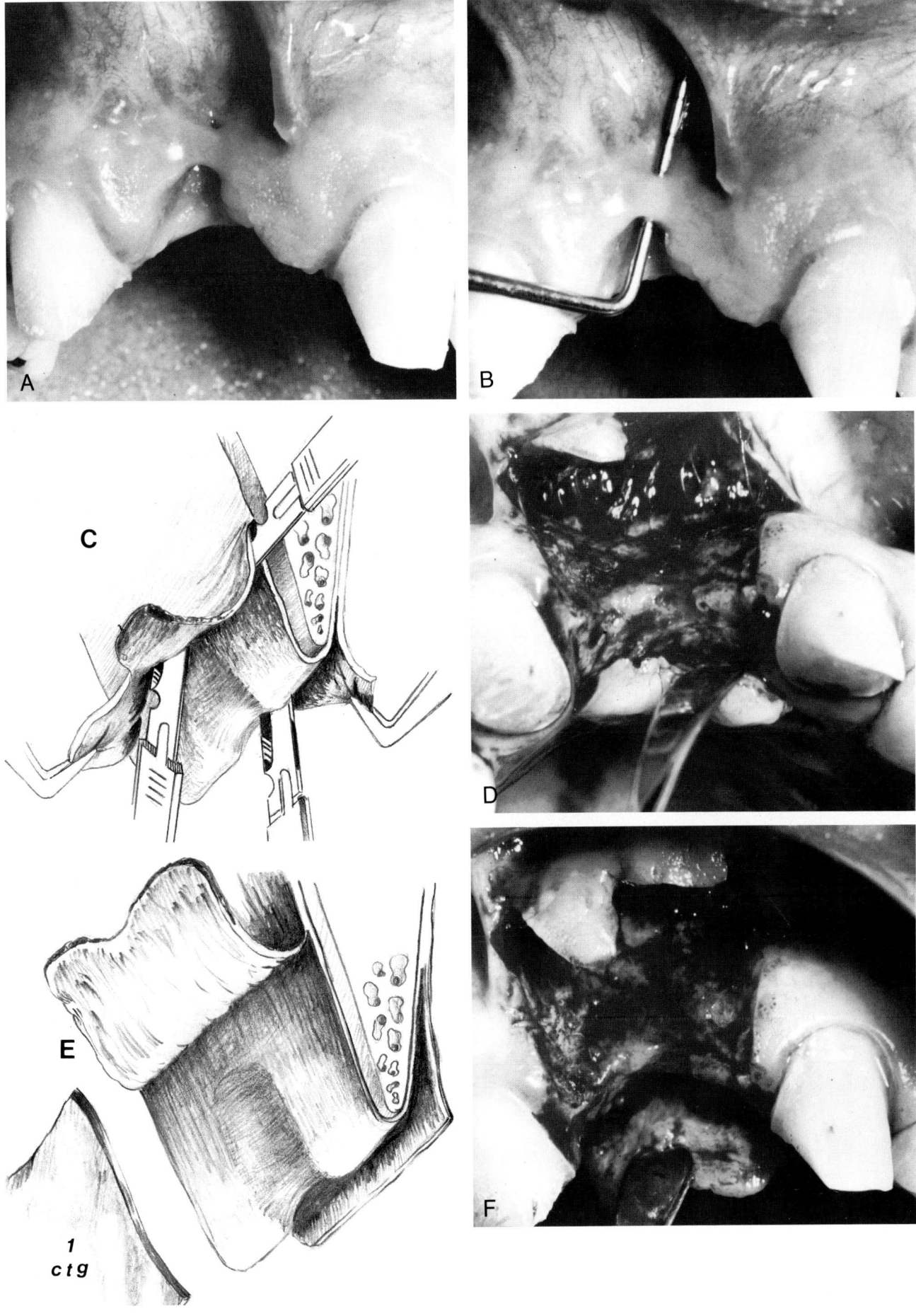

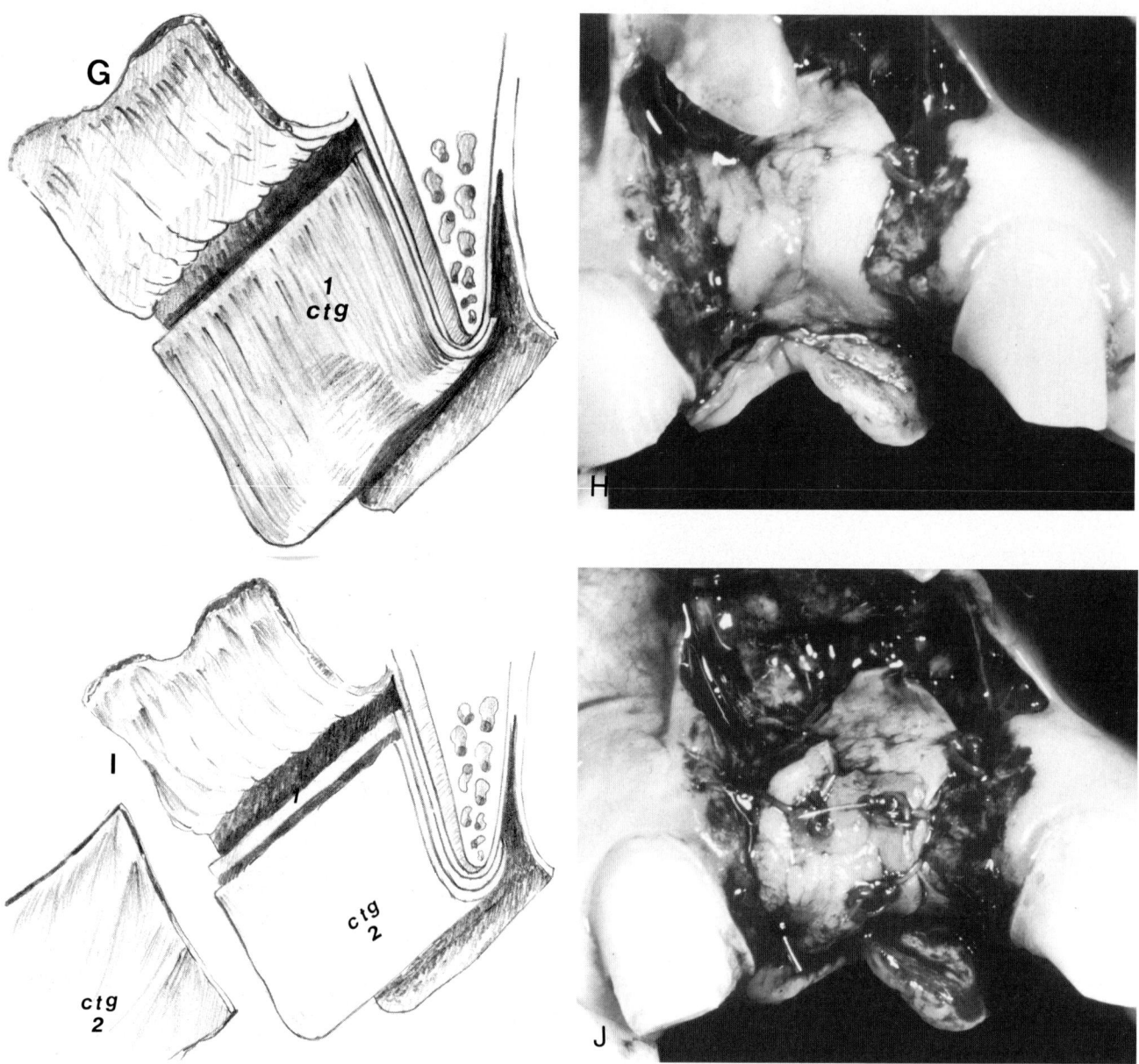

Fig. 10-13. Ridge Augmentation: Subepithelial Connective Tissue Graft. **A, B,** Before treatment. A Class III ridge deformity. **C, D,** Diagrammatic and clinical representation of buccal palatal partial-thickness flaps being reflected. **E,** Partial-thickness flaps being reflected. **F,** Partial-thickness flaps being reflected. **G, H,** Connective tissue graft placed (first piece). **I, J,** Second connective tissue graft placed and sutured over the first.

Ridge Augmentation

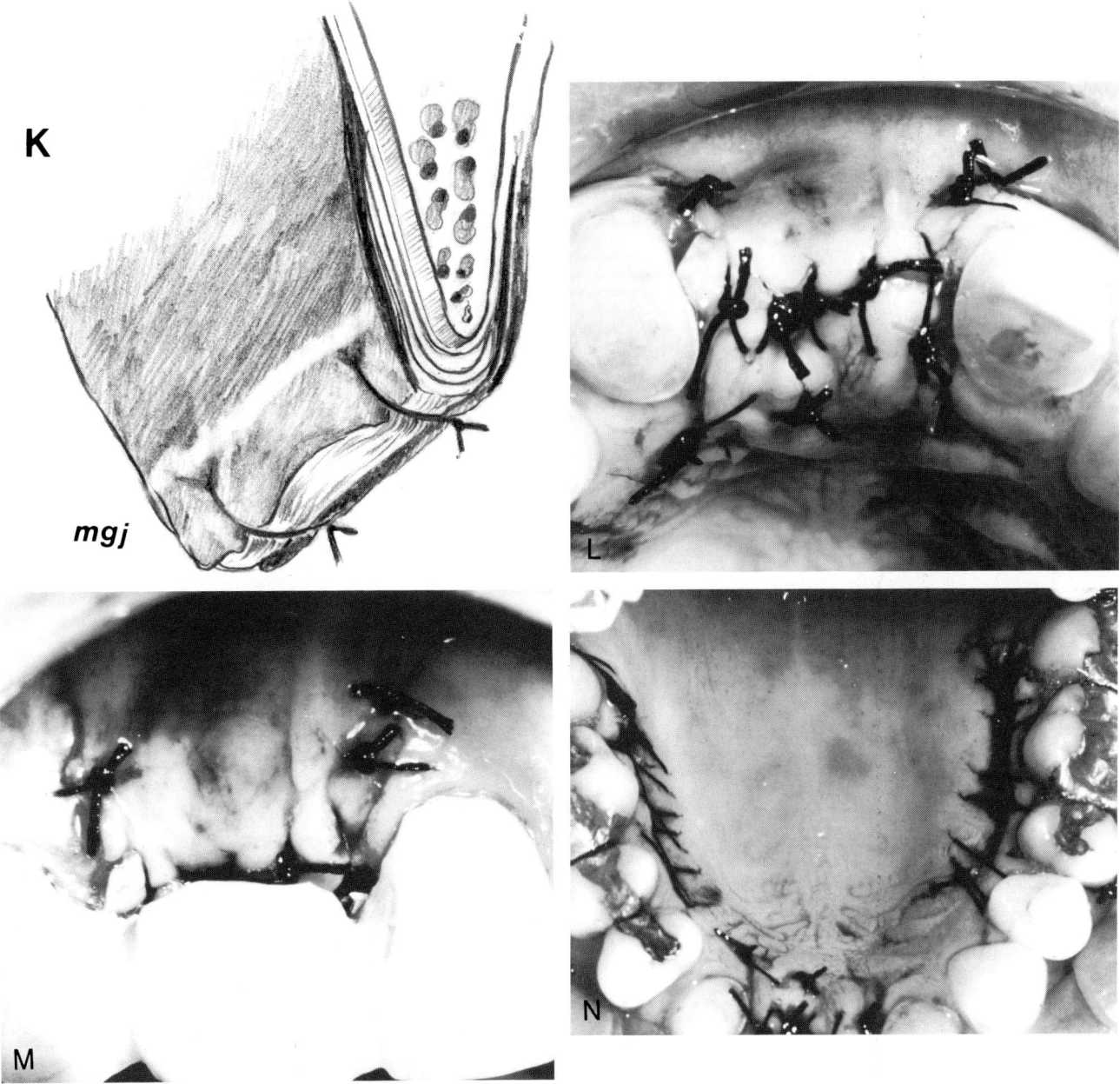

Fig. 10-13 (continued). K, L, Buccal and occlusal views of flaps coronally positioned and sutured. **M,** Temporary bridge recemented with pontic cutback. Note significant increase in ridge height. Compare to A and B. **N,** Palatal view of final suturing with primary coverage.

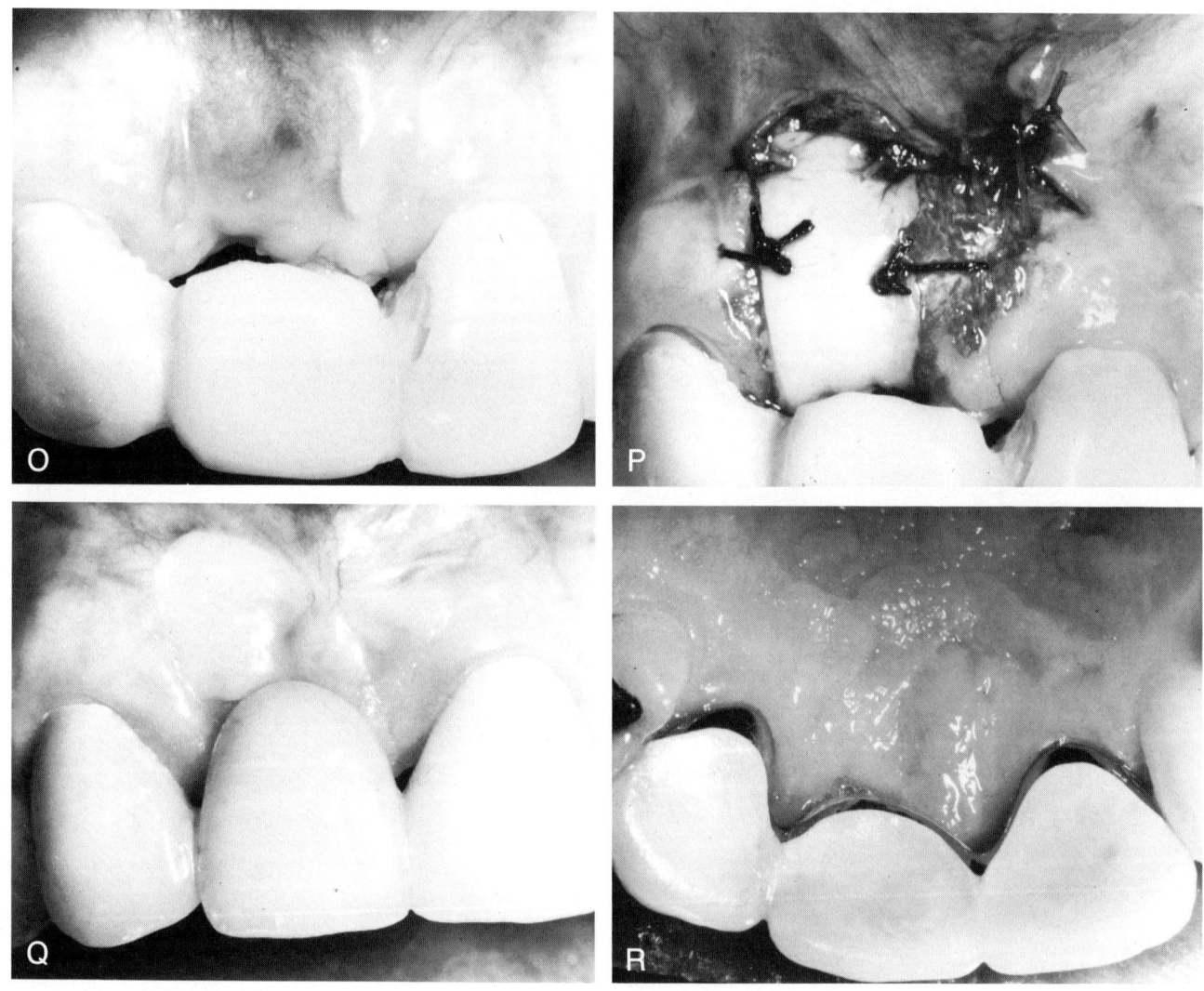

Fig. 10-13 (continued). **O,** Two months later. Note lack of keratinized gingiva over pontic area. **P,** Free gingival graft for increasing zone of keratinization in pontic area. **Q, R,** One year later, buccal and palatal views. (Prosthetics by David Gale, Sharon, OK.)

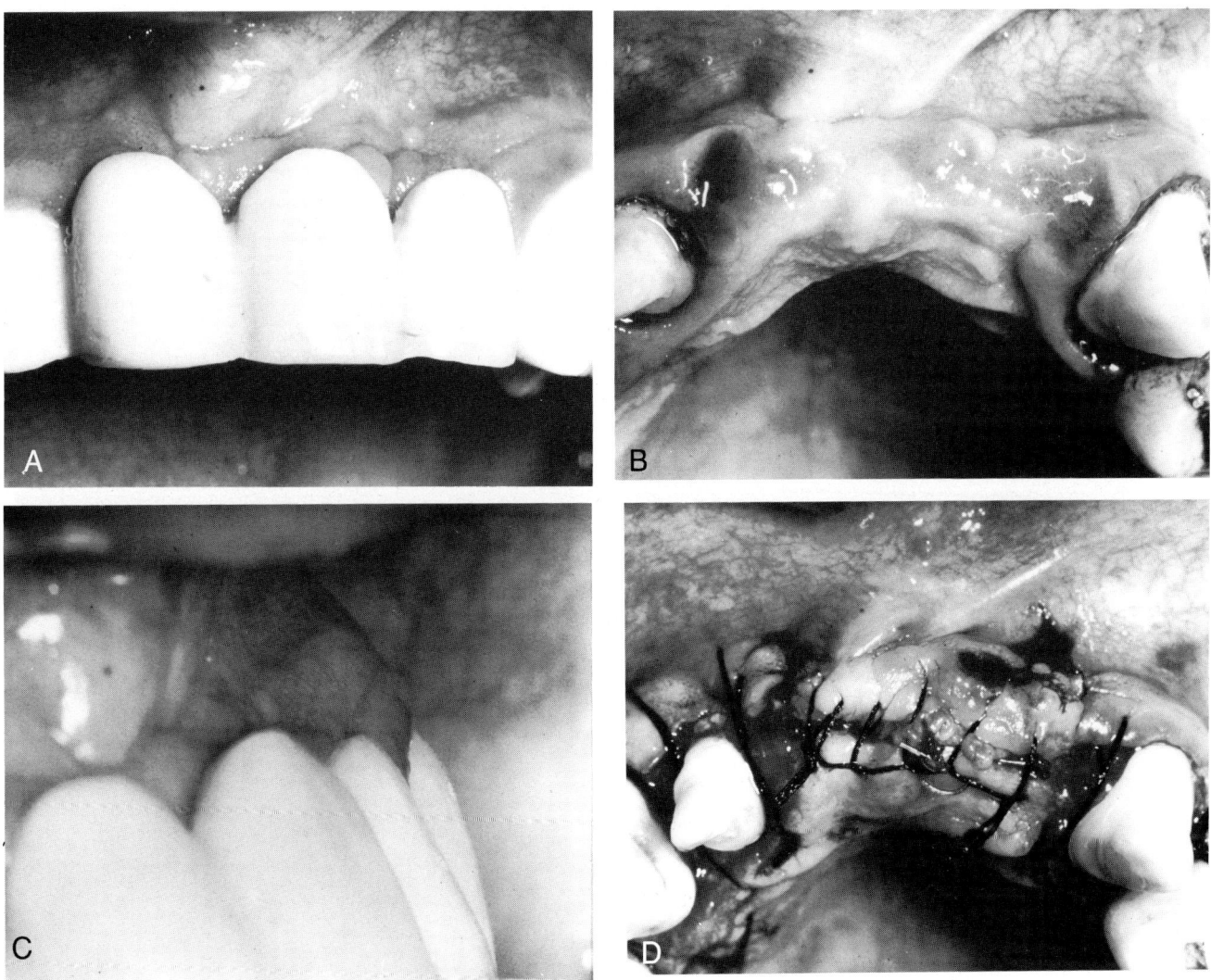

Fig. 10-14. Ridge Augmentation: Subepithelial Connective Tissue Graft. **A, B,** Before treatment. Note on side view that crowns are all anterior to ridge. **C,** Presurgical view of ridge. **D,** Final suturing of augmentation and crown lengthening.

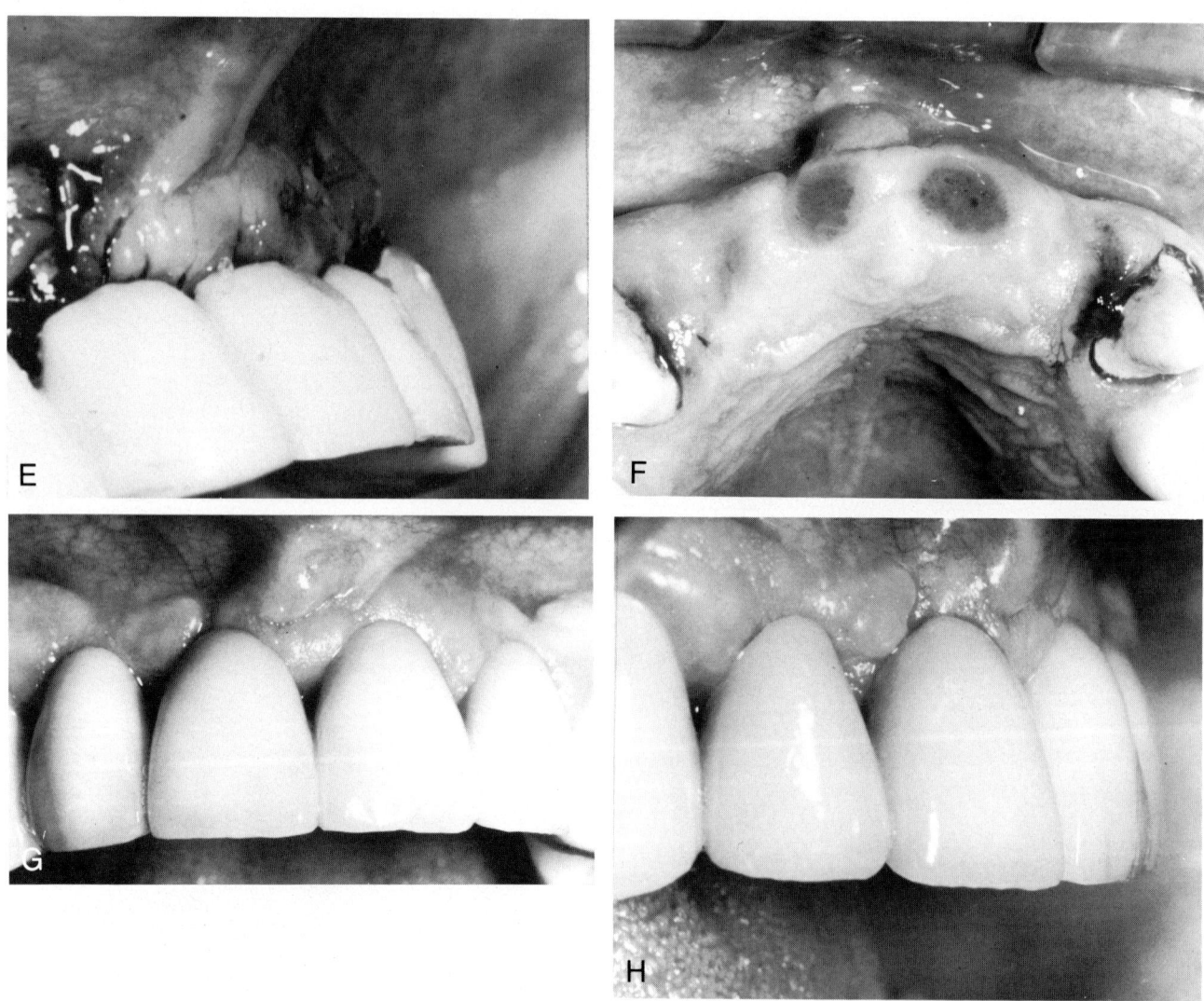

Fig. 10-14 (continued). **E,** Temporaries replaced. Note new position of crowns in relationship to ridge. **F,** 6 to 7 weeks later; note ridge enhancement as compared to C. **G, H,** Final prosthetics, buccal and side views. Compare to A and B. (Prosthetics completed by Michael Katz, Stoughton, MA.)

Ridge Augmentation

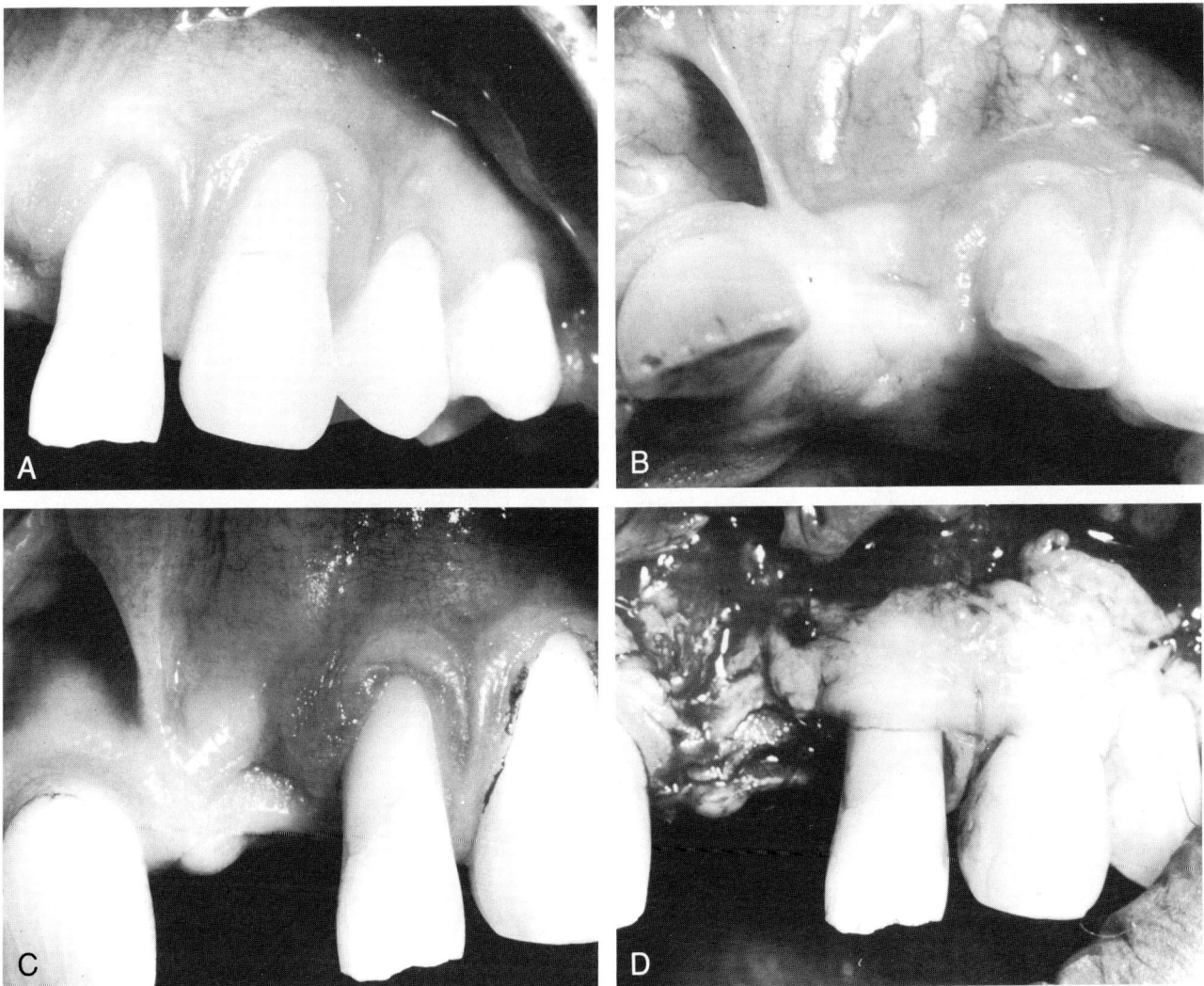

Fig. 10-15. Root Coverage and Ridge Augmentation: A Combination Procedure. **A,** Before treatment. Deep-wide Class III gingival recession on tooth no. 10 and Class II recession on tooth no. 11. **B,** Class II ridge defect in conjunction with gingival recession. **C,** Biomechanical root preparation with citric acid. **D,** Subepithelial connective tissue graft placed.

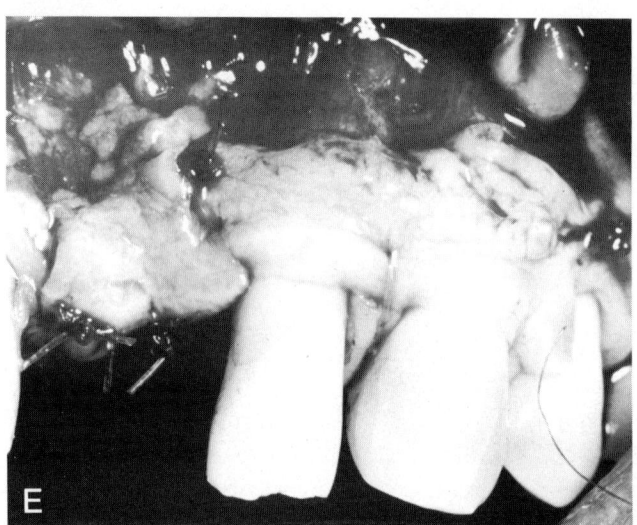
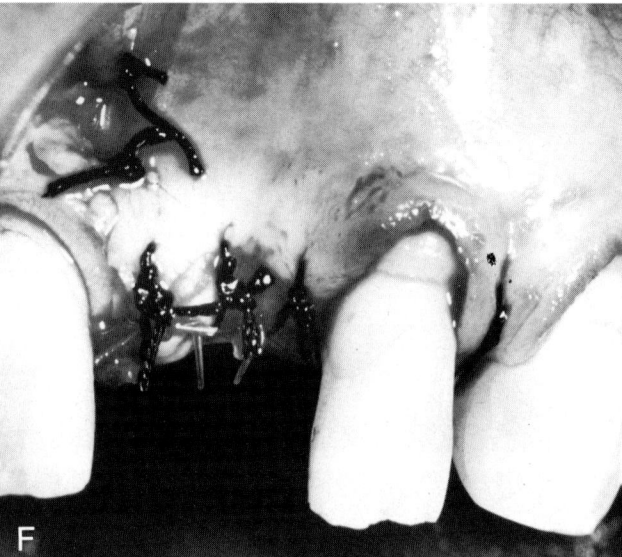
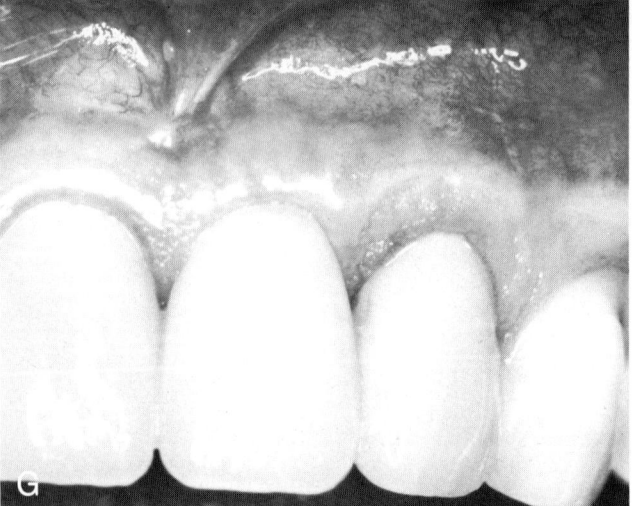

Fig. 10-15 (continued). **E,** Connective tissue graft placed on collapsed ridge. **F,** Suturing complete. **G,** Final prosthetics 6 months later. Note excellent cosmetic result.

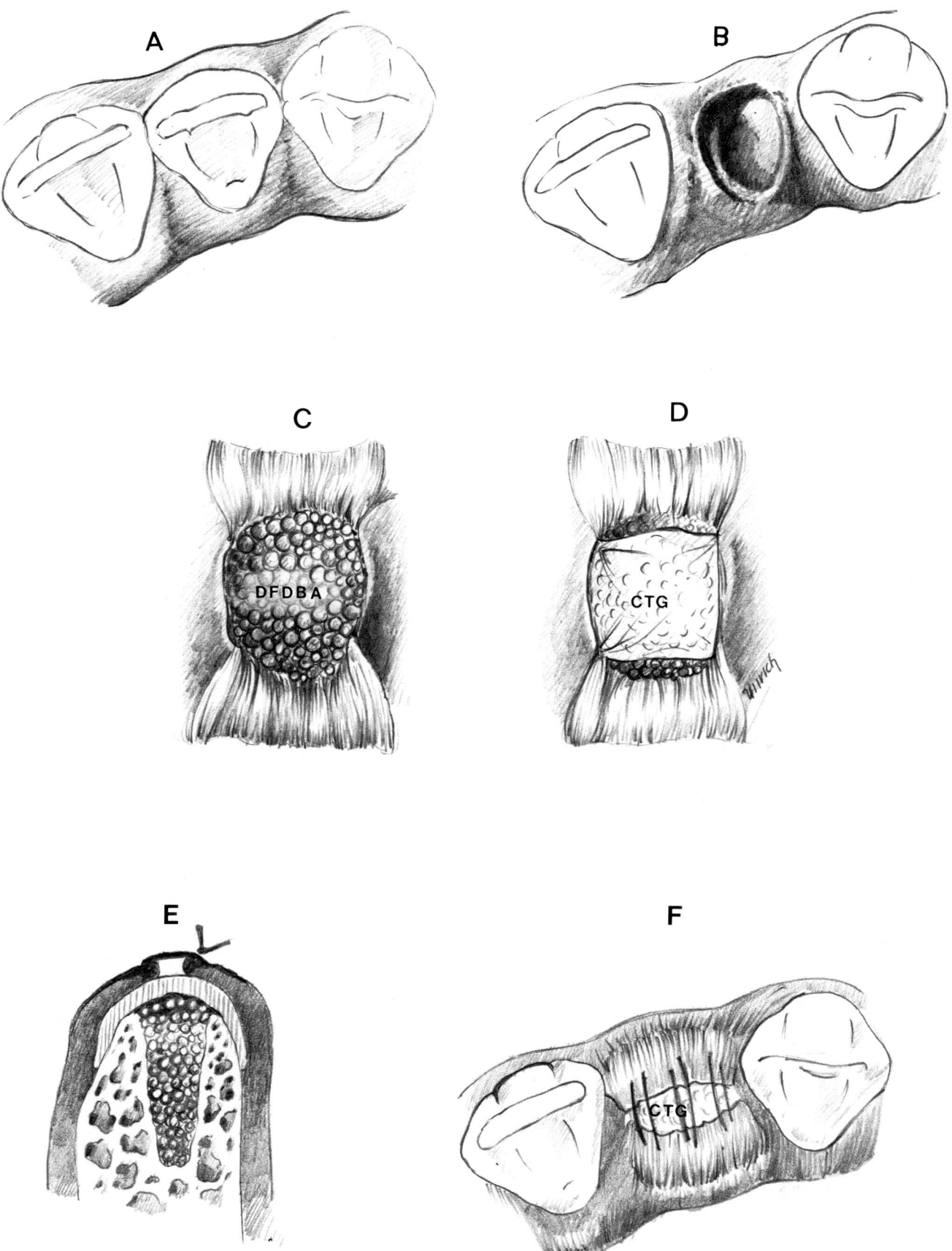

Fig. 10-16. Socket Preservation. **A,** Before lateral (middle) tooth is extracted. **B,** Tooth extracted. **C,** Socket filled with DFDBA or other implant material. **D,** Connective tissue graft placed for biologic cover. **E,** Cross-sectional view of sutured case. **F,** Occlusal view of final suturing.

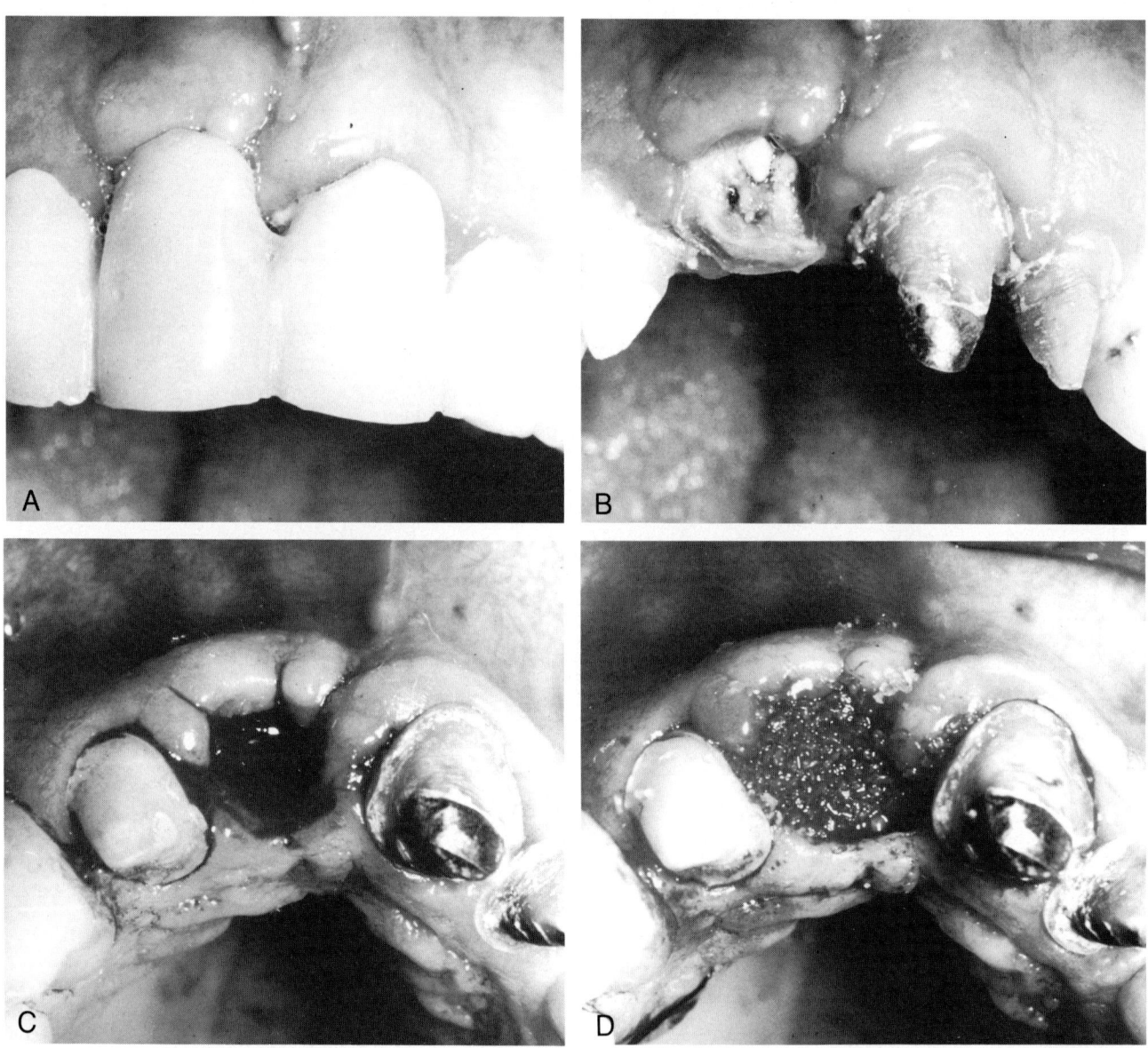

Fig. 10-17. Socket Preservation. **A,** Before treatment, with temporary bridge. **B,** Root to be extracted reduced to gingival crest. **C,** Tooth extracted. **D,** DFDBA placed into socket.

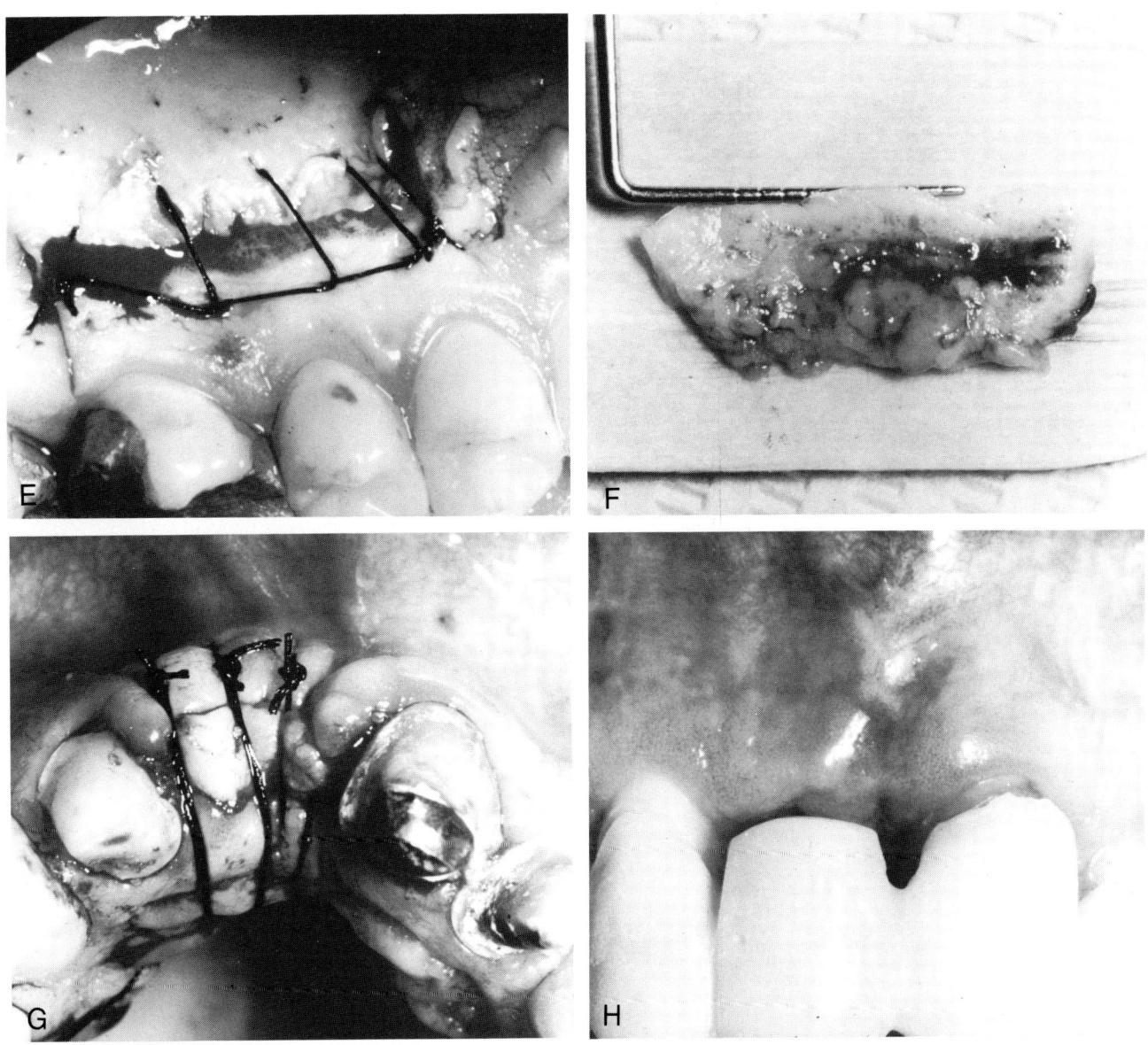

Fig. 10-17 (continued). **E, F,** Subepithelial connective tissue graft taken from palate. **G,** Graft placed over socket and under buccal flaps. **H,** Two months later. Note excellent ridge preservation prior to final prosthetics.

11

RESECTIVE OSSEOUS SURGERY

HISTORICAL REVIEW

Historically, osseous surgery was performed for the primary purpose of eliminating *necrotic or infected bone*. This was the generally held belief until Kronfeld (1935) established that *all bone is healthy*. This led to the modern concepts of osseous resective and inductive surgery, which are based primarily on the work of the following individuals:
1. Goldman (1950): "The Development of Physiologic Gingival Contours by Gingivoplasty"
2. Schluger (1949), "Osseous Resection—A Basic Principle in Periodontal Surgery"
3. Friedman (1955), "Periodontal Osseous Surgery: Osteoplasty and Ostectomy"
4. Prichard (1957), "The Infrabony Technique as a Predictable Procedure"
5. Goldman and Cohen (1958), "The Infrabony Pocket: Classification and Treatment"
6. Ochsenbein (1958), "Osseous Resection in Periodontal Surgery"
7. Ochsenbein (1986), "A Primer for Osseous Surgery"

Their work established the basic guidelines, definitions, terminology, and treatment procedures used today.

RATIONALE AND OBJECTIVES

The basis for performing resective osseous surgery lies in the fact that periodontal disease attacks the underlying or supportive bony architecture. This resorptive process results in an osseous form with sharp, uneven marginal deformities and irregularities. The bone, being hard, maintains these irregularities, while the gingival tissue, being soft, tends to follow a more fluid form. These inherent differences result in deep pockets that can be probed.

Osseous resective surgery has as its primary objectives the removal of osseous deformities and the creation of a *physiologic parabolic contour: A physiologic osseous form that will mimic the final anticipated gingival architecture*. This contour will be conducive for pocket elimination and maintenance of physiologic gingival architecture. The interdental area will be conical and coronally positioned to the buccal and lingual (palatal) plates of bone, which have a parabolic shape and flow smoothly from the interdental area (Fig. 11-1). The interdental area will follow the shape of the cementoenamel junction and have a prominent conical shape anteriorly that tends to become flatter and broader in the molar areas (Fig. 11-2). These factors allow a thin, scalloped, knife-edged gingival architecture with pyramidally shaped papillae that fill the interproximal space.

It is important to note that Ochsenbein (1977) pointed out that the gingival tissues were the dominating factor in establishing the osseous contours. He believed that after surgery the gingival tissues would tend to seek their original architectural form.

TISSUE MANAGEMENT

Treatment of osseous deformities involves the use of a full-thickness, inverse beveled, mucoperiosteal flap. The flap is scalloped. As a general rule, the clinician, *when scalloping the flap, should anticipate the final underlying osseous contour, which is most prominent anteriorly and decreases posteriorly* (see Chapter 5 on flap design and technique). Partial-thickness flaps are generally not indicated because of the limited access and visibility they provide and the fact that osseous surgery results in a torn, lacerated periosteum with little or no protection for the underlying bone.

All granulation tissue and residual connective tissue fibers must be removed prior to osseous surgery. Small bony defects are often hidden or obscured by residual fibers that are not removed. Plaque, calculus, softened cementum, and remnants of the junctional epithelium are all removed from the root surface.

TERMINOLOGY AND METHODS

Osseous resective surgery uses the techniques of *osteoplasty* and *ostectomy* (Friedman, 1955), techniques that are for the reduction and removal of *nonsupporting* and *supporting bone,* respectively.

OSTEOPLASTY

Osteoplasty is defined as a plastic procedure by which **nonsupporting bone** is reshaped to achieve a physiologic gingival and osseous contour for the following purposes (Fig. 11-3):
1. Pocket elimination
2. Tori reduction
3. Intrabony defects adjacent to edentulous ridges
4. Incipient furcation involvement
5. Reduction of thick, heavy ledges and/or exostosis
6. Shallow osseous craters
7. Blunted interdental craters
8. Small intrabony defects associated with the buccal or lingual surfaces
9. Enhanced flap placement with improved alveolar contours

Osteoplasty includes the techniques of **grooving** or **festooning** (Ochsenbein, 1958) and **radicular blending** (Carranza, 1984).

Vertical grooving or festooning is designed to reduce the buccal and lingual thicknesses of bone interdentally. These *vertical depth cuts* or hollowing out provide for greater root prominence on the radicular surface allowing a more favorable gingival architecture, minimal bone removal, and a smooth transition from the radicular to the interradicular space. The vertical grooving often reduces the external walls of small craters, making further osseous contouring unnecessary. For this reason, *osteoplasty usually precedes ostectomy.*

Radicular blending is generally indicated for use on a thicker, heavier bone, following vertical grooving. The procedure is used to establish an even-flowing, thin radicular surface that rises over root prominences and falls in the valleys established by the vertical grooves.

Blunted Interdental Septa and Thick Bony Margins

Two of the most commonly found early osseous deformities are those of *blunted interdental septa* and *thick or heavy bone margins.* They may occur independently, but often occur together. They are treated predominantly by osteoplasty.

Procedure

With the flaps reflected, the osseous topography is viewed bucally, lingually (or palatally), and occlusally. This allows the clinician to develop a three-dimensional mental image of the relationships between the individual teeth and their bony housing, which helps determine a perspective for performing osseous surgery.

Figure 11-4A shows blunting of the interdental septa combined with heavy bony margins. The interproximal area, being blunted, and *not* having a *negative architecture,* may require some osseous resective procedures to produce a more definitive *positive architecture.*

The first step is *vertical interradicular grooving or festooning.* These grooves are carried to the line angles of adjacent teeth and determine the buccolingual width of the bone. Using a round No. 6, 8, or 10 bur in a high-speed handpiece with copious amounts of water, the grooves are cut (Fig. 11-4B).

Once the vertical grooves are completed, *radicular blending* is begun, using the same size bur (Fig. 11-4C). The bur is moved with sweeping strokes as if one were painting, back and forth, rising over the root prominences and falling into the depressions created by the grooves. This is continued until an even-flowing osseous form is created. The round bur sometimes leaves a roughened surface that can be smoothed by using a round diamond stone of similar size.

Upon completion of radicular blending, a flat crest of bone is left interproximally at the same level as the radicular surfaces. Generally, this is not acceptable because the *gingival tissue will inherently form a scalloped contour with a pyramidally shaped papilla regardless of the underlying bony contours.* The end result, if no further osseous surgery is done, will be a residual tissue pocket of 4 to 5 mm.

To determine the amount of osseous scalloping or ostectomy to be done, it is necessary to know the preoperative shape and form of the tissue, because the tissue has a tendency to develop relatively the same shape after surgery. The amount of tissue scalloping necessary will decrease as the interproximal osseous area becomes broader. This is seen as one moves from the incisors to the molars (see Fig.

11-2) or as bone loss increases interproximally. Therefore, as a general rule *the final bony contours should mirror or approximate the healthy preoperative gingival form. Excessive scalloping or grooving should be avoided.*

In Figure 11-4D, a small No. 2 or No. 4 round bur in a high-speed handpiece is used to outline or *scribe* (see ostectomy) the bone at the correct level. Care is taken not to contact the teeth. *Scribing* the bone allows it to be visualized and facilitates removal (with Ochsenbein No. 1 or 2 chisels) (Fig. 11-4E).

The completed osseous form is one with scalloped or parabolic radicular surfaces that gradually rise interdentally to a conically shaped interproximal bone (Fig. 11-4F).

Figure 11-5 shows a clinical example of this procedure.

OSTECTOMY

Ostectomy is the plastic removal of *radicular* and *interradicular supporting bone* to eliminate osseous deformities.

Indications

1. Sufficient bone remaining for establishing physiologic contours without attachment compromise
2. No esthetic or anatomic limitations
3. Elimination of interdental craters
4. Intrabony defects not amenable to regeneration
5. Horizontal bone loss with irregular marginal bone height
6. Moderate to advanced furcation involvements
7. Hemisepta

Advantages

1. Predictable pocket elimination
2. Establishment of physiologic gingival and osseous architecture
3. Establishment of a favorable prosthetic environment

Disadvantages

1. Loss of attachment
2. Esthetic compromise
3. Increased root sensitivity

Contraindications

1. Areas of insufficient remaining attachment or where ostectomy might unfavorably alter the prognosis of the adjacent teeth

2. Anatomic limitations (prominent external oblique ridge or zygomatic arch, etc.)
3. Esthetic limitations (anteriorly, high smile line, etc.)
4. Effective alternative treatment

Ostectomy is done by the technique of *spheroiding* or *parabolizing*. *Spheroiding* or *parabolizing* is the removal of *supporting bone* to produce a *positive gingival and osseous architecture*. An architecture in which the bone is higher interproximally than it is buccally or lingually and has a smooth, even-flowing *scalloped* or *parabolic* shape on the radicular surface is achieved by the following:

1. Horizontal grooving
2. Scribing
3. Hand instrumentation

Horizontal grooving is the technique by which a small round bur in a high-speed handpiece is placed interproximally at the base of the osseous defect and drawn buccally and lingually. This flattens the interproximal area in a buccolingual direction but not in a mesiodistal direction.

Scribing is the technique by which high-speed rotatory instrumentation is used to outline on the radicular bone, that bone which is to be removed by hand instrumentation. This *scribing* provides a visual outline that facilitates the use of hand chisels for final bone removal. High-speed rotatory instruments are not to be used for the removal of bone adjacent to teeth for fear of *nicking* and damaging the teeth.

Craters and Hemisepta

The most common type of intrabony defects are *craters* and *hemiseptae*. These are caused by the inflammatory lesion's following the blood vessels into the interproximal area, resulting in loss and hollowing of the interproximal bone. The end result produces a *negative osseous architecture* in which the base of the interproximal bone is below that of the buccal and/or lingual (palatal) radicular surfaces. Without resective osseous procedures for treatment of these defects, tissue pockets will immediately re-form.

The osseous resective techniques employed are the same for craters, hemisepta, and intrabony defects.

Procedure

Figure 11-6A represents small interproximal osseous defects or *craters* in which there is a central loss of interproximal bone while the buccal and lingual radicular walls remain intact. Technically, this is classified as a two-wall intraosseous defect.

Figure 11-6B depicts *horizontal grooving*. The largest round bur (No. 2, 4, or 6) that can safely fit interproximally without coming in contact with the teeth is placed in the most apical portion of the intrabony defect. It is drawn in a straight line both buccally and lingually (palatally) to flatten and in effect remove the interproximal defect in a buccolingual direction.

It is important to note that horizontal grooving, while reducing the interproximal defect, produces a **negative osseous architecture,** in which the interproximal bone is more apical than the buccal or lingual radicular bone. As a general rule, *osseous resective surgical procedure ideally should result in a **positive osseous architecture,** with the interproximal bone coronal to the buccal and lingual radicular bones.*

In Figure 11-6C, the negative osseous architecture is produced by the horizontal grooving. Spheroiding or parabolizing is begun with *osseous scribing* along the dotted line. A small No. 2, 4, or 6 round bur is used to scribe the bone. As a rule, scribing should follow the anticipated final desired gingival architecture.

Hand chisels are used to remove bone facially and lingually (Fig. 11-6D). This produces the desired scalloped or parabolic osseous form capable of supporting a similar gingival architecture.

The final osseous contouring is performed at the line angles of the teeth to remove small bony spicules often referred to as *widow peaks* (Schluger, 1949) (Fig. 11-6E). These *widow peaks* are residual pieces of cortical bone left over from the horizontal grooving that form a crater in a mesiodistal direction. They will not be absorbed and will result in immediate postoperative tissue pocketing. Hand instrumentation with Ochsenbein chisels as well as various bone files is recommended to remove these residual bony spurs interproximally.

The completed osseous form is shown in Figure 11-6F. Note the positive osseous architecture that rises and falls gradually with a coronally placed, conically shaped, interproximal crest of bone.

The procedure is clinically outlined in Figures 11-7 and 11-8.

Management of Deep Craters

In treating craters, it is not always possible to make the center portion of the interproximal bone the most coronal portion (Fig. 11-9a,a'), because, in deep craters, too much buccal and/or lingual bone would have to be sacrificed. In these cases, the bone is ramped either buccally or lingually, with only one of the walls totally removed while the other is only partially reduced (Fig. 11-9b,b'). Sometimes, the defect is positioned either buccally or lingually, favoring removal of only one wall and therefore ramping the bone in that direction (Fig. 11-9c,c').

OSSEOUS MANAGEMENT OF TEETH WITH FURCATIONS

Osseous resective procedures in areas of furcations often have to be managed with an understanding of the anatomic interrelationships among the following:
1. Length of root trunk
2. Location and form of bony defect
3. Furcation involvement and location
4. Alveolar housing
5. Tooth position

The most critical factors are the length of the root trunk and the position and depth of the osseous defect. These two factors ultimately determine the direction (buccal, lingual, or palatal) and amount of osseous corrective procedures necessary to create a positive architecture without involving the furcations.

Maxillary Molars

The maxillary buccal furcation is the primary area of concern in performing osseous resective procedures. Excessive removal of buccal bone (ostectomy) to create a positive gingival architecture may unnecessarily involve this furcation. For this reason, a palatal approach has been recommended (see Chapter 6). Ramping of bone toward the palate will minimize reduction of buccal bone, maintain esthetics, and most importantly, preserve the integrity of the buccal furcation.

If buccal resective procedures are required, a scalloped or parabolic form should be created over the mesial and/or distal roots. The buccal furcation should be untouched and allowed to remain coronally positioned. This permits the gingival tissues to rise and fall in a gradual manner as it does between any two teeth with roots in close approximation.

Mandibular Molars

Tibbetts et al. (1976) and Ochsenbein (1986) have noted the importance of the lingual axial inclination of the first and second mandibular molars, as a result of which the lingual gingival architecture is usually flat regardless of the buccal gingival contours. Ochsenbein states that "since the base of the crater is vertical to the contact area . . . shallow and medium depth crater types generally have their bases located lingually. . . ." Tibbets et al. and Ochsenbein concluded that the defects should therefore be ramped primarily lingually without attempting to achieve a scalloped or parabolic form over the roots. They also pointed out the need for osteoplasty on the lingual aspect, especially in the second molar area, to reduce the prominence of the mylohyoid ridge, permitting pocket elimination and adequate gingival form.

Clinical management of complex osseous deformities is shown in Figures 11-10, 11-11, and 11-12.

Edentulous Ridge

Defects often occur posteriorly adjacent to edentulous ridges (Fig. 11-13A). These defects are easily corrected by reducing the edentulous ridge down to the base of the defect (Fig. 11-13B). This results in a minimal amount of supporting bone being removed.

Ideally, the molar shown in Figure 11-13 would be uprighted orthodontically, which might reduce or eliminate the need for extensive osseous surgery. It would also promote a more favorable axial inclination for prosthetic rehabilitation.

BIOLOGIC WIDTH

Restoration of fractured (traumatized), severely decayed, partially erupted (delayed passive eruption), worn, or poorly restored teeth is often difficult, if not impossible, for the dentist. Periodontal exposure or prophylactic lengthening of these teeth must adhere to certain biologic principles and an adequate biologic width must be maintained.

Biologic width is the term applied to the dimensional width of the dentogingival junction (epithelial attachment and underlying connective tissue) (Fig. 11-14). Garguilo et al. (1961) quantified this as almost a constant 2.04 mm (the epithelial attachment is 0.97 mm; and connective tissue is 1.07 mm) with a sulcus depth of 0.69 mm.

Nevins and Skurow (1984) defined biologic width as the sum of the combined supracrestal fibers, the junctional epithelium, and the sulcus. This was over 3 mm when measured from the crest of bone. Wagenberg et al. (1989) concluded that at least 5 to 5.25 mm exposed tooth structure above the crest was required for adequate crown preparation. This was supported by Bragger et al. (1992), who showed that creating a distance of 3 mm from the alveolar crest to the future reconstruction margin was stable periodontally for up to 6 months.

Tooth lengthening procedures (Figs. 11-15, 11-16, and 11-17) often employ some combination of tissue removal, osseous surgery, and orthodontics. The amount of tooth structure exposed (about 4 mm) must be enough to permit proper tooth preparation, and account for an adequate marginal placement, thus ensuring a good marginal seal with retention for both provisional and final restorations (Saadoun et al. 1983), while still providing for the biologic width of tissue. *Impingement on the zone* (biologic width) *results in bone absorption.*

Rosenberg and Garber (1980) have outlined the factors that should be taken into account prior to tooth lengthening procedures:
A. Etiologic Factors
1. Caries
2. Trauma/fracture
3. Altered passive eruption
4. Restorative requirements
B. Restorative Considerations
1. Esthetics
2. Form
3. Function
4. Retention
5. Marginal seal
C. Limiting Factors
1. Crown-to-root ratio
2. Maintainability
3. Esthetics
4. Location of furcations
5. Predictability
6. Tooth-arch relationship
7. Comparison of adjacent periodontium

BASIC RULES OF OSSEOUS SURGERY

In the descriptions of osteoplasty and ostectomy certain basic principles were noted. These are reviewed here as a checklist for the clinician to follow:

Rule 1: A full-thickness mucoperiosteal flap should be used whenever osseous resective surgery is contemplated.

Rule 2a: The scalloping of the flap should anticipate the final underlying osseous contour, which is most prominent anteriorly and decreases posteriorly.

Rule 2b: The scalloping of the flap should reflect the patient's own healthy gingival architecture.

Rule 2c: The degree of tissue and bone scalloping is reduced as the interproximal area becomes broader as a result of bone loss.

Rule 3: Osteoplasty generally precedes ostectomy.

Rule 4: Osseous resective surgery should whenever possible result in a *positive osseous architecture.*

Rule 5: High-speed rotary instrumentation should never be used adjacent to the teeth and should always be used with a generous spray.

Rule 6: The final bony contours should approximate the expected healthy postoperative gingival form *with no attempt to improve upon it.*

FORCED ERUPTION

Crown lengthening often results in the apical positioning of marginal tissue with or without removal of bone. This will compromise both esthetics and periodontal support, resulting in an unsightly long clinical crown with associated loss of interproximal tissue. To avoid this situation, Ingber (1974) developed the concept of forced orthodontic eruption. This technique permits extension of the tooth and leveling of the intrabony defect at the same time. The end result is orthodontic correction of a periodontal problem, minimizing or eliminating the need for corrective periodontal surgery (Fig. 11-18).

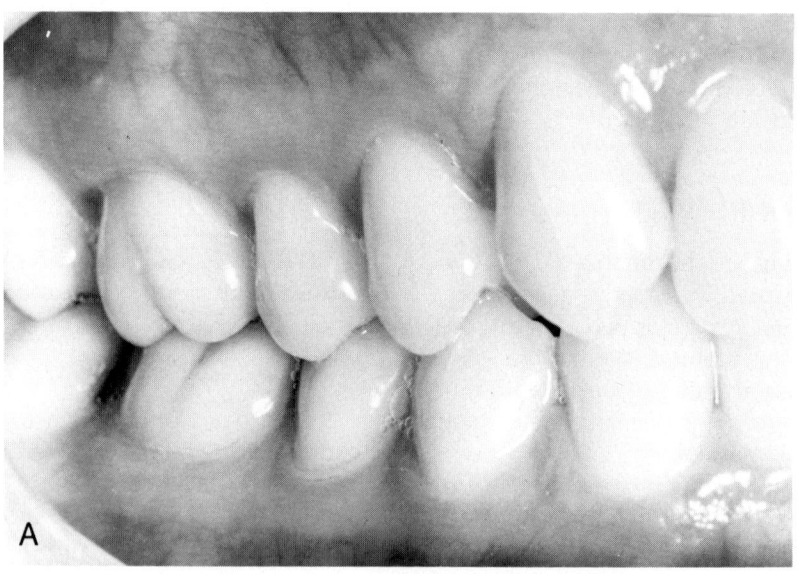

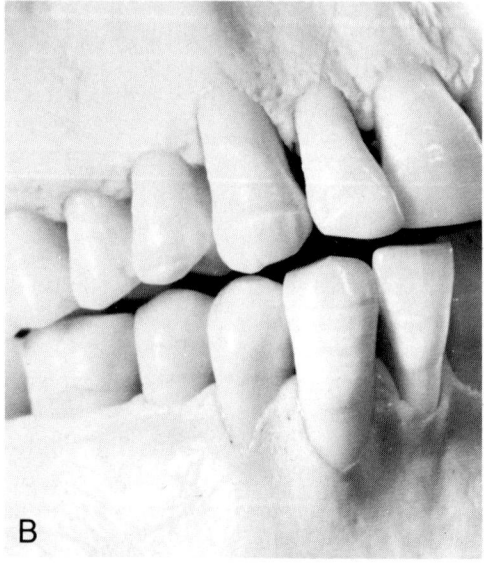

Fig. 11-1. Ideal Gingival and Osseous Contours. **A,** Gingival contours showing a scalloped, parabolic architecture with a pyramidally shaped conical papilla. **B,** Underlying osseous architecture with scalloped parabolic contours that mimic gingival form.

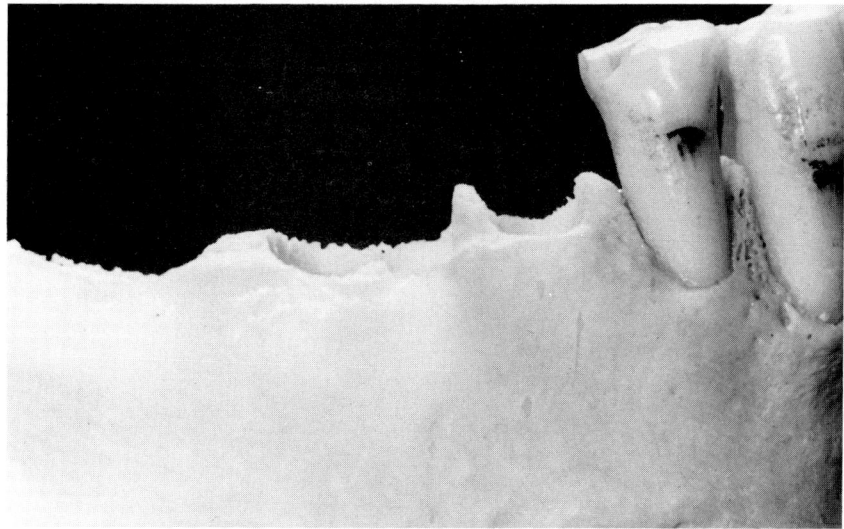

Fig. 11-2. Interdental Osseous Form. The interdental osseous form tends to be thinner and more conical anteriorly, becoming flatter and broader in the molar areas.

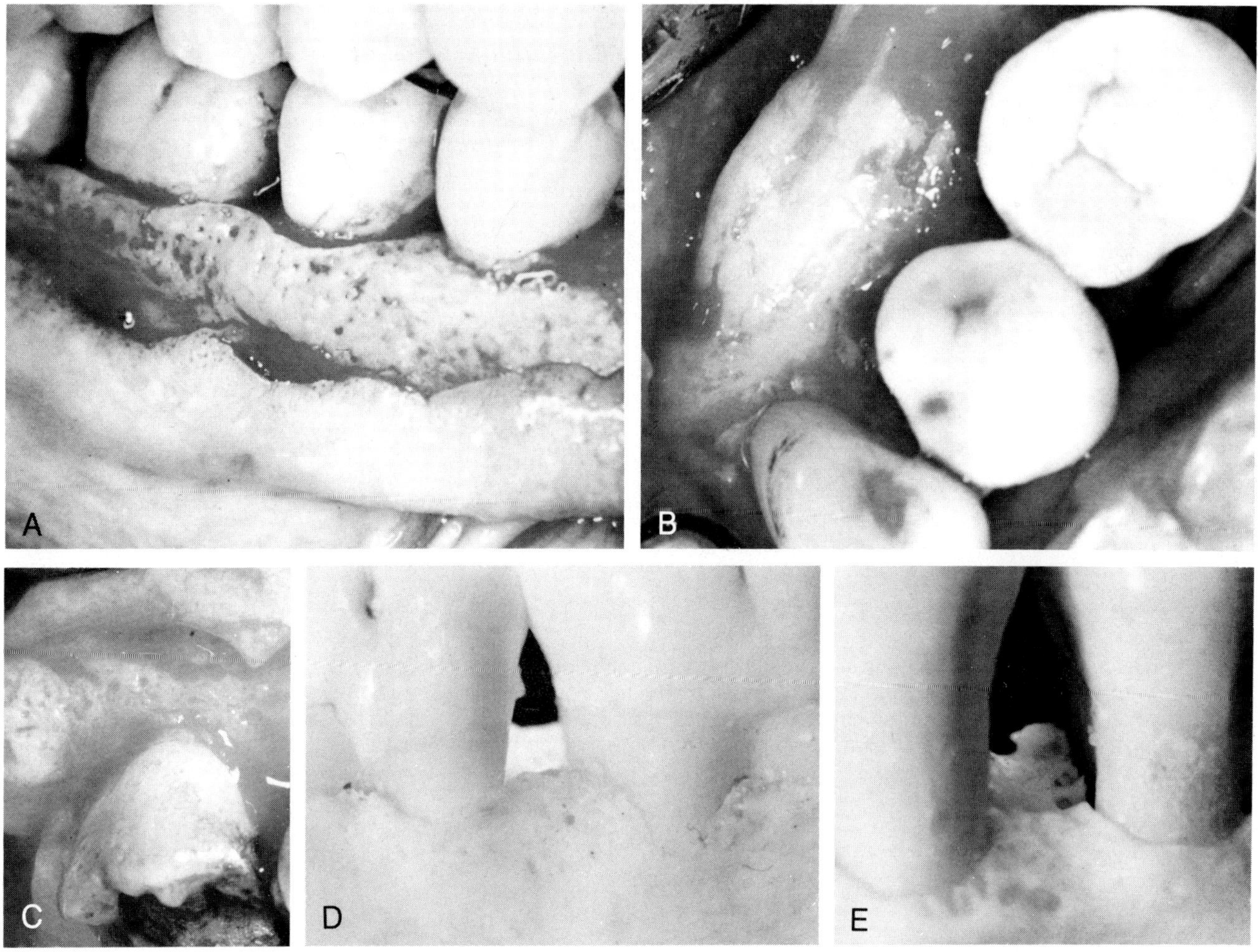

Fig. 11-3. Indications for Osteoplasty. **A,** Thick bony margins. **B,** Tori. **C,** Exostosis. **D,** Small craters. **E,** Blunted interdental septa.

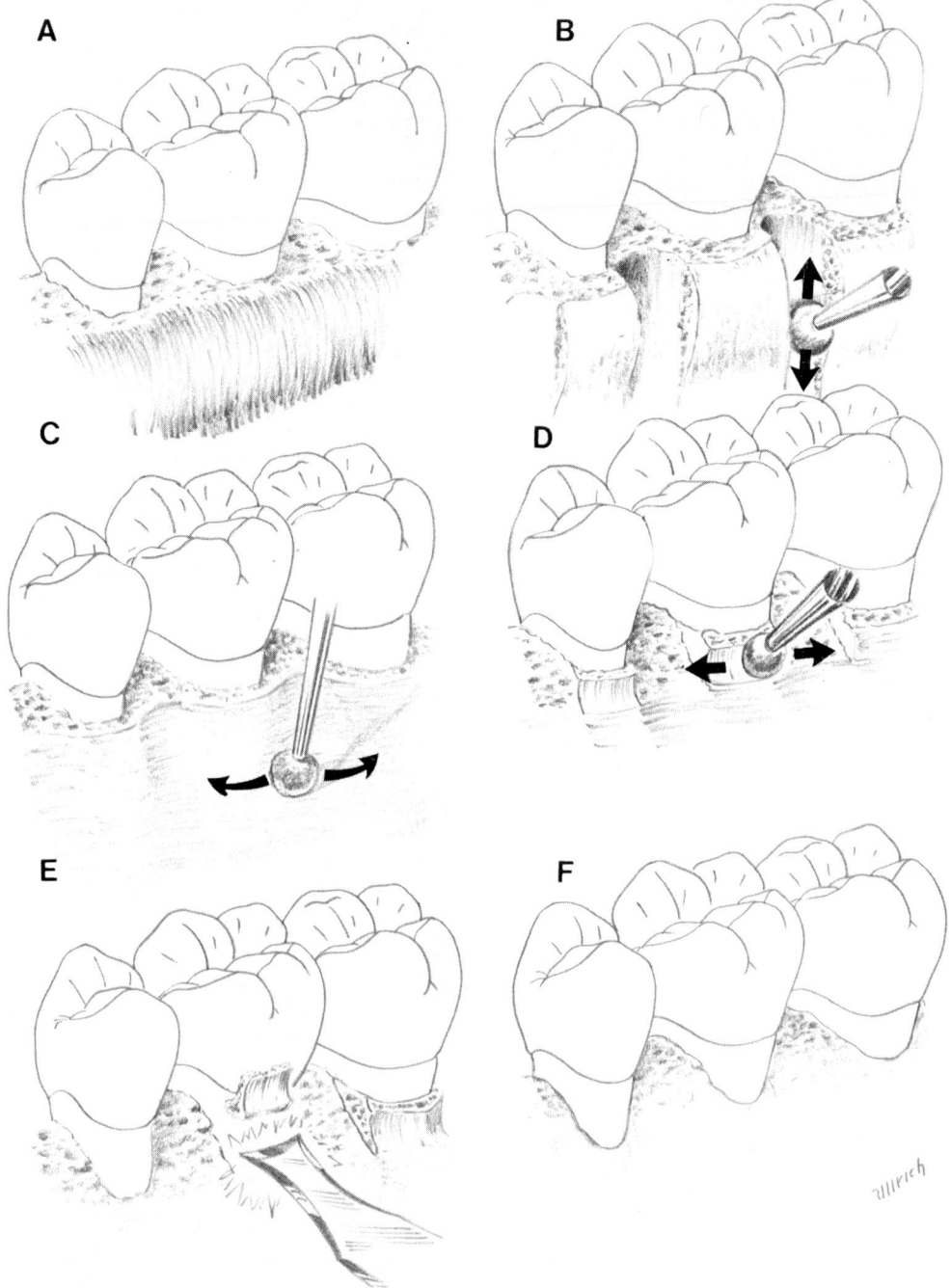

Fig. 11-4. Osteoplasty for Heavy Ledges, Thick Margins, or Blunted Interproximal Septa. **A,** Depicts thick margins and blunted interproximal septa. **B,** *Vertical grooving* to establish width and thin bone interdentally. **C,** *Festooning* or *radicular blending* to reduce thick bony margins and establish physiologic form. **D,** *Scribing* for outlining bone to be removed. **E,** Minor *ostectomy* for final physiologic *parabolic* contour. **F,** Completed reshaping. Note thinned bone with ideal interproximal contour.

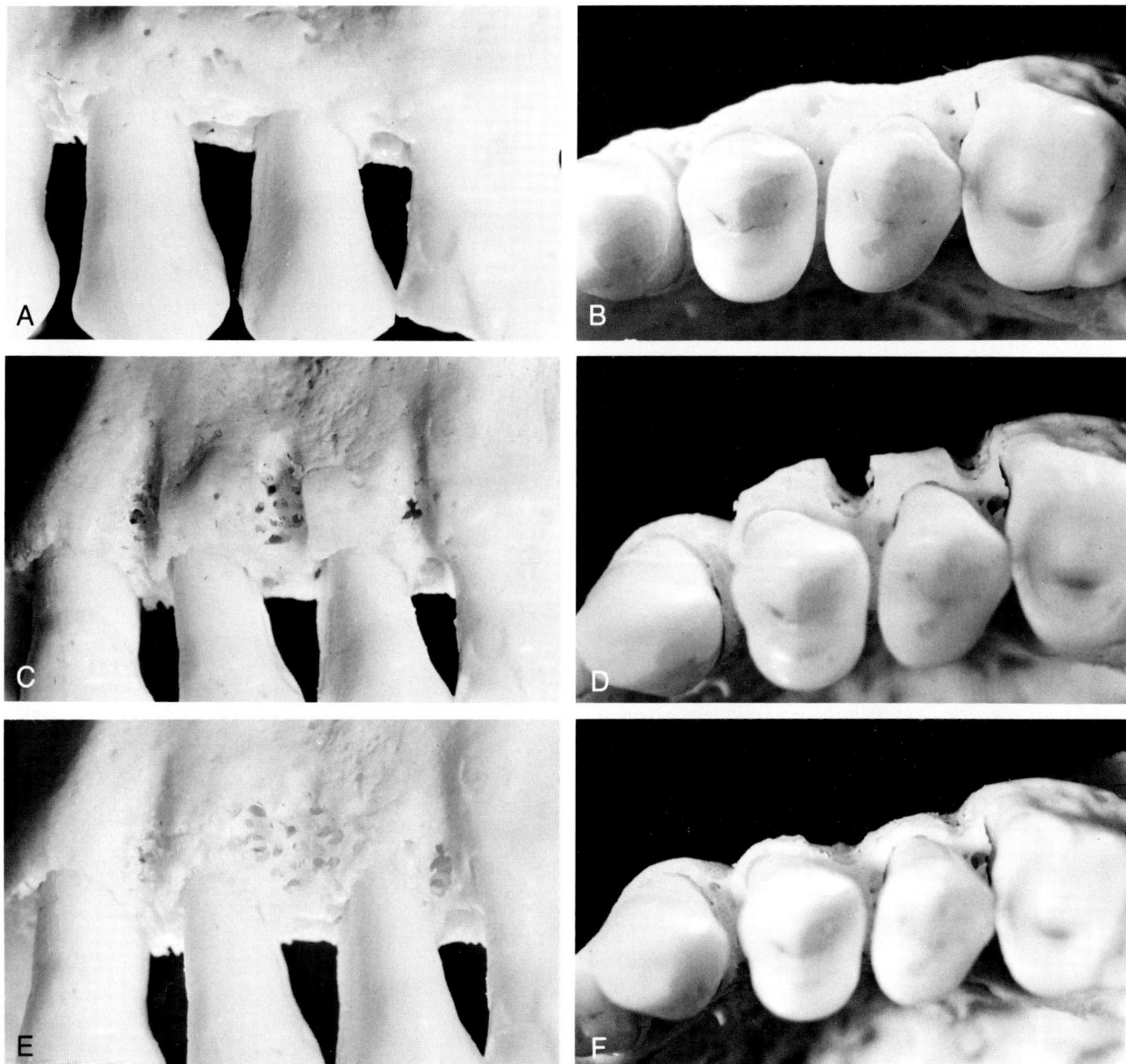

Fig. 11-5. Osteoplasty for Reduction of Bulbous Bone and Thick Margins. **A, B,** Buccal and occlusal views before treatment, showing thick margins and a bulbous osseous contour. Note the blunted interdental septa with no bony defects. **C, D,** Vertical grooving or festooning from buccal and occlusal views. Note that grooves are carved to the line angles of the teeth. Vertical grooves establish the buccolingual width of the alveolus. **E, F,** Radicular blending completed. Note the even-flowing, scalloped, parabolic contours. Some ostectomy was done on the facial aspect. Compare with A and B.

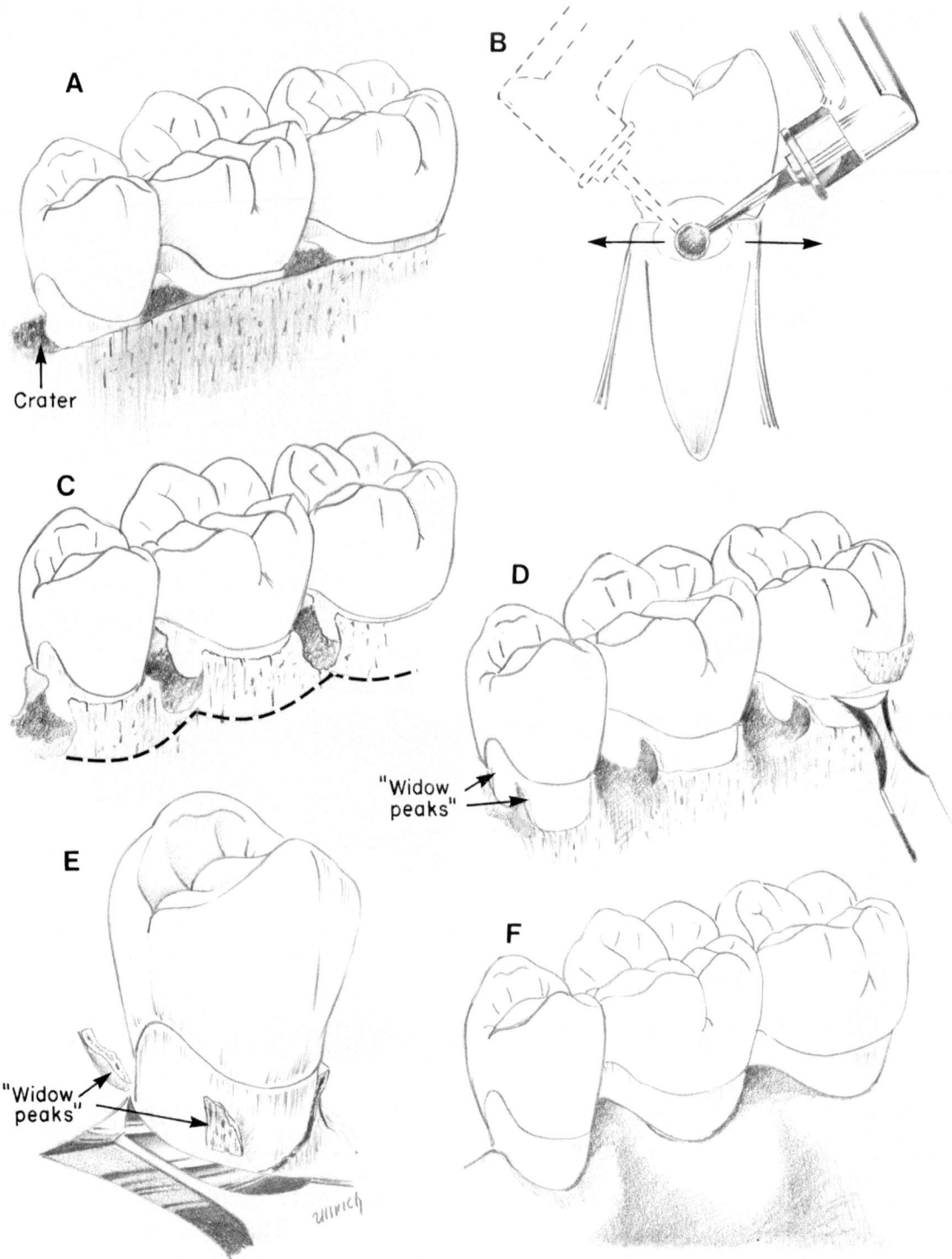

Fig. 11-6. Ostectomy for Osseous Deformities: Craters, Hemisepta, and Intrabony Defects. **A,** Represents interproximal craters. **B,** *Horizontal* grooving. A small round bur is used to reduce the buccal and lingual crater walls. **C,** Dotted line outlines bone to be *scribed* prior to removal to establish a physiologic form. **D,** Bone removal with Ochsenbein chisels (after scribing). Note small spicules of residual bone or *widow peaks* (WP). **E,** Removal of residual bone or *widow peaks* left at line angles and interproximally. **F,** Ostectomy completed and physiologic form established.

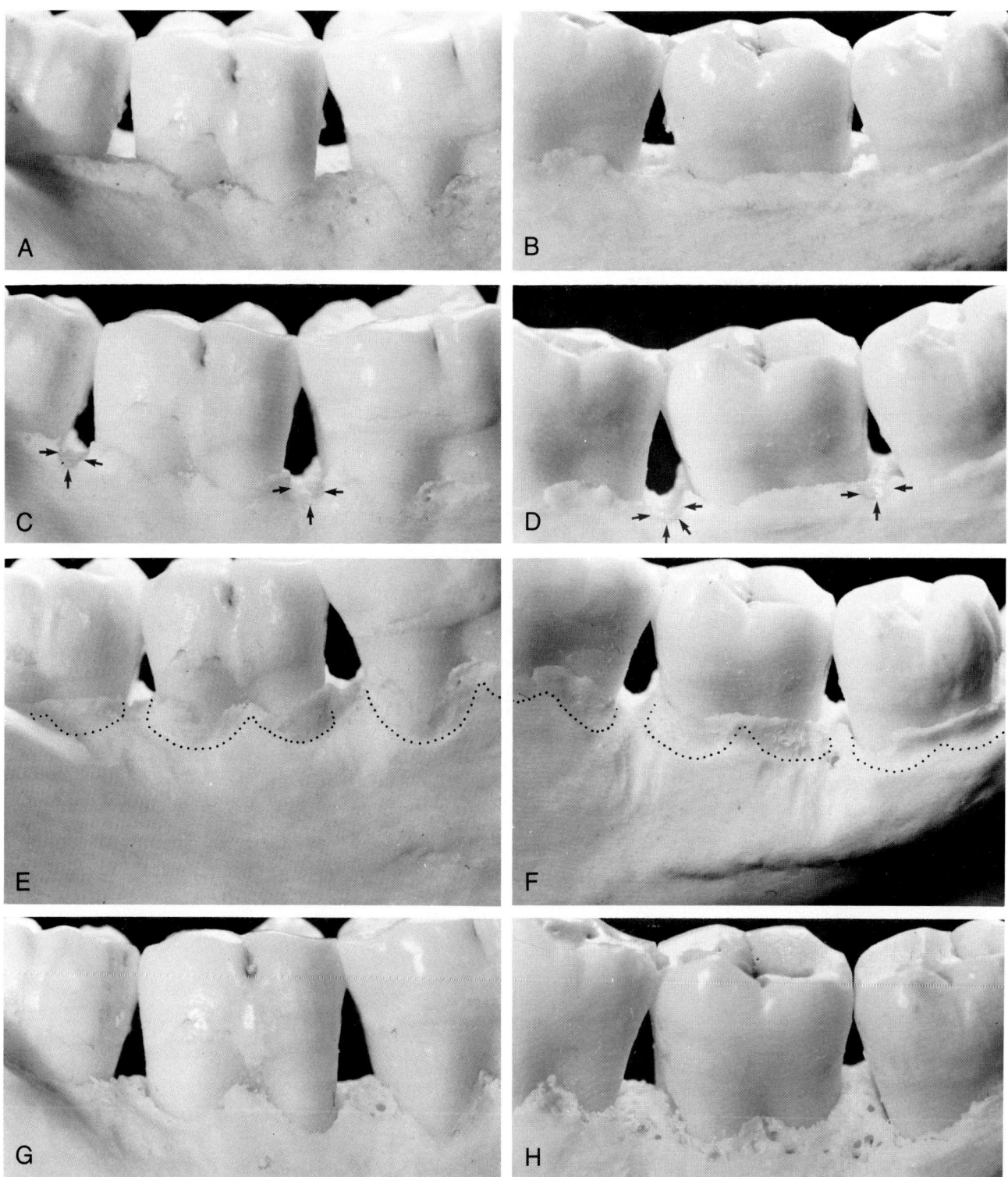

Fig. 11-7. Osseous Surgery (Ostectomy and Osteoplasty) for Treatment of the Osseous Crater—Example I. **A,** Buccal view showing small interdental craters. **B,** Lingual view. Note heavier lingual ledges and small craters. **C, D,** Buccal and lingual views of horizontal grooving; note that the interproximal areas are leveled off buccolingually but a small crater is formed mesiodistally (see arrows). **E,** The bone is *scribed* (outlined areas) prior to removal. **F,** Lingual view of *scribed* bone. Some vertical grooving and radicular blending have also been completed. **G,** Final buccal osseous contour. Note even-flowing contours; compare with A. **H,** Final lingual contours. Note scalloped parabolic contours; compare with B.

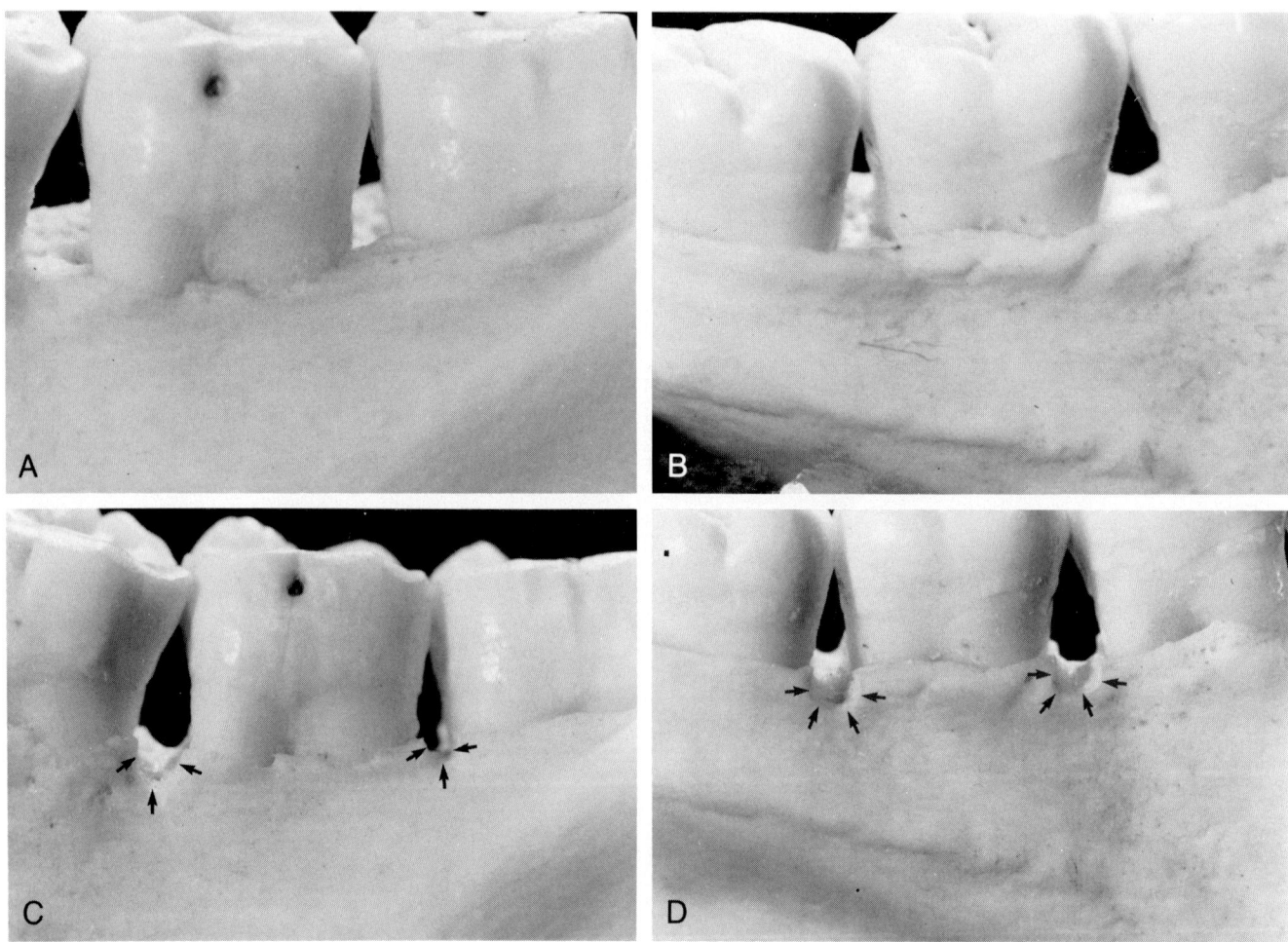

Fig. 11-8. Osseous Surgery (Ostectomy and Osteoplasty) for Treatment of the Osseous Crater—Example II. **A, B,** Buccal and lingual views showing small interdental craters. Note the lack of positive osseous architecture. **C, D,** Horizontal grooving, buccal and lingual views. Arrows indicate residual mesiodistal crater and negative osseous architecture.

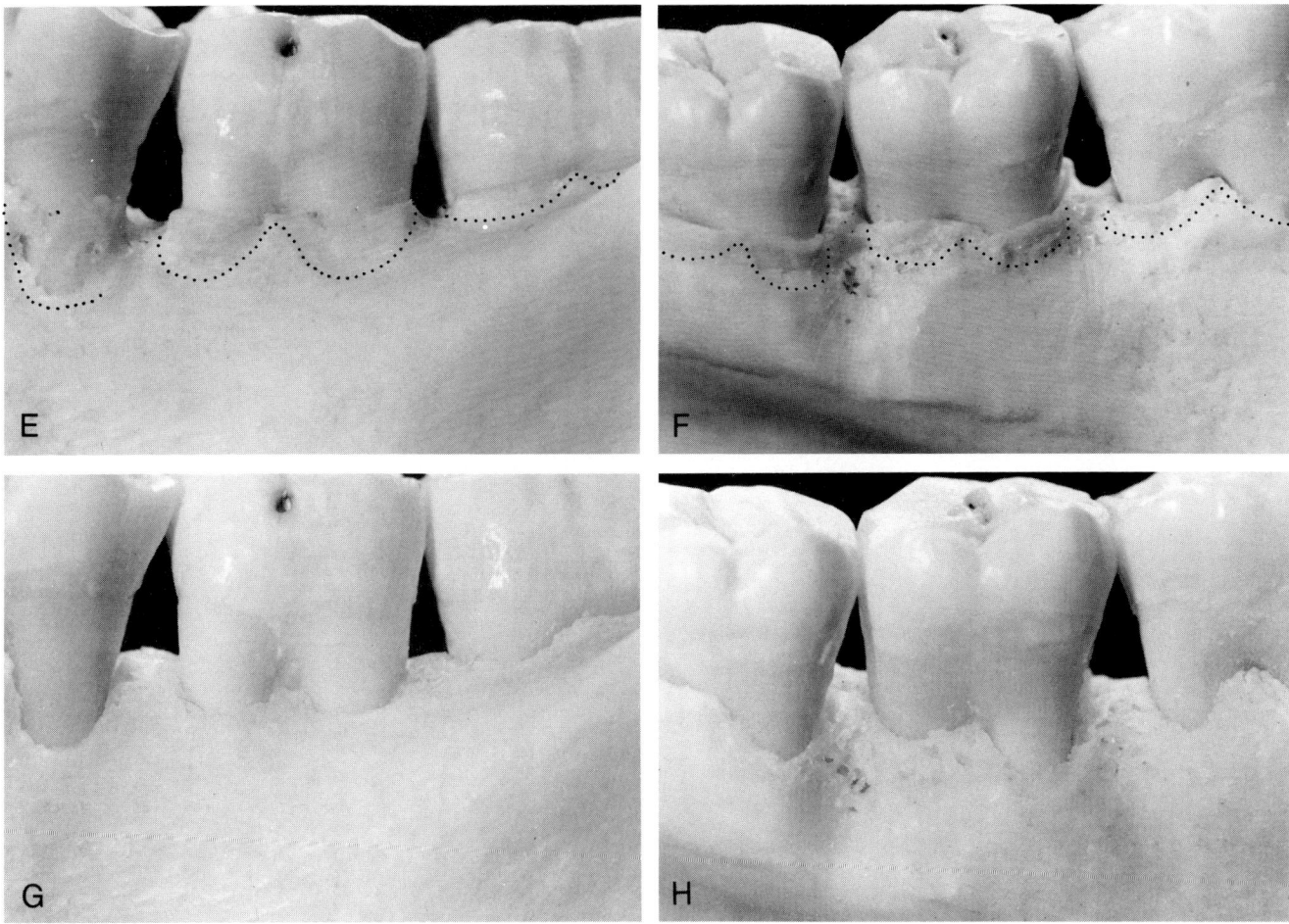

Fig. 11-8 (continued). **E,** Scribing (outlined area) carried to line angles to assure removal of widow peaks. **F,** Scribing (outlined area) completed on lingual surface. **G, H,** Osseous surgery completed. Note fluid parabolic contours, especially when compared with A and B, respectively.

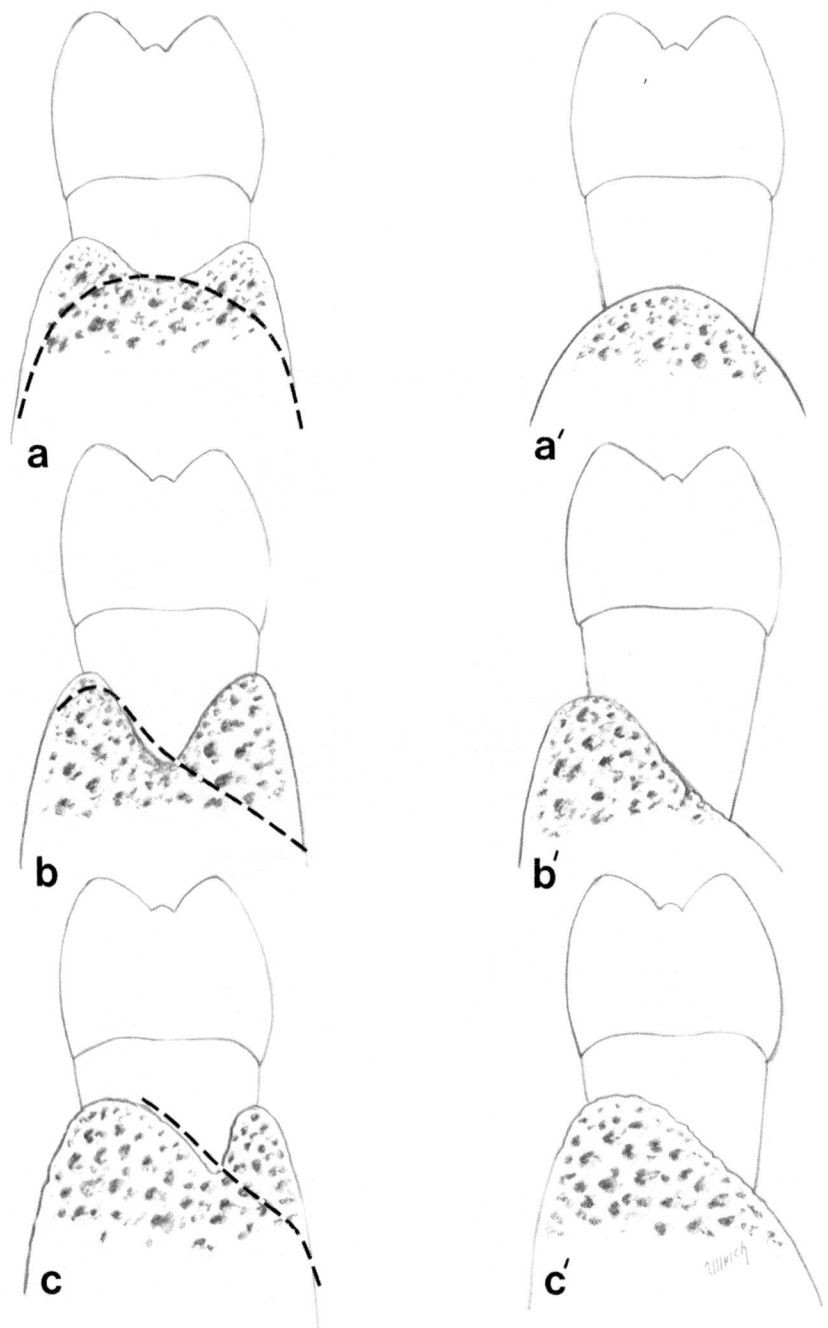

Fig. 11-9. Osseous Correction of the Interproximal Crater. **a,a′**, Ideal correction of osseous crater. **b,b′**, Treatment of deep interproximal crater. **c,c′**, Treatment of buccally positioned crater.

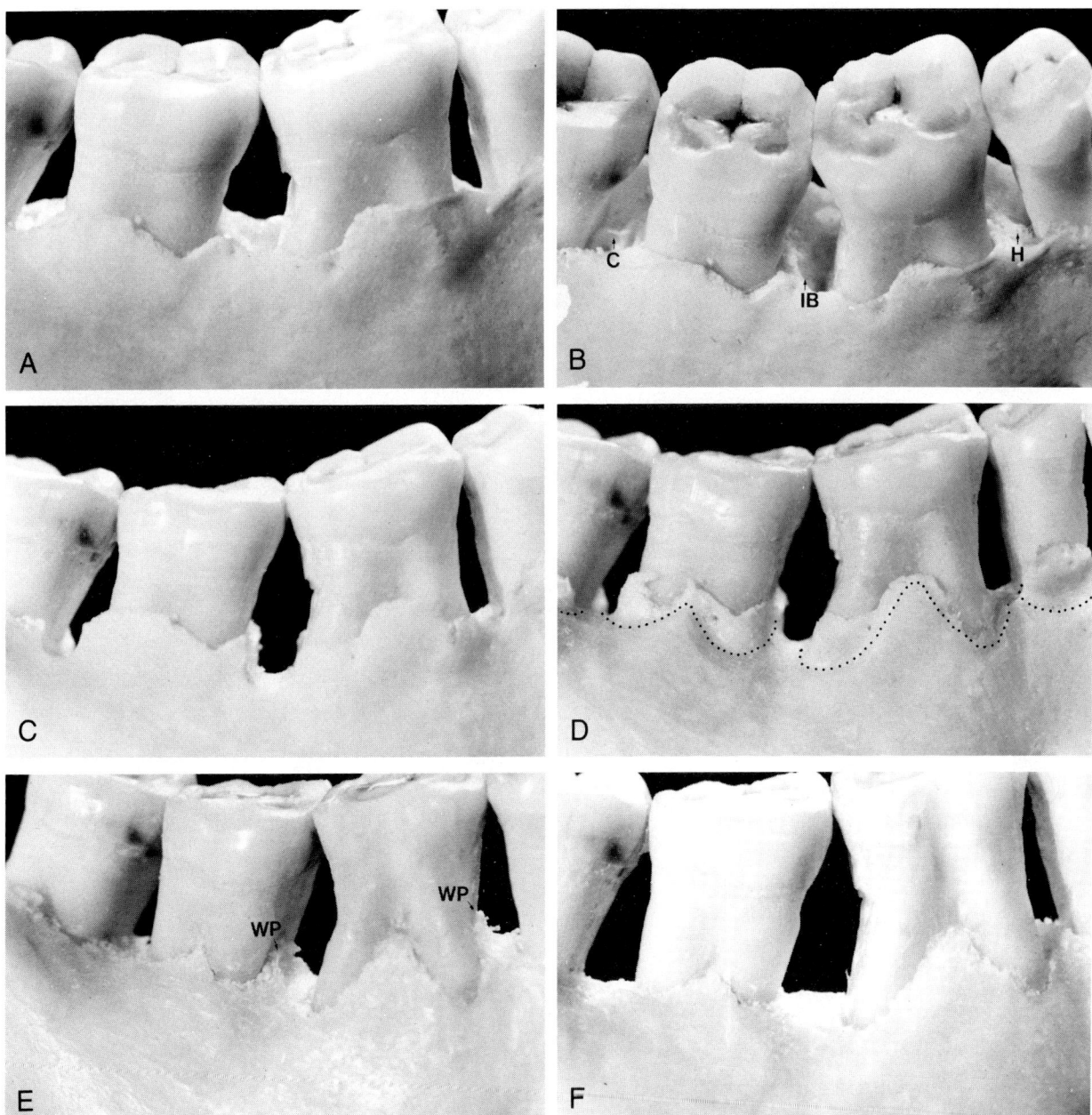

Fig. 11-10. Osseous Surgery for Multiple Complex Intraosseous Lesions—Example I. **A,** Buccal view of irregular marginal osseous contour. **B,** Occlusal view. Note deep intraosseous defects. C, crater; IB, intrabony defects; H, hemiseptum. **C,** Horizontal grooving. Note interdental osseous contour is level. **D,** *Scribing* (outlined area) is used to outline the bone to be removed during ostectomy. **E,** Ostectomy completed buccally; small spicules or *widow peaks* (WP) still remain interproximally. **F,** Osseous contouring completed with interproximal smoothing of bone and no furcation involvement.

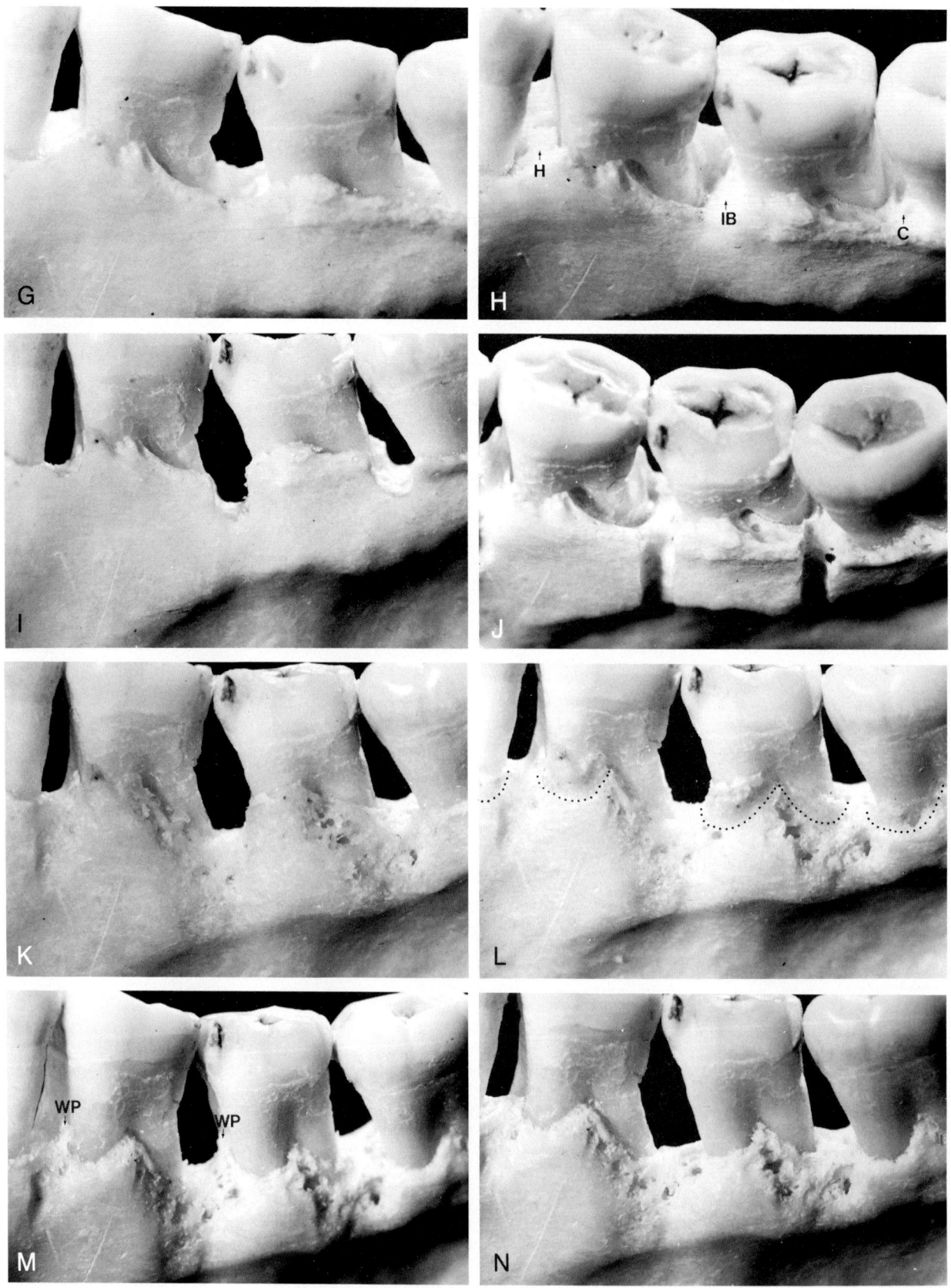

Fig. 11-10 (continued). G, Lingual view with irregular osseous margins. **H,** Occlusal view of defects. H, hemiseptum; IB, intrabony defect; C, crater. **I,** Horizontal grooving. Note level interproximal bone, negative bony architecture, and mesiodistal crater formation. **J,** Vertical grooving. Note how thick lingual plate of bone is. Grooves establish buccolingual width. **K,** Radicular blending completed. **L,** Scribing for final contour completed (outlined areas). **M,** Ostectomy completed lingually but *widow peaks* (WP) remain. **N,** Case complete with smooth-flowing contours and no involvement of furcation areas.

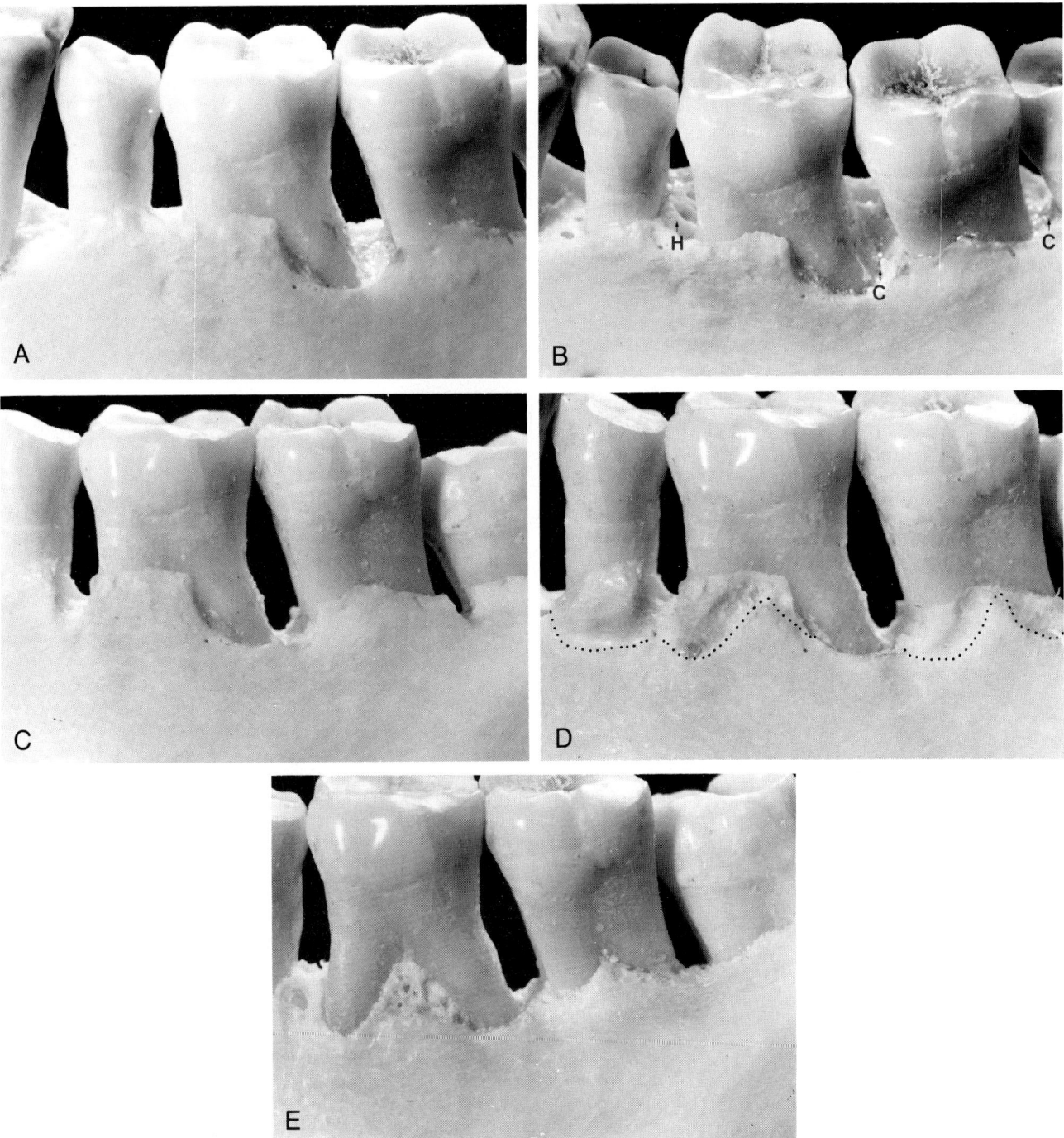

Fig. 11-11. Osseous Surgery for Multiple Complex Intraosseous Lesions—Example II. **A,** Buccal view with irregular margins. **B,** Occlusal view showing irregular interproximal contours. H, hemiseptum; C, craters. **C,** Horizontal grooving. **D,** Scribing to outline final contour. **E,** Osseous contouring completed. Note scalloped parabolic form without furcation involvement. Compare with A.

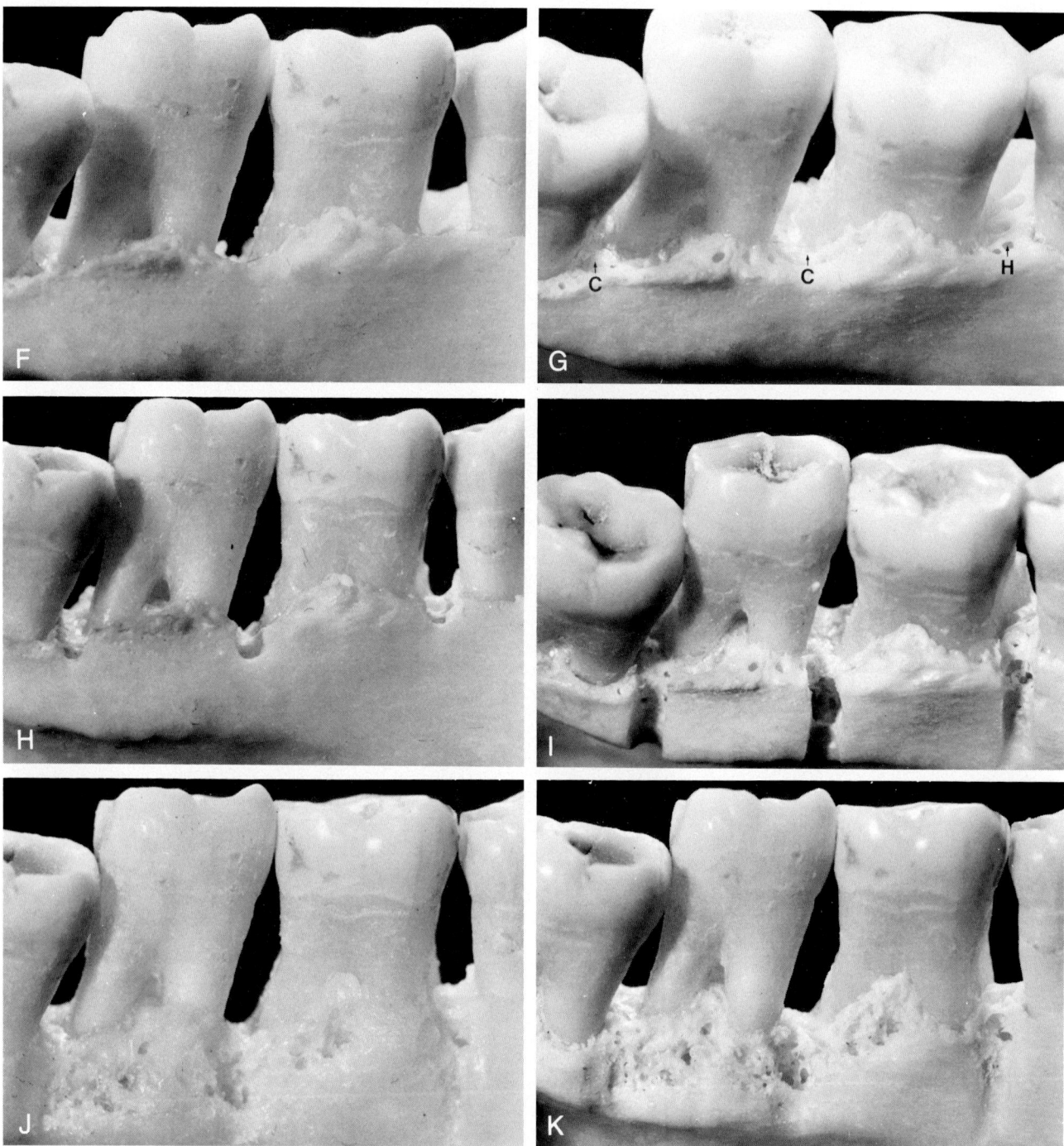

Fig. 11-11 (continued). **F,** Lingual view showing irregular bone margin. **G,** Occlusal view of interproximal defects. C, craters; H, hemiseptum. **H,** Horizontal grooving to level defects. **I,** Vertical grooves or depth cuts prior to thinning alveolus. **J,** Radicular blending or festooning complete. **K,** Case completed after ostectomy, with even-flowing, parabolic contours. Compare with F.

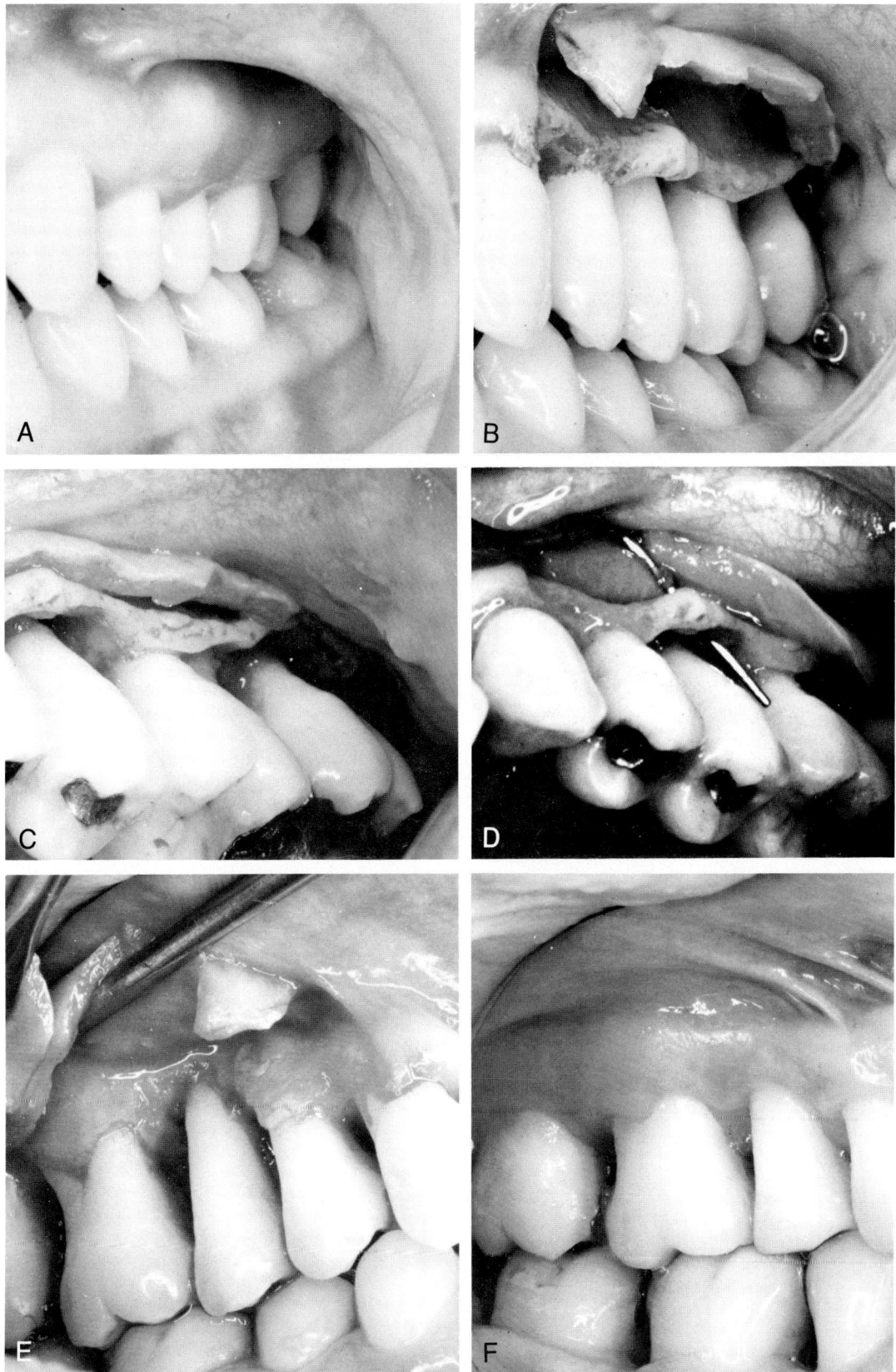

Fig. 11-12. Osseous Surgery for Reduction of Bulbous Bone and Intraosseous Defects. **A,** Before treatment. Note the bulbous contour of the bone. **B,** Mucoperiosteal flap reflected, showing uneven buccal contour with prominent ledges. **C,** Occlusal view showing hollowed-out bulbous bone with deep intraosseous defects. **D,** Probe in place, showing bone fenestration. **E,** Osseous contouring, ostectomy, and osteoplasty completed. **F,** Eight months later, case completed. (Originally contributed by Edward S. Cohen, D.M.D., to Glickman's Clinical Periodontology and reprinted by permission of W.B. Saunders Co.)

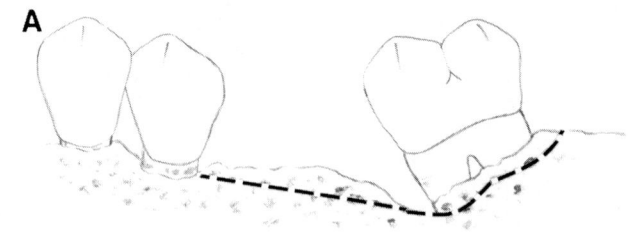

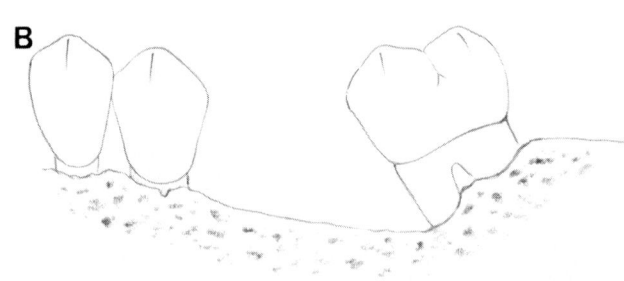

Fig. 11-13. Osseous Resection of Edentulous Ridge Area. **A,** Note defect approximating tilted molar. Dotted line outlines bone to be removed to create physiologic parabolic architecture. **B,** Osseous surgery completed.

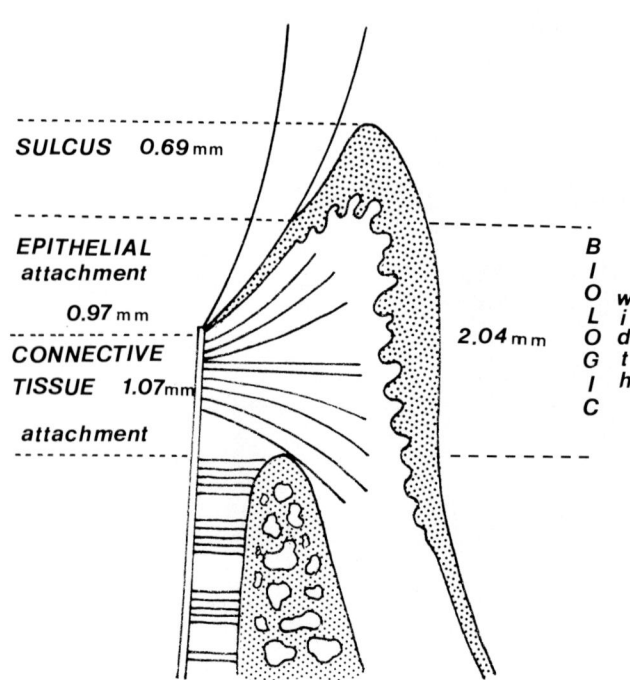

Fig. 11-14. Biologic Width. Representation of the average dimensions of the connective tissue and epithelial attachment above the bone.

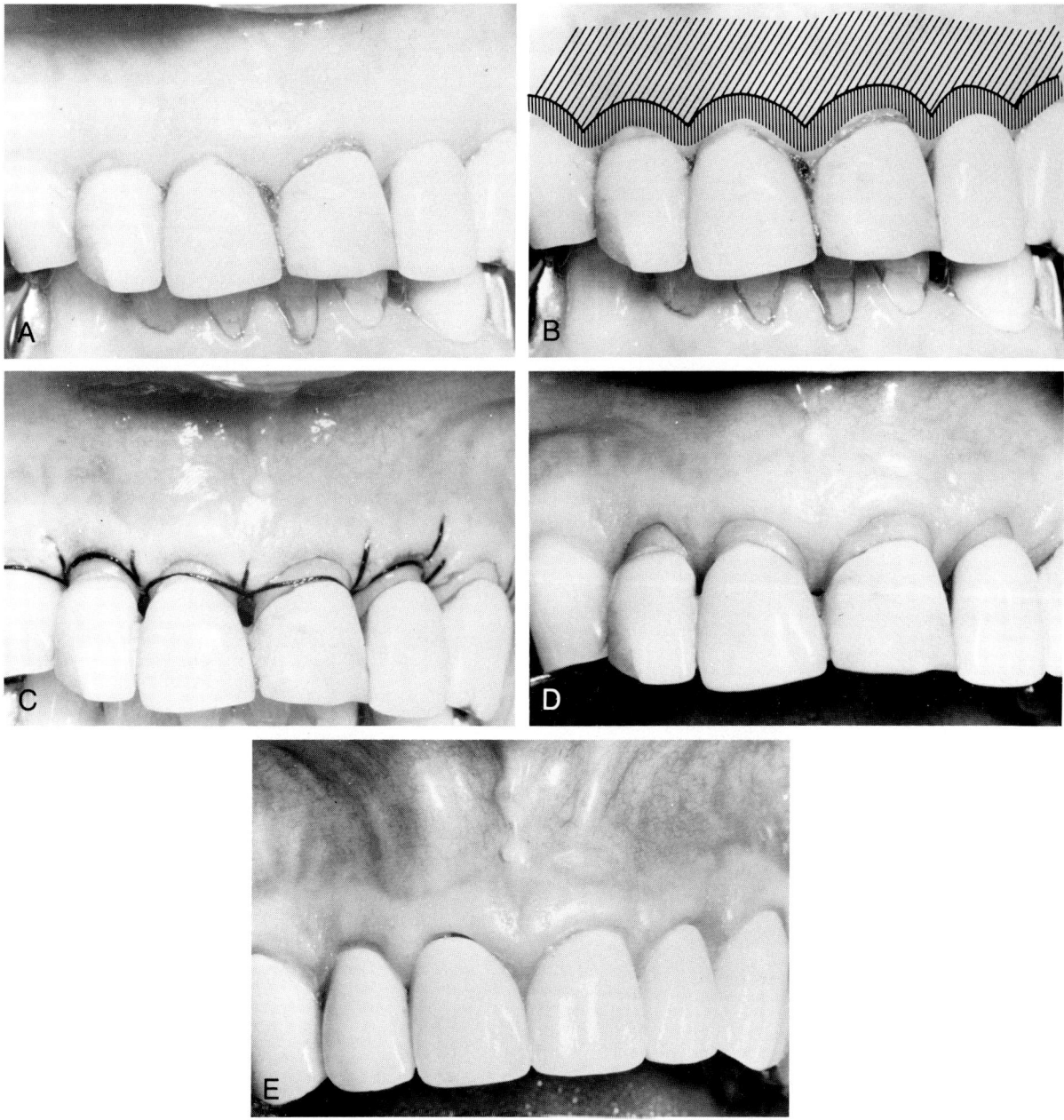

Fig. 11-15. Apically Positioned Full-Thickness Flap for Prosthetic Lengthening. **A,** Before. **B,** Incisions outlined. A modified flap without vertical incisions was utilized. **C,** Flaps reflected and sutured apically after osseous surgery. **D,** Two months later. Note excellent contour. **E,** Case completed 5 months later. (Prosthetics done by Dr. David Edwards, Bridgewater, MA.)

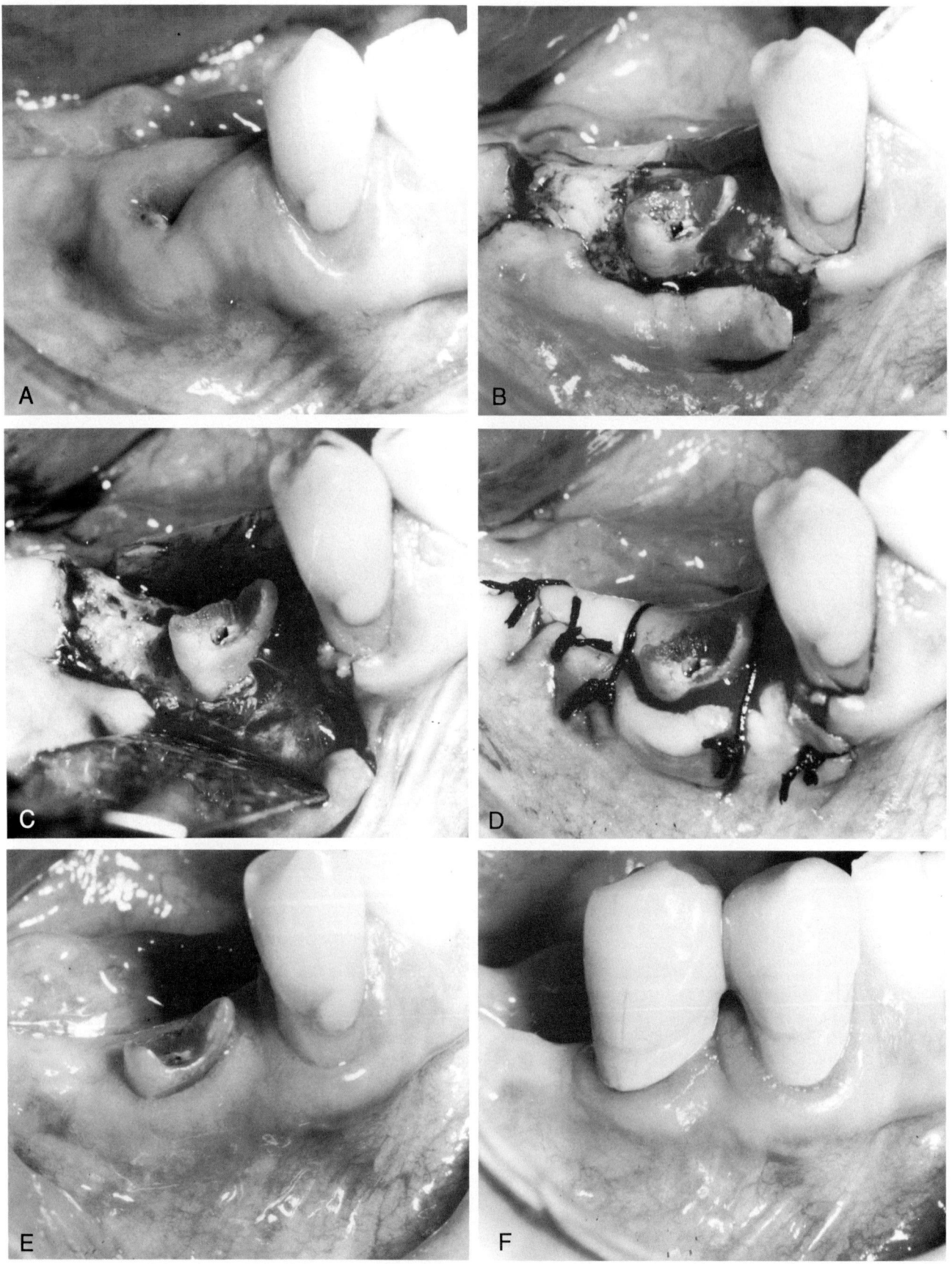

Fig. 11-16. Osseous Surgery for Crown Lengthening Prior to Prosthodontics: Fractured Tooth. **A,** Before surgery showing tooth fractured below the gum. **B,** Flaps reflected and tooth exposed. **C,** Osseous surgery for a minimum of 3 to 4.5 mm of root exposure. **D,** Flaps positioned and sutured. **E,** Tissue healed. Note that enough tooth structure has been exposed so that the biologic width will not be impinged upon. **F,** Six months later, case completed. (Prosthetics done by Dr. David Gale, Sharon, MA.)

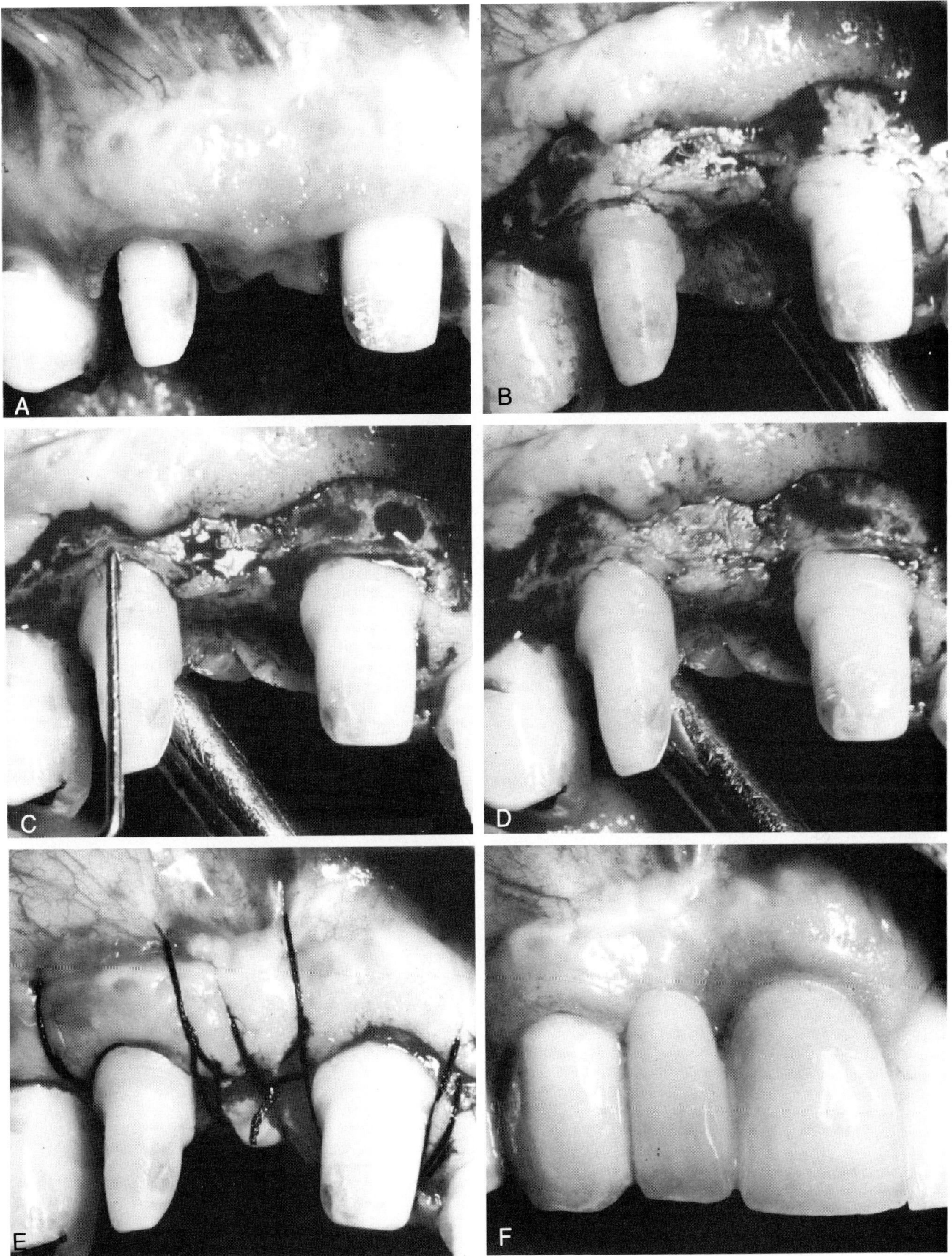

Fig. 11-17. Osseous Surgery for Crown Lengthening Prior to Prosthodontics: Subgingival Margins. **A,** Before surgery the old bridge was removed. **B,** Flaps reflected. Margins approximate bone and impinge on biologic width. **C,** Cuspid lengthened 3 mm below margins. **D,** Central lengthened 3 mm below margins. **E,** Flaps apically positioned and sutured. **F,** Eight months later, case complete.

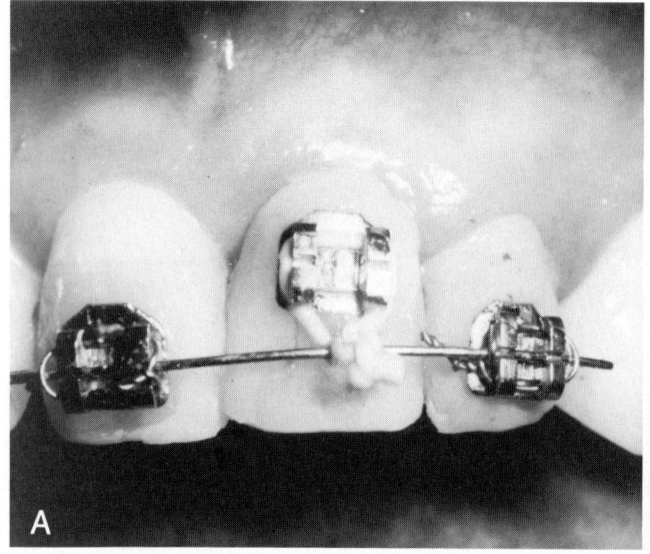
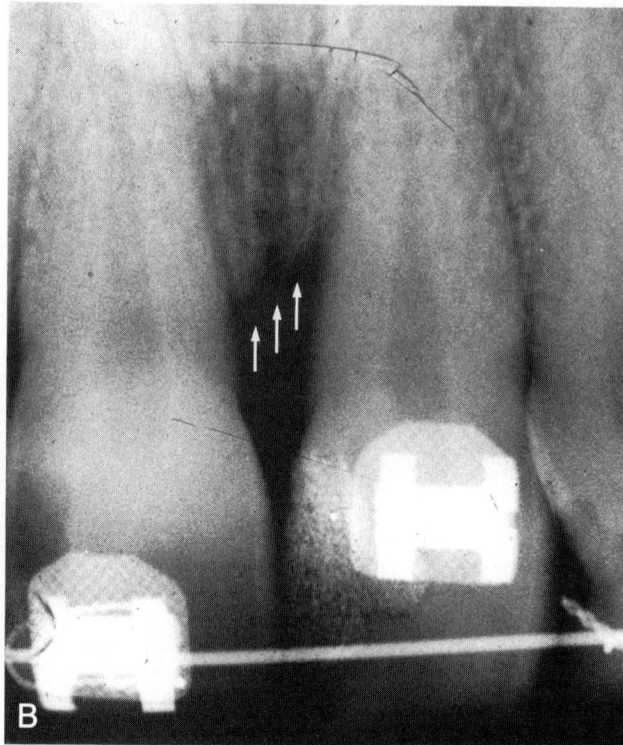
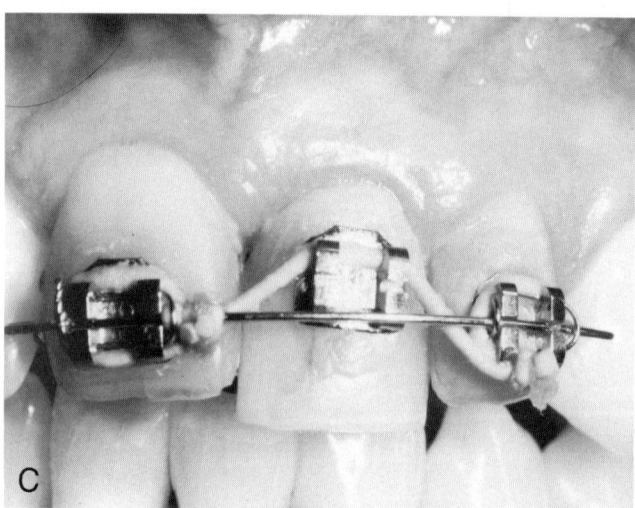
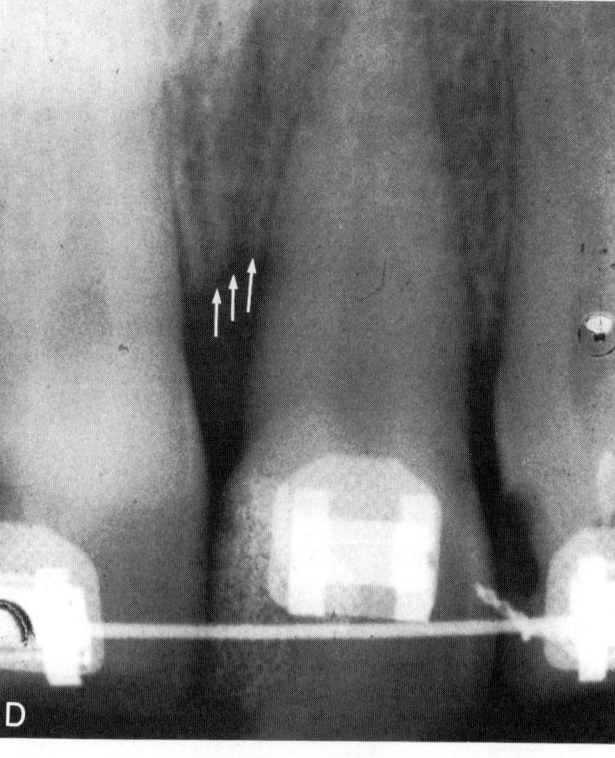

Fig. 11-18. Forced Eruption. **A, B,** Pretreatment clinical and radiographic views. Note mesial intrabony defect on central incisor. **C,** Four weeks later; note extrusion of tooth. **D,** X ray (1 month) with slight radiographic change.

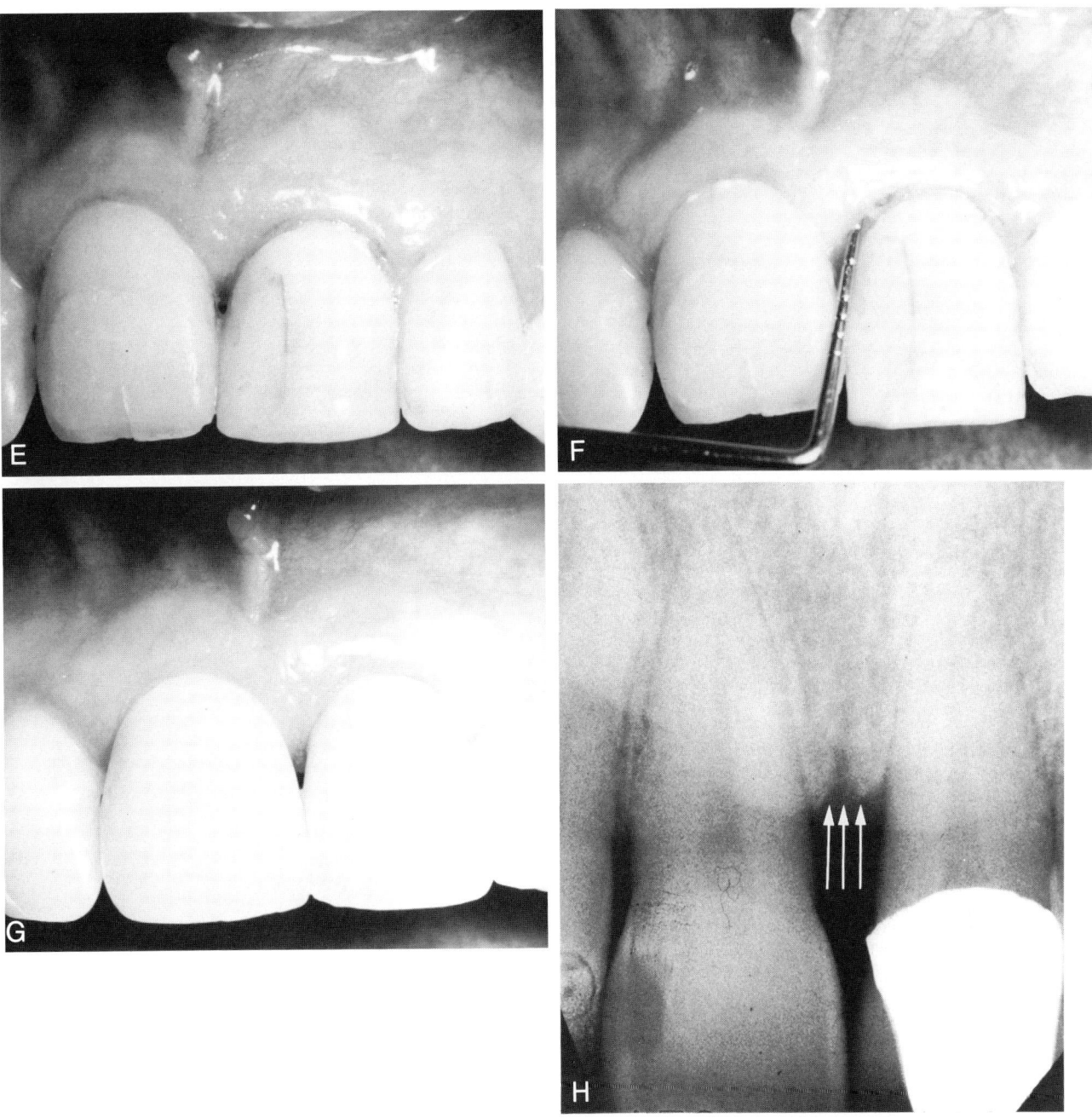

Fig. 11-18 (continued). E, F, Three months later with coronal movement of CEJ completed and pocketing reduced. **G, H,** One year later; final prosthetics completed. X ray showing complete resolution of intrabony defect.

12

INDUCTIVE OSSEOUS SURGERY

Periodontal therapy ideally would reconstruct or reconstitute all gingival and osseous structures lost through disease. In an attempt to achieve this, clinicians have long tried with varying degrees of success to induce osseous regeneration, cementum formation, and fibrous attachment in order to achieve new attachment (reattachment).

The intrabony (infrabony) pocket, which Goldman (1949, 1958) identified, classified (Fig. 12-1), and outlined treatment for, offers the greatest chance for regenerative techniques. This is especially true of two- and three-wall deep, narrow intrabony defects and deep intraosseous craters (Ellegaard and Loe, 1971). They offer an osseous topography that will hold a blood clot, with or without graft material, and that will permit ingrowth of primordial vascular and osseous cells from the bony lateral walls. On the other hand, if the osseous deformity is not amenable to regenerative or inductive procedures, as in the case of one-wall intrabony defects, or is small, as in the case of shallow craters, osseous resective surgery may be the treatment of choice.

DEFINITIONS

The following definitions are from the *Proceedings of World Workshop in Periodontics* (1989):

Repair

Healing of a wound by tissue that does not fully restore the architecture or function of the part, as in the case of a long, junctional epithelium or ankylosis.

Reattachment

The reunion of connective tissue with a *healthy* root surface on which viable periodontal tissue is present *without* new cementum, as in the case of trauma or after a supracrestal fiberotomy.

New Attachment

The reunion of connective tissue with an *unhealthy* or *previously diseased* root surface that has been deprived of its periodontal ligament. This reunion occurs by formation of *new cementum* with inserting collagen fibers, as in the case of guided tissue regeneration (GTR).

Linkage

The reunion of connective tissue with an *unhealthy* or *previously diseased* root surface *without* new cementum (Stahl, 1979). This is thought to occur after root demineralization.

Regeneration

Reproduction or reconstitution of the lost or injured parts by restoration of new bone, cementum, and periodontal ligament (reunion of connective tissue) on an *unhealthy* or *previously diseased* root surface. Ideally, complete restoration would also restore total function.

INTRABONY DEFECTS

Preparation for Bone Regeneration and New Attachment

Figure 12-2 graphically portrays the three critical zones to which treatment is applied (Ratcliff, 1966; Glickman, 1972; Wirthlin, 1981):

1. The root surface (Fig. 12-2,A1).
2. The granulomatous tissue of the defect (Fig. 12-2,A2a) and the residual trans-septal and periodontal fibers covering the bone (Fig. 12-2,A2b).
3. The underlying bone (Fig. 12-2,A3).

Treatment of all intraosseous defects is the same and involves the following:
1. Removal of plaque, calculus, softened cementum, and the junctional epithelium from the root surface (Fig. 12-2B).
2. Removal of all granulation tissue from the bony defect (Fig. 12-2C).
3. Removal of all connective tissue and periodontal ligament fibers covering the bone (Fig. 12-2A, B).
4. Decortification of dense or sclerotic bone (Fig. 12-2D).

Procedure for Treatment of Intrabony Defects

1. Sufficient local anesthesia for hemostasis and greater visualization.
2. The final osseous topography is now determined by sounding for the underlying bone with a periodontal probe (Fig. 12-3A).
3. A full-thickness mucoperiosteal flap is raised using sulcular incisions (Fig. 12-3 B through E). Maximum conservation of interproximal tissue is attempted so that primary closure can be achieved. Figure 12-4 shows differing interproximal incisions for increasing the chances of maintaining primary root coverage interproximally. It is an attempt to reduce or minimize "dove-back" of the papilla during healing, thus further exposing graft and defect.

    Additional biomechanical root preparation (citric acid, tetracycline) may now be employed as the final step prior to intramarrow penetration.

    Takei et al. (1985) published a procedural technique that permits total interproximal coverage that may be useful in certain situations, especially with anterior defects (see Chapter 7, Figs. 7-5 through 7-7).
4. The flap is extended at least one tooth mesial and distal to the defect for exposure of at least 2 to 3 mm of surrounding sound bone (Fig. 12-3F).
5. Vertical releasing incisions are optional.

Once the flaps are reflect the three zones—root surface, soft tissue, and bone—are addressed.

Zone 1: The Root Surface

The root surface must be meticulously scaled and root planed, which is probably the most difficult aspect of treatment (Figs. 12-2,B1 and 12-3G). Scaling alone is not sufficient, because it will not remove softened or necrotic cementum, bacterial endotoxins, remnants of the junctional epithelium, or residual calculus. Enamel finishing burs are often used to remove residual calculus and smooth the root surface. If thorough root preparation is not carried out, the root surface may not be amenable to cementogenesis (Stahl, 1977) or able to sustain the growth of fibroblasts (Aleo et al., 1975). Some clinicians (Prichard, 1983) on the other hand believe that root planing is contraindicated and will prevent cementogenesis.

Zone 2: The Soft Tissue

With the flaps reflected, large curettes are used against the bony surface to remove all granulation tissue and residual fibers attached to the bone (Figs. 12-2,C2a, b and 12-3H, I). The tissue is difficult to remove, and the process is tedious. Small curettes and ultrasonic instruments are used in the apical recesses and in the periodontal ligament space for curettage and lavage. *All fibers must be removed to open the marrow spaces and permit intimate contact between graft material and bone* (Fig. 12-3J, K).

Zone 3: The Bone

The bone is gone over with fine curettes to remove any residual fibers and to open the marrow spaces. *Chronic wounds are often associated with a dense or sclerotic bone that is poorly vascularized* and therefore less osteogenic than freshly created defects. For this reason *decortification* is performed. Small holes are made in the bone with a sharp curette or small round bur (No. 1/4 to 1/2), permitting (1) rapid proliferation of granulation tissue with undifferentiated mesenchymal cells, (2) rapid regeneration of bone, and (3) rapid anastomosis of graft and bone (Fig. 12-2D). The holes are made into areas of anticipated vascularity. Finally, the periodontal ligament is scraped with the tip of an explorer to promote bleeding and stimulate cell proliferation (Fig. 12-3C).

6. Selection of the graft material(s) (autograft, allograft, alloplast, GTR) to be placed will vary by individual clinical preference, nature of the defect to be filled (intrabony versus furcation) and final results sought (regeneration, new attachment, or repair) (Fig. 12-3M).
7. The graft material is placed in small increments, care is taken to pack each increment down adequately while also removing excessive fluid (Fig. 12-3N).
8. The graft material may be overfilled, underfilled, or neutrofilled (Fig. 12-5). Overfilling will compensate for some loss of graft material but will make primary closure difficult.
9. The flaps are reapproximated with digital pressure over the defect. If there is not 100% defect coverage the flaps can be further scalloped with a sharp No. 15 scalpel blade on the buccal and/or lingual surfaces to accommodate total coverage (Fig. 12-6). *Note:* Limited osteoplasty may also help in flap closure.

10. Vertical mattress or intrapapillary suturing is ideally recommended using monofilament, Gore-Tex, or Vicryl sutures (Fig. 12-3P). This prevents the *wicking* of bacteria into the graft site, reduces suture inflammation, and at the same time permits suture retention for 14 days. The longer suture retention increases flap tensile strength and assures adequate implant coverage.
11. Postoperatively the patient is placed on doxycycline 100 mg b.i.d. or tetracycline 250 t.i.d. for 10 to 14 days. The packing is changed after 7 days, and sutures are removed in 14 days. Peridex mouth rinse is recommended for 3 weeks.

The clinical procedure outlining the steps in achieving successful root coverage are seen in Figure 12-3.

Upon completion of the individual steps, and if no graft is to be used, all that remains to be done is flap closure.

The positive results sometimes obtainable by the basic intrabony technique are shown in Figure 12-7.

Bowers, Schallhorn, and Mellonig (1982), in their literature review of *human* histologic material on regeneration in intrabony defects, concluded that in areas adjacent to bone implants cementogenesis and osteogenesis appeared to be enhanced. This was as opposed to nongrafted sites, which tended to show less bone fill, less cementogenesis, and greater likelihood of healing by a long-junctional epithelium.

Factors Affecting Success or Failure of Regeneration Procedures

According to Mellonig (1992), the following factors affect success or failure of regeneration procedures:
1. Plaque control
2. Underlying system disease (diabetes, etc.)
3. Root preparation
4. Adequate wound closure
5. Complete soft-tissue approximation
6. Periodontal maintenance, short term and long term
7. Traumatic injury to teeth and tissues
8. Defect morphology
9. Type of graft material
10. Patient's repair potential

Failure to Achieve Bone Regeneration

Failure often is not attributable to preparation but to rapid epithelial downgrowth (Ramfjord, 1971). Epithelial proliferation apically, being more rapid than that of connective tissue or bone regeneration, will continue along the root until it encounters granulation tissue and then stop, a process known as *contact inhibition*.

Prichard (1983), who has had a great deal of success with regeneration, in describing his successful technique states that "Epithelial must be prevented from growing into the defect. Replacing the flap over the orifice of the defect is probably the most common cause of failure." As a means of avoiding this error, he counsels that "The gingiva must be removed to the vestibular and oral margins of the bony walls of the defects." In effect, he allows for healing by secondary intention and *stunting* of epithelial downgrowth by bone exposure. His results have been confirmed by Becker et al. (1986).

Ellegaard et al. (1974) and Karring and Ellegaard (1976), using free soft-tissue grafts to cover the orifice of intraosseous defects, found that they could achieve epithelial retardation and greater bone fill than in similar defects covered with flap tissue. (See the section on Guided Tissue Regeneration.) They hypothesized that the grafts prevented epithelial proliferation while allowing granulation tissue to develop adequately.

In order to prevent failures, and at the same time increase the bone's capacity to regenerate attachment, osseous enhancement and inductive procedures have been developed.

Grafting for New Attachment

Rationale, Objectives, Selection

The primary rationale for using graft materials in intrabony defects is to enhance the regenerative capability of bone and achieve a new attachment apparatus. In the process we seek to achieve most, if not all, of the following objectives (Goldman and Cohen, 1979):

1. *Osteoinduction* (Urist and McLean, 1952): A process by which the graft material is capable of promoting
   a. Osteogenesis
   b. Cementogenesis
   c. New periodontal ligament
2. *Osteoconduction* (Urist et al., 1958): The graft material acts as a *passive matrix*, like a *trellis* or *scaffolding* for new bone to cover over.
3. *Contact inhibition* (Ellegaard et al., 1976): The process by which the graft material prevents apical proliferation of the epithelium.

Advantages of Grafting

The overriding advantage is the potential regeneration of noncorrectable periodontal defects.

288   Inductive Osseous Surgery

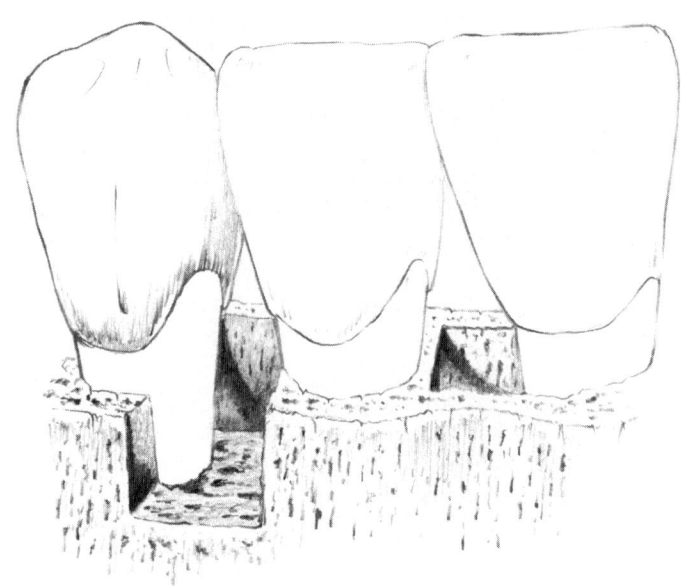

Fig. 12-1. Classification of Intrabony Defects. Intrabony defects are classified by the remaining walls and the root surfaces involved.

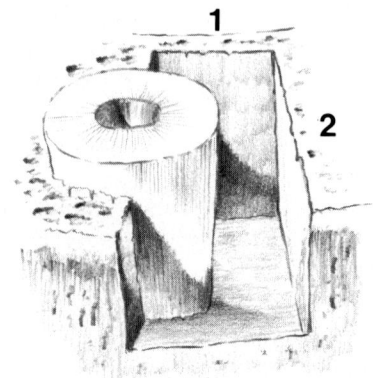

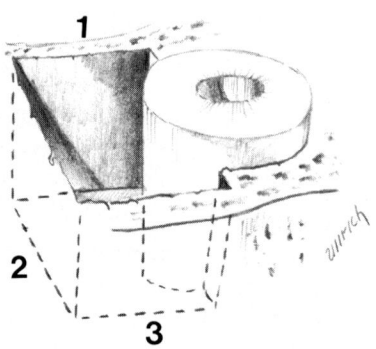

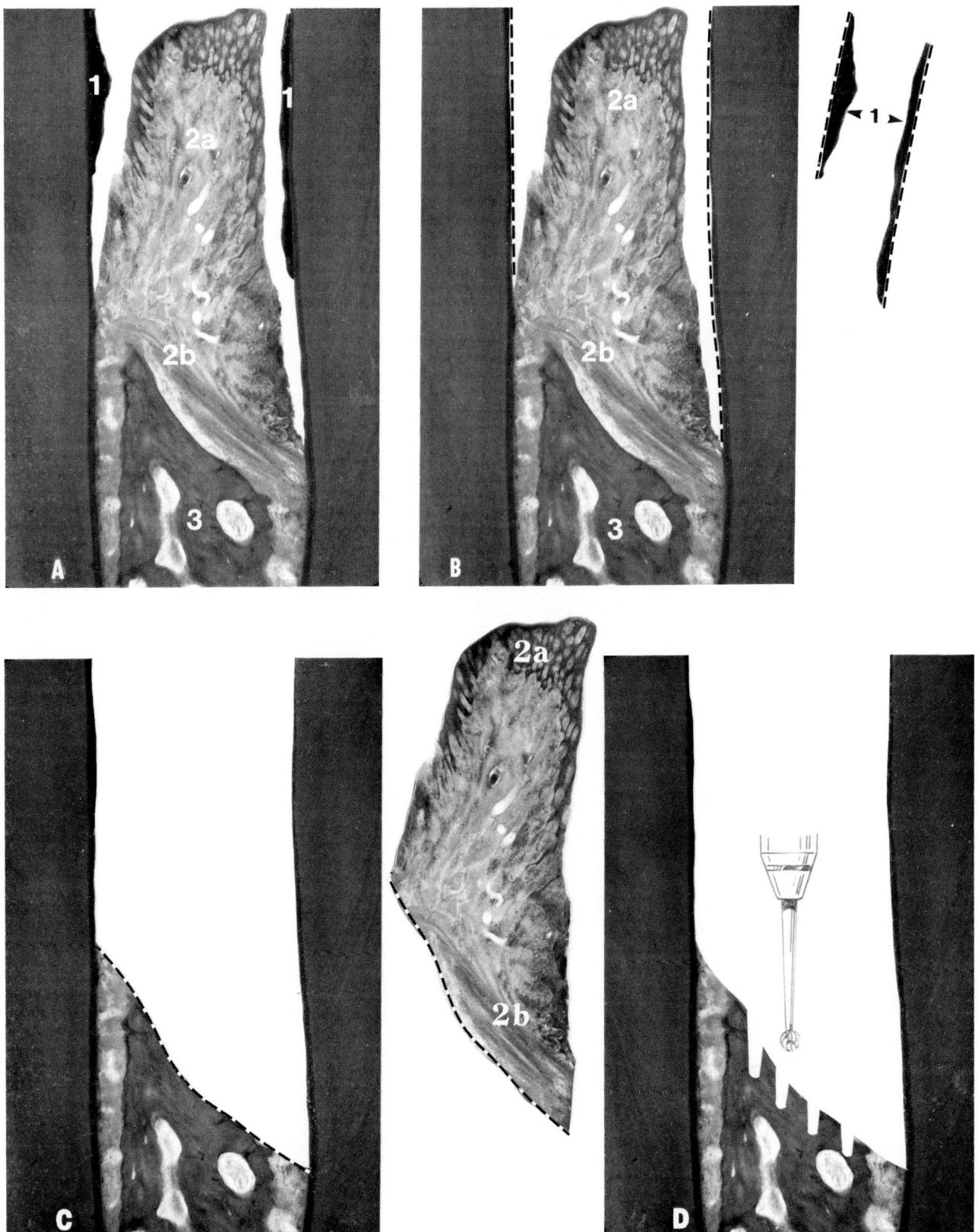

Fig. 12-2. Three Zones for Treatment of Intrabony Defects. **A,** (1), the root surface; (2a), the soft tissue of the pocket; (2b), the connective tissue fibers covering the bone. (3) The bony defect. **B,** The plaque, calculus, and soft cementum. (1) is removed. **C,** Removal of the soft-tissue pocket (2a) and underlying periodontal fibers (2b). **D,** Intramarrow perforation of bony housing.

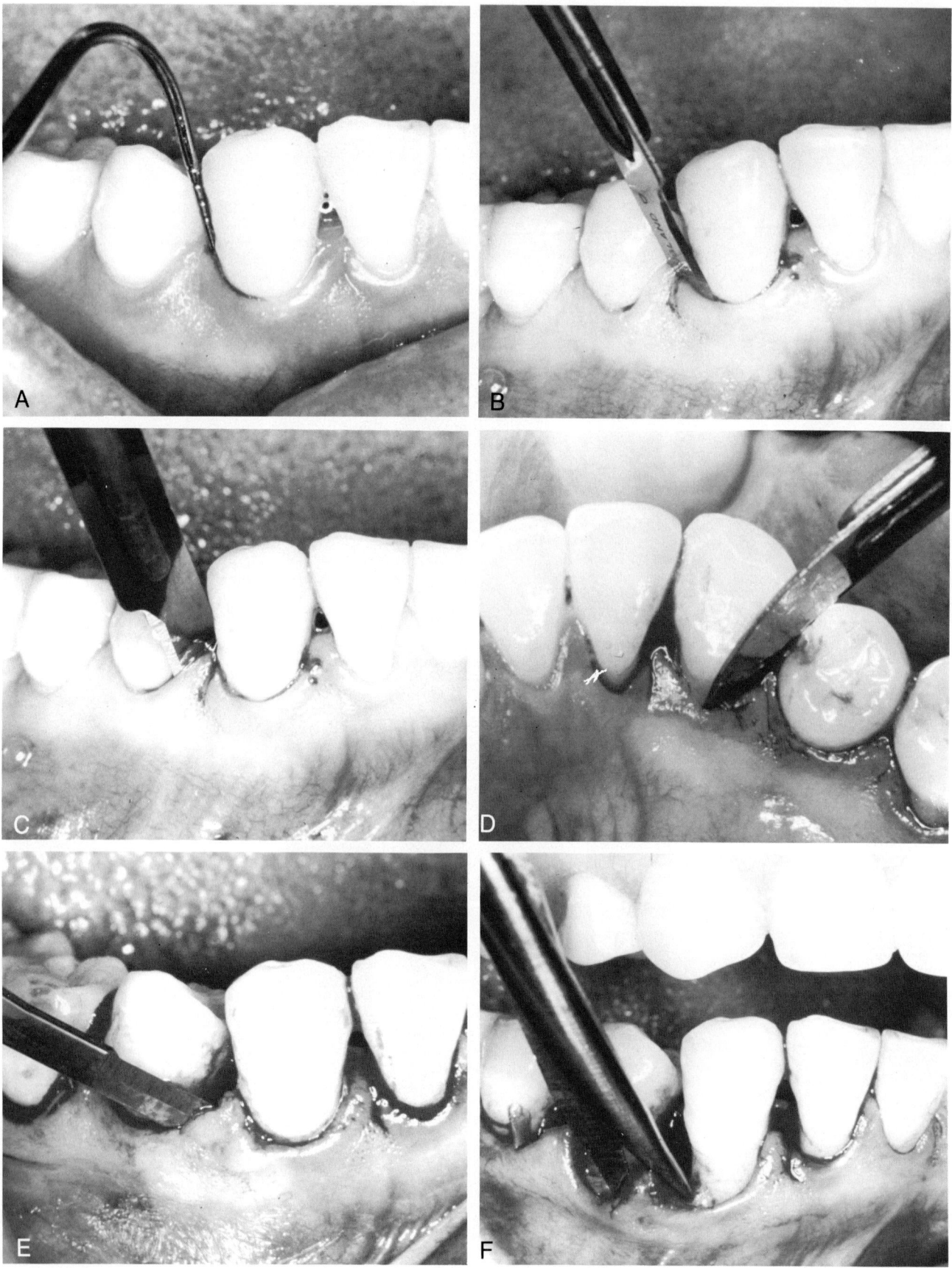

Fig. 12-3. Surgical Technique and Placement of Demineralized Freeze Dried Bone Allograft (DFDBA). **A,** Before surgery with probe in place delineating 7-mm pocket and intrabony defect. **B, C, D,** Buccal and lingual sulcular incisions for minimum preservation of interproximal tissue. **E,** Papilla being freed from underlying tissue. **F,** Periosteal elevator for flap reflection.

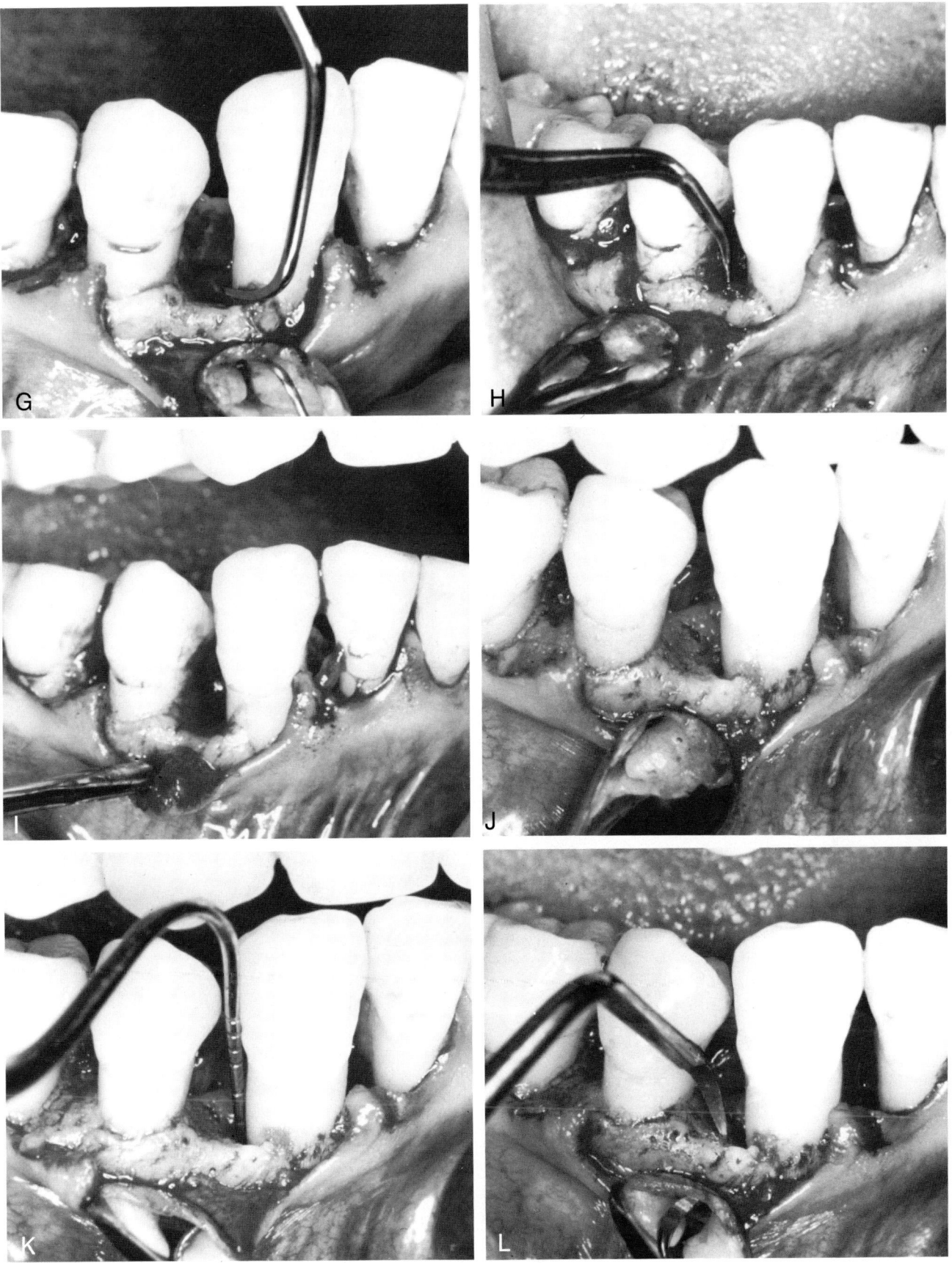

Fig. 12-3 (continued). **G,** Teeth scaled and root planed. **H,** Interproximal granulation tissue removed. **I,** Gross granulation tissue removed. **J,** Scaling continued for complete osseous debridement. Note complete removal of tissue overlying the bone and exposure of defect. **K,** Probe in small apical three-wall defect. **L,** Bone decortification and periodontal ligament stimulation.

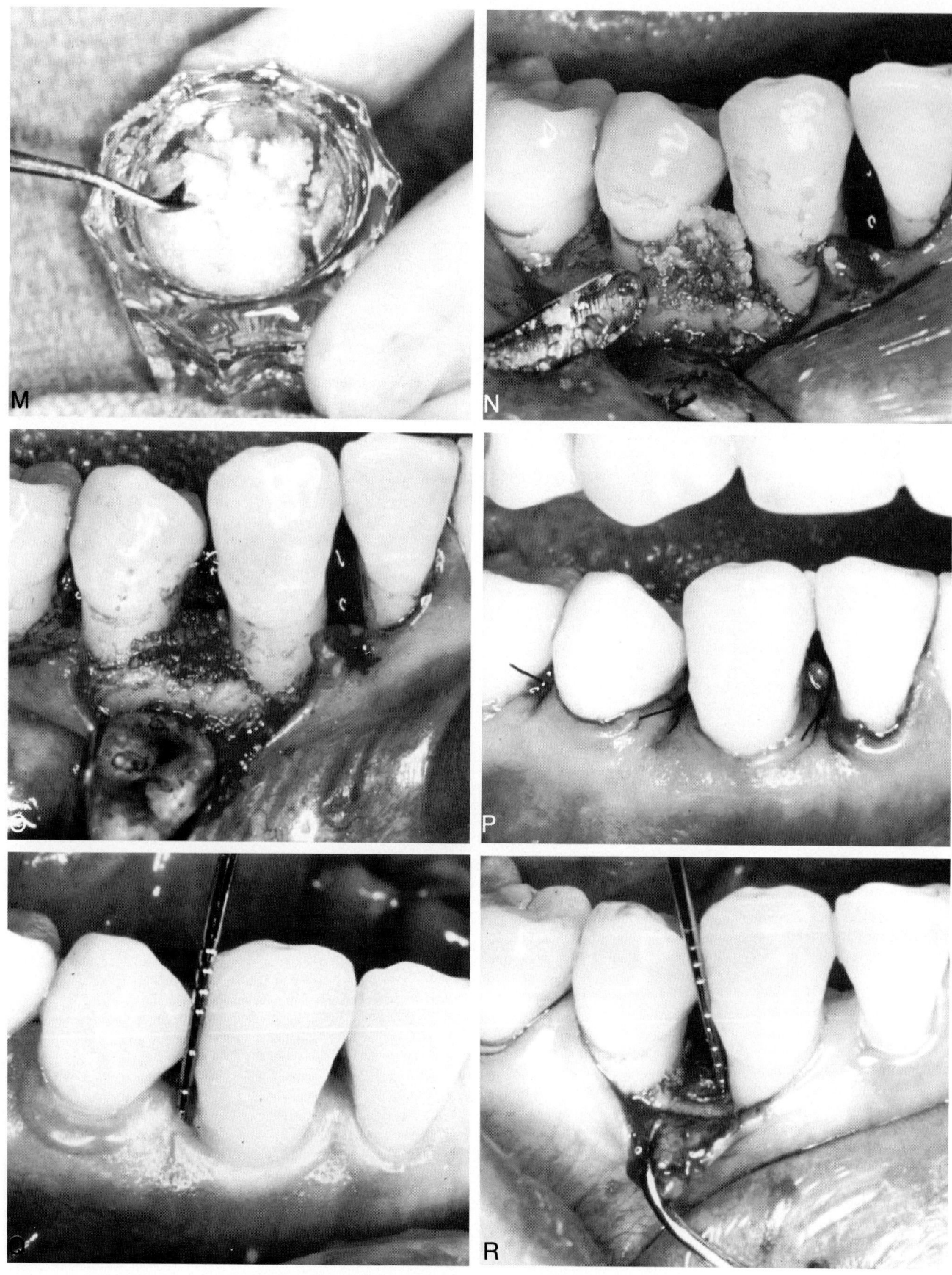

Fig. 12-3 (continued). **M,** DFDBA rehydrated in sterile dappen dish. **N,** DFDBA placed with sterile plastic instrument. **O,** Defect completely filled. **P,** Flaps completely replaced and sutured for 1° coverage. **Q,** One year later. Note reduction in pocket depth. **R,** Re-entry showing bone regeneration. (Contributed by Dr. James Mellonig, San Antonio, TX.)

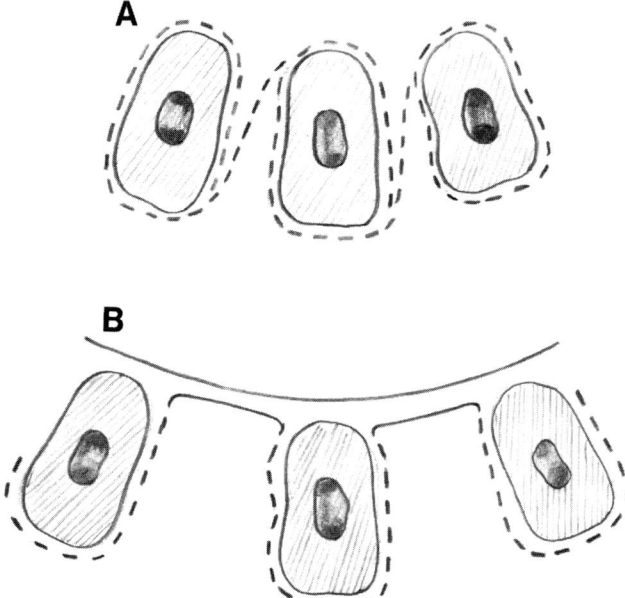

Fig. 12-4. Interproximal Incisions for Implant Coverage. **A,** Diagonal incision is made when interdental space is narrow. This will permit greater surface contact when sutured. **B,** Wide embrasures permit a *"trap door"* incision to provide complete interdental coverage.

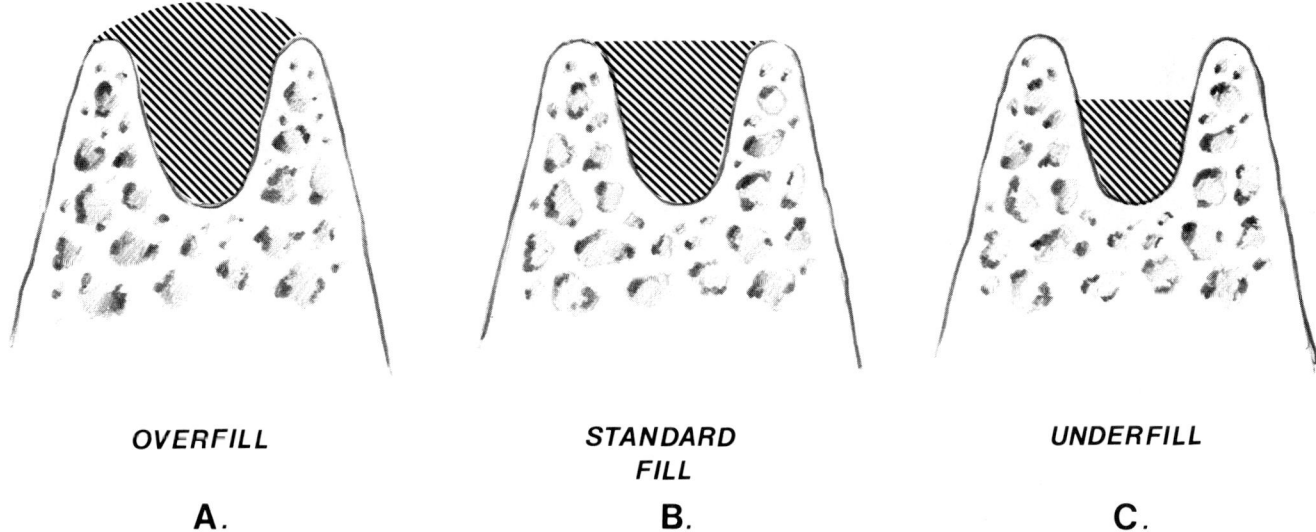

OVERFILL　　　　　STANDARD　　　　　UNDERFILL
　　　　　　　　　　　　FILL
A.　　　　　　　　　**B.**　　　　　　　　　**C.**

Fig. 12-5. Intrabony Defect Size versus Quantity of Implant Material. **A, B, C,** various amounts of implant material that may be placed into defects.

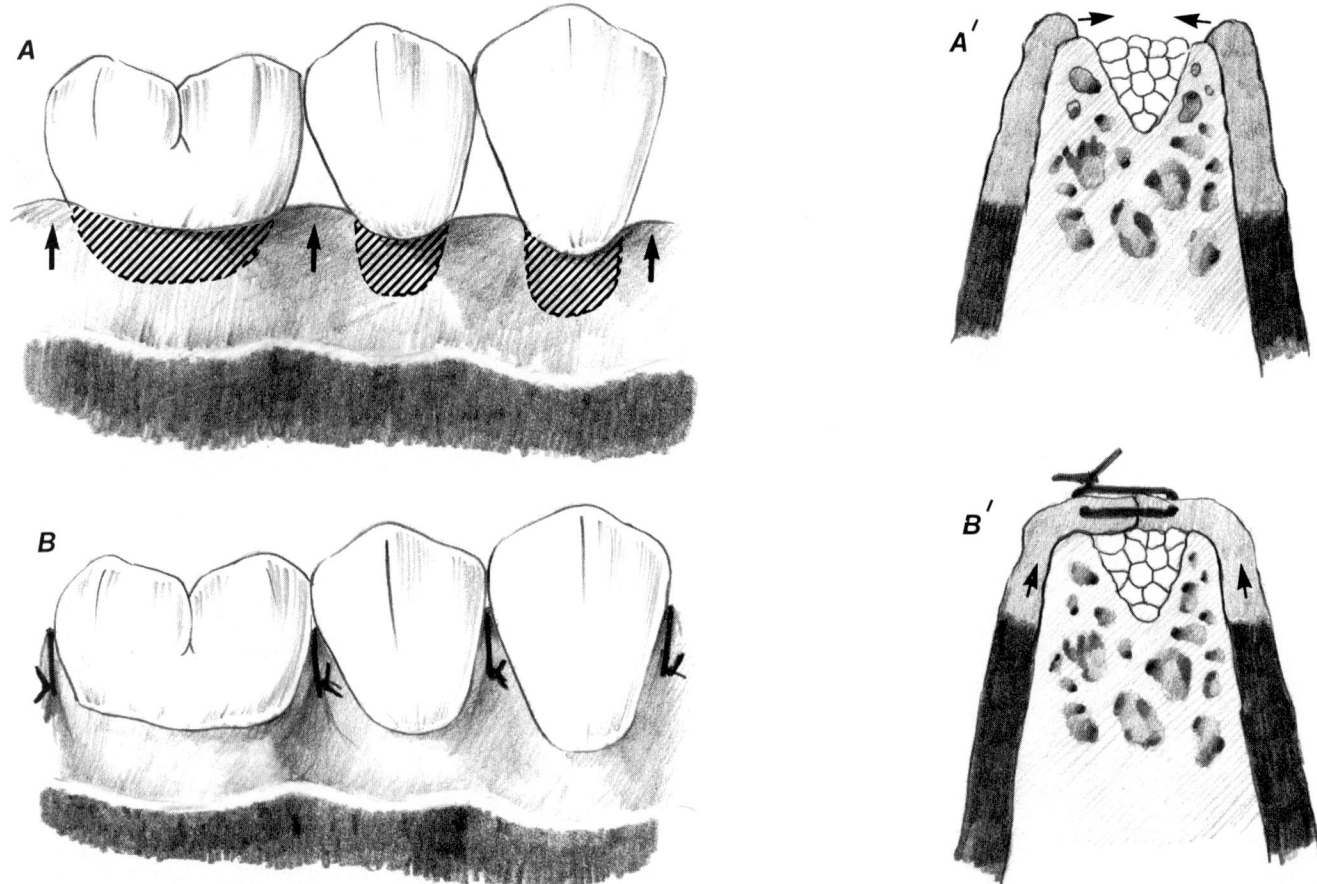

Fig. 12-6. Flap Modification for Graft Coverage. **A, A′,** Incomplete interproximal flap coverage of defect. Shaded areas delineate additional scalloping for increasing interproximal coverage. **B, B′,** Additional scalloping has been completed and 100% implant coverage is achieved.

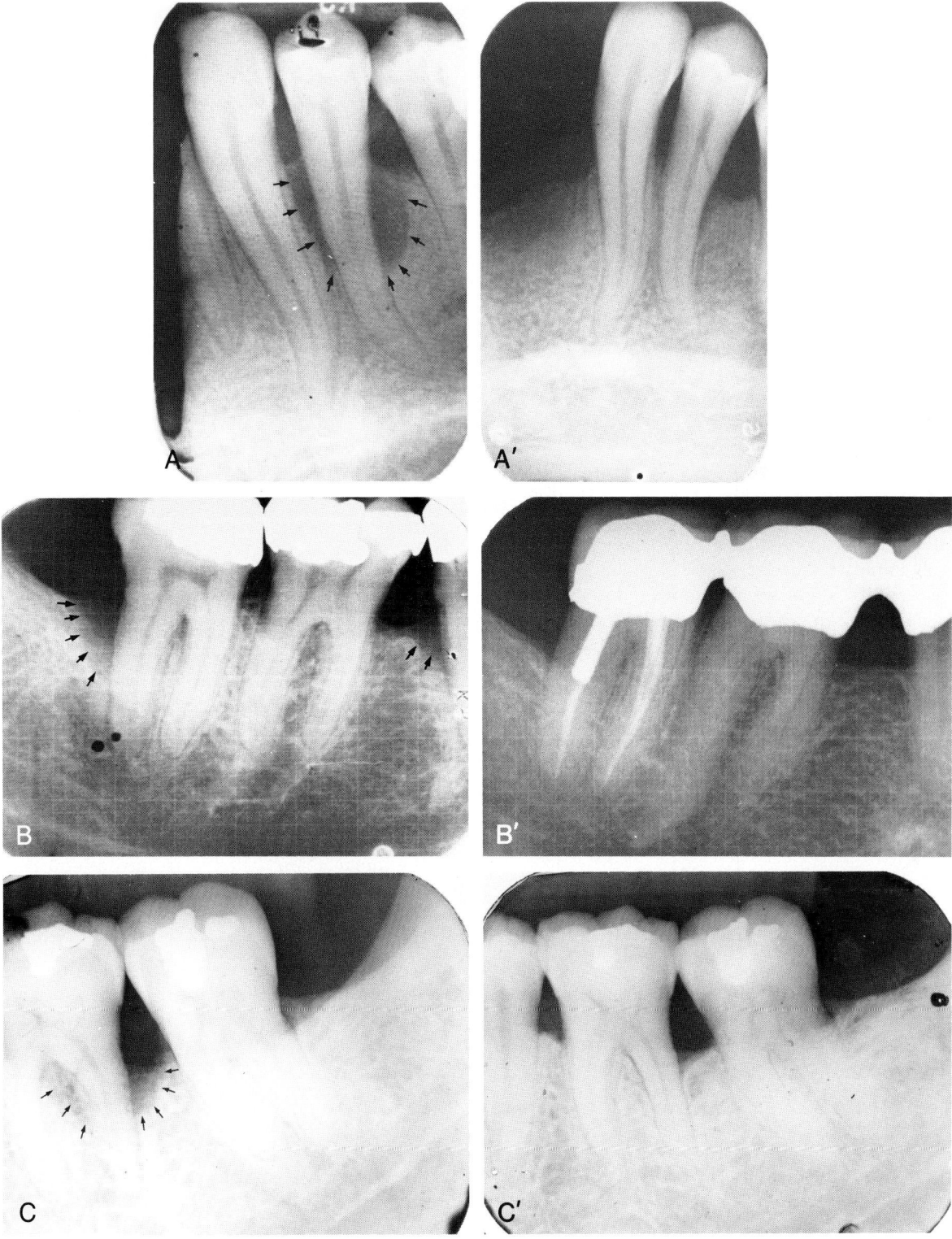

Fig. 12-7. Results Obtained by Open-Flap Curettage of Intrabony Defects. **A, B, C,** Before-treatment x-ray studies. **A', B', C',** Post-treatment x-ray studies. Note significant increase in bone obtainable by conservative treatment.

Disadvantages of Grafting

According to Mellonig (1992) the following are disadvantages of grafting:
1. Increased treatment time
2. Longer postoperative treatment
3. Autografts require two sites
4. Increased postoperative care
5. Variability in repair and predictability
6. Need for multistep therapy—secondary surgeries
7. Greater expense
8. Availability of graft material

SELECTION OF GRAFT MATERIAL

Selection of the specific grafting material is based on a number of factors, each of which must be evaluated. The following are some of the determining factors used in the selection process (Bell, 1964; Schallhorn, 1976):
1. Osteoinductive potential
2. Predictability
3. Accessibility—ease of obtaining material
4. Availability—quantity of material obtainable
5. Safety
   a. Biologic compatability
   b. Immunologic acceptability
   c. Minimal sequalae—preoperatively and postoperatively
6. Rapid vascularization

Classification

This classification of graft material is based on the degree of inductive potential. The materials are listed in decreasing order of inductive potential under each heading.
I. OSTEOINDUCTIVE IMPLANTS: Implants that induce or promote bone growth
   A. Autogenous bone grafts
      1. Extraoral—hip marrow
         a. Fresh
         b. Frozen
      2. Intraoral
         a. Osseous coagulum—bone blend
         b. Tuberosity
         c. Extraction sites
         d. Osseous coagulum
         e. Contiguous autograft
   B. Allografts
      1. Demineralized freeze-dried bone allografts (DFDBA)
      2. Freeze-dried bone allografts (FDBA)/Autogenous bone grafts (ABG)
      3. Freeze-dried bone allografts (FDBA)

It is important to note that the DFDBA and the FDBA/ABG have greater inductive potential than the intraoral grafts but less than the hip marrow (Bowers et al. 1985).
II. OSTEOCONDUCTIVE IMPLANTS: Implants that are *passive* and serve only as a *lattice* to be covered over with new bone and replaced.
   A. Allografts
      1. Freeze-dried bone allografts (FDBA)
      2. Demineralized freeze-dried bone allografts (DFDBA)
   B. Alloplasts
      1. Porous hydroxyapatite
III. OSTEONEUTRAL IMPLANTS: Implants that are totally inert and serve only as *space fillers*. They have been categorized by Froum et al. (1982) as biocompatible foreign bodies within the gingival tissue that do not provide a framework for new bone to cover.
   A. Alloplastic materials
      1. Resorbable—β-tricalcium phosphate
      2. Nonresorbable—durapatite, hydroxyapatite, (HTR)
IV. GUIDED TISSUE REGENERATION (GTR): An epithelial exclusionary technique that promotes new connective tissue attachment without use of any implant material. (See the section on Guided Tissue Regeneration.)

Autogenous Bone Marrow Grafts

Extraoral Sites

Schallhorn (1967, 1968), in an attempt to get adequate osteogenic donor material for grafting, chose hip marrow, which has the highest inductive potential, to treat periodontal defects. The marrow cores were obtained using a Turkell bone trephine and either immediately inserted into the prepared osseous defect or placed in Minimum Essential Media and kept cool or frozen. Storage does not seem to decrease significantly the osteogenic potential.

The obtained grafted material is packed firmly into the intraosseous defect, at or slightly above the marginal lip of bone. The flap (full- or partial-thickness) is closed tightly over the defect to permit primary-intention healing. A partial-thickness flap is used if a free soft-tissue graft is to be used for coverage (Fig. 12-8).

Hip marrow implants, although offering excellent results in two- and three-wall intraosseous defects and even providing supracrestal apposition (Hiatt and Schallhorn, 1973; Dragoo and Sullivan, 1973 A,B), displayed such negative factors as ankylosis and root resorption, which preclude their routine use in periodontal surgery (Ellegaard et al., 1976).

Intraoral Sites

OSSEOUS COAGULUM. Robinson (1969) devised a technique for obtaining bone grafting donor material consisting of a mixture of bone shavings and blood from the surgical field, termed *osseous coagulum*. The concept was based on the fact that mineralized substances can induce osteogenesis; it appears to be an extension of the technique, developed by Nabers and O'Leary (1965).

The shavings were obtained during osteoplasty. They were collected on a large retractor or mirror and mixed with the patient's blood in a sterile dappen dish (Fig. 12-9). The most suitable sites for obtaining bone shavings are exostoses, tori, heavy marginal ridges, and adjacent sites undergoing osseous correction.

In summarizing his technique, Robinson claimed significant fill in three-wall defects, but unpredictable repair of one- and two-wall osseous defects. Freeman (1973) questioned the ability and use of osseous coagulum to enhance bone regeneration.

OSSEOUS COAGULUM—BONE BLEND. Diem et al. (1972) modified Robinson's original osseous coagulum technique to permit easier access and collection of donor material, a procedure termed *osseous coagulum—bone blend*. He used a sterile capsule and pestle to mix or blend the bone obtained from extraction sites, exostoses, tori, or edentulous ridges. The bone spicules (cancellous and cortical), obtained with chisels and rongeurs, were triturated for 60 seconds to produce a homogenous mass, which could easily be placed in a bony defect and firmly packed inside.

Froum et al. (1975A,B, 1976) found that *osseous coagulum—bone blend provided the same regenerative potential as did iliac marrow and significantly greater than that of open debridement*. He further noted that the amount of bone fill may depend more on *available osseous* surfaces than on the *number of osseous walls*.

TUBEROSITY SITES. Hiatt and Schallhorn (1973), in seeking alternative sources to iliac crest implants, chose the tuberosity as a potential source for residual red marrow or primitive reticular cells that have a pluripotential competence. At the very least, they believed, cancellous bone was a potential source of large numbers of osteoblasts. The cancellous bone was obtained after careful removal of the cortical plate by use of rongeurs and cone curettes (Fig. 12-10).

After treating 166 intrabony defects with cancellous bone implants from the tuberosity, extraction sites, and edentulous ridges, they noted that total regeneration was obtained in three-wall defects but only partial fill of two-wall defects. They summarized their results with the following formulation: "The degree of regeneration in an osseous defect . . . varies directly with the adequacy of the soft tissue coverage and with the surface area of the vascularized bony walls lining the defect; it varies inversely with the root surface area."

Extraction Sites

Halliday (1969), in an attempt to provide adequate procurement of autogenous cancellous bone, developed a two-stage surgical procedure. The technique used a bone trephine to create artificial defects in the mandible; 6 or 7 weeks later, the area was reentered, and the new bone was removed and transplanted to the intraosseous defect.

The concept of using newly formed bone from artificial defects has been extended to include bone from extraction sites. If extractions are required, they are timed to coincide with treatment of the intraosseous defects so that reentry can take place 6 to 8 weeks later (Fig. 12-11).

BONE SWAGING. Ewen (1965) introduced the contiguous or *bone swaging* technique for treating bony defects, in which bone from an edentulous area was moved next to the tooth to get rid of the defect. This required that the bone be fractured, without completely severing it to maintain the blood supply, and at the same time be moved next to the tooth (Nabers and O'Leary, 1967).

For practical purposes, *this is a difficult, impractical technique, the results of which have not been borne out by research*. It is further limited by the need for an adjacent edentulous ridge and bone quality that permits bending without fracturing.

ALLOPLASTS—CERAMICS

Ceramic materials, although convenient, readily available, and economical, have not been shown to function in any capacity other than that of an inert space filler. They have no significant osteoinductive capacity but have been shown to have some osteoconductive capacity (porous hydroxyapatite) (Louise, 1992). They serve well as biologic expanders (tricalcium phosphate) when sufficient autogenous bone is unavailable (Figs. 12-12 and 12-13).

In a series of studies comparing FDBA, DFDBA, and porous hydroxyapatite (Interpore) in intrabony defects (Kennedy et al., 1985, 1988; Barnett et al., 1989; Bowen et al., 1989; Oreamuno et al., 1980) no significant differences in probing attachment levels and probing bone levels were found. Egelberg (1992), in reviewing their results, found one out of two

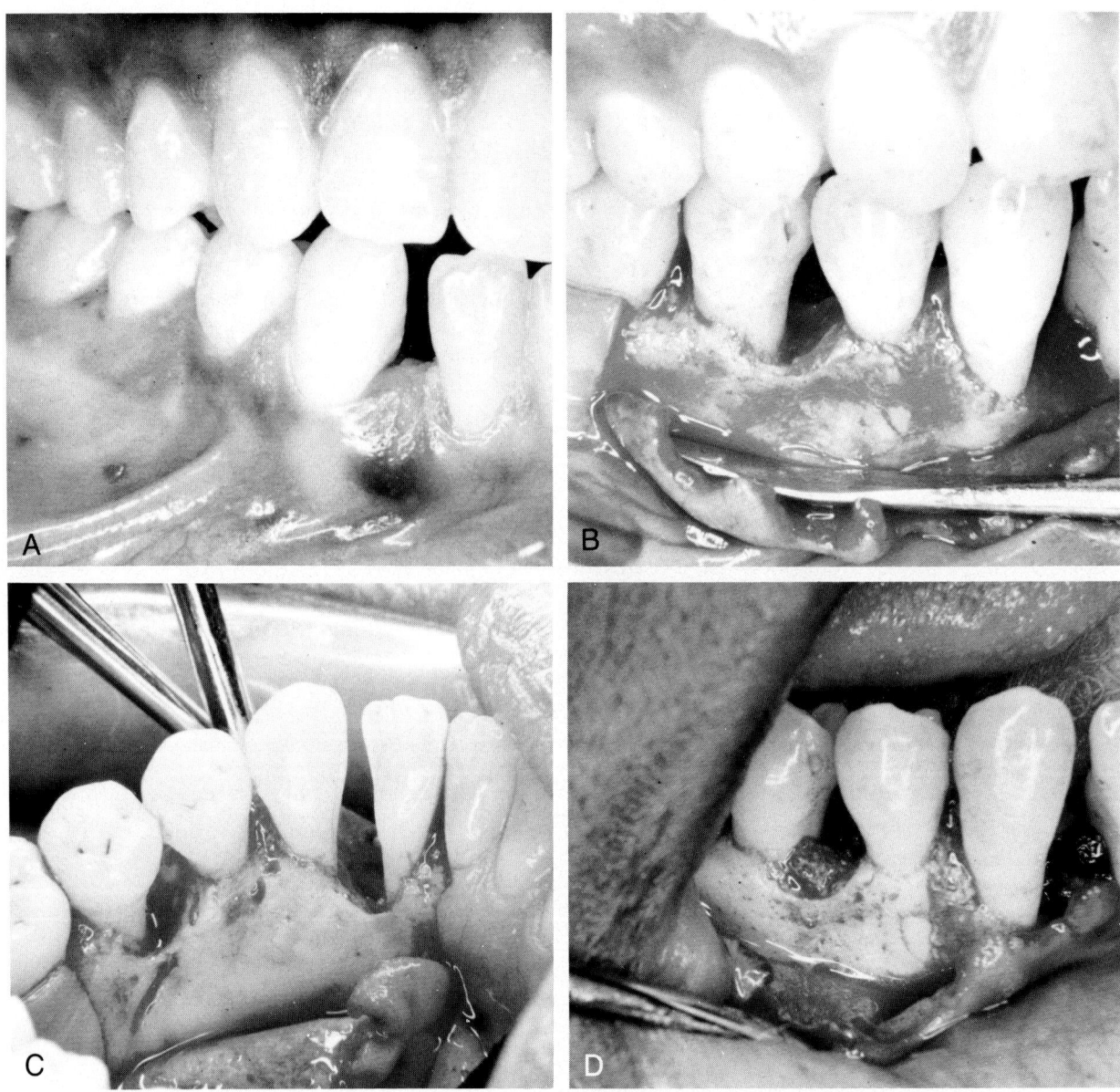

Fig. 12-8. Autogenous Hip Marrow Implant. **A,** Before treatment. **B,** Mucoperiosteal flap reflected, showing defect on second premolar. **C,** Lingual view of intrabony defects. **D,** Hip marrow placed in defect between premolars.

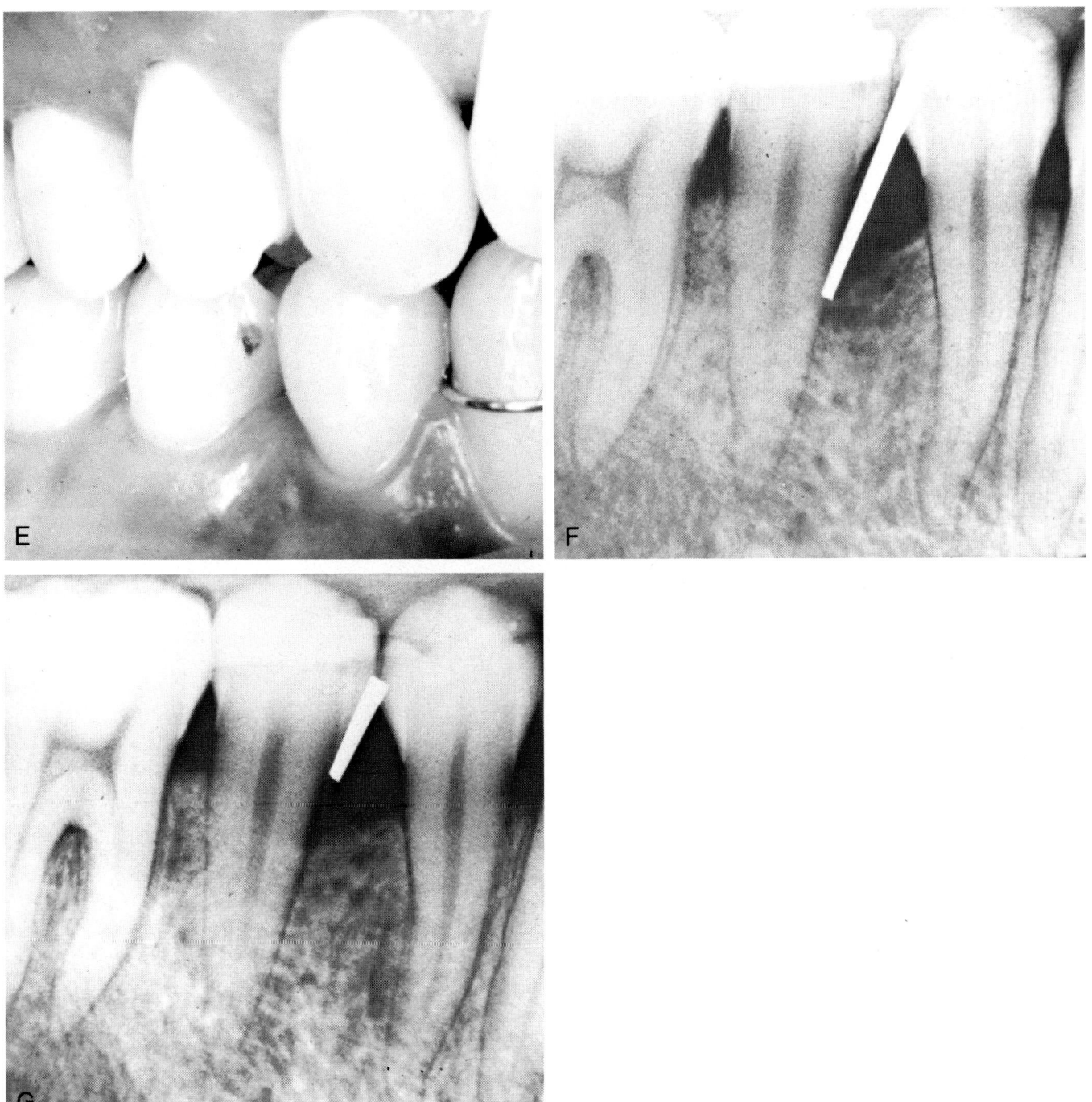

Fig. 12-8 (continued). E, Seven months later. **F,** Osseous defect with metal point at base of pocket prior to treatment. **G,** Seven months later, metal point at base of pocket and bone repaired. (Originally contributed by Edward S. Cohen, D.M.D. to Glickman's Periodontology and reprinted with permission of W. B. Saunders Co.)

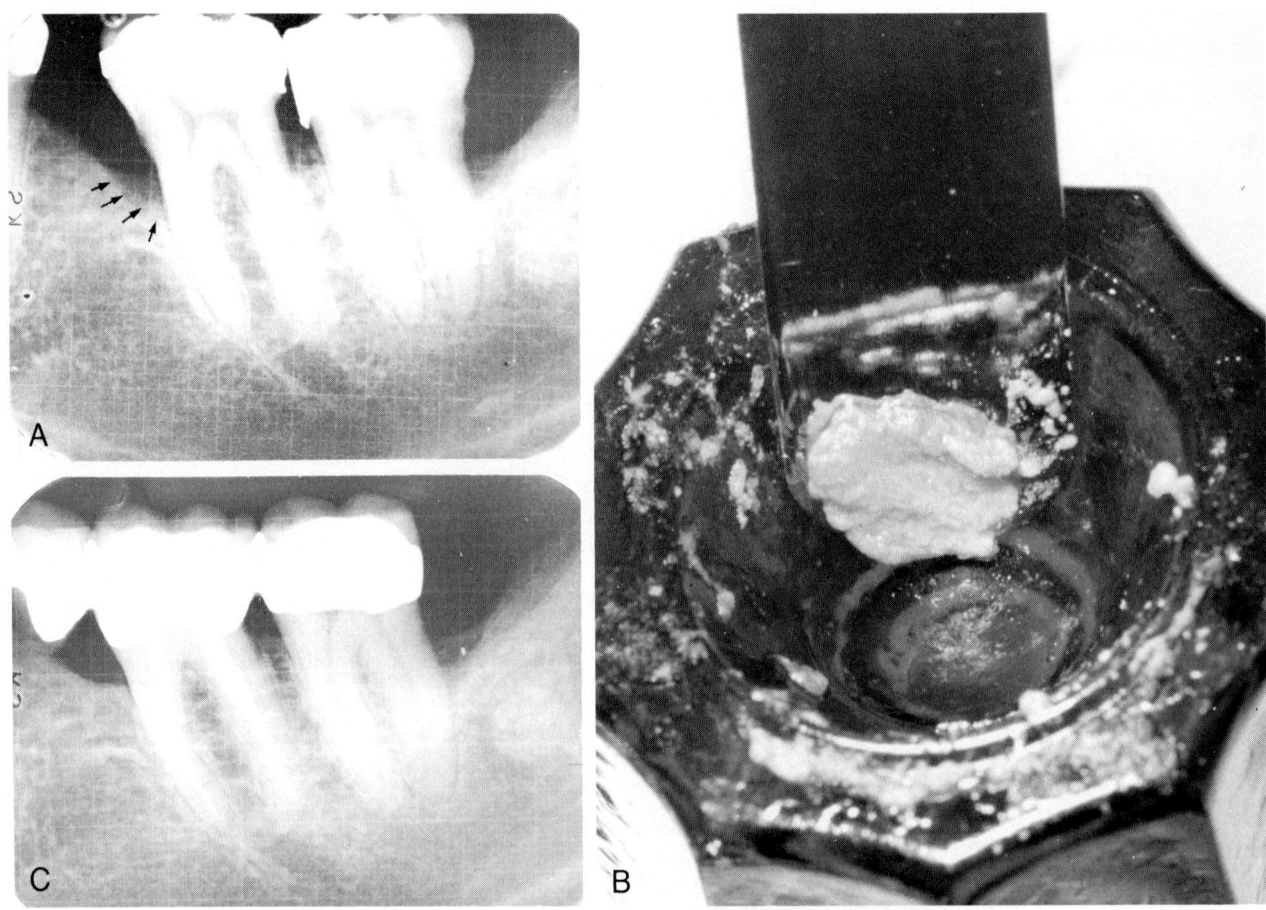

Fig. 12-9. Osseous Coagulum Bone Implant. **A,** Pretreatment x-ray study showing osseous defect on mesial of first molar. **B,** Osseous coagulum collected on large spoon retractor and placed into defects. **C,** Five-year post-treatment x-ray study showing complete bone fill.

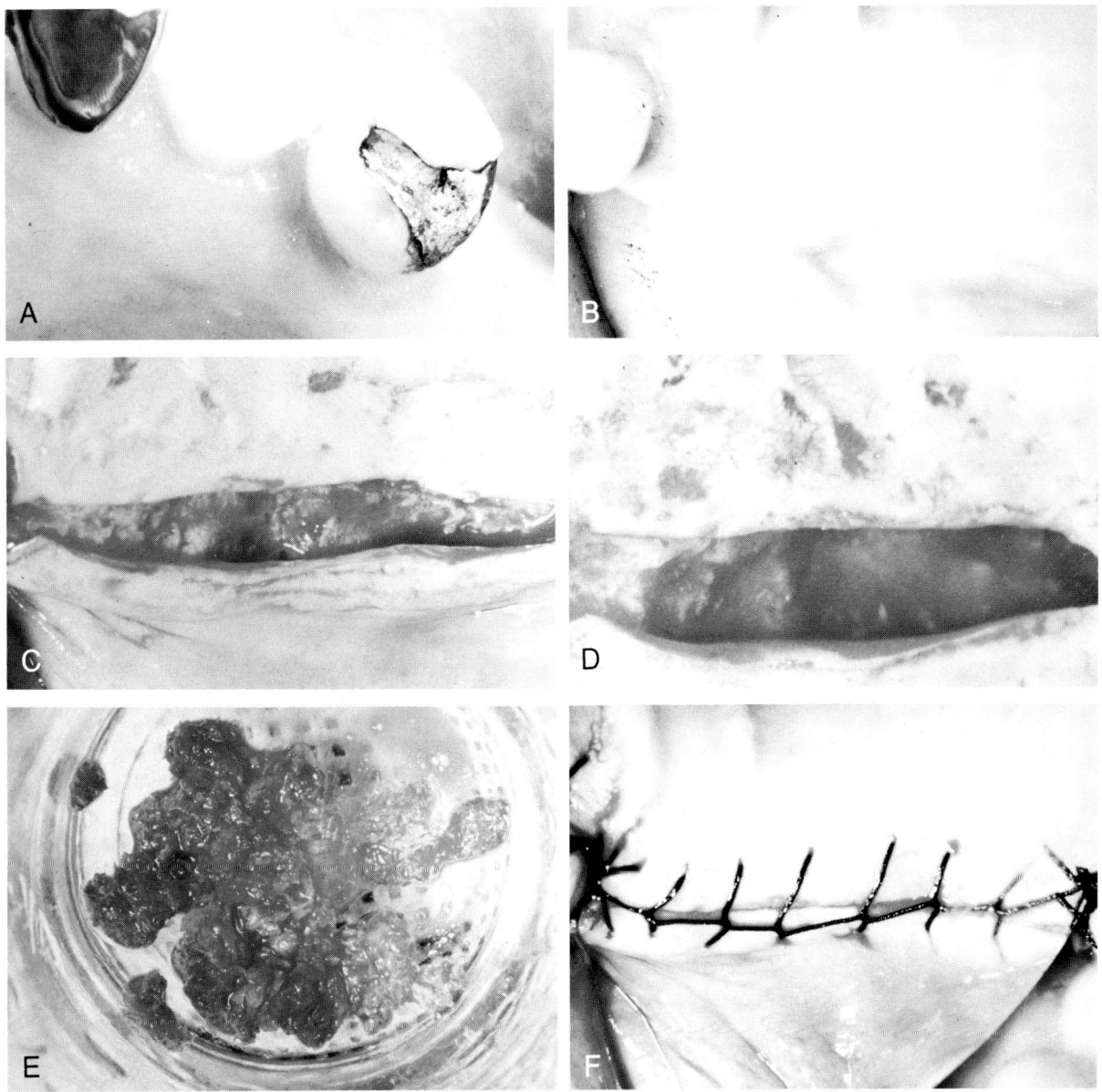

Fig. 12-10. Autogenous Tuberosity Bone Implant. **A,** Before treatment. **B,** Maxillary edentulous ridge and tuberosity. **C,** Mucoperiosteal flaps reflected. **D,** Autogenous cancellous bone removed. **E,** Cancellous bone placed in sterile container. **F,** Ridge and tuberosity sutured.

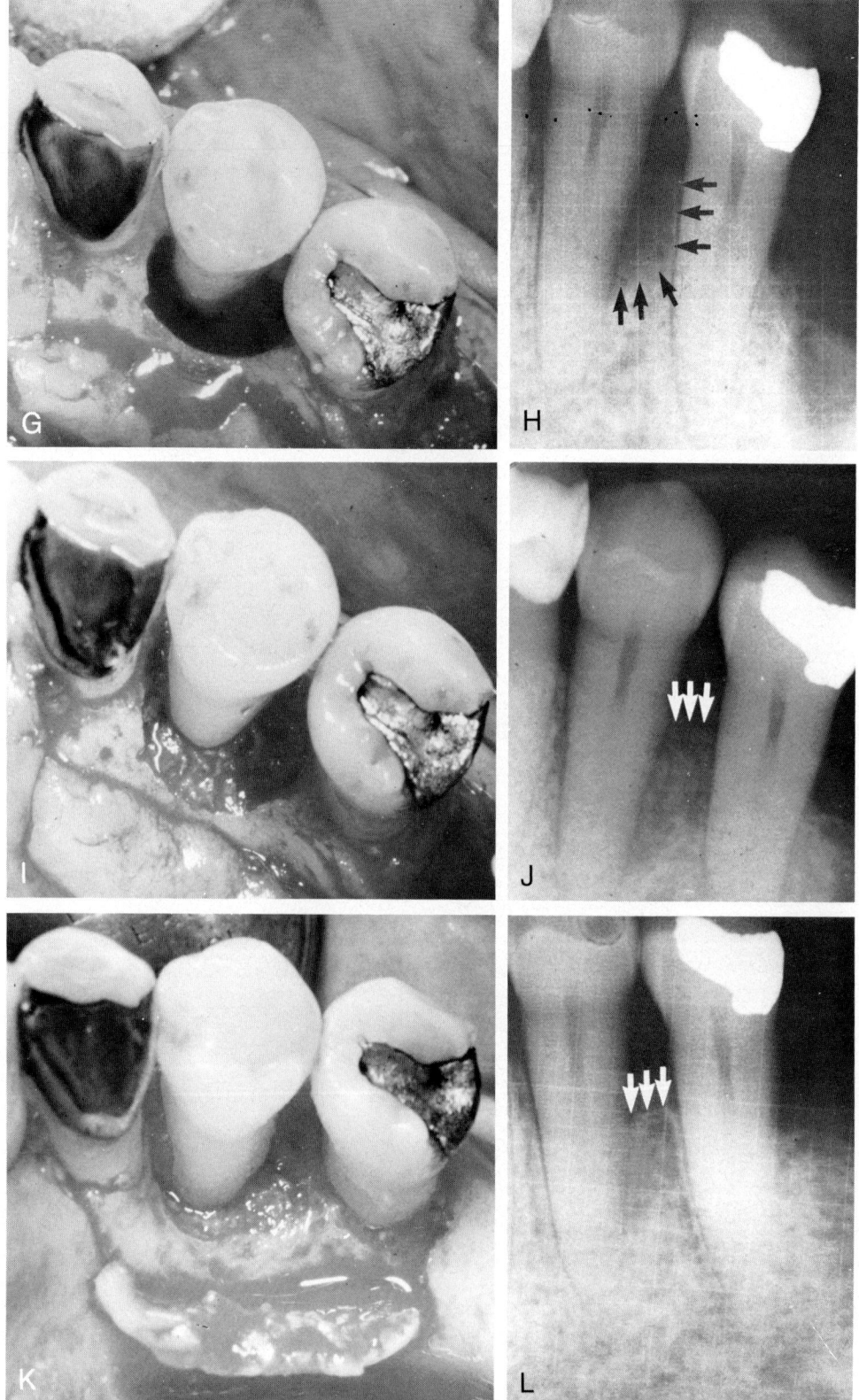

Fig. 12-10 (continued). **G,** Lingual flap reflected and deep intraosseous defect visualized. **H,** Before-treatment x-ray study. **I,** Autogenous cancellous bone placed. **J,** X-ray study done at time of graft placement. **K,** Re-entry 6 months later, showing bone regeneration. **L,** X-ray study showing bone regeneration.

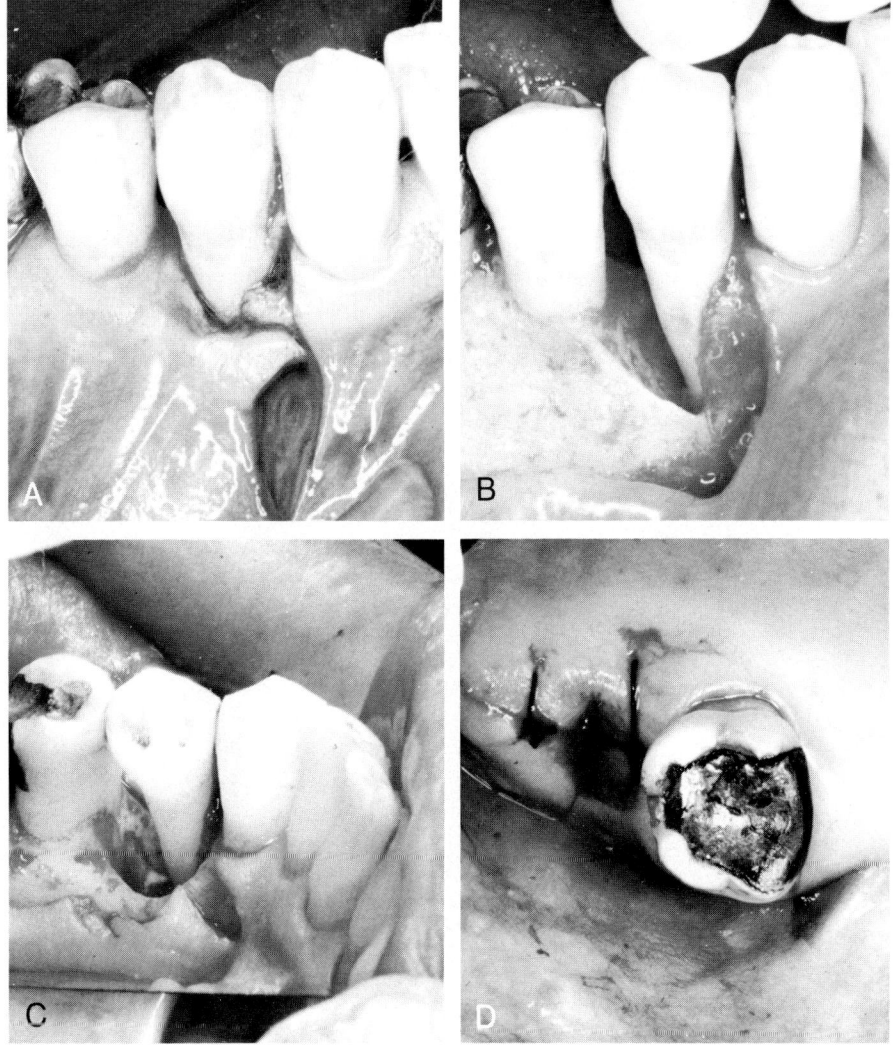

Fig. 12-11. Autogenous Bone Implant from Extraction Site. **A,** Mucoperiosteal flap preparation. **B,** Buccal view of angular intraosseous defect **C,** Lingual view of same defect. **D,** Autogenous bone taken 8 to 10 weeks after tooth extraction.

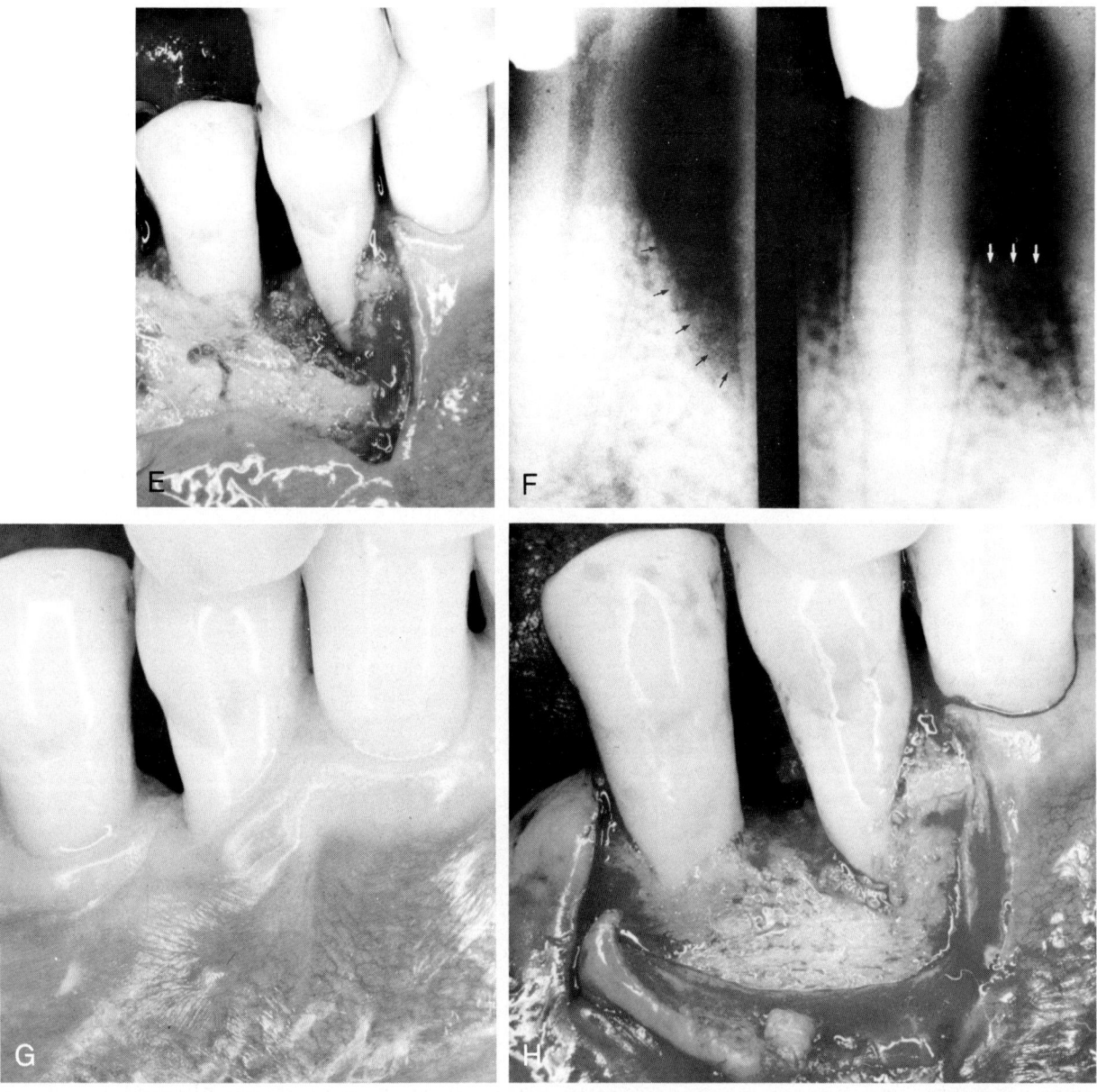

Fig. 12-11 (continued). **E,** Graft placed at or slightly above crest of defect. **F,** Preoperative (left) and postoperative 6-months x-ray studies. Note osseous regeneration (arrows). **G,** Six months later, at time of re-entry. **H,** Re-entry, showing bone regeneration. Compare with B. (Originally contributed by Edward S. Cohen, D.M.D. to Glickman's Clinical Periodontology and reprinted by permission of W. B. Saunders.)

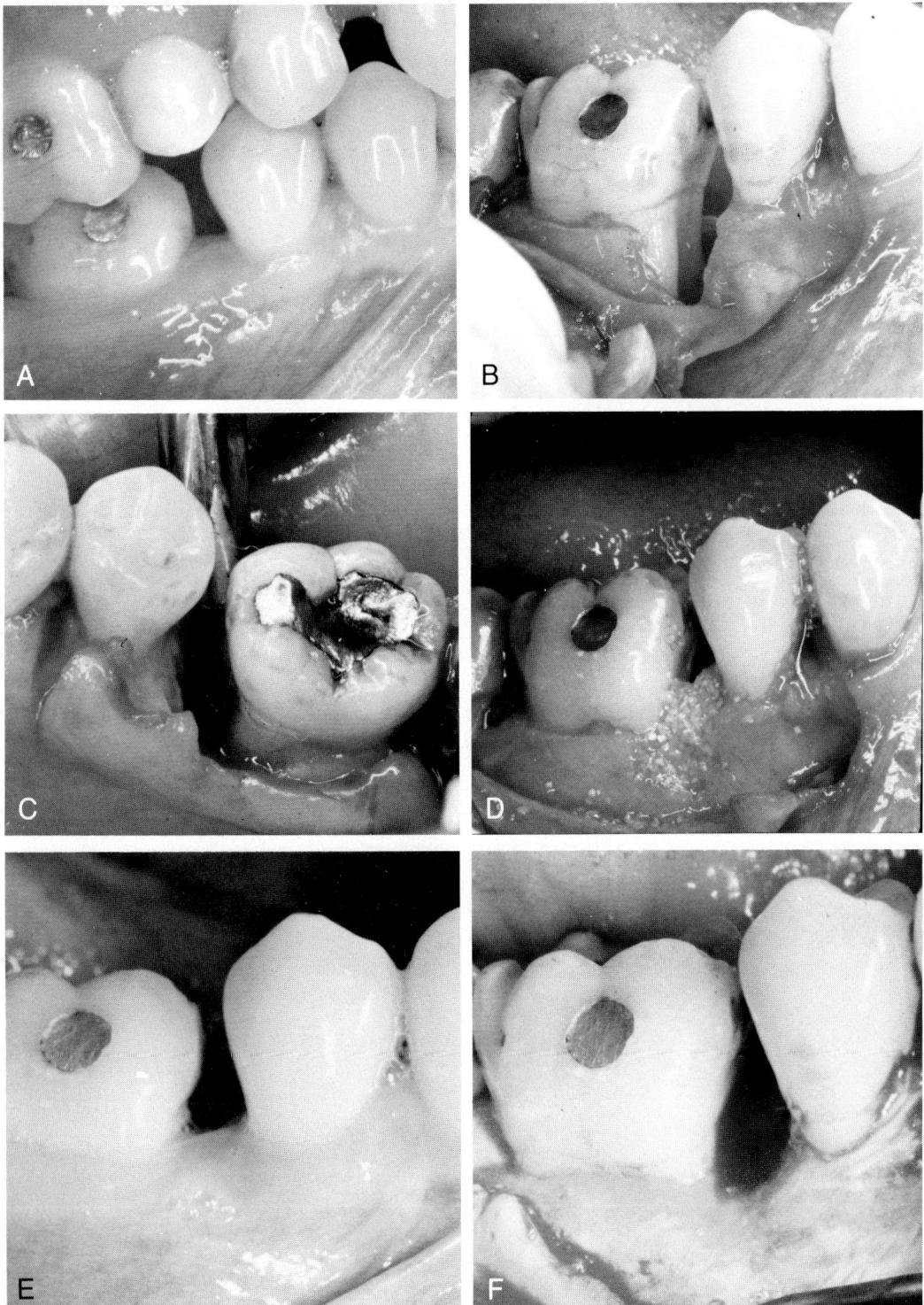

Fig. 12-12. Hydroxyapatite (Perigraft) Implant. **A,** Before treatment. **B,** Buccal view, showing intrabony osseous defect. **C,** Lingual view of osseous defect. **D,** Hydroxyapatite graft placed. **E,** Five months later. **F,** Re-entry 5 months later, showing restoration of buccal defect. Compare with B.

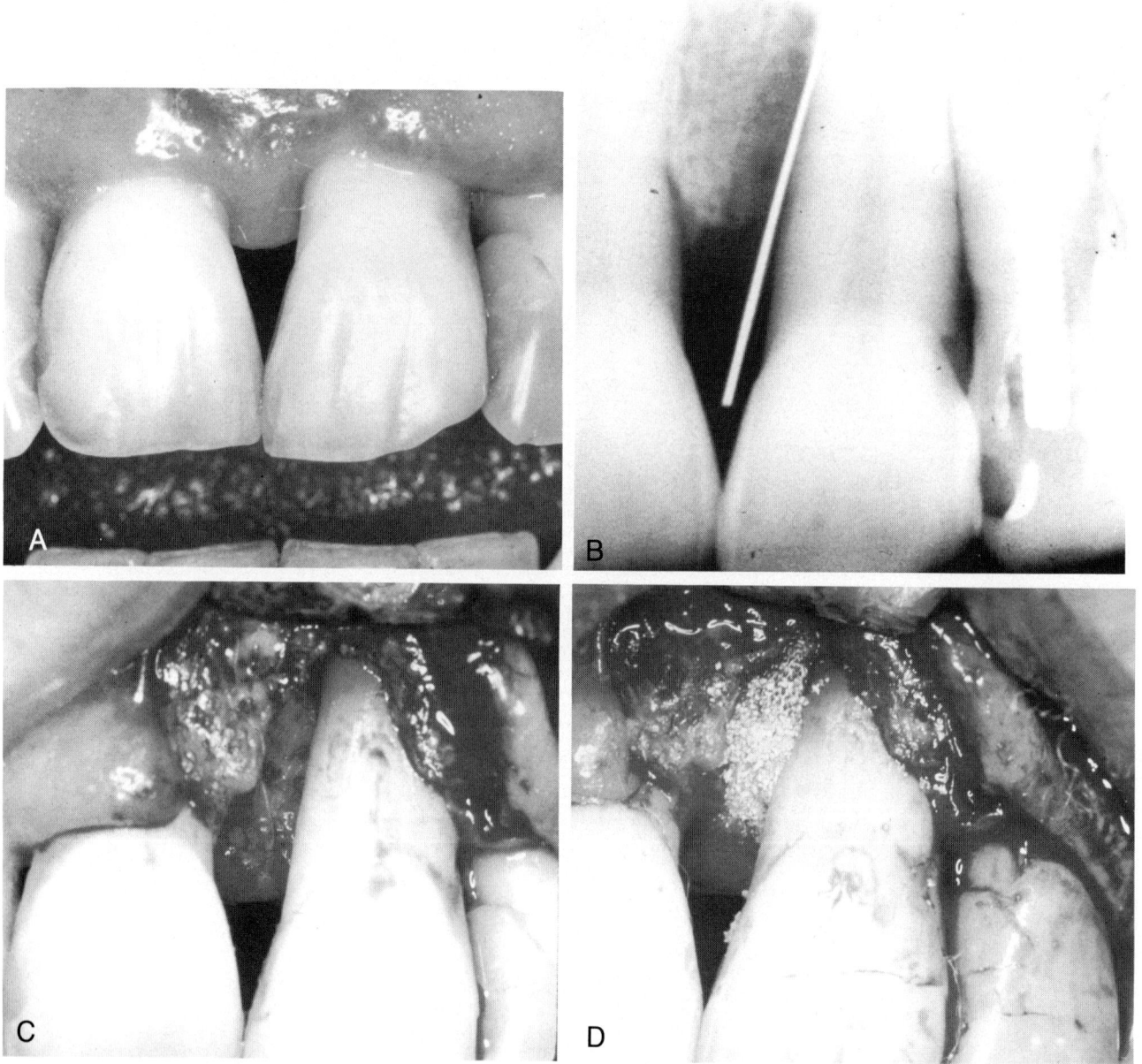

Fig. 12-13. Hydroxyl (Interpore) Implant Material. **A,** Pretreatment view. **B,** X-ray study with gutta-percha to base of defect. **C,** Osseous intrabony defect exposed. **D,** Hydroxyapatite placed in defect.

Inductive Osseous Surgery

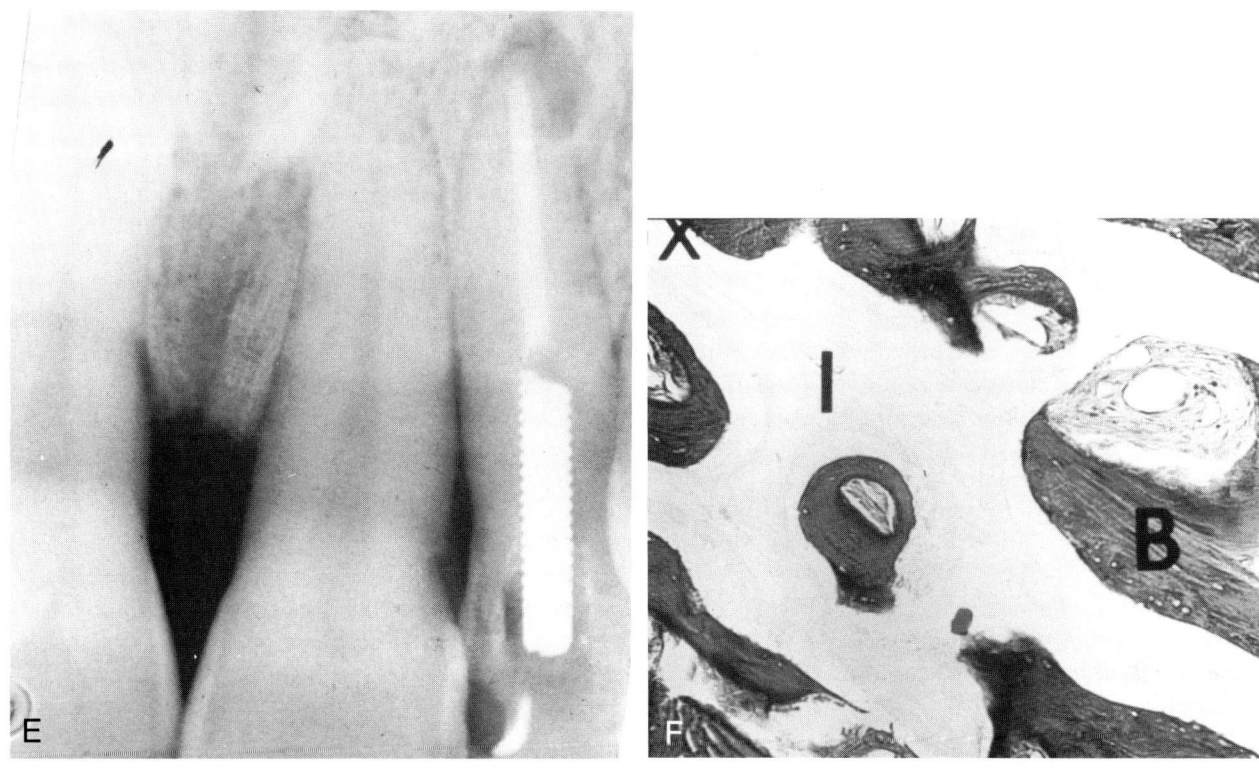

Fig. 12-13 (continued). **E,** X-ray view 7 months later. **F,** Histologic view (sample) showing bone growing over implant material. (Contributed by Dr. Theodore West, Englewood, NJ.)

defects *had a gain* of 2 mm or more in bone and one out of three defects had a gain of 3 mm or more in bone (Figs. 12-14 and 12-15).

Kennedy et al. (1988) using porus hydroxyapatite (Interpore 200) in Class II furcations on mandibulars found significant gains in attachment levels (1.82 mm; $p \leq 0.001$) and horizontal (1.56; $p \leq 0.001$) bone fill. Corsair (1990) obtained 51% fill of intrabony defects with a resorbable hydroxyapatite (Osteogen) with a predictable controlled resorption rate. In his 5-year evaluation of durapalite (Periograf) Yukna (1980) found that grafted sites improved or stayed the same 86% of the time compared to only 62% for debridement (DEBR) and that 38%, or three times as many, of DEBR areas failed as opposed to HA-grafted sites. Yukna (1990) in analyzing the results using a synthetic (HTR) polymer found 71% of the participants had an overall positive ($\geq 50\%$) response as compared to only 24% for the control sites, which had flap debridement alone. Shahmiri (1992), on the other hand, found no significant differences between the control and HTR-treated intrabony sites.

Saffar et al. (1990) in biopsies of human intrabony defects, found that tricalcium phosphate (TCP) was progressively modified and resorbed and eventually replaced by bone. He concluded that TCP has osteogenic potential. Pepelassi et al. (1991), using a combination of doxycycline-tricalcium phosphate and sterile plaster of paris three to seven times with a likelihood of 50% as greater defect fill in Class II furcations when compared to the nongrafted controls. Class III furcation showed even more pronounced changes.

It is important to note that histologically, healing is by a long-junctional epithelium (repair) with the hydroxy-, hydroxyl-, durapatite and HTR being well tolerated but surrounded by and encapsulated by connective tissue.

ALLOGRAFTS

Demineralized Freeze-Dried Bone Allografts (DFDBA)

Urist (1965, 1968, 1971, 1980) has shown the inductive capabilities of demineralized freeze-dried bone allografts (DFDBA). He and his co-workers have isolated a *bone morphogenic protein* (BMP) that is capable of osteogenic induction by inducing primordial cells to differentiate into osteoblasts. Demineralization exposes the collagen matrix that harbors the inductive proteins (BMP), thereby permitting greater inductability. The ideal particle size is between 250 and 500 μm. This small size permits

1. High inductive potential
2. Easy resorption and replacement
3. Increased surface area for primordial mesenchymal cell interaction.

Particles smaller than 250 μm are absorbed too quickly; and the larger ones are inadequately utilized.

DFDBA at present is the only nonautogenous material that meets all the criteria for the ideal grafting material (Table 12-1).

1. Availability
2. Predictability
3. Biocompatibility
4. Osteoinductive
5. Osteoconductive
6. Cost effective
7. Safety

Mellonig (1984) has shown significant bone regeneration using the DFDBA. He showed a 64.7% increase with DFDBA as opposed to 37.8% for the controls ($p < 0.01$). Furthermore, his results showed a 78% fill for all types of intrabony defects with 90% for two-wall defects. More recently Bowers et al.

Table 12-1. Criteria for an Ideal Implant Material

	Bone Marrow	Intraoral Bone	DFDBA	Ceramics
Osteoinductive	+++	+	++	−
Osteoconductive	+++	++	++	+
Immediately osteogenetic	+++	+	++	−
New cementum induction	+++	+	++	−
Safety	+	+++	+++	+++
Stability to remain in position	+++	+	++	+
Replacement	+++	+++	++	−
Adequate supply	+	+	+++	+++

(1985), in a preliminary report, showed DFDBA capable of producing not only bone fill in intrabony defects but also new attachment both clinically and histologically. Bowers (1989A,B) completed the histologic evaluation of new attachment utilizing DFDBA in 32 grafted versus 25 nongrafted sites. The DFDBA group showed significantly greater new attachment ($p < 0.005$), new cementum ($p < 0.005$), new connective tissue ($p < 0.05$), and new bone ($p < 0.001$) in intrabony defects grafted with DFDBA than in nongrafted sites. Nongrafted defects showed no new cementum or periodontal ligament regeneration.

The clinical results can be seen in Figures 12-15, 12-16, 12-17, and 12-18.

Freeze-Dried Bone Allografts (FDBA)

FDBA, a material readily obtainable from various bone banks, has been shown to be osteoconductive. When FDBA is combined with an autogenous bone graft (ABG), it may become osteoinductive (Saunders et al., 1983).

Sepe et al. (1978) and Mellonig (1980, 1981) have shown that you can achieve a 50% or greater bone fill in various types of defects 60% of the time. More recently, Saunders et al. (1983) have shown that when FDBA is combined with ABG, there is an 80% chance of achieving 50% or greater bone fill in all defects.

Yukna and Sepe (1982) used a combination of tetracycline and FDBA in a 4:1 ratio in 62 defects and were able to achieve complete fill in 22 sites, greater than 50% in 39 sites, and less than 50% in only 1 site. These results appear to be better than those when FDBA is used alone.

FDBA, being readily available, appears to be an ideal material for use as a biologic expander when ABG material is insufficient alone (Fig. 12-19).

TREATMENT OF PERIODONTAL FURCATIONS WITH CORONALLY POSITIONED FLAPS AND CITRIC ACID

Conventional periodontal therapy has often met with limited success in treating Class II and Class III furcation lesions. Martin et al. (1988), Gantes et al. (1988, 1991), and Garrett et al. (1990) devised a surgical procedure that was designed to gain adequate wound closure and clot stabilization. The technique uses citric acid for contact inhibition of epithelial downgrowth and a coronally positioned flap for wound closure and clot retention. Stahl and Froum (1991) have recently confirmed histologically the ability to achieve new attachment using this technique.

This technique has provided one of the most successful bone fill results of Class II furcations. In separate studies (1988, 1990) they found an average of 67 to 70% bone fill by volume with 43 to 56% displaying 100% bone fill. Results were not enhanced by use of DFDBA or resorbable membranes (collagen or dura matter). Bone fill results in Class III furcation were limited to only 15%.

It is important to note that these favorable results do not carry over to treatment of intrabony defects. Egelberg (1992), in reviewing a series of studies comparing intrabony defects with and without citric acid (CA) (Renvert et al., 1981, 1985A, 1985C; Chamberlin, 1985) and CA versus osseous grafting (Renvert et al., 1985B) found no significant differences in probing attachment level (1.1 mm to 2.0 mm) or probing bone levels (0.6 mm to 1.3 mm).

Indications

1. Class II or Class III mandibular furcations
2. Class II maxillary buccal furcations

Advantages

1. Simple
2. Predictable
3. Cost effective

Disadvantage

Complicated suturing for coronal flap position.

Procedure

1. An orthodontic bracket or tube is cemented to the buccal or lingual surface above the furcation to be treated (Fig. 12-20A).
2. Vertical incisions are made on the mesial and distal aspects of the tooth *dissecting the interdental papilla*. Each incision is approximately 15 mm in length and made down to bone (Fig. 12-20B).
3. An intrasulcular incision is now made joining the two vertical incisions (Fig. 12-20B).
4. Upon reflection of a mucoperiosteal flap, the exposed roots are scaled and root planed with hand and ultrasonic scalers and all granulation tissue is removed. Enamel projections are removed with high-speed pear-shaped finishing burs (Fig. 12-20C).
5. Osseous surgery is *not* performed.
6. The apical portion of the mucoperiosteal flap is fenestrated to permit coronal positioning (Fig. 12-20D).

7. A saturated solution of citric acid (pH 1.0) is applied with cotton pellets for 3 minutes, followed by saline irrigation (Fig. 12-20E).
8. Bleeding in the furcation is stimulated by *scratching* the periodontal ligament with an explorer.
9. The authors recommend the following suturing techniques to assure flap placement: "A 4-0 silk suture is passed through the tube starting from the mesial aspect; the suture is continued with a horizontal mattress in the distal part of the flap margin; subsequently the suture is passed interdentally on the distal aspect of the tooth, swung around the tooth, passed interdentally on the mesial aspect of the tooth, followed by a horizontal mattress in the mesial flap margin; the suture is tied with the flap margin in a coronal position and with a tight apposition of the flap over the entire mesiodistal extension of the crown" (Fig. 12-18F).
10. Tetracycline ointment (aureomycin 3%) is placed over the flap margins. A periodontal dressing is now placed.
11. The patient is placed on tetracycline 250 Q.I.D. for 2 weeks. One week later the dressing is removed, the area debrided, tetracycline ointment reapplied, and the area repacked. The sutures and dressings are removed in 2 weeks.

The clinical procedure is depicted in Figures 12-21 and 12-22.

GUIDED TISSUE REGENERATION

Prichard (1967, 1983) and Ellegaard et al. (1974) showed the benefits of epithelial retardation and exclusion in promoting bone regeneration. Yet, it was not until Nyman et al. (1982A,B) devised a predictable method for epithelial exclusion that the concept gained acceptance.

Using first a Millipore filter and later a Teflon Gore-Tex membrane under the flap to exclude epithelial downgrowth, they were able to get new connective tissue attachment in furcations and angular defects. New bone was achieved only in the angular defects.

This technique appears most suitable for Grade I and Grade II furcations and intrabony defects, where implants do not seem to work and where resective osseous surgery is limited. The main drawback to the technique is the need to remove the filter in a second surgical procedure 4 weeks later (see Chapter 13).

Inductive Osseous Surgery

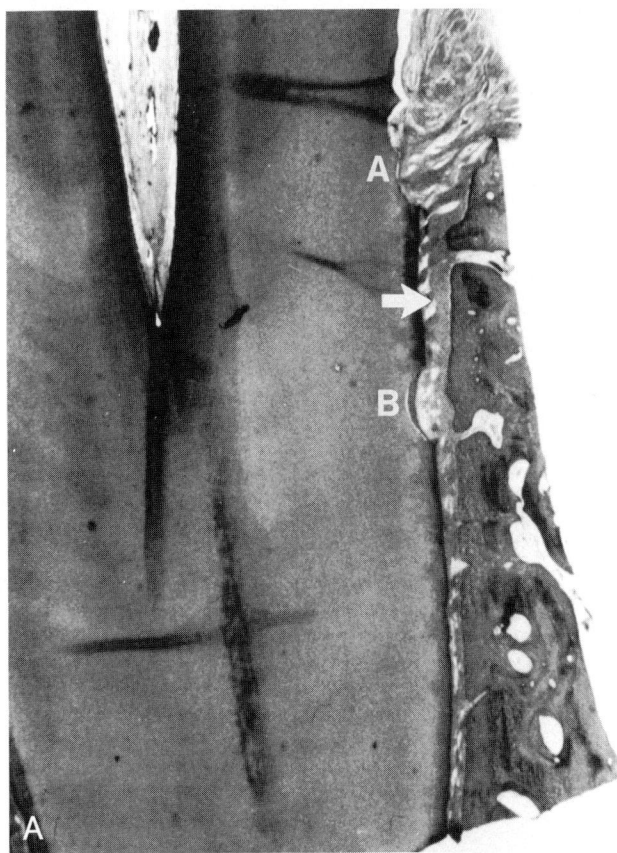

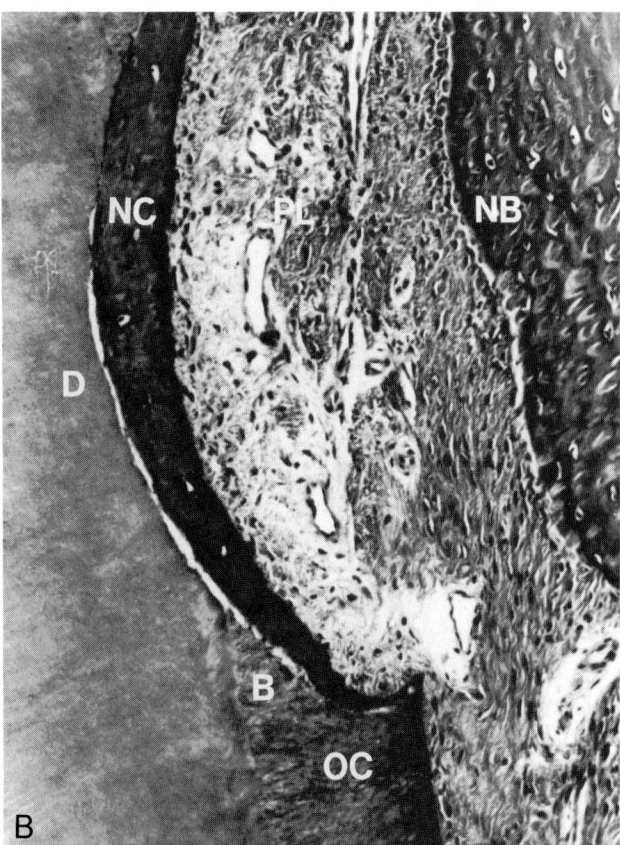

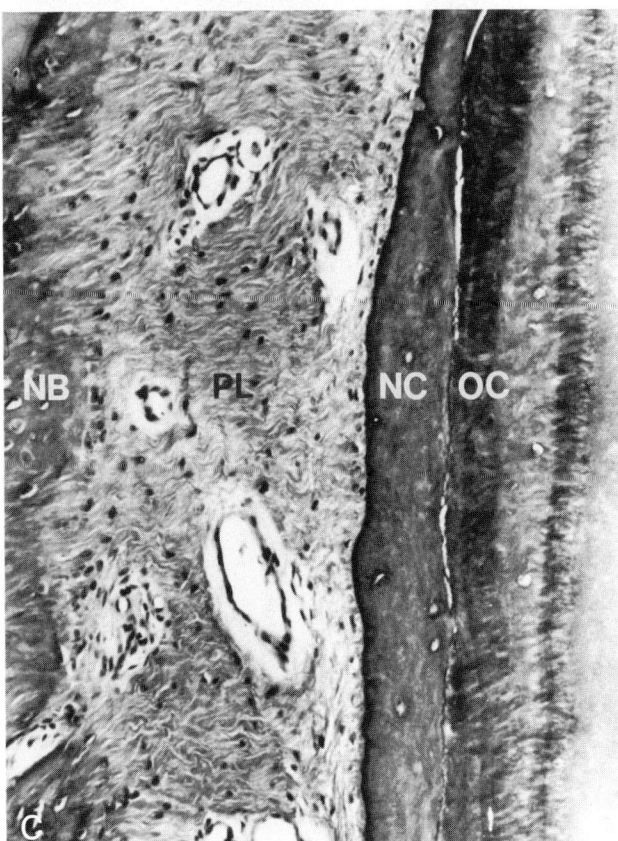

Fig. 12-14 **A,** Grafted defect demonstrating new attachment apparatus formation from calculus reference notch (B) to reference notch (A). New cementum formed over both dentin and old cementum. The junctional epithelium is located approximately level with the alveolar crest at reference notch (A) (H&E, original magnification 4x). **B,** Higher magnification of calculus notch (B) in A demonstrating the formation of a new attachment apparatus. Note that new cellular cementum (NC) has formed over old cementum (OC) and over dentin (D). Periodontal ligament fibers appear to be oriented both parallel and perpendicular at this level. (H&E, original magnification 40x). **C,** Higher magnification of region of arrow in A. Note new cellular cementum formation (NC) over old cementum (OC). Also note perpendicular arrangement of periodontal ligament fibers (PL) at this level. (H&E, original magnification 40x). (Contributed by Gerald M. Bowers, Baltimore, Maryland.)

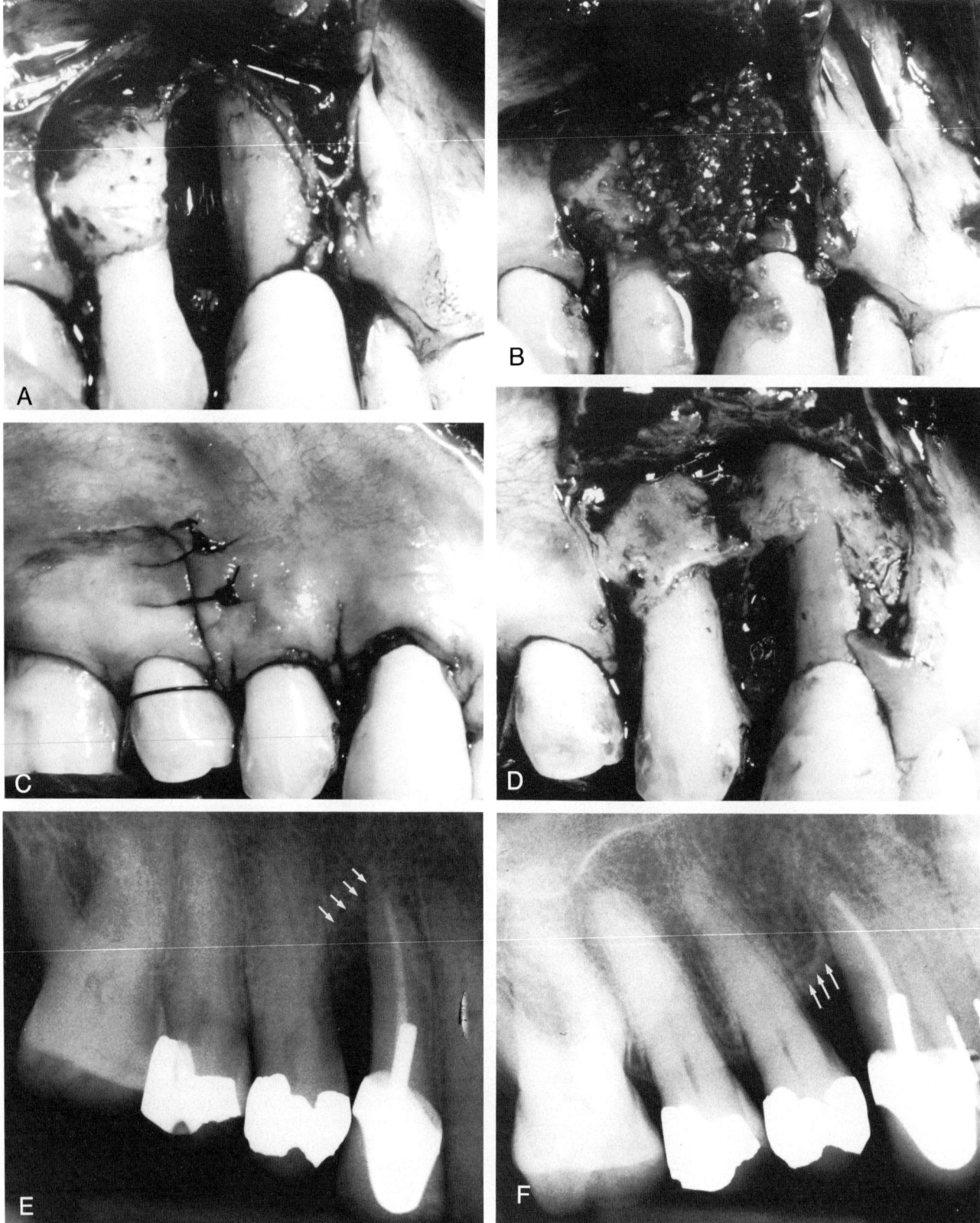

Fig. 12-15. Demineralized Freeze-Dried Bone Allograft. **A,** Initial view of defect: 2-wall with buccal dehiscence. **B,** DFDBA placed. **C,** Flaps sutured. **D,** Re-entry 1 year later. Note significant bone increases compared to A. **E,** X-ray study taken before surgery. **F,** X-ray study taken at time of re-entry.

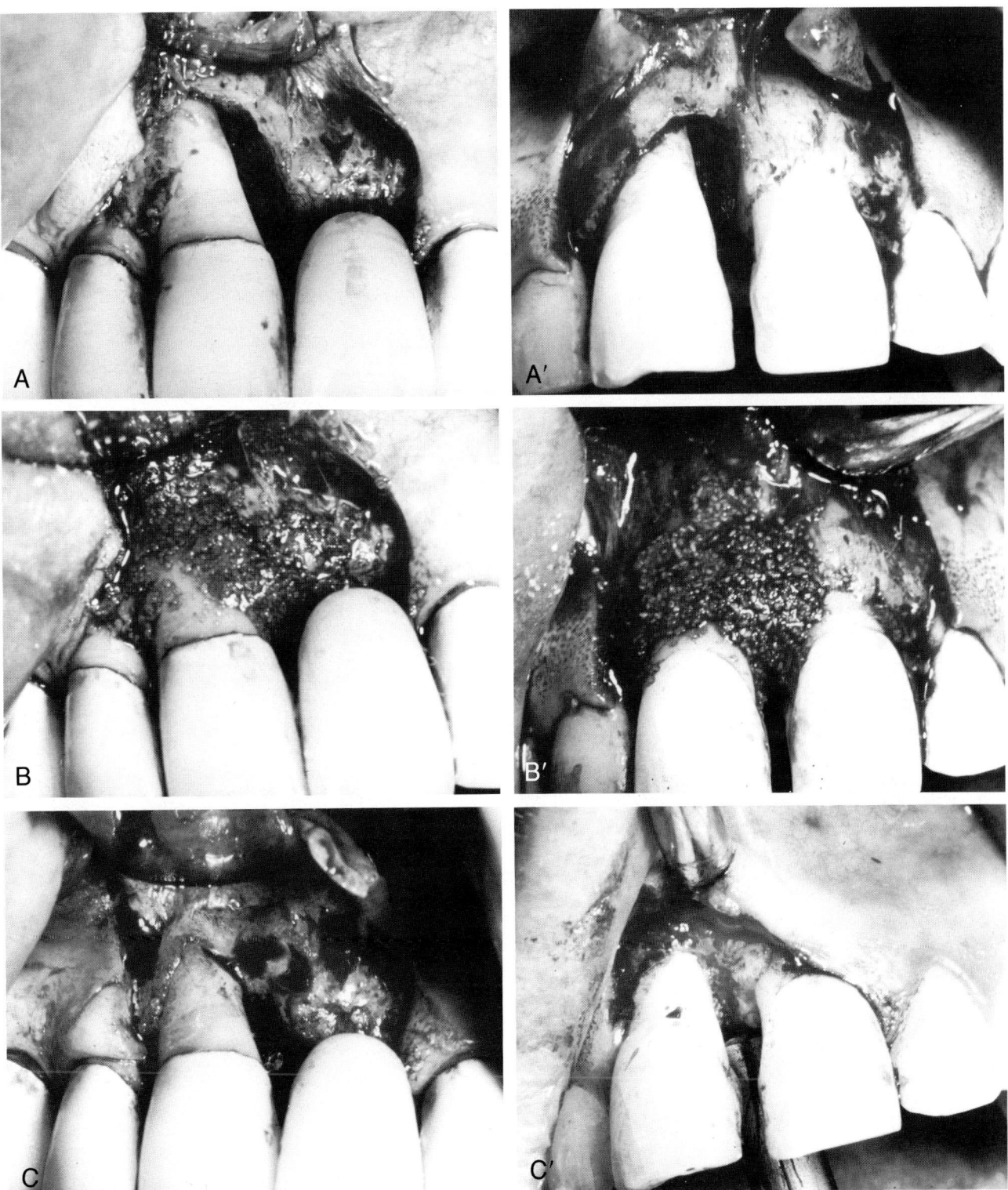

Fig. 12-16. Demineralized Freeze-Dried Bone Allograft on *Two Different* Central Incisors. **A, A′**, Defects exposed. **B, B′**, DFDBA placed. Note placement of graft material over exposed root surface. **C, C′**, Re-entry after 1 year. Note defect fill and some coverage of root dehisencies.

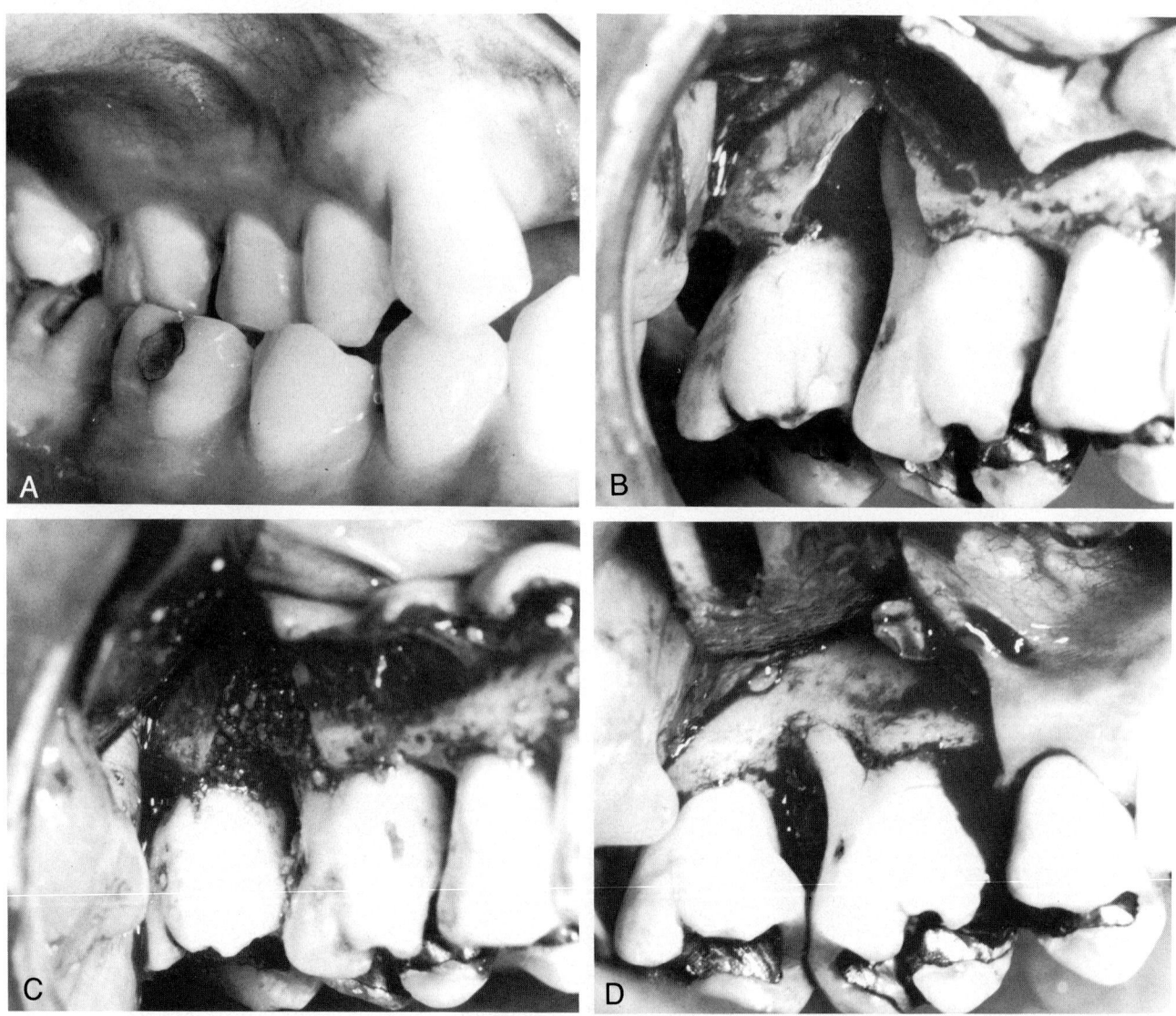

Fig. 12-17. Demineralized Freeze-Dried Bone Allograft (DFDBA). **A,** Before surgery. **B,** Defect exposed. Note loss of buccal plate, DB root dehiscence, and interproximal defect. **C,** DFDBA placed. **D,** Re-entry after 1 year. Note bone regeneration (compare with B).

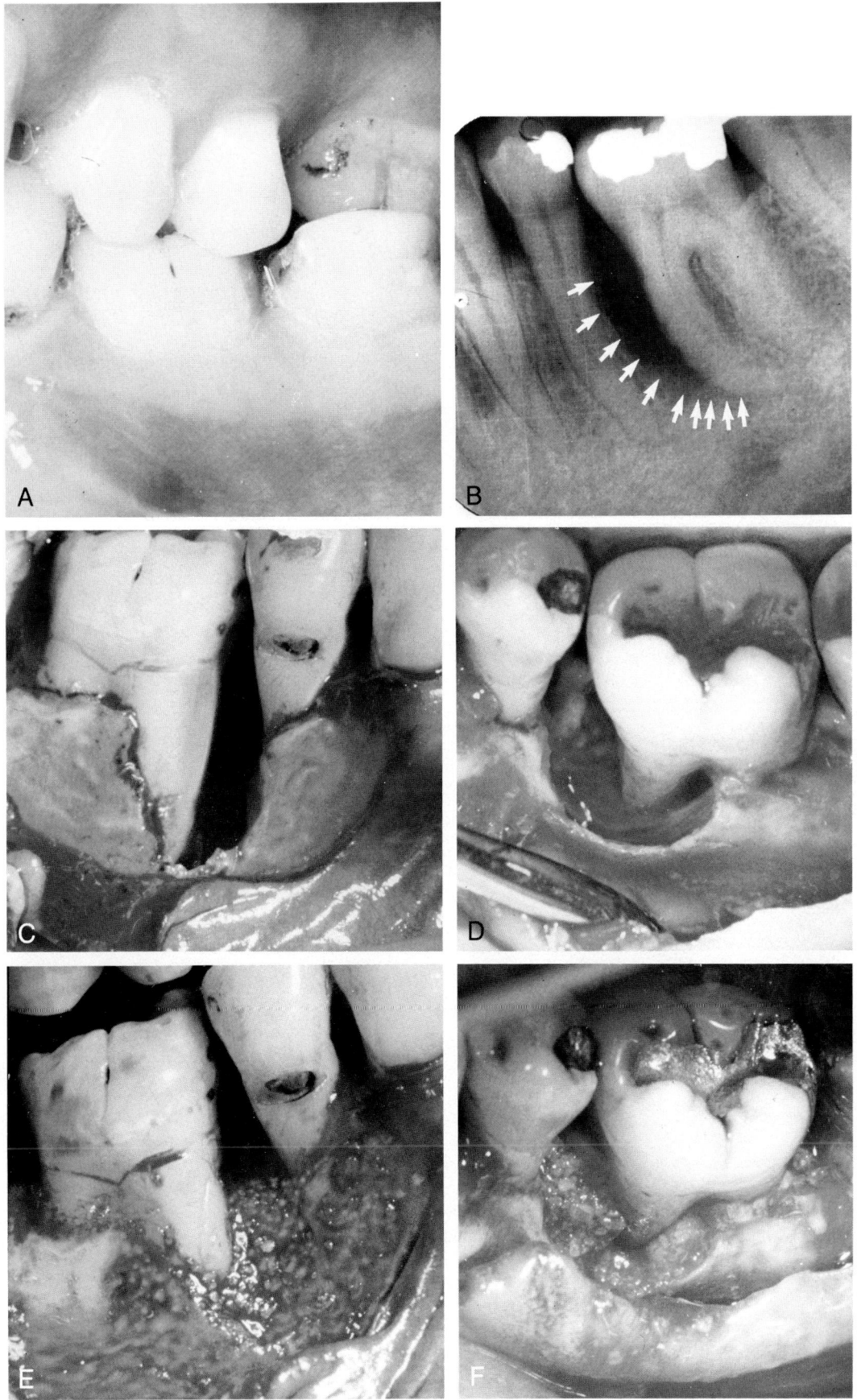

Fig. 12-18. Demineralized Freeze-Dried Bone Allograft (DFDBA). **A,** Before treatment. **B,** Pretreatment x-ray study. Arrows show extent of defect. **C,** Buccal view of defect. **D,** Lingual view of defect. Note circumferential nature of defect, with furcation involvement. **E,** DFDBA placed; buccal view. **F,** Lingual view of implant.

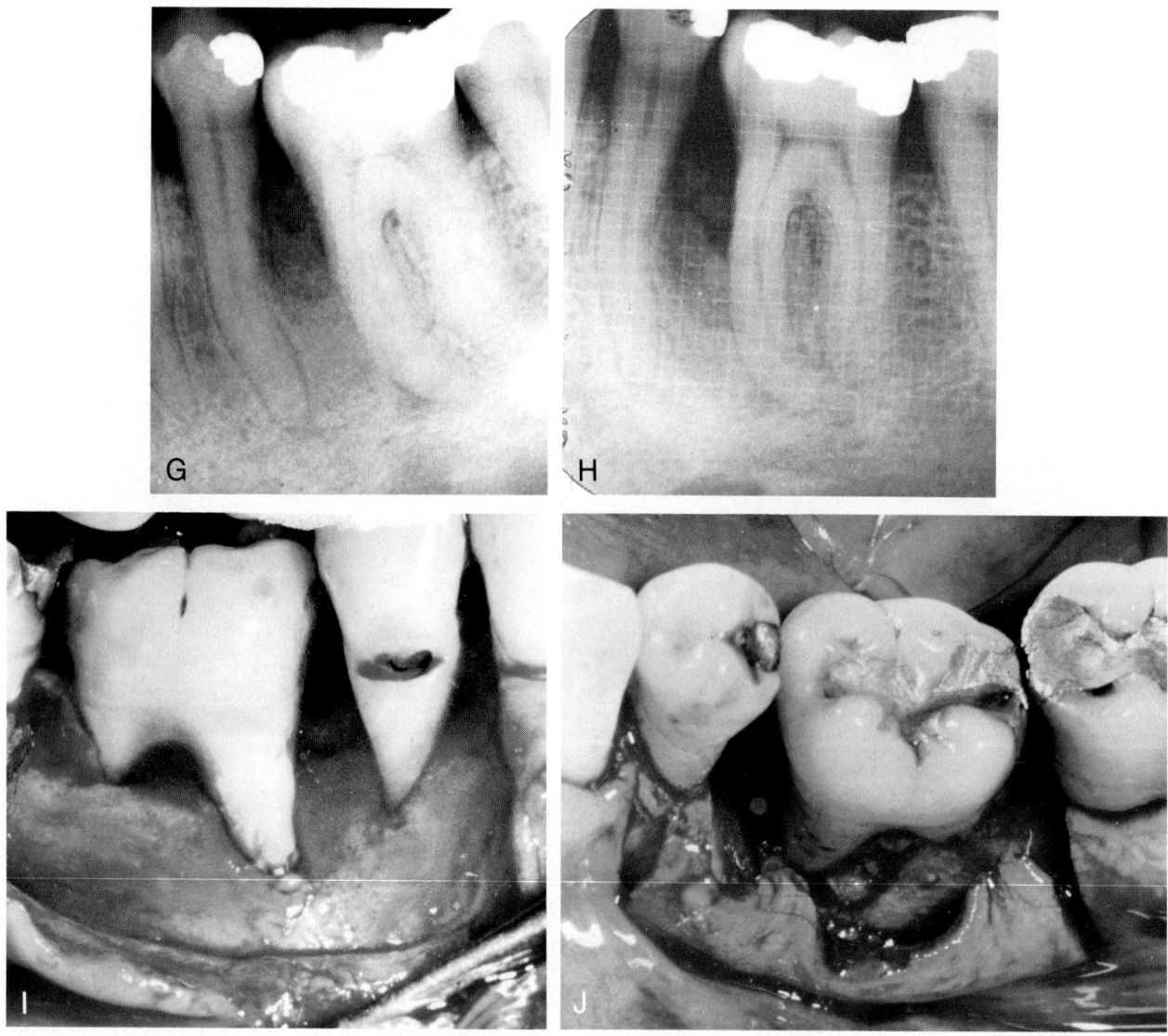

Fig. 12-18 (continued). **G,** X-ray study done at time of graft placement. **H,** X-ray study done 6 months later. **I,** Re-entry at 6 months; buccal view. **J,** Lingual view. Note bone-fill in furcation.

Inductive Osseous Surgery

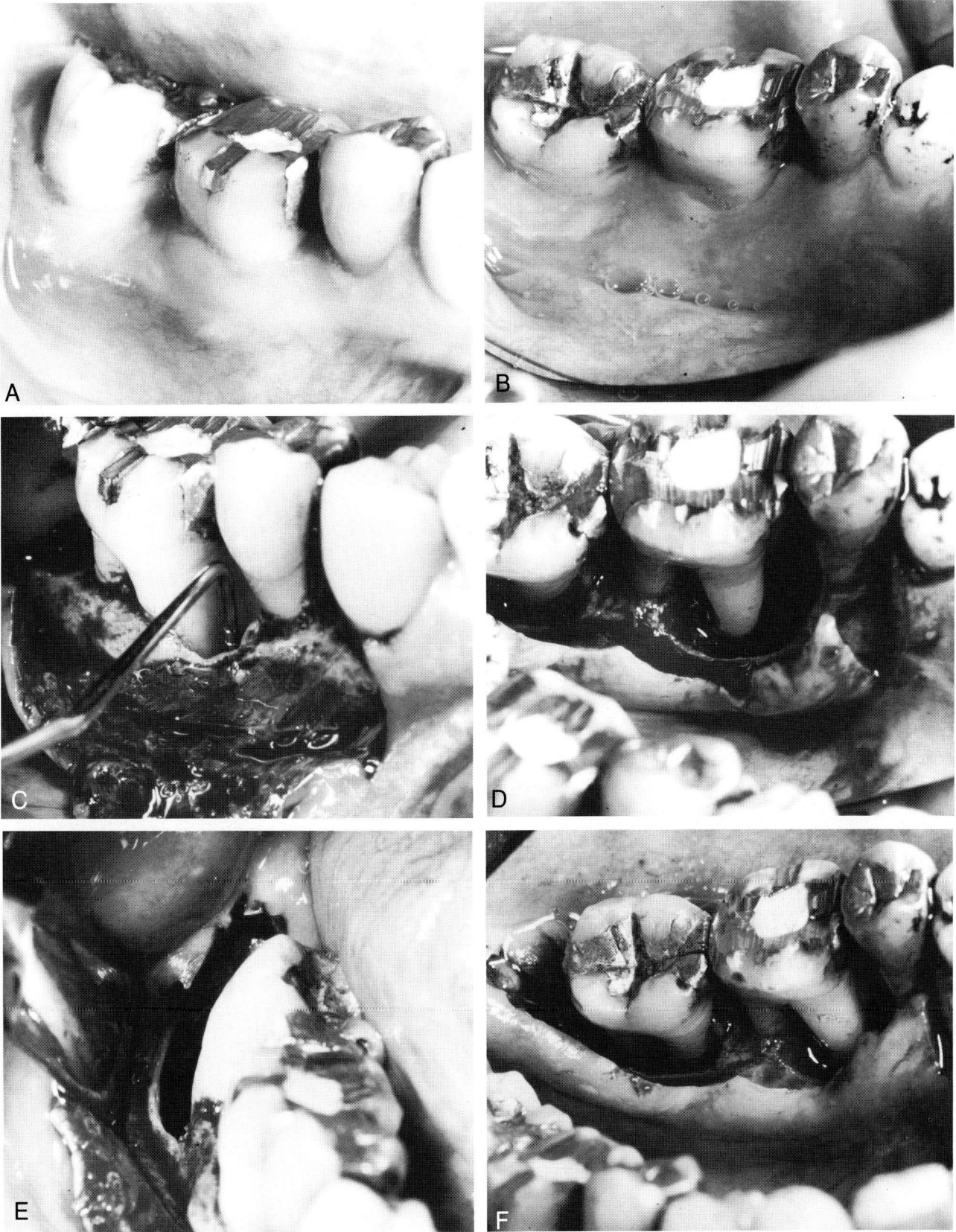

Fig. 12-19. Demineralized Freeze-Dried Bone Allograft (DFDBA). **A, B,** Before surgery; buccal and lingual views. **C, D,** Buccal and lingual views of deep circumferential intrabony defect about mesial root of first molar with lingual Grade II furcation. **E, F,** Buccal and lingual views of deep circumferential defect about second molar.

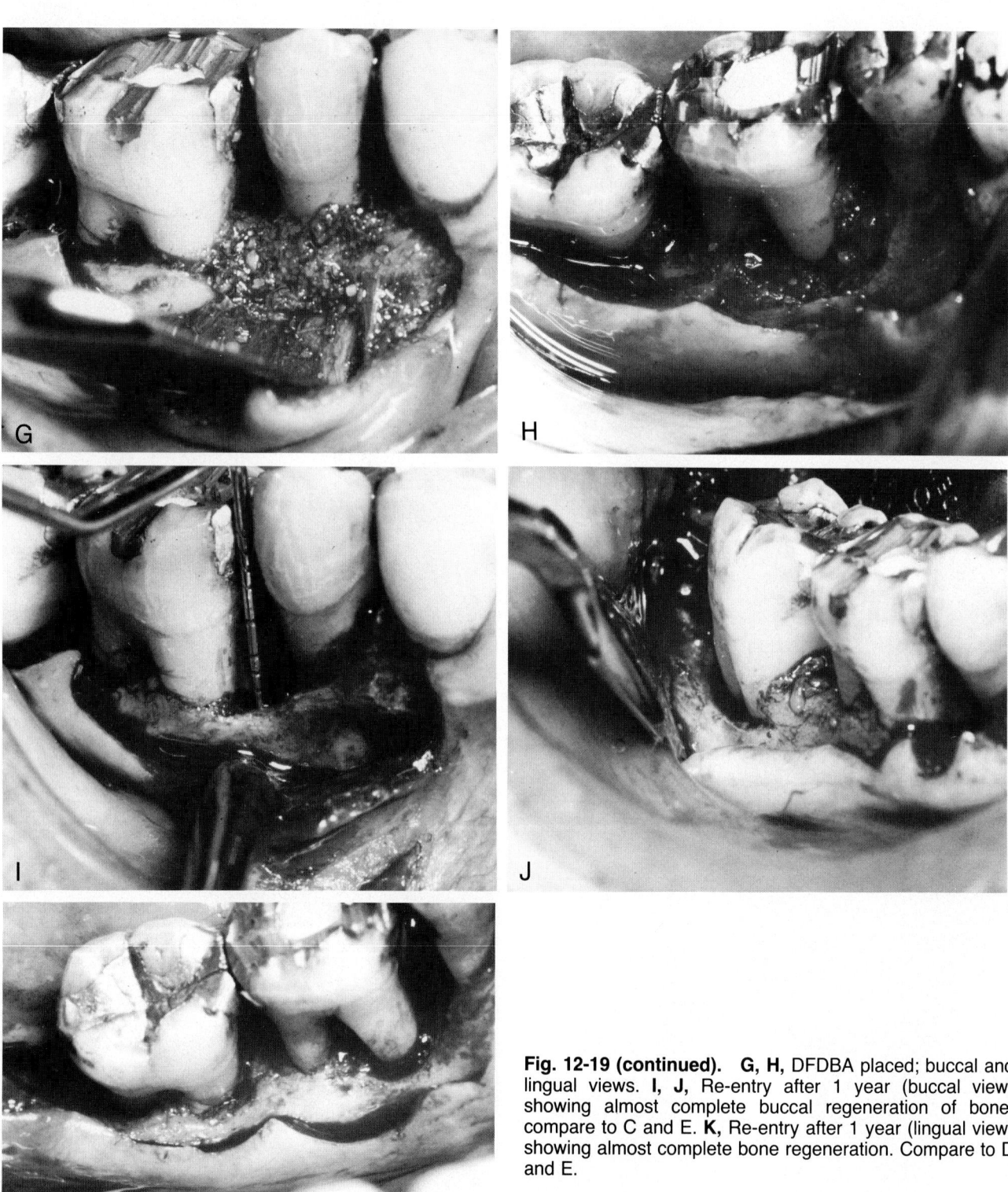

Fig. 12-19 (continued). **G, H,** DFDBA placed; buccal and lingual views. **I, J,** Re-entry after 1 year (buccal view) showing almost complete buccal regeneration of bone; compare to C and E. **K,** Re-entry after 1 year (lingual view) showing almost complete bone regeneration. Compare to D and E.

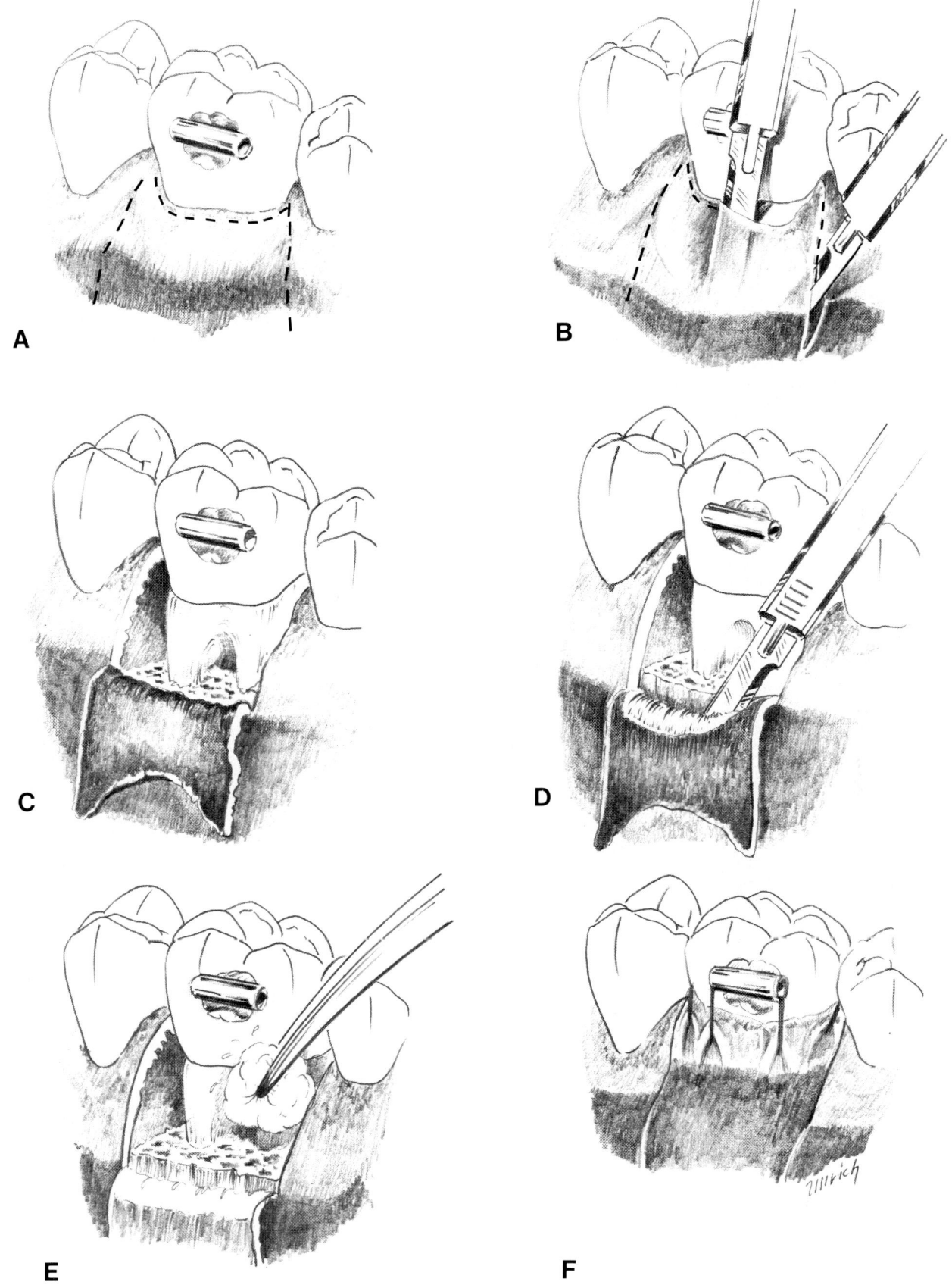

Fig. 12-20. Citric Acid and Coronally Positioned Flaps. **A,** Before treatment with incisions outlined. **B,** Vertical and sulcular incision being made. **C,** Flap reflected with furcation exposed. **D,** Apical periosteal fenestration for flap release for coronal positioning. **E,** Citric acid application (pH 1.0 for 3 min). **F,** Flap coronally positioned and sutured.

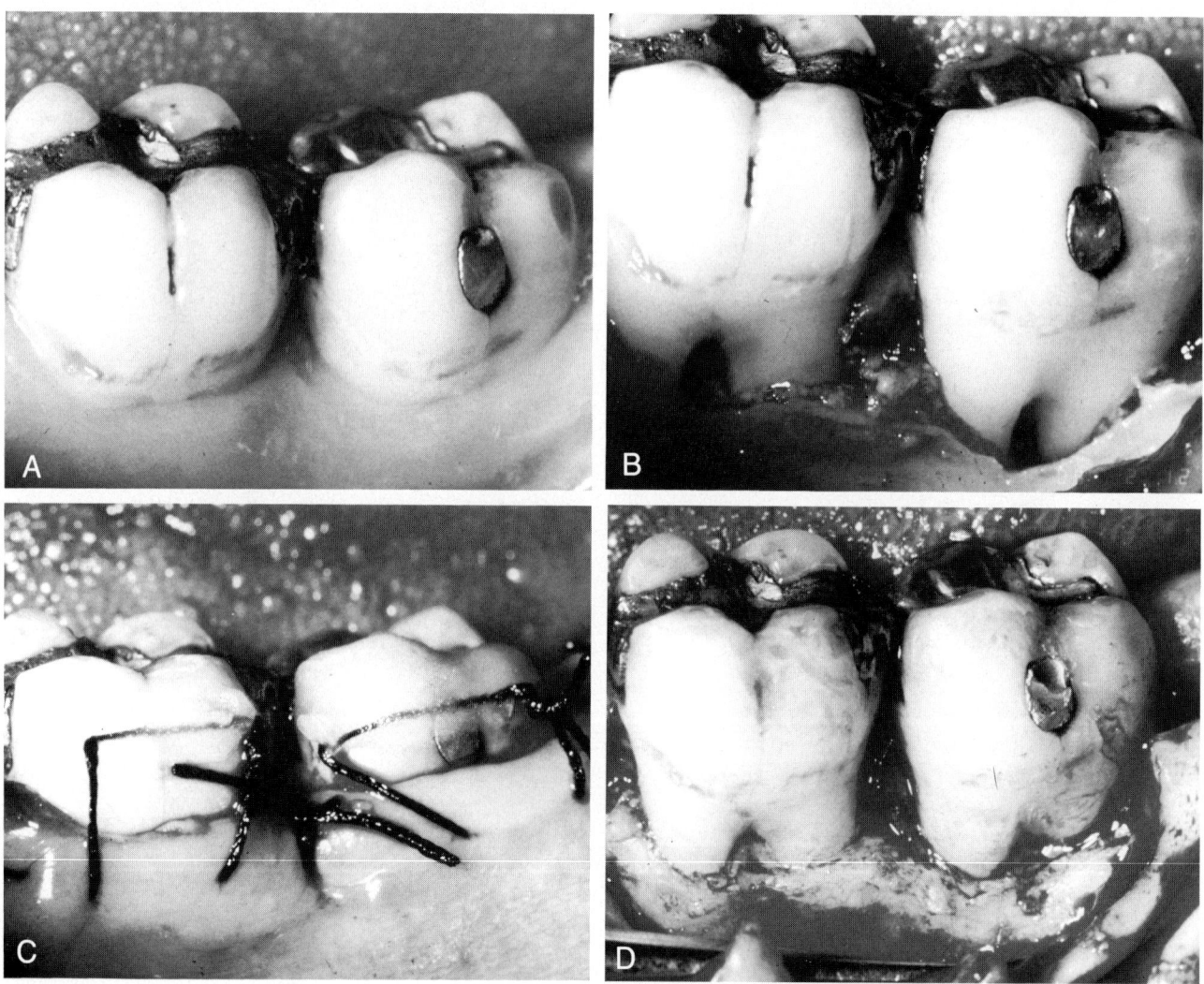

Fig. 12-21. Citric Acid and Coronally Positioned Flaps. **A,** Before surgery. **B,** Grade II furcations exposed. **C,** Flaps sutured coronally. **D,** Re-entry 1 year later. Complete bone regeneration; compare to figure B. (Contributed by Dr. Bernard Gantes.)

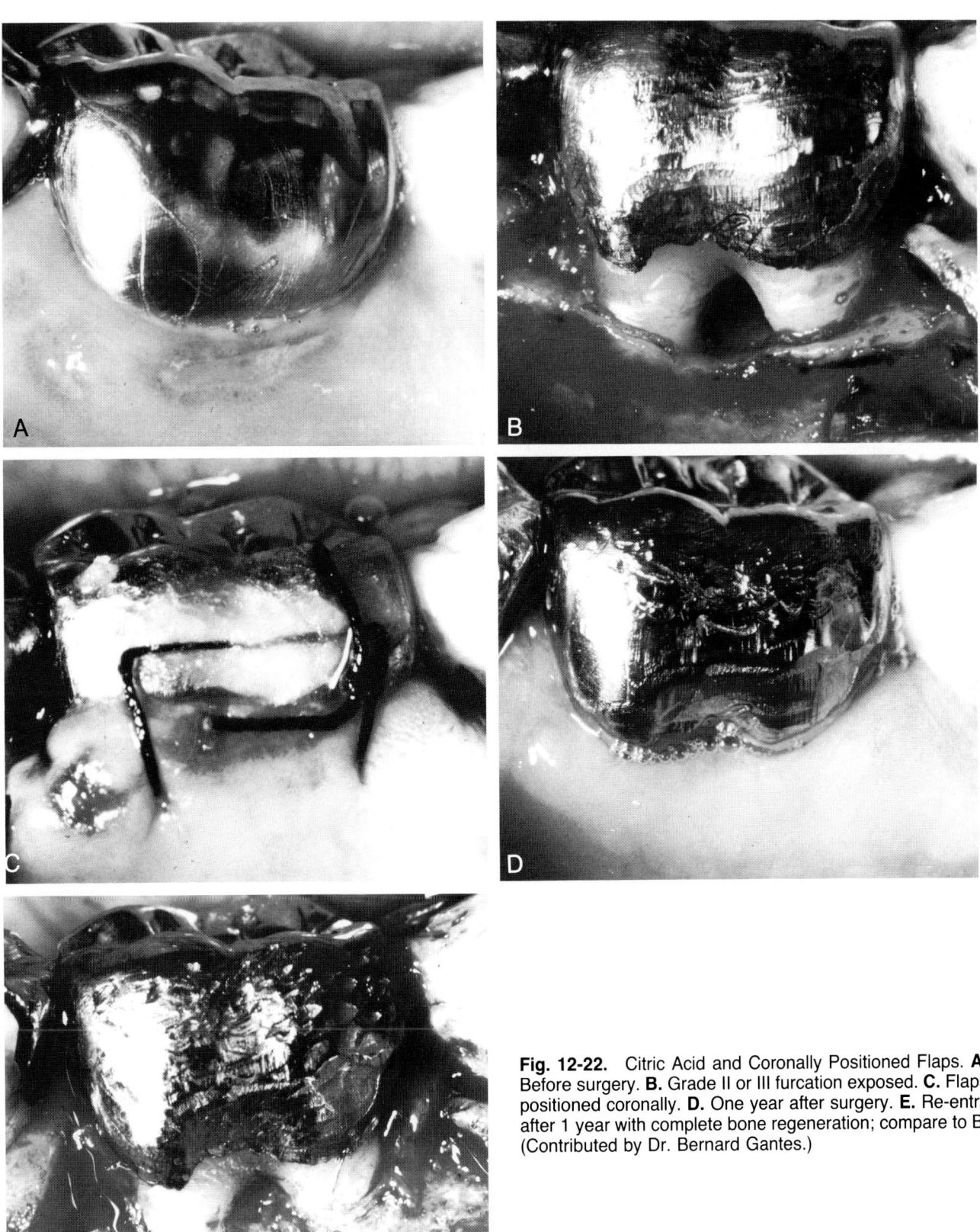

Fig. 12-22. Citric Acid and Coronally Positioned Flaps. **A,** Before surgery. **B.** Grade II or III furcation exposed. **C.** Flaps positioned coronally. **D.** One year after surgery. **E.** Re-entry after 1 year with complete bone regeneration; compare to B. (Contributed by Dr. Bernard Gantes.)

13

GUIDED TISSUE REGENERATION

INTRODUCTION

If the ultimate goal of periodontal therapy is regeneration of the lost supporting tissues (bone, cementum, and periodontal ligament) the apical proliferation and migration of the epithelium must be prevented (Stahl, 1977, 1986). For it is the rapid apical proliferation that results in healing by a long junctional epithelia (LJE), which precludes regeneration and results in repair (Melcher, 1976; Aukhil et al., 1988). The concept of guided tissue regeneration (GTR) is one which attempts to exclude or prevent this apical proliferation of epithelium in favor of other cells that will increase the likelihood of regeneration—bone and periodontal ligament (PDL) (McHugh, 1988).

The true nature of the attachment achieved can be determined only histologically. Even with regeneration of bone one cannot be sure that healing is not by a LJE. Caton (1980) analyzed the results from four different types of surgical procedures—scaling and root planing; modified Widman flaps with either debridement alone or in conjunction with autogenous or synthetic bone grafts—and found that all healed by LJE. This was also confirmed by others. The only exception to this is when various bone grafting materials are used (Bowers et al., 1982, 1985, 1989B).

Ellegaard et al. (1974) used free gingival grafts to cover osseous defects that had received implants in order to retard the rapid apical migration of the epithelium. They found a significant gain in new attachment with and without bone grafts. Histologically (Ellegaard, 1983), the apical proliferation of the epithelium was shown to be delayed 10 to 12 days, resulting in less pocketing and greater connective tissue attachment.

Melcher (1976) postulated four different connective tissues that compete for the root surface during healing: (1) the *lamina propria* of the gingiva with the gingival epithelium, (2) the *periodontal ligament*, (3) the *cementum,* and (4) the *alveolar bone.* Which cell phenotype succeeded in repopulating the root surface determined the nature and quality of the attachment and regeneration (Fig. 13-2).

The biologic basis for GTR was borne out of this type-specific cell repopulation theory. Melcher (1962, 1976) and Aukhil, et al. (1988) have shown that each cell type results in a specific type of repair or regeneration *gingival epithelium: long junctional epithelium; bone ankylosis; gingival connective tissue-root resorption; periodontal-ligament regeneration (bone, cementum, and periodontal ligament)* (Fig. 13-2). Aukhil, et al. (1988) have demonstrated that although the PDL and bone compartments are individual, they do blend together to help in regeneration and new attachment.

ANIMAL STUDIES

A number of studies were undertaken to determine the nature and quality of the attachment when the root surface was repopulated by different selected cell types. Karring et al. (1980) found that roots submerged in the bone resulted in ankylosis. Nyman et al. (1980) submerged roots between the gingival connective tissue and the bone. They found resorption adjacent to the gingival connective tissue and ankylosis next to the bone. Neither tissue appeared capable of producing a true connective tissue attachment. Nyman et al. (1982) used a millipore filter over a window created in the bone and found that only when cells from the PDL were allowed to repopulate the wound was total regeneration achieved. Gottlow et al. (1984) used both a millipore filter and a Gore-Tex membrane (W.L. Gore and Associates, Inc.) over submerged roots in monkeys to demonstrate

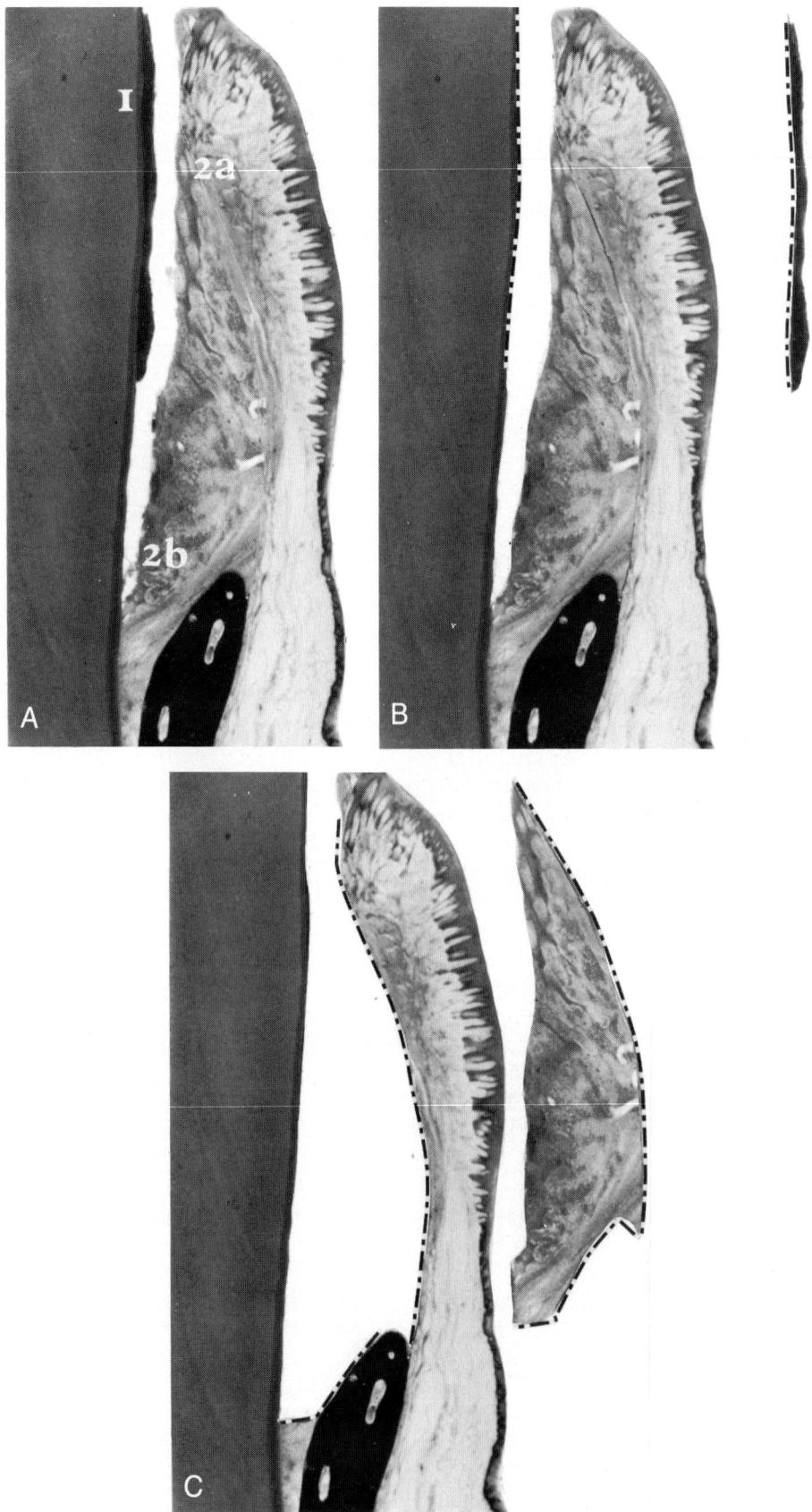

Fig. 13-1. Guided Tissue Regeneration. **A,** Periodontal disease: calculus, pocket formation, inflammation, bone loss. **B,** Calculus removal and root planing. **C,** Removal of inflamed undersurface of flap.

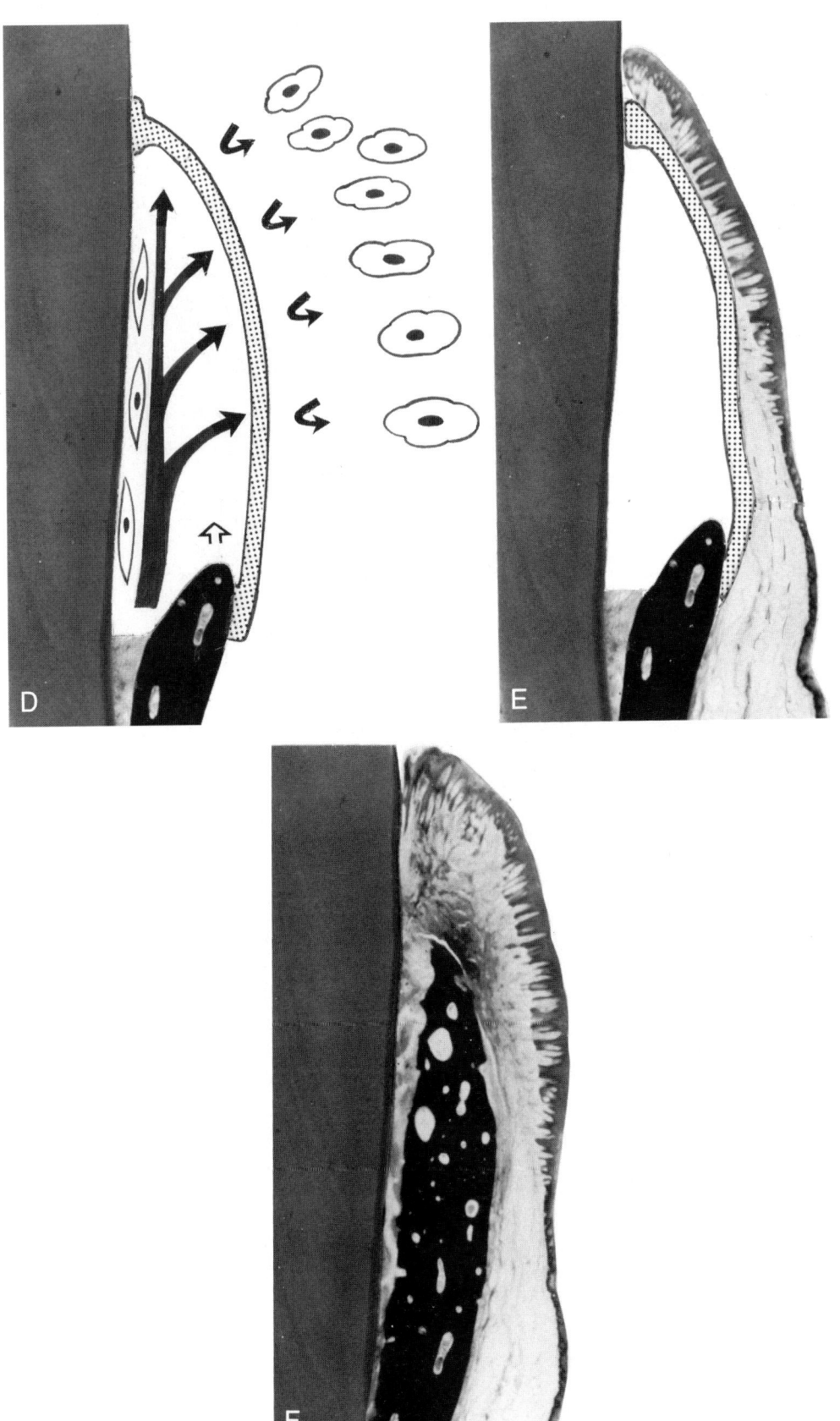

Fig. 13-1 (continued). **D,** Membrane positioned to prevent epithelial cell migration and promote cellular growth from PDL and bone. **E,** Flap positioned over membrane. **F,** Regeneration.

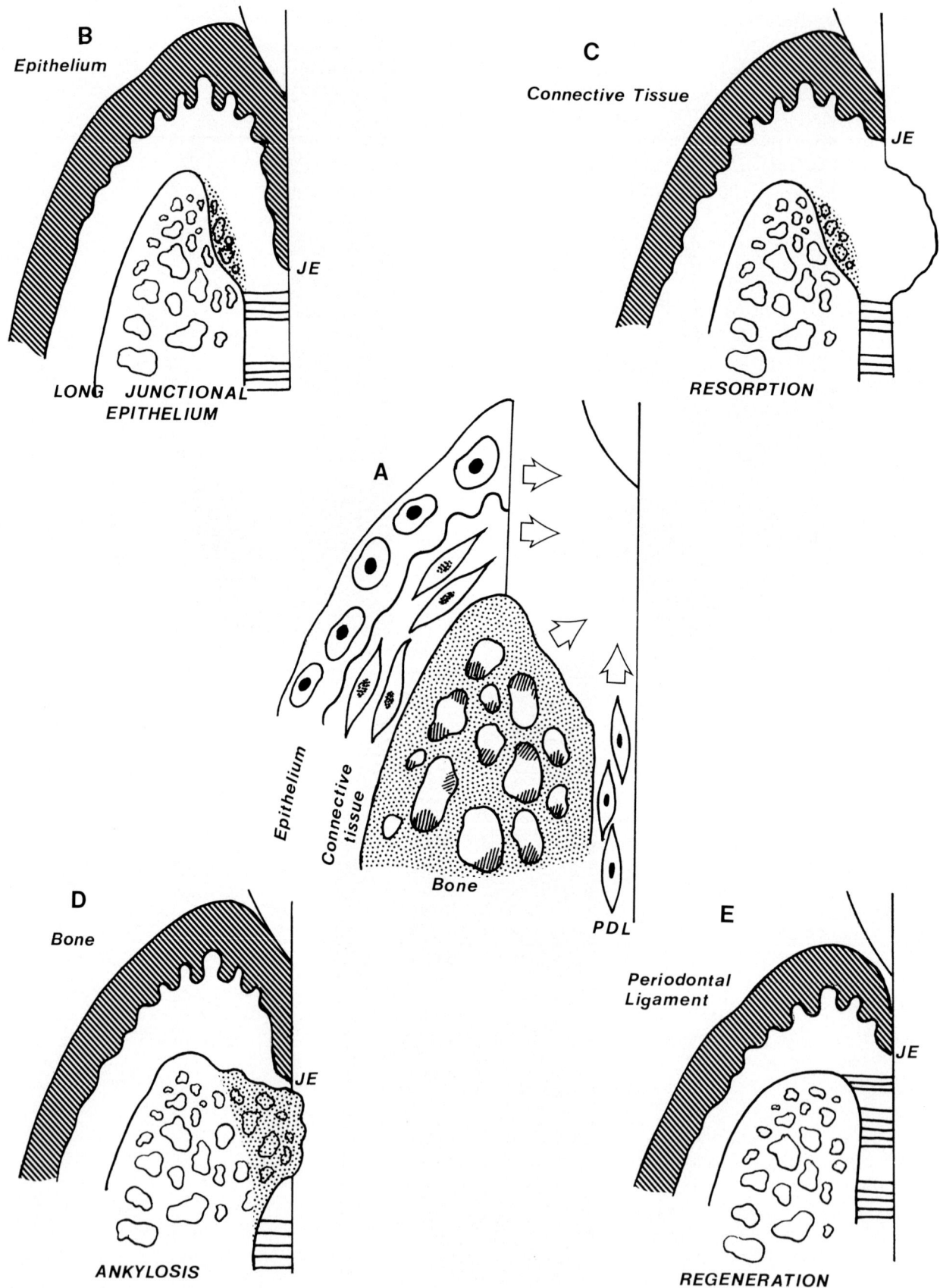

Fig. 13-2. Type-Specific Cell Repopulation Theory of Healing. **A,** Different competing cell types for wound repopulation. **B,** Epithelium and long junctional epithelium. **C,** Connective tissue and resorption. **D,** Bone and ankylosis. **E,** Periodontal ligament and regeneration.

repopulation of the wound by cells of the PDL resulting in a considerably greater increase in new attachment of test teeth. The need for selective repopulation from the PDL was confirmed by Karring et al. (1986). Utilizing a combination of tight and loose elastics about the roots to prevent or permit cell repopulation from the PDL. They found that *regeneration happened only when cells from the PDL were allowed to populate the root.*

HUMAN STUDIES

The successful use of barriers in the animal model led to their use in human clinical trials. Nyman et al. (1982) tested the hypothesis of GTR on a single mandibular incisor using a millipore filter (Fig. 13-1). He was able histologically to show 5 mm of new attachment above the alveolar crest 3 months later. Gottlow et al. (1986) studied 12 teeth (5 histologically) in 10 patients in whom mucoperiosteal flaps were used with underlying teflon membranes. The results indicated *"that a regenerative surgical therapy based on the principles of guided tissue regeneration predictably results in connective tissue attachments"* in both intrabony defects and furcations, and that variations in results may be due to morphological differences in defects allowing for greater or lesser amount of periodontal ligament cells. Gottlow (1984) postulated that because ankylosis did not occur "the migration rate of the periodontal ligament cells is at least as high as that of bone cells." Caffesse et al. (1991), on the basis of his previous research, postulated that "repopulation of the treated root surfaces by cells originating from the periodontal ligament is needed to prevent root resorption and dentoalveolar ankylosis." He and others (Gottlow et al., 1984; Boyle et al., 1983; Lindhe et al., 1984; Houston et al., 1985) also found CA and TTC did not enhance the effectiveness of the membrane.

Intrabony Defects

A number of studies have shown that in intrabony defects significant new connective tissue attachment gains can occur without similar increases in alveolar bone and that the amount of new attachment versus the amount of bone regeneration varies with the specific site when the GTR technique is used (Gottlow et al., 1984; Bogle et al., 1983; Lindhe et al., 1984; Houston et al., 1985). *This connective tissue and bone variance has been interpreted to mean that bony tissue regrowth and PDL regeneration are unrelated.* Gottlow et al. (1986) notes that bony regeneration may be restricted to angular as opposed to horizontal defects because of a combination of the greater surface area, which provides more osteogenic cells, and the walls of the defect, which provide a potential space for cells to migrate into.

These findings are in opposition to those of Becker et al. (1988) and Handelsman et al. (1991), who found that bone fill in intrabony defects correlated closely to attachment gains. Cortellini et al. (1993A, 1993B) and Tonetti et al. (1993) recently found a mean bone regeneration of 4.3 mm ± 2.5 mm one year following treatment of 40 deep vertical defects. Overall, they achieved 100% fill in 32.5% of the cases, ≥ 50% fill in 57.5% of the cases, and only < 50% only 10% of the time. They concluded that the combination of GTR and a strict plaque control program resulted in clinically significant and highly predictable bone regeneration.

Furcations

Becker et al. (1988) studied Grade II, Grade III, and intrabony defects in 27 patients and found a gain in new attachment of 2.3 and 1.5 mm for Grade II and Grade III furcations, respectively, with a 3.7 mm gain for vertical defects ($p < 0.01$). It is important to note that the authors coined the term *"open probing attachment"* to describe a tissue that was not bone but was firm, resistant to probing forces, and had the consistency of rubber dam. No radiographic changes were evident.

In a series of studies Pontoriero (1987, 1988, 1989, 1992) studied Grade II and Grade III defects in humans using e-PTFE (Gore-Tex periodontal material). Using a calibrated probe with a standardized pressure he found 90% of Grade II and 25 to 35% of Grade III furcations were nonprobeable as opposed to the controls, for which only 20% of Grade II and 0% of Grade III furcations were nonprobeable. Partial fill was achieved in 50 to 60% of the Grade III test sites. Finally, it was noted that in Grade III furcations having an entrance height of over 3 mm he was unable to obtain complete defect closure. Complete closure occurred only when entrance height was less than 3 mm.

Metzler et al. (1991) found that GTR had limited application as a therapeutic modality for mesial and distal Grade II furcations of maxillary molars. In a re-entry study Lekovic et al. (1989) found no difference in the bone level between test and controls, although there were significant improvements in pocket depth of 4.09 mm at the test sites.

Selvig (1990) postulated that successful membrane results were achieved due to the fact that the membrane potentiates or contributes to clot stability and protection by protecting the clot from the disruptive movements of the overlying flap.

Gottlow and Karring (1992) studied the maintainability of new attachment gains by GTR for 5 years and concluded that *"the results demonstrated that the attachment gain obtained as a result of the GTR treatment could be maintained over periods of up to 5 years."*

Combination Grafts

In an attempt to overcome this bone–connective tissue variance a number of different osteogenic (inductive, conductive, neutral) materials have been employed under the barrier. Schallhorn and McClaine (1988) used an e-PTFE membrane (Gore-Tex periodontal material) with demineralized freeze dried bone allografts (DFDBA) or tricalcium phosphate (TCP) and CA versus e-PTFE membrane alone. They found that *although attachment gains were similar between the two groups, 72% (33 of 46) of the furcations having the combined treatment had complete furcation bone fill as opposed to 31% (5 of 16) for the membrane alone. In the* **vertical furcation defects** *the respective attachment gains were 5.3 mm versus 4.5 mm for the membrane and graft and membrane alone, and gains of 4.2 mm to 3.1 mm were seen for horizontal furcal probing. CA appeared to increase the favorable results in both vertical defects and furcations.*

Kerstein et al. (1992) found that the use of CA did not enhance the positive effects. They concluded that "the barrier membrane procedure apparently gave a healing result beyond which further improvement could not be achieved by root surface conditioning."

McClaine and Shallhorn (1993) found membrane-only site regression after 53 to 70 months such that the membrane and graft group now became statistically significant for clinical probing attachment levels ($p=0.005$) and for horizontal probing depth ($p=0.003$). In Grade II furcations initially showing complete furcation fills with the membrane alone, 2 of 5 (40%) remained completely filled in the long term. There was no such change in the membrane and graft group. Overall, they found a 31% regression for the sites treated by membrane alone. This was opposed to Gottlow and Karring (1992), who found no significant changes after 4 to 5 years.

In a re-entry study Anderegg et al. (1991) compared DFDBA with the e-PTFE (Gore-Tex periodontal material) membrane to the membrane alone. He found that although both techniques showed significant improvement in bone and probing attachment levels, the combination of graft plus membrane resulted in a significant ($p=0.05$) increase of both vertical and horizontal bone fill as compared to the membrane alone. This was in spite of the fact that the probing attachment gains were not statistically different between the two groups. Lekovic (1990) used porous hydroxyapatite in combination with an e-PTFE membrane and found that those cases treated by the combination technique showed a "gain in clinical attachment and horizontal and vertical bone fill while the lesions with the membrane only gained probing attachment with less bone fill."

Stahl and Froum (1991) histologically showed new attachment and bone regeneration when membranes were combined with either DFDBA or hydroxyapatite implants in humans.

Conclusions

The Proceedings of the World Workshop in Clinical Periodontics (1989) defines **guided tissue regeneration** *as a procedure that attempts regeneration through differential tissue responses. It concluded that GTR was not an experimental procedure and that it showed predictability for connective tissue attachment in intrabony defects and in Grade II furcation involvement. Bone regeneration was less predictable. Finally, they differentiated* **new connective tissue attachment** *from* **regeneration** *in that the former does not show evidence of coronal growth of bone, while the latter does.*

NONRESORBABLE MEMBRANES

Gore-Tex Barrier

At present the only nonresorbable material available for GTR is expanded polytetrafluoroethylene (e-PTFE), made by W.L. Gore and Associates. It is a biocompatible porous material possessing two unique microstructures. One is the *open microstructure* of its collar, which is designed to retard or inhibit the apical proliferation of epithelium through contact inhibition. The other is the *occlusive membrane,* which acts as a barrier to the gingival connective tissues and the underlying root surface while still allowing them to integrate with it, and this further retards epithelial downgrowth. It comes in various sizes (Fig. 13-3).

Procedural Guidelines

Patient Selection

In the medically compromised patient (heart murmur, mitral valve prolapse, rheumatic heart disease, uncontrolled diabetes, heart or other prosthetic devices, etc.) the addition of a prosthetic device such as Gore-Tex periodontal material may increase the risk for complications.

Indications

1. Patients with *good oral hygiene.*
2. Adequate keratinized gingiva; the material should be covered with a thick, heavy keratinized gingiva.

Defect Selection

Defect selection may have the greatest impact on the predictability of the regenerative result.

A. Most predictable
1. For Grade II furcations on teeth with high interproximal bone, a large vertical component, spacemaking morphology, long root trunks, and good evidence of loss in a furcation. Furcations opening at the CEJ make coverage and closure difficult.
2. 2-3 wall intrabony vertical defects ≥ 4-5 mm measurable defects.

B. Moderate predictability
1. Two wall defects.
2. Maxillary medial or distal Class II furcations.

C. Low predictability
1. One wall defect
2. Class III furcation with high interproximal bone, long root trunks, large vertical component, space-making morphology.

D. Least predictability
1. Horizontal bone loss.
2. Class III furcations with horizontal bone loss.

Contraindications

1. In cases where flap vascularity will be compromised
2. Very severe defects—minimal remaining periodontium
3. Horizontal defects
4. In case of flap perforation

Surgical Procedure

Primary Incisions

1. Intrasulcular incisions are made in preparation for a full mucoperiosteal flap. Maximum conservation and preservation of the interdental papilla ensures total material coverage and primary-intention healing (Fig. 13-4A).
2. All residual pocket epithelium is removed after flap reflection to permit integration between the e-PTFE and the flap connective tissue (Fig. 13-4B).
3. Incisions should extend 1 to 2 teeth mesial and/or distal of the area being treated to permit adequate visualization.
4. Vertical incisions should be placed mesially where necessary.

Defect preparation

1. Degranulation of defect. *Without thorough defect debridement, predictable regenerative results cannot be expected.*
2. Scaling and root planing for removal of all tooth deposits (Fig. 13-4C, D).
3. Use of additional high-speed rotary instrumentation for defect and/or root refinements.
4. Decortification of bone for increased vascularity and scratching of the PDL to stimulate cell and vascular proliferation. Without a clot in the defect space, regeneration cannot occur.
5. Optional use of biochemical root surface modifiers: citric acid or tetracycline.
6. Optional use of a bone augmentation material: DFDBA.

Selection of Gore-Tex Periodontal material

1. Maintain sterility of material
2. Choose a size that offers the most ideal design for defect coverage (Fig. 13-4E, F).
3. Shape material with scissors. Avoid leaving sharp edges.
4. Enough material should be left to permit lateral and interproximal suturing while leaving at least 3 mm apical and lateral overextension of defect margin (Fig. 13-4E, F).
5. Do not remove the open microstructure or coronal portion of the material. It can be trimmed on the lateral aspects.
6. The material should fit smoothly, avoiding folds, overlaps, and protrusions, which may compromise the overlying gingival tissue.
7. *In either periodontal or bony ridge defects, the amount of space beneath the material determines the maximum potential regeneration.* **Without space maintenance, regeneration is not possible.**

Suture Material

1. Gore-Tex Suture (provided with material) is recommended for placing the material and flap closure (Fig. 13-4G, H).
2. Silk or monofilament sutures may be used in areas away from the material.
3. Bioabsorbable sutures are not recommended.

Suturing Technique

1. Sling sutures are used to approximate material over the defect without engaging the flap or tissue (Fig. 13-4G).
2. The material must fit tightly against the tooth surface at all points to prevent epithelial prolif-

eration between tooth and material and to help in stabilizing the wound.
3. The flap margin should ideally be 2 to 3 mm coronal to the material.
4. Tight flap apposition is desired to avoid premature flap opening and material exposure.
5. An apical horizontal periosteal releasing incision may enhance material coverage. Do not compromise blood supply.
6. Interproximal incisions approximating the material are closed first.

Material Removal

1. Removal should be 4 to 8 weeks after placement or any time a serious complication occurs.
2. If the material cannot be removed with a gentle tug, sharp dissection is recommended. A sulcular incision is made to extend one tooth mesially and distally (Fig. 13-4I).
3. Extreme care should be used to avoid damaging the underlying new granulation tissue. Sharp dissection is used to reflect the overlying tissue (Fig. 13-4J).
4. A small tissue forceps is used to remove the material (Fig. 13-4K).
5. Light curettage of the inner flap surface is recommended for removal of any epithelial remnants.
6. The flap is reapproximated over the new tissue and sutured with silk sutures (Fig. 13-4L).

Postoperative Considerations

1. Peridex mouthwash should be for 10 days. If the material becomes exposed, Peridex should be used until removal.
2. Tetracycline 250 q.i.d. or Doxycycline 100 mg b.i.d. should be used for 7 to 10 days. *Note:* Gore does not recommend this at this time.
3. Periodontal dressing may or may not be used depending on the clinician's discretion.
4. Gentle brushing is recommended.
5. Flossing at the treated site is to be avoided while the material is in place.
6. The patient should be seen biweekly if there is no exposure, and weekly if exposure is present.
7. Do not attempt to cover previously exposed material.
8. The material should be removed immediately should any complications develop.

The clinical procedures are depicted in Figures 13-5, 13-6, 13-7, and 13-8.

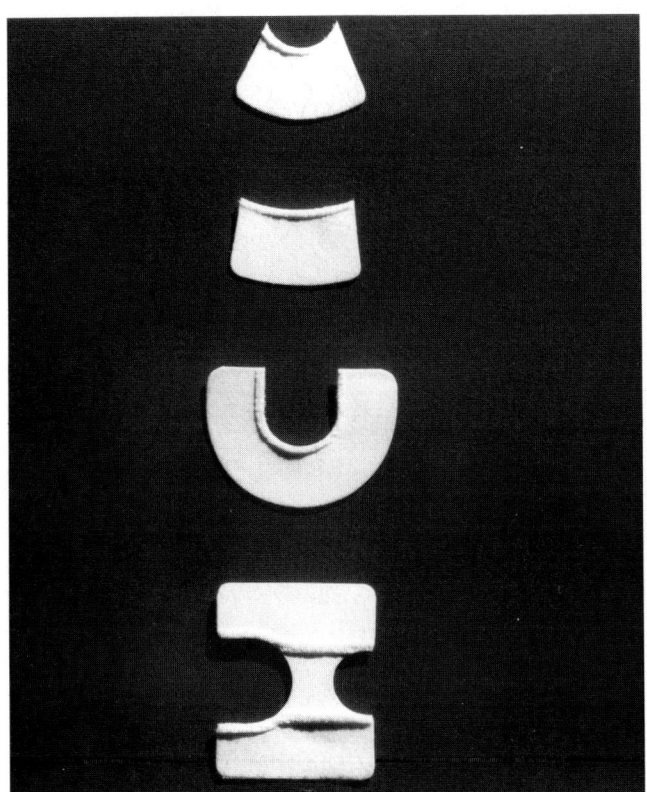

Fig. 13-3. Different sizes of e-PTFE material (Gore-Tex).

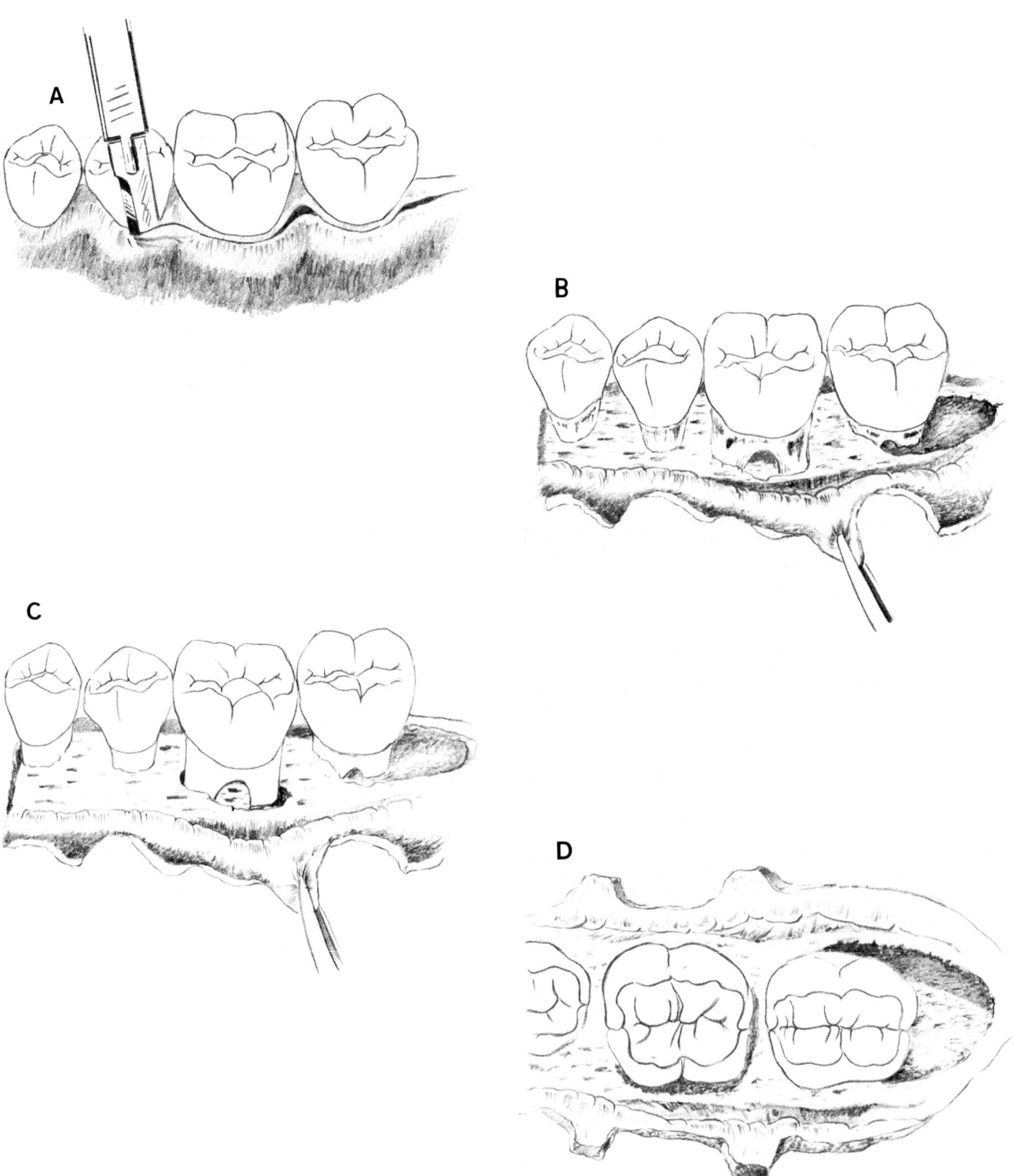

Fig. 13-4. Guided Tissue Regeneration Surgical Technique. **A,** Incisions outlined. Sulcular incisions with maximal preservation of interproximal tissue. **B,** Flaps reflected. **C, D,** Meticulous scaling, root planing, and tissue debridement so that defects are completely devoid of tissue.

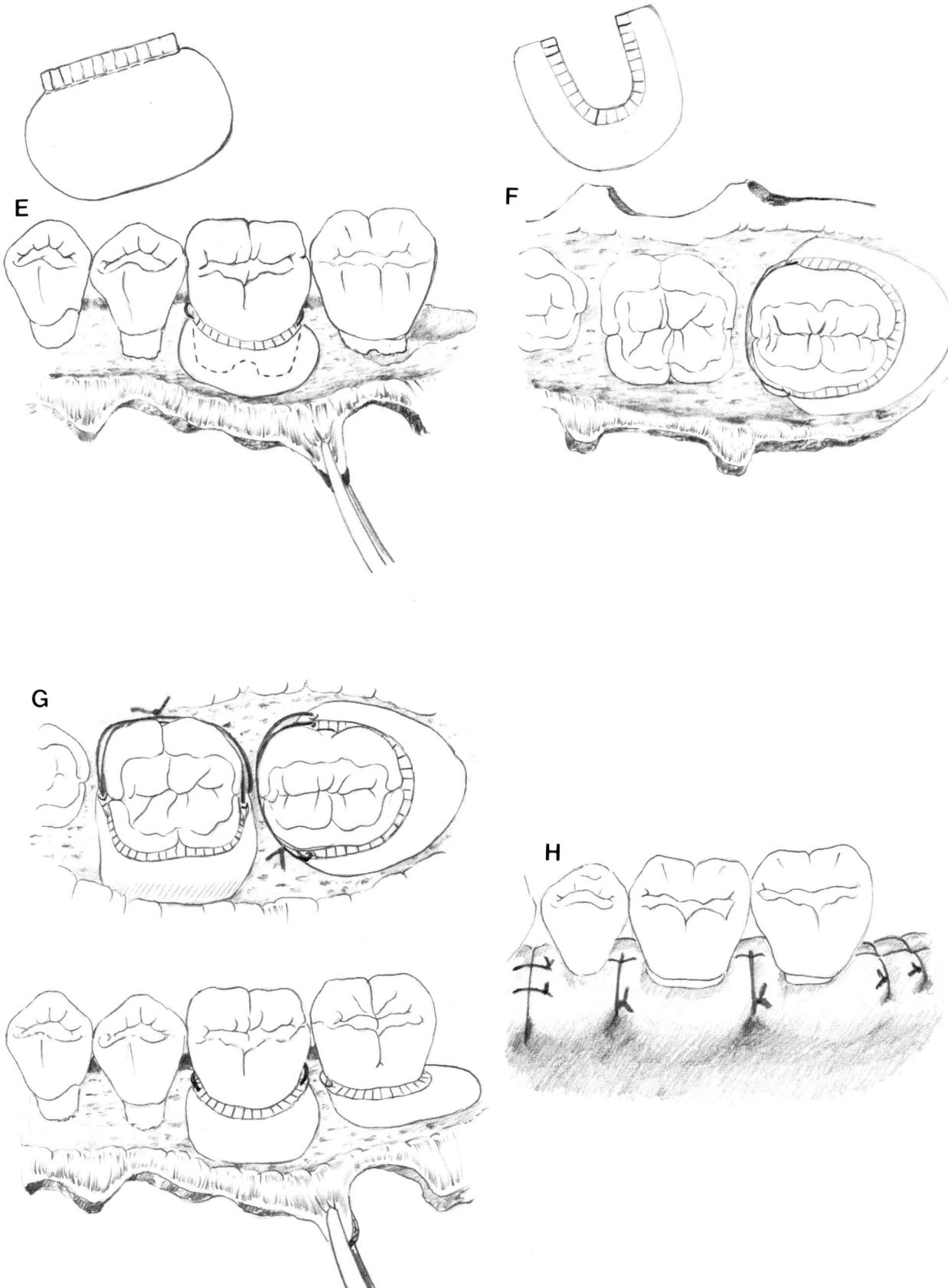

Fig. 13-4 (continued). E, Membrane placed over furcation area. **F,** U-shaped membrane placed over distal defect. **G,** Membranes sutured with Gor-Tex sutures: occlusal and buccal views. **H,** Suturing completed with interrupted sutures.

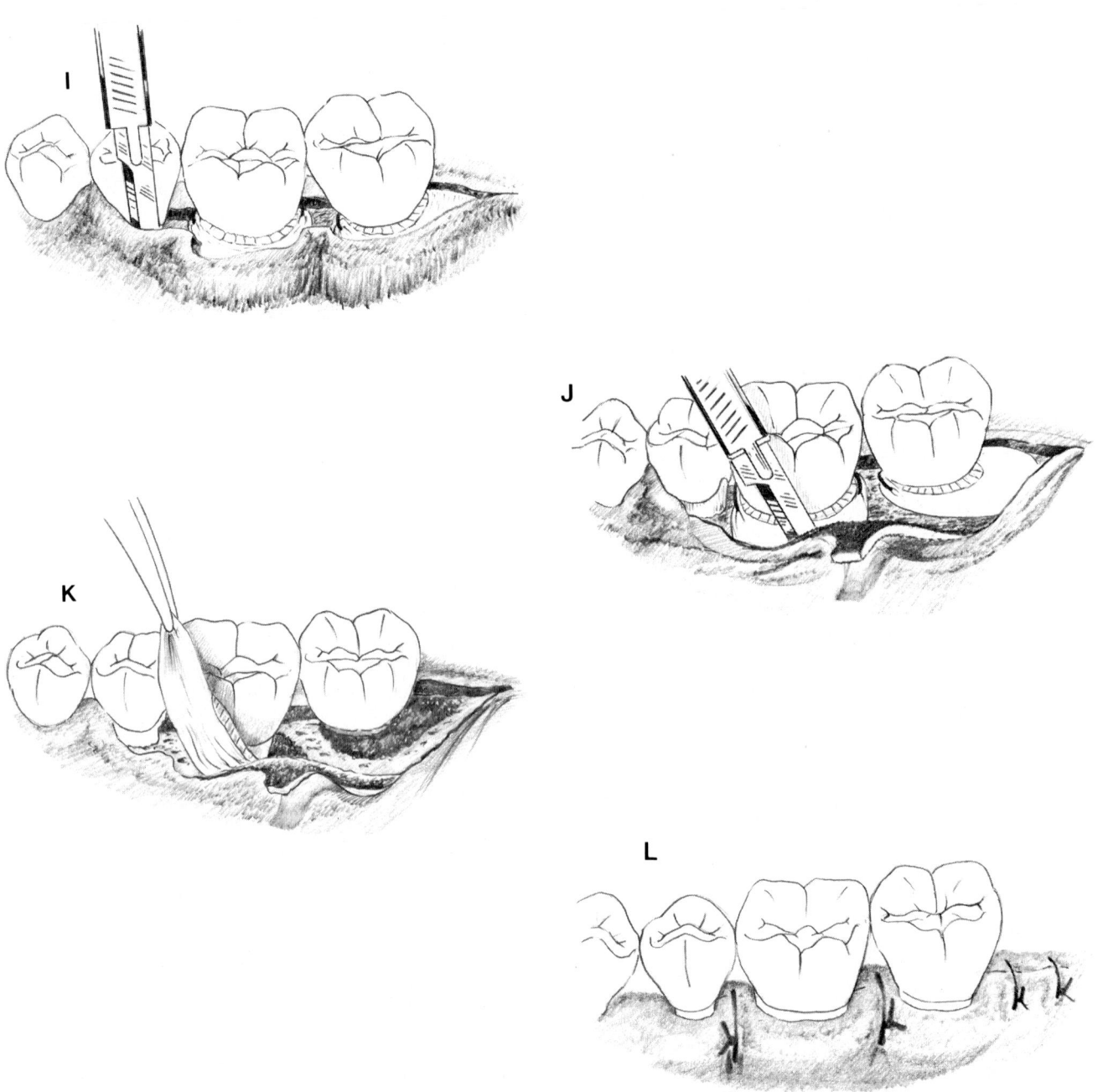

Fig. 13-4 (continued). **I, J,** Membrane removal. Flaps are reflected by sharp dissection for removal of ingrown tissue and epithelium from under the flap. **K,** Membranes are removed. **L,** Final suturing with interrupted sutures.

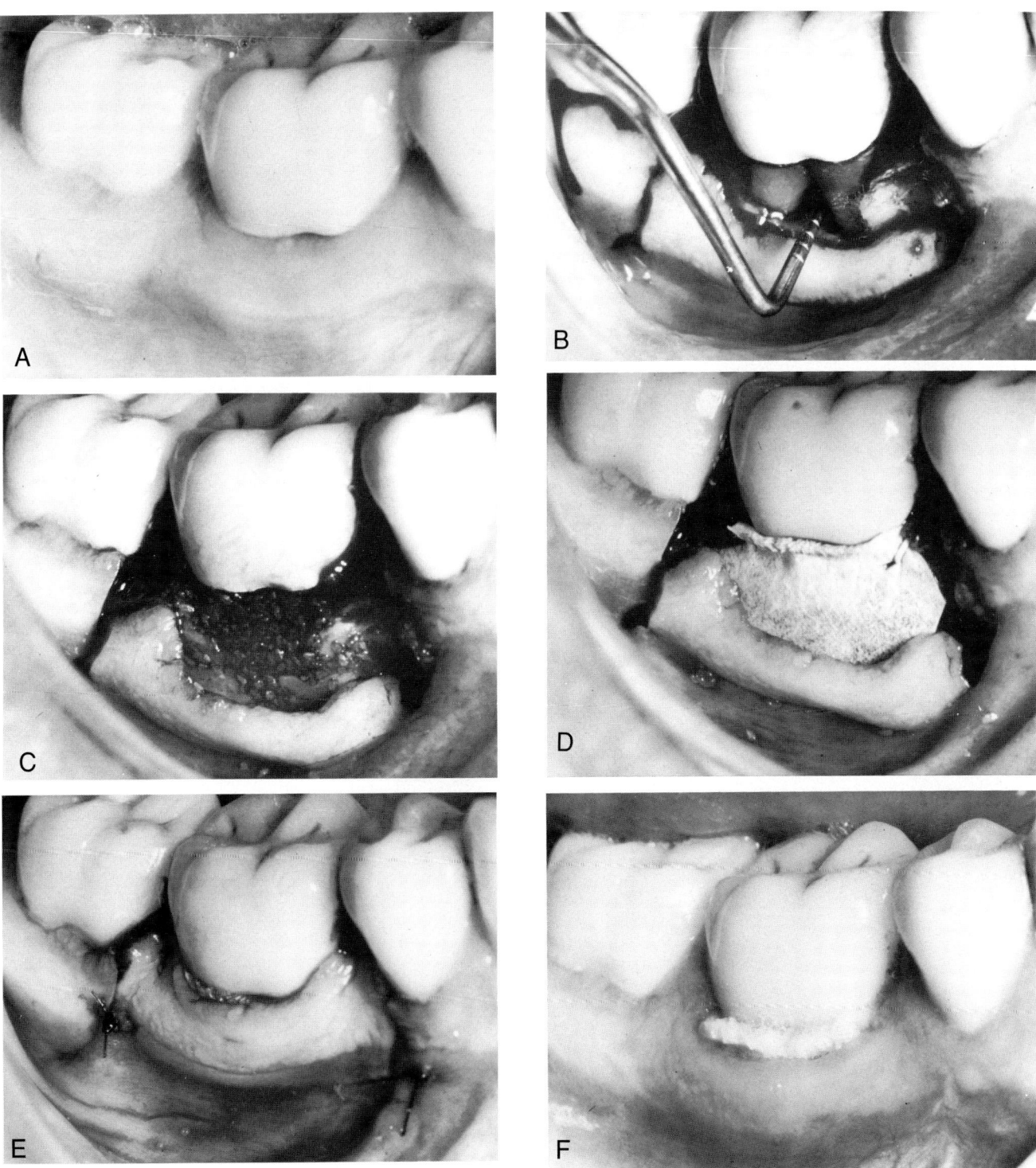

Fig. 13-5. Guided Tissue Regeneration (Grade II Furcation). **A,** Before treatment. **B,** Furcation exposed with 7 mm horizontal probability. **C,** DFDBA placed. **D,** e-PTFE membrane placed. **E,** Flap sutured. **F,** Seven weeks later.

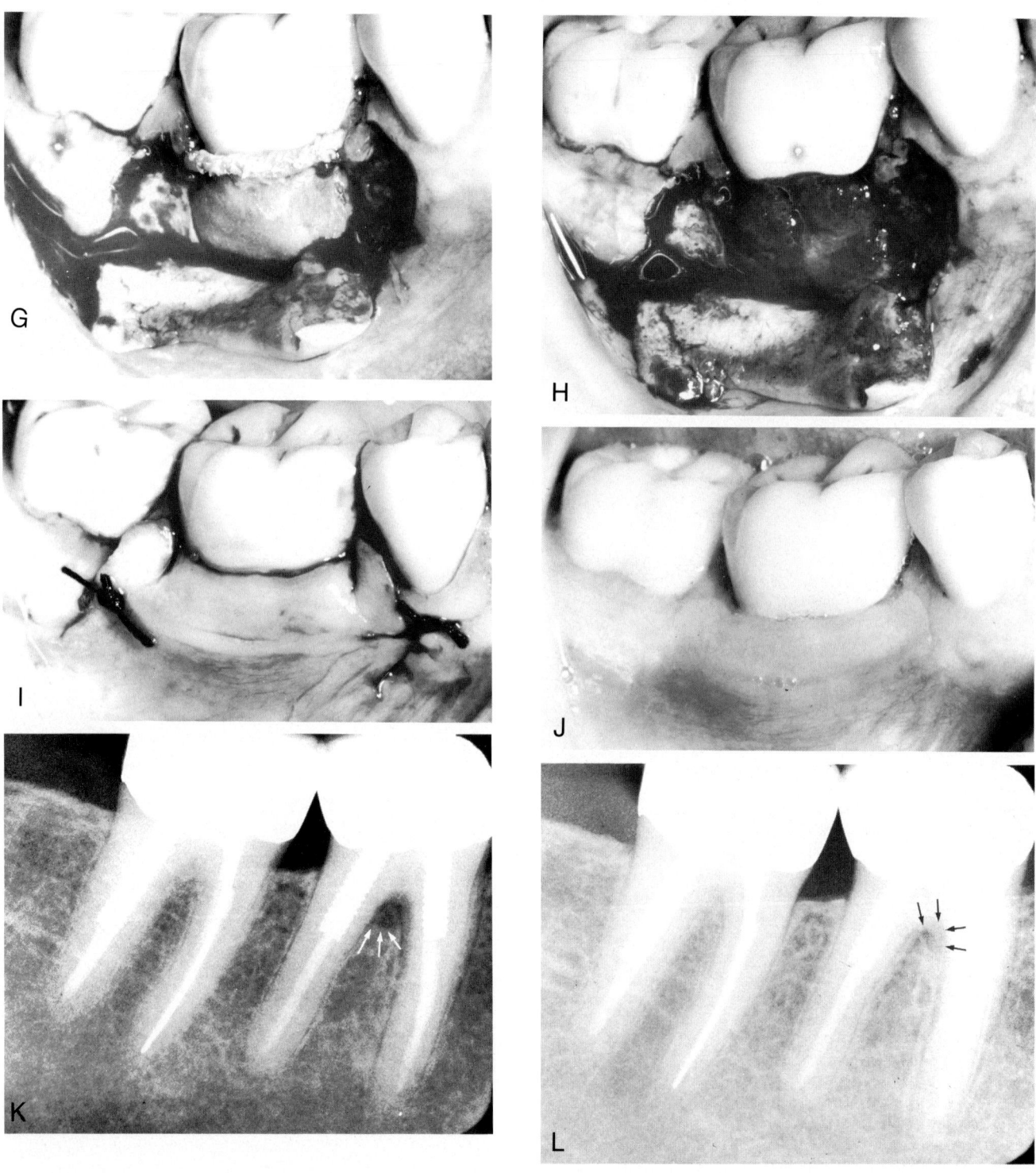

Fig. 13-5 (continued). G, Membrane exposed at time of removal (7 weeks). **H,** Healing granulation tissue. **I,** Flaps repositioned. **J,** Final healing after 3 months. **K,** Preoperative x-ray study shows obvious furcation involvement. **L,** Healed furcation 1 year later.

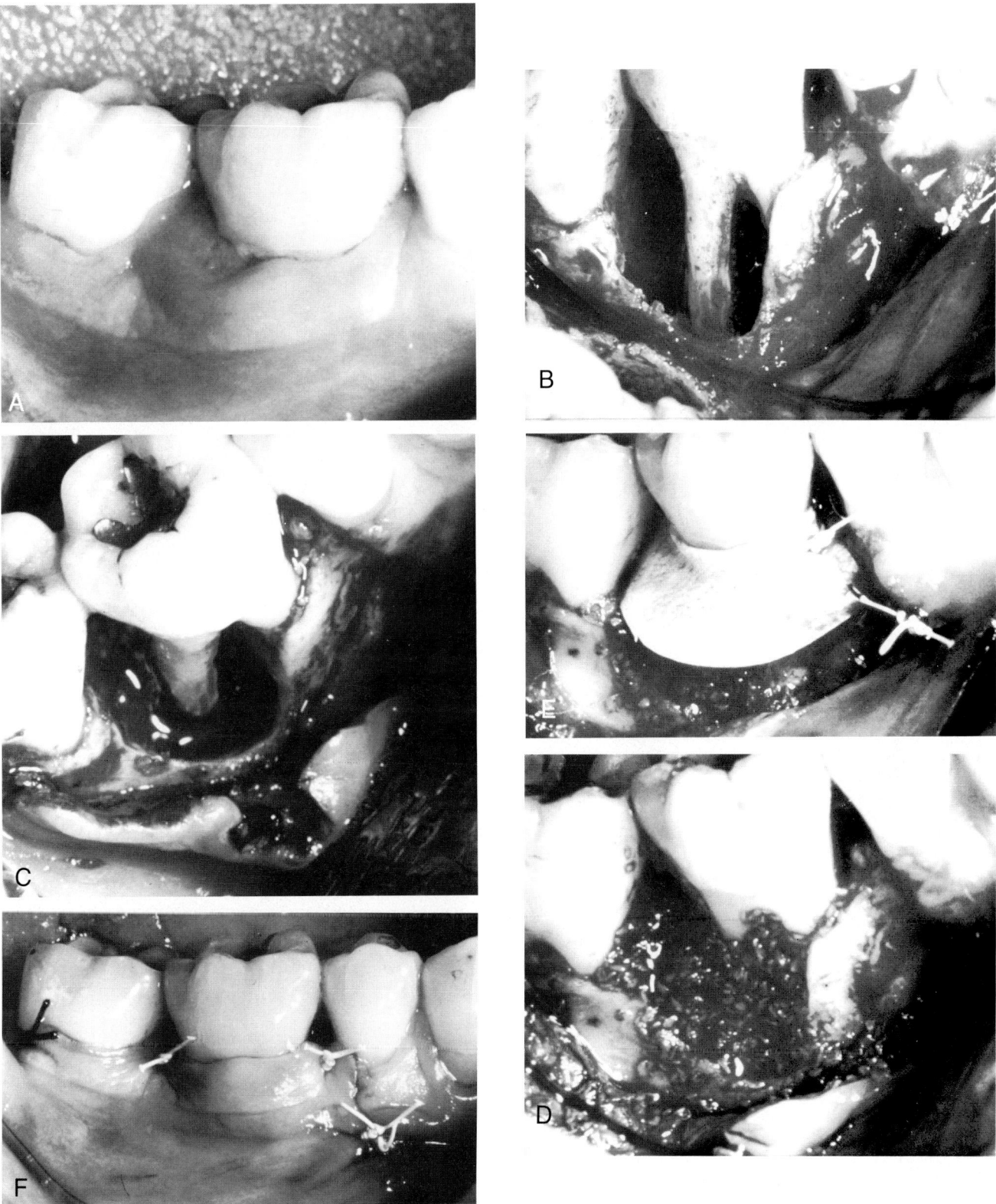

Fig. 13-6. Guided Tissue Regeneration (Grade III Furcation). **A,** Before treatment. **B,** Grade III furcation and distal defect exposed. **C,** Occlusal view of circumferential defect about distal root. **D,** DFDBA placed. **E,** U-shaped e-PTFE membrane placed. **F,** Flap repositioned with Gore-Tex sutures.

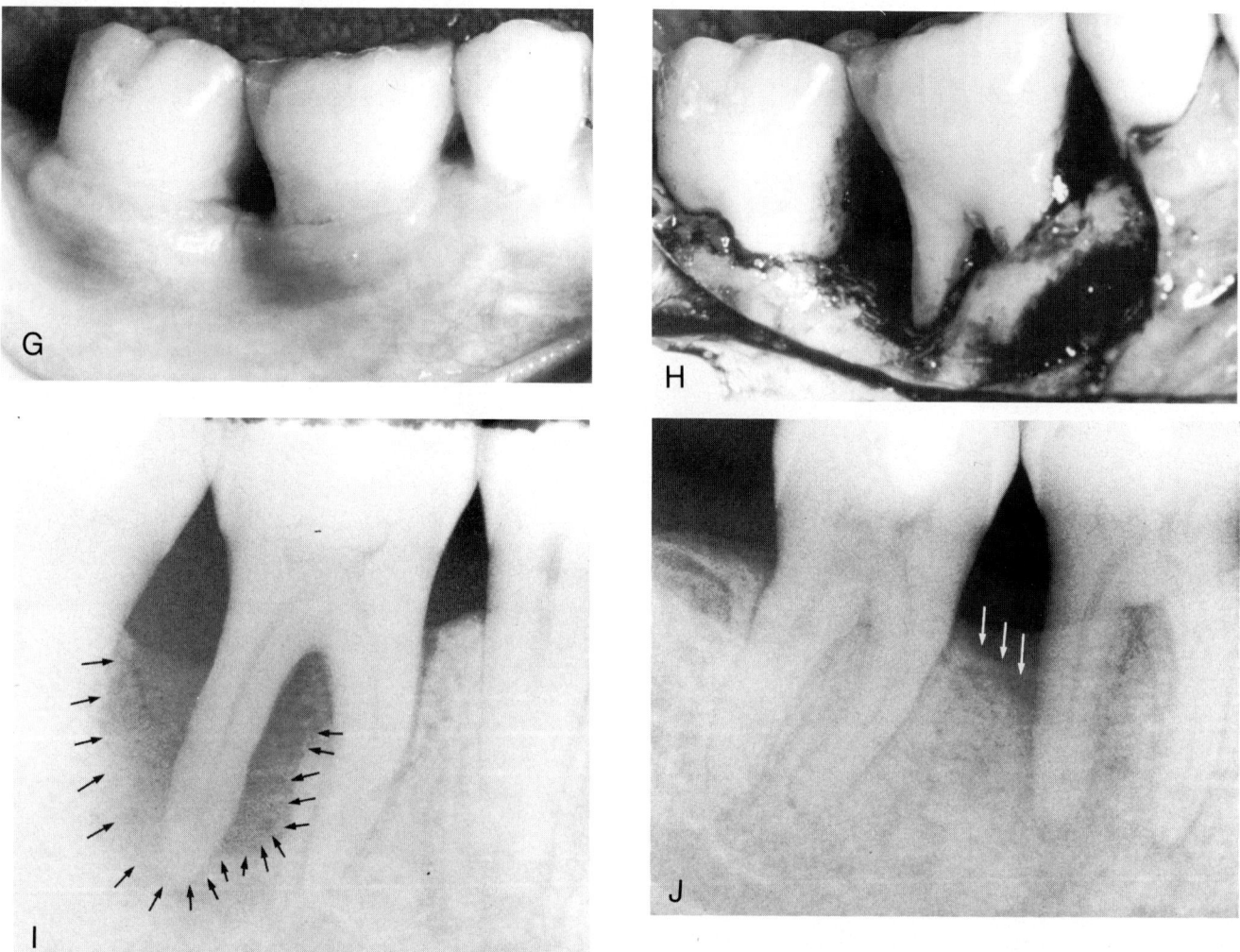

Fig. 13-6 (continued). **G,** One year later. **H,** Re-entry after 1 year. Note complete fill of furcation and significant coverage of distal root with bone. **I,** Before treatment x-ray study. **J,** X-ray study showing bone regeneration of furcation. Small residual distal defect remains.

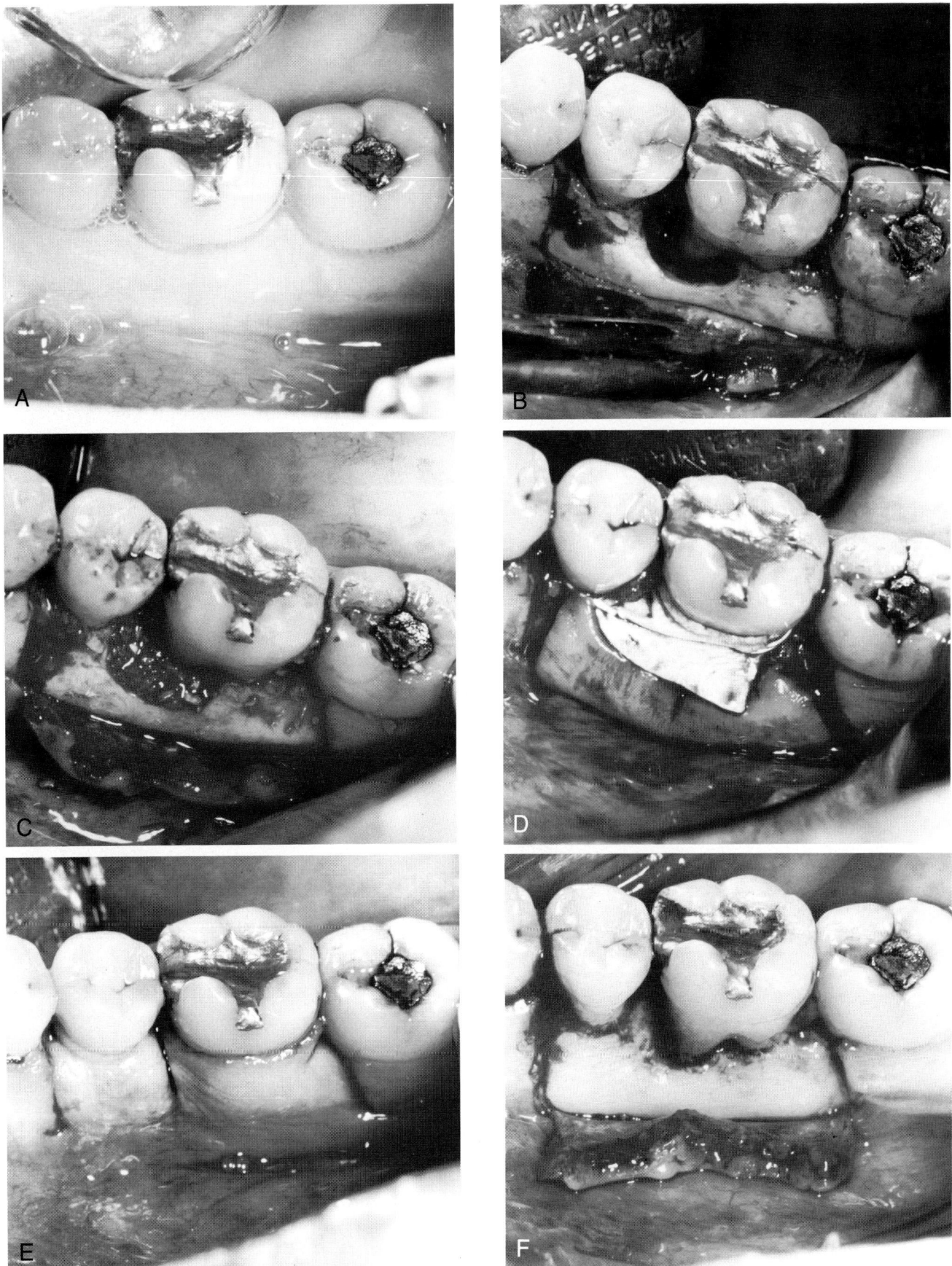

Fig. 13-7. Guided Tissue Regeneration of Intrabony Defect and Incipient Furcation. **A,** Before treatment. **B,** Two-surface three-wall defect exposed with incipient furcation. **C,** DFDBA placed. **D,** e-PTFE membrane placed. **E,** Flap repositioned. **F,** Re-entry after 1 year. Note complete fill of defect and incipient furcation.

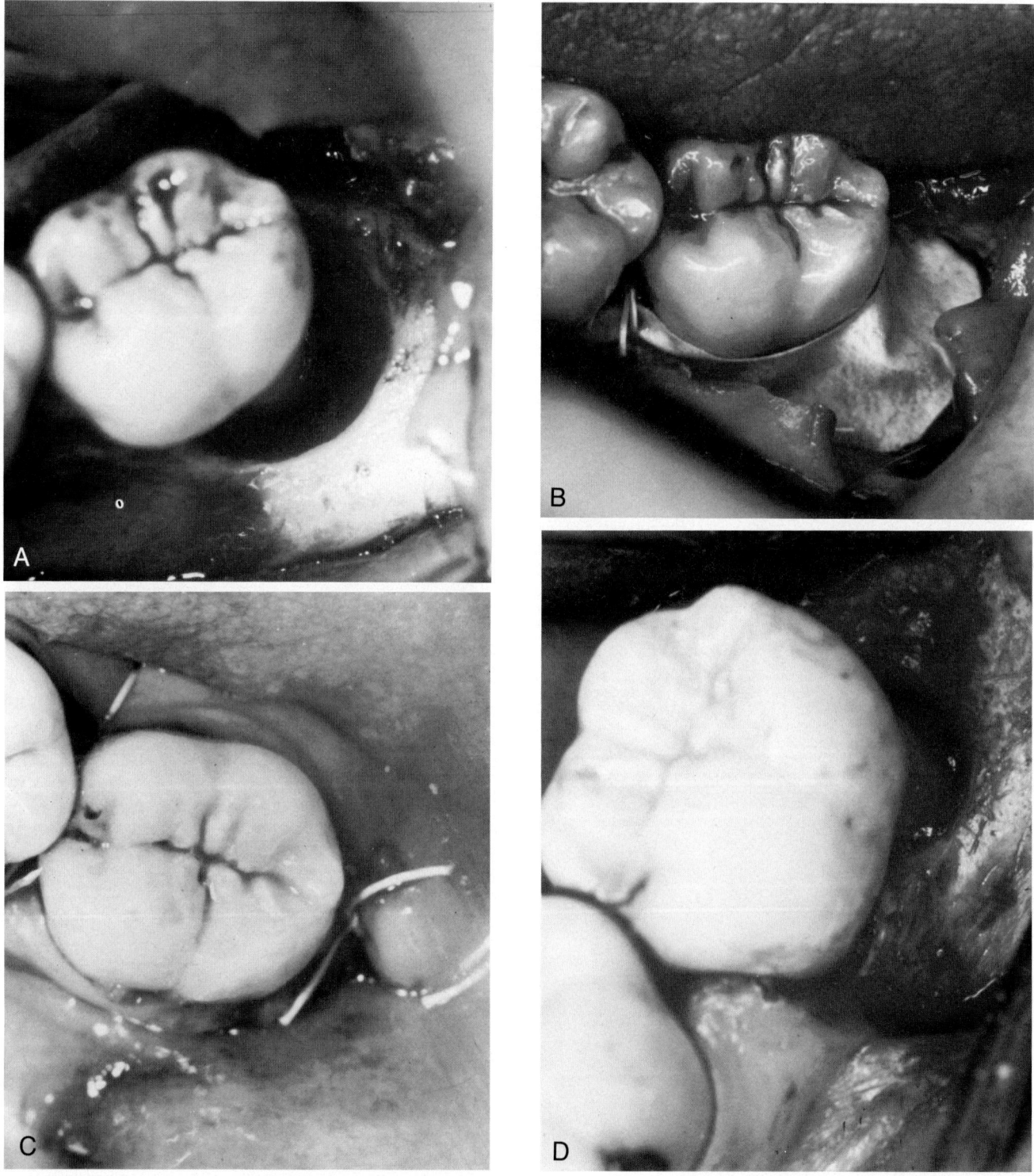

Fig. 13-8. Guided Tissue Regeneration of Intrabony Defect. **A,** Defect exposed. **B,** e-PTFE membrane positioned. **C,** Flaps repositioned. **D,** Re-entry after 11 months. Note bone fill without use of graft material.

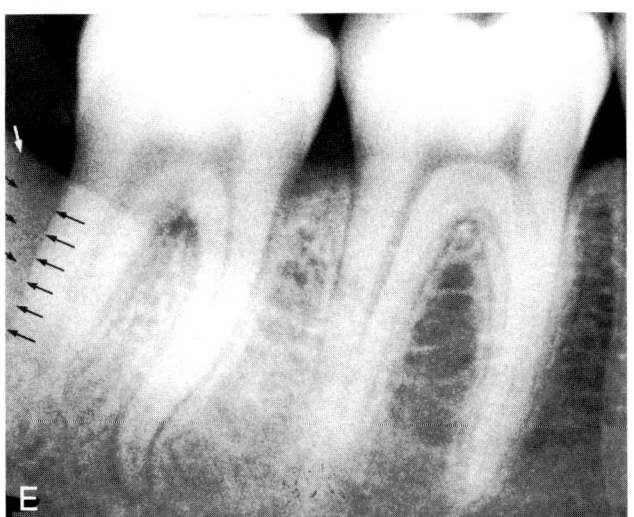
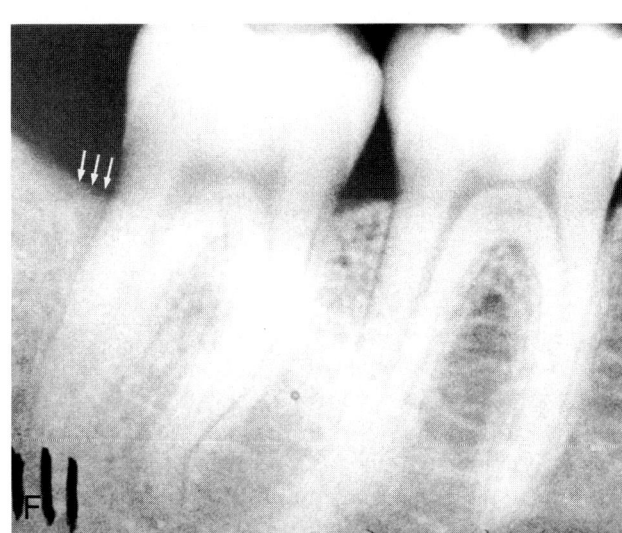

Fig. 13-8 (continued). **E,** Before treatment x-ray study. **F,** 11 month x-ray study showing bone regeneration. (Courtesy of Dr. Berton Becker, Flagstaff, Arizona.)

BIORESORBABLE MEMBRANES

BIODEGRADABLE MEMBRANES

The ideal membrane barrier is one that will permit GTR to occur while being physiologically compatible and biodegradable. Studies have shown a number of different materials to hold promise—woven vicryl/mesh (Johnson and Johnson), Periogen, cross-linked bioresorbable Type I collagen (Perio-Barrier), and oxidized cellulose mesh (Surgical). Different studies (Blumenthal and Steinberg, 1990; Blumenthal, 1988; Pitaru, et al., 1988; Magnusson, et al., 1990; Chung, et al., 1990; Galgut, 1990; and Lekovic, et al., 1991) have shown these various materials to hold promise. Guidor (John O. Butler Co.), a polylactic acid resorbable material was recently the first resorbable membrane barrier approved by the FDA for use specifically for guided tissue regeneration.

It is important to note that the surgical principles and procedures that now apply to nonresorbable membranes will be applicable to resorbable barriers. The main differences will be in postoperative considerations and lack of need for a secondary removal surgery in most cases.

Bioresorbable Guidor Matrix Barrier

Guidor (John O. Butler Company) is a new *single-step* bioabsorbable material composed of polylactic acid blended with a citric acid ester. It is designed to provide initial barrier function during the early stages of healing for a minimum of 6 weeks. During this time, both design shape and polymer matrix stability are maintained; during the later stages of healing, the barrier is slowly resorbed and replaced by the periodontal tissues (Fig. 13-9).

Recent studies (Laurell et al., 1992; Laurell et al., 1993) have shown that Guidor is well tolerated clinically with minimal tissue recession, matrix exposure, and gingival pathology. As a bioabsorbable membrane for guided tissue regeneration, it has been shown to result in significant gains in clinical attachment in infrabony defects and Grade II furcations (Gottlow et al., 1992A, 1992B; Gottlow et al., 1993A, 1993B). *Note: As a new material extensive research is limited but very promising.*

Design

Guidor is designed as a double-layered matrix with two distinct perforated layers (Fig. 13-10). The *external* layer has large *rectangular perforations*, for easy penetration of the outer gingival tissues. This rapid influx of gingival corrective tissues prevents epithelial downgrowth and minimizes gingival recession, matrix exposure, pocket formation, infection, and inflammation. The *internal* layer has minute *circular perforations* that retard tissue penetration but still allow for nutrition. Alveolar bone and periodontal ligament can enter these small perforations to eventually merge with the gingival connective tissue. The two layers are separated by many *inner spacers* forming a compartment into which tissue can grow. The coronal portion of the matrix has a preplaced *ligature*. A *bar* is positioned on top of the internal layer to function as a seal between the matrix and root surface.

Guidor is also designed to be *pliable or malleable* with no memory. Once shaped, it "does not" tend to return to its original form, thus preventing undue flap pressure. The matrix design makes inadvertent exposure of the material less problematic because the perforation pattern permits integration with adjacent tissues the entire length of the matrix. Exposed material will disappear in 6 to 8 weeks. Resorption is by hydrolysis (Fig. 13-11).

Indications

1. Class II furcation
2. Infrabony defects
3. Recession defects

NOTE: Guidor has not been tested clinically for use in regeneration of alveolar bone, either by itself or in conjunction with implants.

Contraindications

Guidor is contraindicated in situations in which periodontal surgery should not be performed.

Placement of Material

As previously noted, all bioabsorbable materials are single-step procedures that do not require material removal. Except for that, **the surgical technique for bioresorbable membranes is identical to that outlined for nonresorbable membranes.**

TRIMMING. The peripheral borders of Guidor may be trimmed to the desired shape (Fig. 13-12A, B). Interproximal configurations should be trimmed peripherally to take into account the shape of the adjacent teeth (Fig. 13-12B).

The internal *coronal or bar* area requires special attention.

1. Remove all necessary material closely approximating the bar to that which is desired. *Be careful not to cut the coronal bar* (Fig. 13-12C).
2. Holding the bar tightly with cotton pliers, *pull the ligature laterally* until it is free of the coronal portion to be removed (Fig. 13-12D).
3. Cut the empty coronal bar portion (Fig. 13-12E).

ADAPTATION. Overextension of the material is not a problem and, in some cases, the additional stability may prevent collapse into the defect.

Flap placement over the material prior to tying will permit matrix softening and increasing malleability. This results in greater matrix adaptability to the bone around the defect and facilitates final ligature tying.

LIGATURE TYING. A single *square knot* is used to tie the ligature around the tooth (Fig. 13-13A). Additional throws are not recommended because they may not unlock the suture (Fig. 13-13B). All blood and clots should be rinsed away with sterile saline prior to knot finalization (Fig. 13-13C).

Final tightening of the knot is best achieved if placed at the line angle (Fig. 13-13D). The ends or *ears* should be cut 5 to 10 mm from the end of the knot to facilitate subgingival placement (Fig. 13-13E).

FLAP SUTURING. A modified mattress suture is recommended for coronal flap positioning. Sutures are to be maintained for *2 to 4* weeks with nonresorbable or slowly resorbing sutures (Fig. 13-14).

Postoperative Considerations

1. A periodontal dressing *is not* recommended.
2. Sutures are to remain for 2 to 4 weeks.
3. For the first 6 weeks, oral hygiene procedures are to be avoided in the surgical site.
4. Peridex mouthwash is to be used during the first 6 weeks.
5. The patient should be seen every other week.
6. Antibiotics are at the discretion of the clinician.

The clinical procedure is seen in Fig. 13-15.

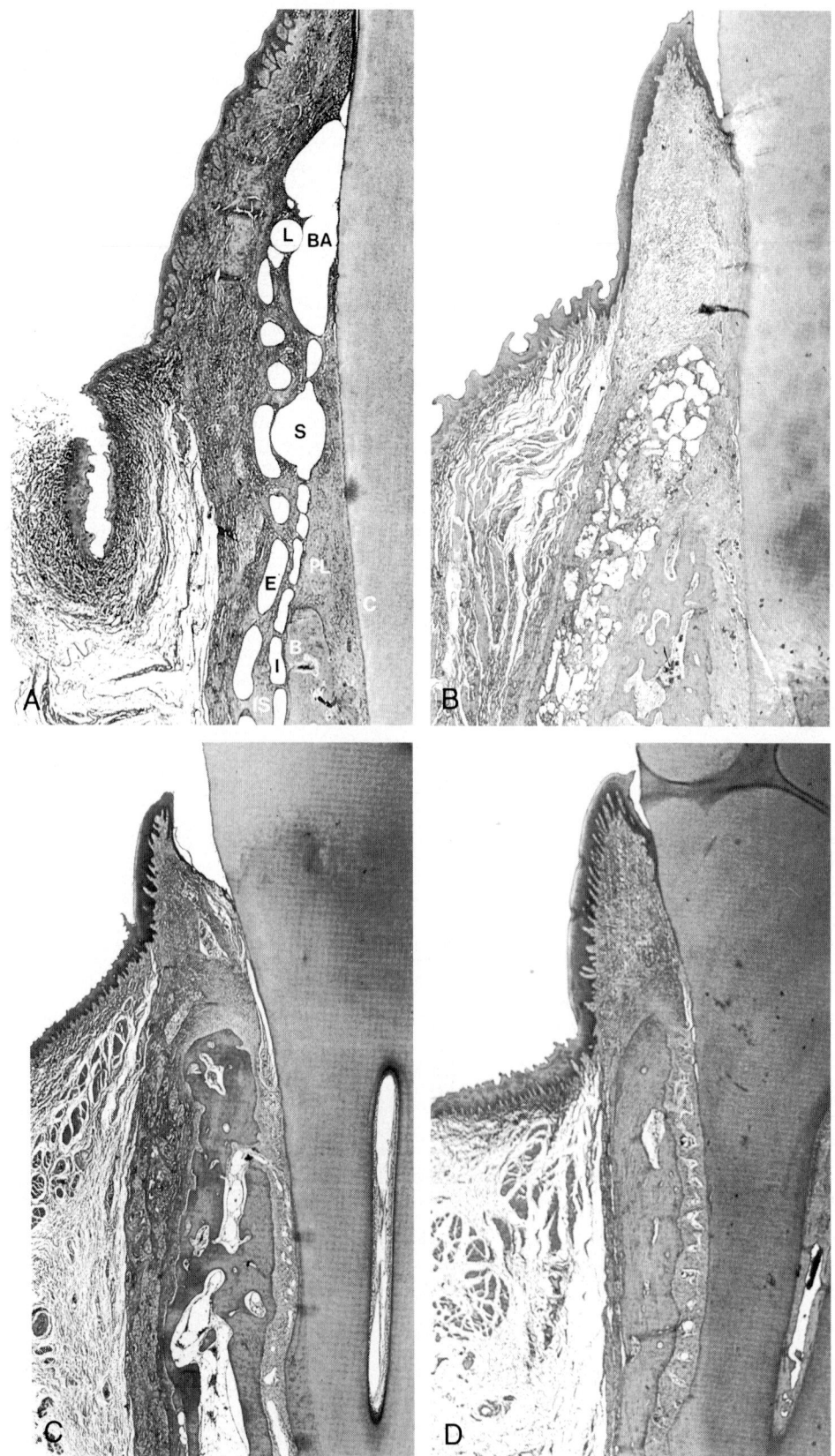

Fig. 13-9. Histologic healing 6 weeks to 24 months—monkeys. **A,** 6 weeks displaying nonresorbed matrix without fragmentation. Ligature (L); coronal bar (BA); spacers (S); external matrix layer (E); inner matrix surface (I); inner space between external and internal layers (IS). Note extensive formation of cementum (C), periodontal ligament (PL), and bone (B). **B,** 3-month section showing outline of matrix material with new bone, collagen, and cementum formation. **C,** 6-month section showing complete resorption of material and replacement with connective tissue. Note regeneration of bone, cementum, and PDL. **D,** 24-month section with healing completed and restoration of tissue complete. (Contributed by Guidor AB, Gothenburg, Sweden.)

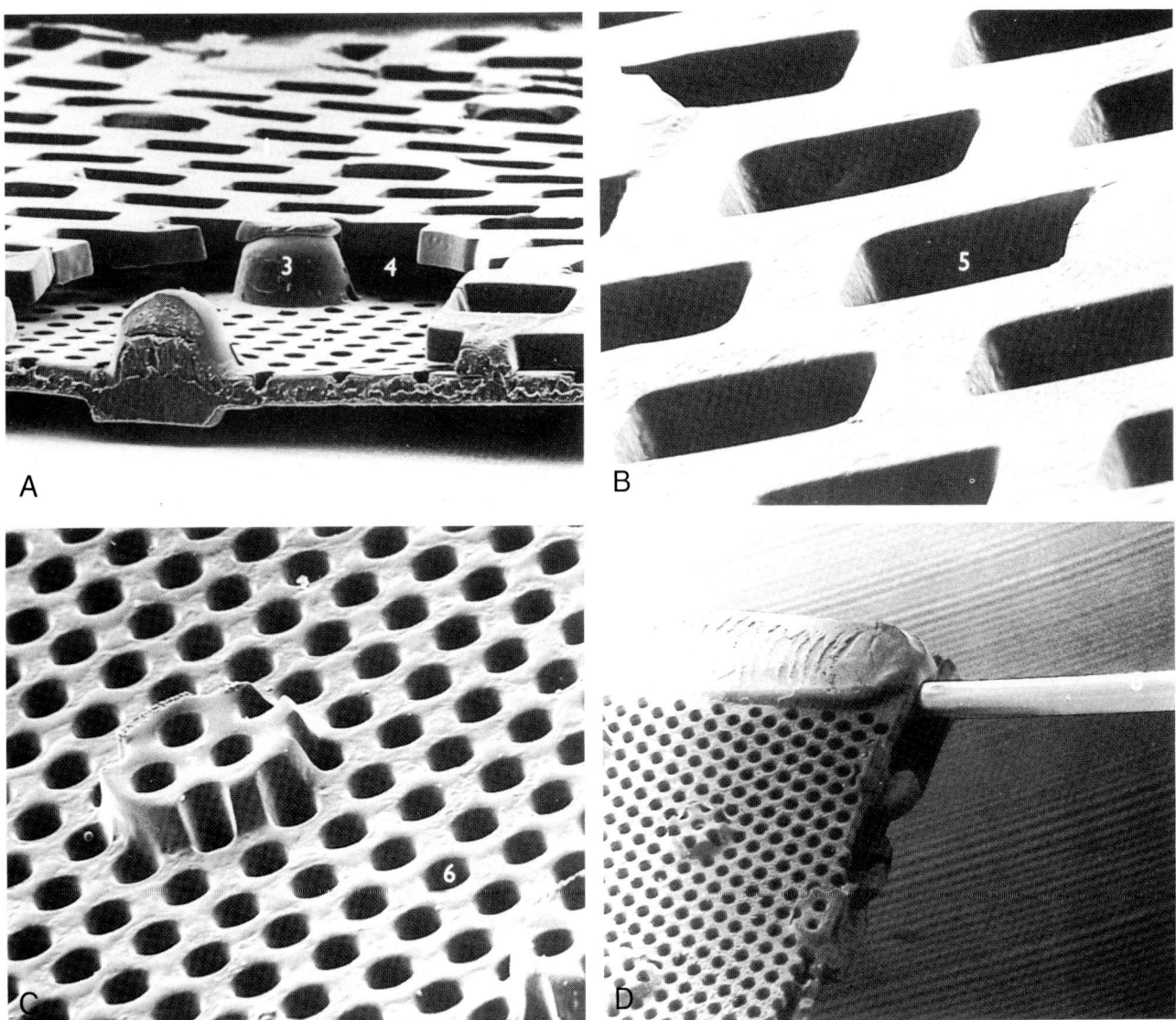

Fig. 13-10. Scanning electron microscope of matrix barrier. **A,** Two layers—1. external layer; 2. internal layer; 3. inner spaces; 4. inner space or compartment. **B,** Large rectangular perforations (5) in the external layer. **C,** Internal layer showing minute perforations (6) and outer spaces facing the root (7). Interportion showing incorporated suturing material, ligature (8), and coronal-bar portion (9). (Contributed by Guidor AB, Gothenburg, Sweden.)

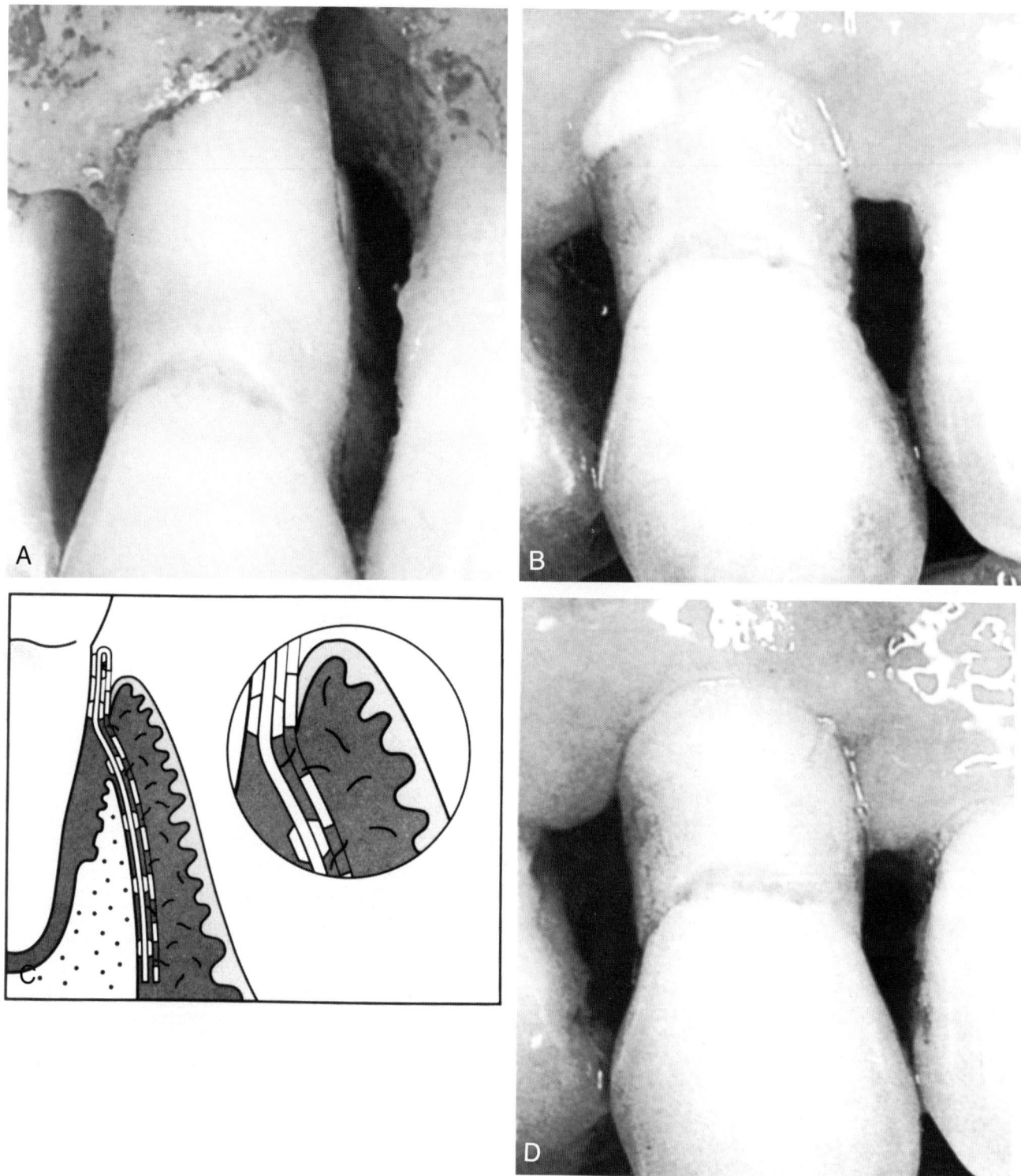

Fig. 13-11. Initial exposure of matrix material. **A,** Defect exposed at time of surgery. **B,** Material exposed. **C,** Diagrammatic representation of exposed material. The material is fully integrated on the external layer *inhibiting* epithelial downgrowth, pocket formation, and infection. **D,** 6 weeks after surgery the exposed material is fully resorbed. (Contributed by Guidor AB, Gothenburg, Sweden.)

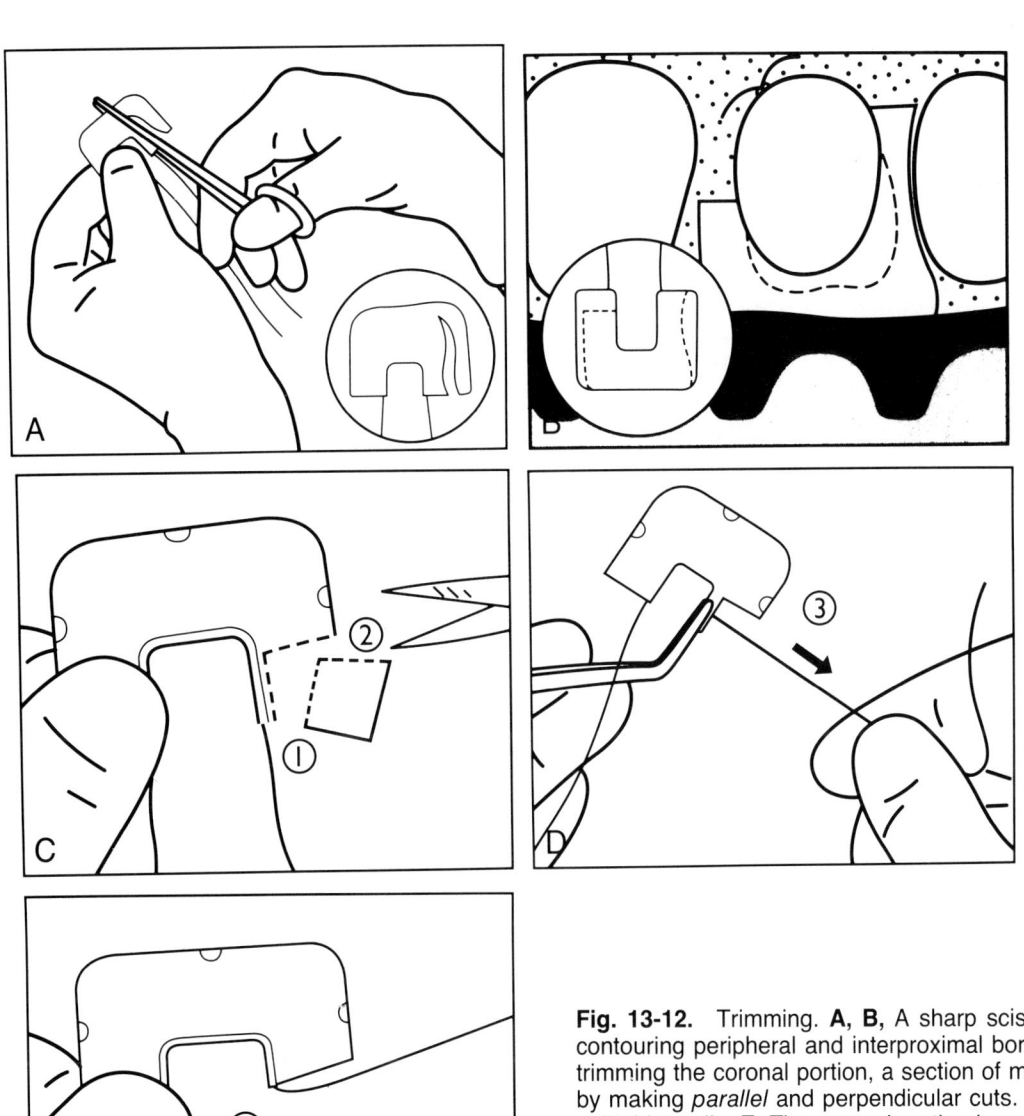

Fig. 13-12. Trimming. **A, B,** A sharp scissors is used for contouring peripheral and interproximal borders. **C,** Prior to trimming the coronal portion, a section of matrix is removed by making *parallel* and perpendicular cuts. **D,** The suture is pulled laterally. **E,** The coronal portion is removed. (Contributed by Guidor AB, Gothenburg, Sweden.)

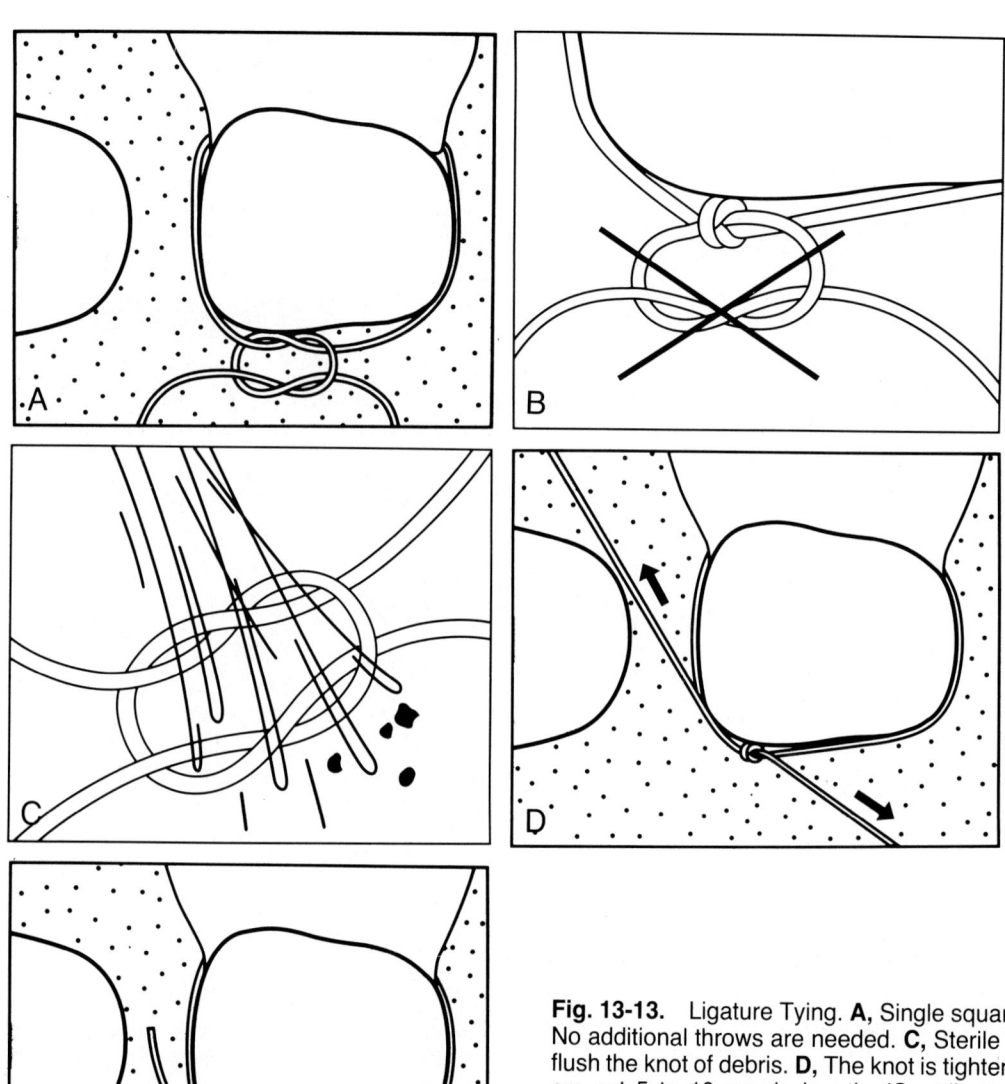

Fig. 13-13. Ligature Tying. **A,** Single square knot is tied. **B,** No additional throws are needed. **C,** Sterile saline is used to flush the knot of debris. **D,** The knot is tightened. **E,** The ends are cut 5 to 10 mm in length. (Contributed by Guidor AB, Gothenburg, Sweden.)

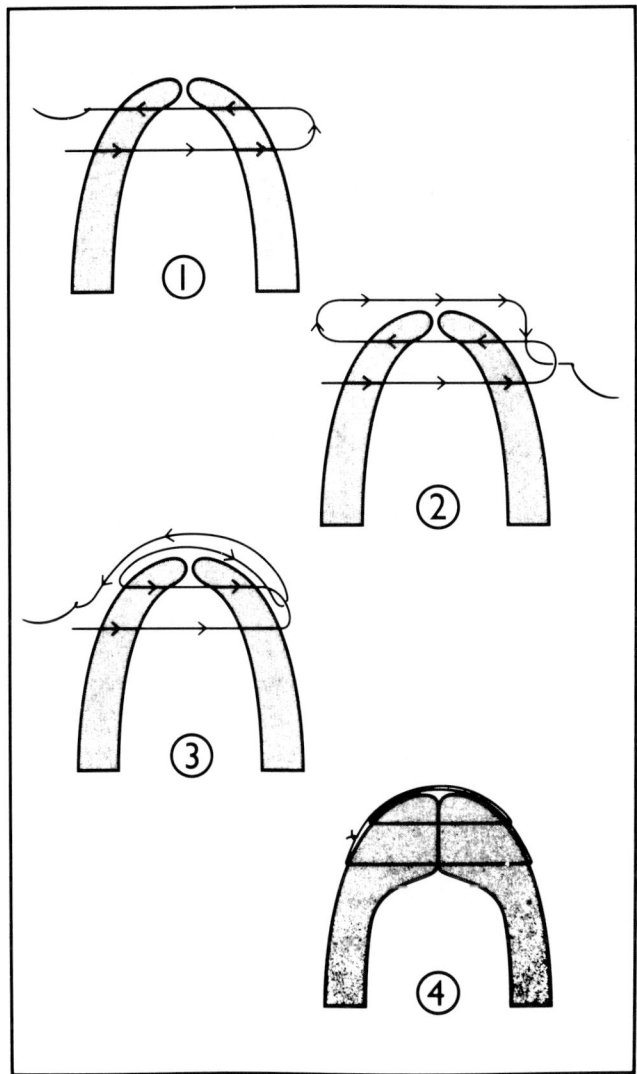

Fig. 13-14. Modified mattress suture for coronal flap positioning. 1. Start buccally to the undersurface of the lingual flap and then through the outer surface of the lingual flap through the undersurface of the buccal flap. 2. The suture is brought lingually over the coronal aspect of the flap and through the loop. 3. The suture is returned buccally above the papilla. 4. The suture is tied buccally. (Contributed by Guidor AB, Gothenburg, Sweden.)

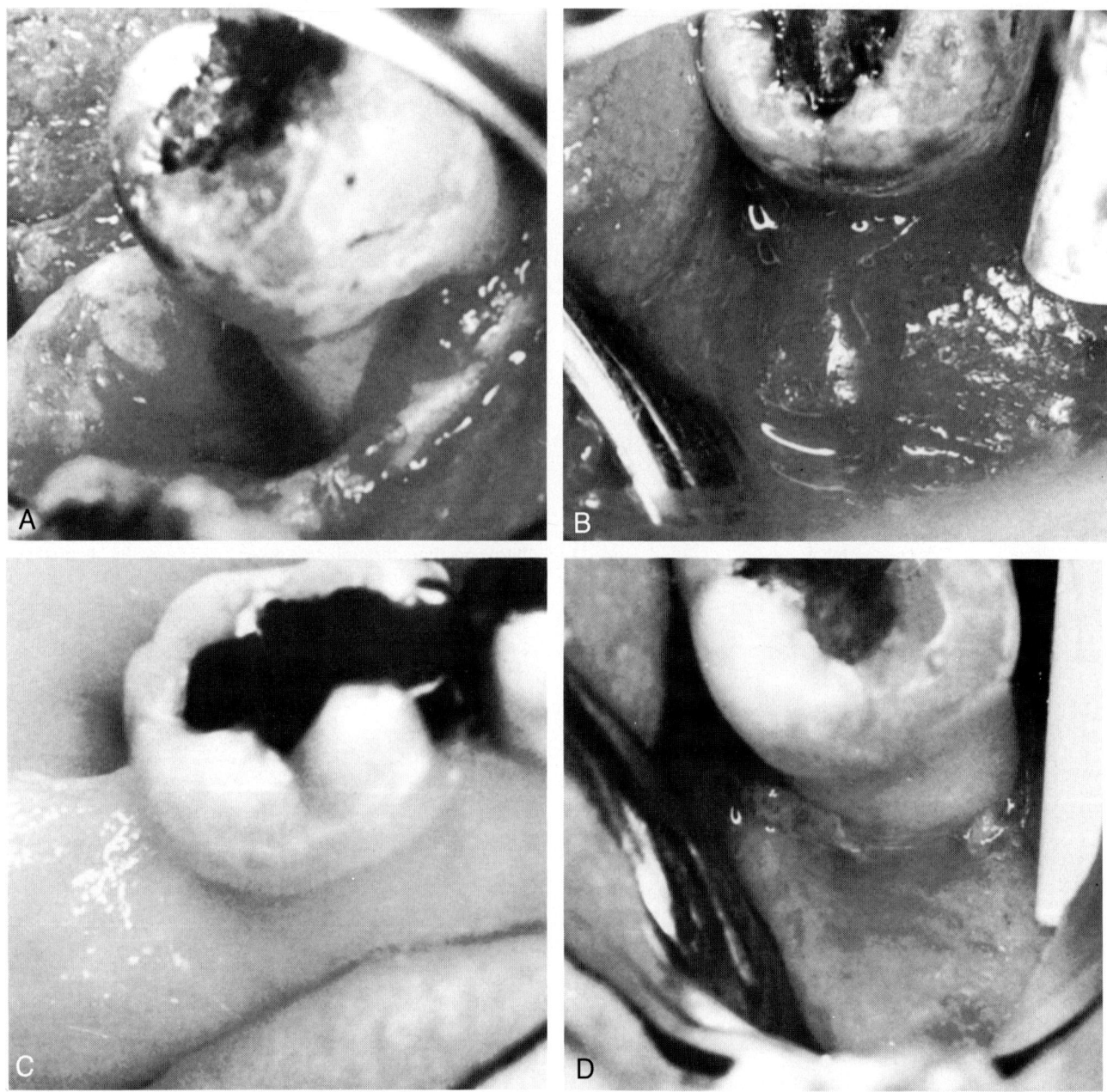

Fig. 13-15. Treatment of infrabony defect. **A,** Flap elevated and defect exposed. **B,** Guidor material placed. **C,** 12-month post surgery. **D,** 12-month reentry showing complete bone fill. (Contributed by Guidor AB, Gothenburg, Sweden.)

RIDGE AUGMENTATION

The success of osseointegrated (endosseous) implants has created not only a need for adequate bony support of edentulous areas but also the need to be able to regenerate bone about implants where dehiscences and/or fenestrations are present. Today the most effective technique for achieving bony ridge augmentation is through the use of e-PTFE (Gore-Tex Augmentation Material, GTAM).

GTAM has been shown to have the ability for ridge preservation and enhancement following extractions (Nevins and Mellonig, 1992) and enhancement both in height and width prior to implant placement (Buser et al., 1990). A number of clinicians (Lazzara, 1989; Becker and Becker, 1990; Nyman et al., 1990; Dahlin et al., 1991A, B; Shanaman, 1992; Wilson, 1992; Werbitt and Goldberg, 1992; Mellonig and Triplett, 1993) have shown significant regeneration of bone about titanium implants that have been placed into immediate extraction sockets. Most recently GTAM has proved effective in sinus bone augmentation and implant placement (Jensen and Greer, 1992; Jensen et al., 1992) (Fig. 13-16).

Material

GTAM has two distinct portions: (1) An inner occlusive portion, which is sufficiently stiff to permit spacemaking, and (2) an outer portion, which allows for greater connective tissue integration promoting clot stability and epithelial inhibition (Fig. 13-17).

Defect Selection

The defects selected may or may not be associated with implants.

Osseous Defects

1. Residual defects
2. Extraction sockets

Peri-implant Defects

1. Fenestration
2. Dehisence
3. Intraosseous
4. Extraction sockets—fresh and residual
5. Peri-implantitis (Gore does not consider this a current application)

Predictability

Predictable success is based on achieving and maintaining adequate space between the defect and e-PTFE. This is achieved naturally in intraosseous defects or by a space filler such as DFDBA (Figs. 13-20, 13-21). Buser (1991, 1993) has recently advocated the use of stainless steel screws for material stabilization and shape maintenance (Fig. 13-23).

1. Most predictable: defects within the bone envelope.
   a. Dehisence
   b. Fenestration
   c. Fresh extraction sites
   d. Localized ridge augmentation
2. Moderate predictability: defects outside of bone envelope.
3. Low predictability: loss of crestal bone height.

Contraindications

Placement is contraindicated in the presence of active infections. Defect debridement and treatment of chronic infections are necessary precursors.

Surgical Procedure

The surgical procedure may be a primary ridge augmentation procedure or in conjunction with implant placement (Fig. 13-18).

1. A full thickness mucoperiosteal flap is used for defect exposure. Flap overthinning is to be avoided.
2. Incisions are extended mesially and distally far enough to assure adequate site exposure (Fig. 13-18A, A').
3. Vertical incisions (if needed) are to be positioned away from and never over the material. On the maxilla the incisions should be made on the palatal aspect so as to assure proper coverage of GTAM material (Fig. 13-18A').
4. Defects, if present, are debrided of all granulation tissue and decorticated where indicated.
5. DFDBA is recommended as a spacer or filler for the defect (Fig. 13-18D,D') (Shallhorn and McClaine, 1988, 1993).
6. The material is sized and shaped so that sharp edges are avoided. The material should extend a minimum of 3 mm beyond the defect margins. The inner portion should lie over the defect (Fig. 13-18E,E').
7. Material contact with adjacent teeth is to be avoided so as to permit sulcus development without material exposure (Fig. 13-18E).
8. The GTAM should be properly adapted to assure coverage of bone and graft. It should fit smoothly, avoiding folds or overlaps.
9. Stabilization is achieved by proper shaping and contouring of the material followed by good flap closure or by using implant cover screws

(Becker and Becker, 1990) or mini screws (Buser et al., 1990, 1993).
10. Simple interrupted nonabsorbable Gore-Tex Sutures are recommended, and primary closure is desired (Fig. 13-18F,F').
11. If unexposed, the material may remain in place from 1 to 9 months or until the time of implant exposure or placement.
12. Material exposure will require weekly supervision, and immediate removal if any complications or infections develop. No attempt should be made to re-cover the material due to bacterial contamination.

The clinical procedures are depicted in Figures 13-19, 13-20, 13-21, 13-22, 13-23, and 13-24.

GTAM Postoperative Considerations

It is important to note that the postoperative considerations differ markedly from those utilized for periodontal applications.

A. Immediate follow-up care
  1. Maintain good oral hygiene.
  2. Avoid denture wear if possible for the first 2 weeks.
  3. In patients who wear dentures, the denture should be adequately relieved to avoid undue pressure, thus preventing material collapse into the defect space and avoiding unnecessary flap perforation and material exfoliation.
  4. Sutures are maintained for as long as they are needed.
  5. The patient is monitored on a biweekly basis.
  6. The patient is given a chlorhexidine mouthwash and on tetracycline 250 mg Q.I.D. for 10 to 14 days. This will help prevent bacterial infection, especially if the material becomes exposed.
B. GTAM removal
  1. The material is removed immediately if complications develop or the edge of the material becomes exposed. Exposure of the material edge may permit bacterial wicking into the defect.
  2. GTAM has been designed to act as a temporary barrier to the epithelium and connective tissue with an optimum removal time of 1 to 9 months.
  3. Early versus late removal: Early removal, although having the advantages of less patient follow-up, easier compliance, and less potential for complications, has the disadvantages of the regeneration being less mature, a need for an additional surgery, and the possibility of implant compromise.

  Late removal has the advantages of a longer regeneration time, avoidance of additional surgery, and that the result can be better evaluated. The main disadvantages are a longer patient monitoring time and that the material is more difficult to remove.
C. Material exposure: If the material becomes exposed the following steps should be taken:
  1. Monitor patient weekly.
  2. Use a chlorhexidine mouthwash.
  3. Have patient gently swab area.
  4. Avoid mechanical trauma, as movement may disrupt regenerating tissues.
  5. Remove material immediately if the edge becomes exposed.
  6. Do not attempt to re-cover material.

Note: Once the material is exposed, it is to be removed at 2 months maximum.

C. Complications: The clinician must decide at the time of any complication if removal is indicated and if removal will facilitate resolution of the complication.
  1. Infection
  2. Flap slough
  3. Perforation
  4. Abscess formation
  5. Bone loss
  6. Pain
  7. Soft-tissue irregularities
  8. Flap perforation
  9. Material exfoliation
E. Evaluating results
  1. Radiograph 6 to 12 months postoperatively
  2. Clinical evaluation at time of material removal (if early) or at second stage implant procedure

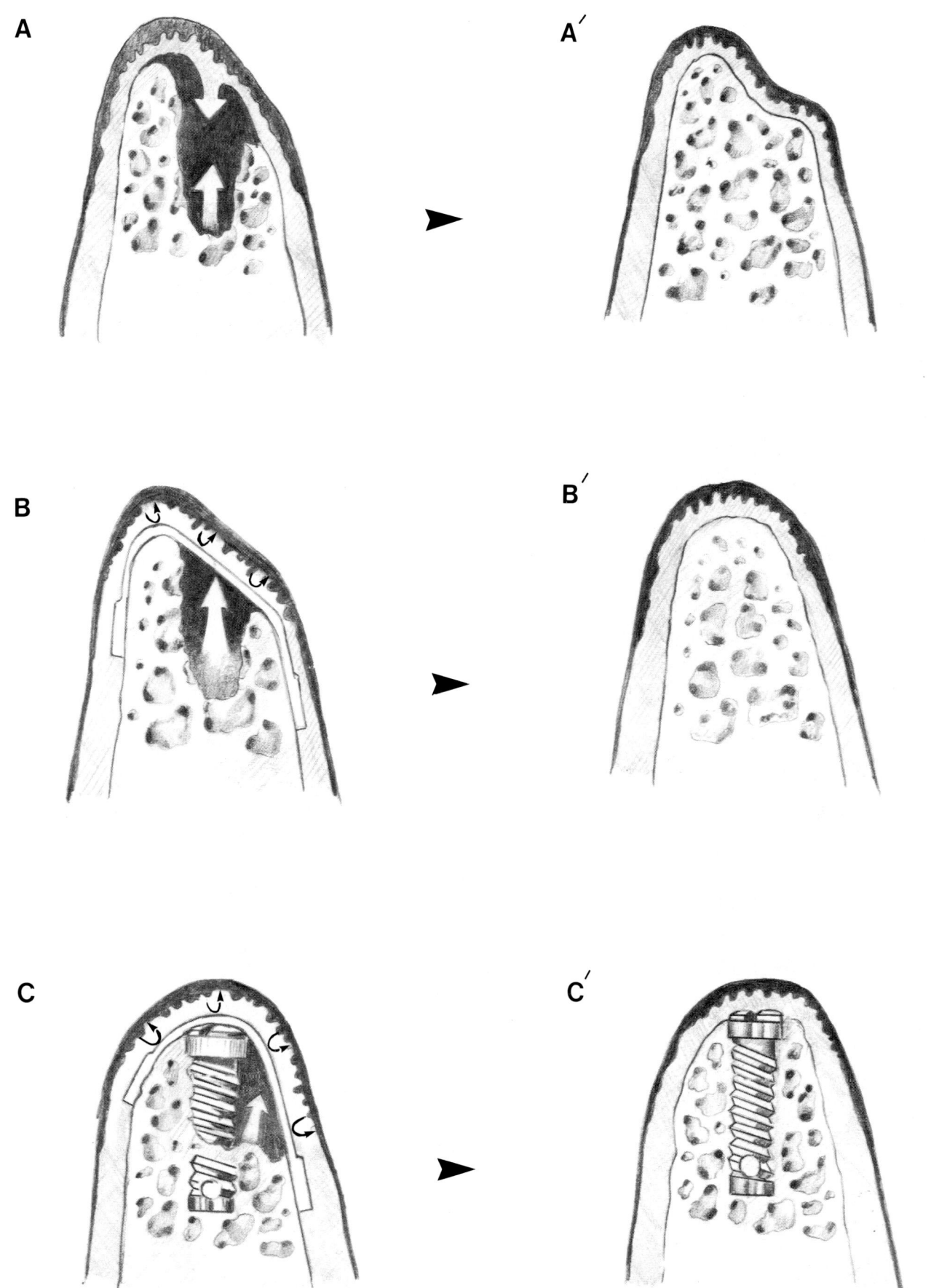

Fig. 13-16. Guided Regeneration for Ridge Augmentation. **A, A′,** Partial ridge regeneration after tooth extraction. **B, B′,** Complete ridge regeneration with membrane placement. **C, C′,** Regeneration of fenestrations, dehisences, and sockets about immediate or delayed implant placement.

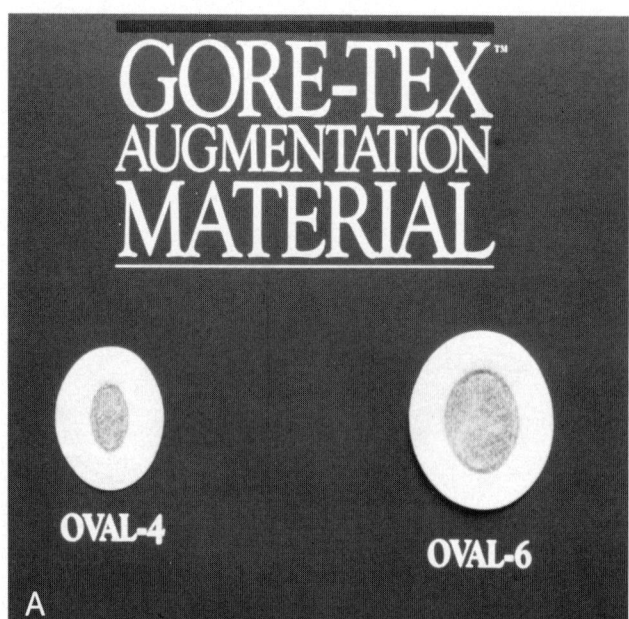
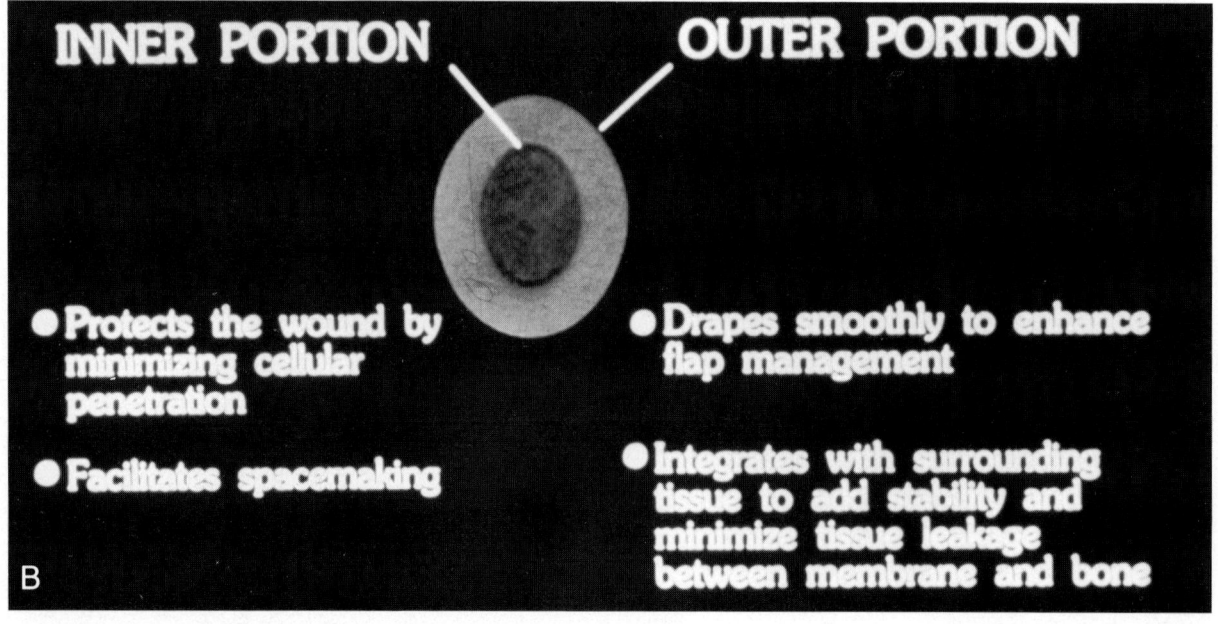

Fig. 13-17. Gore-Tex Augmentation Material (GTAM). **A,** Different sizes of material available. **B,** The zones of GTAM.

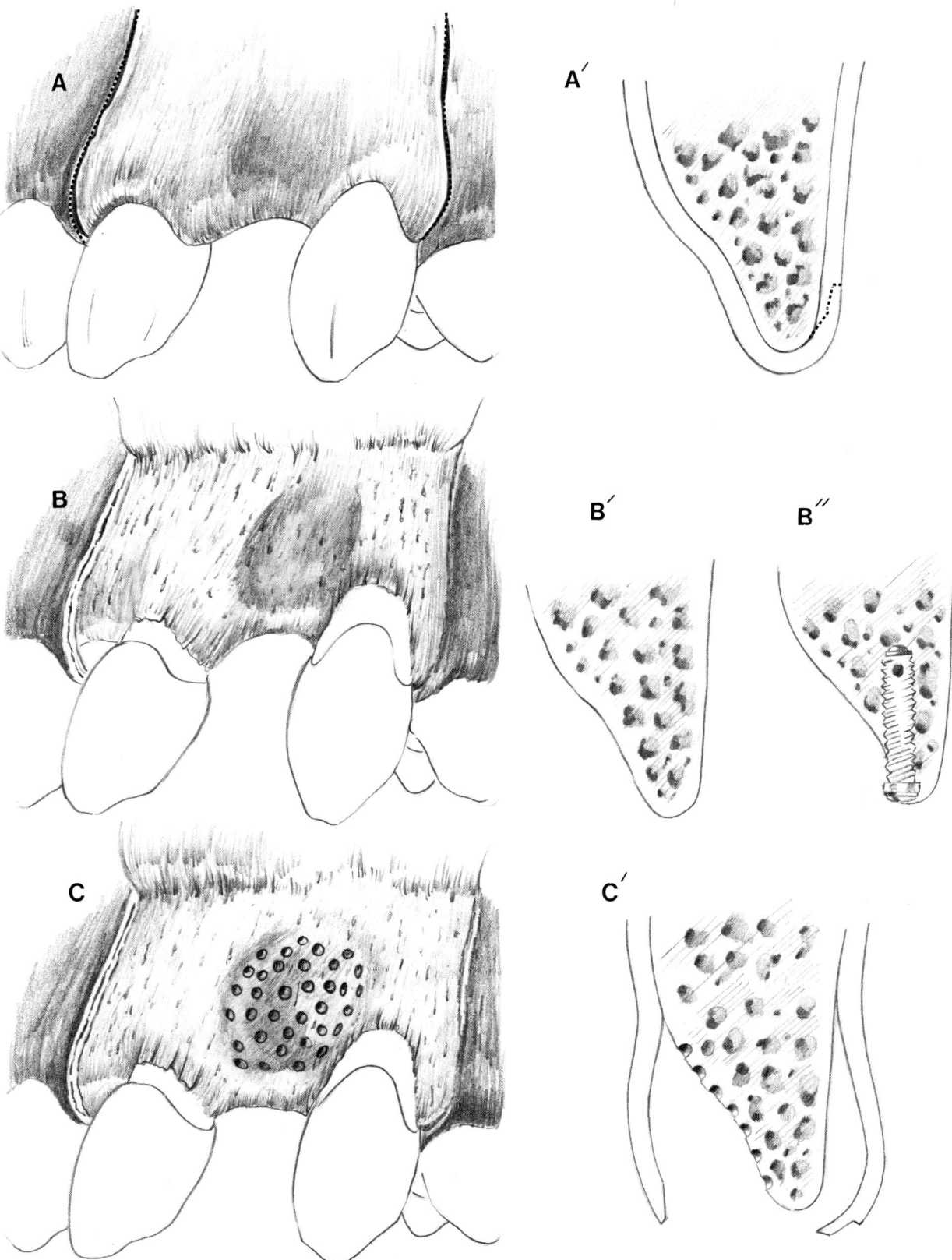

Fig. 13-18. Ridge Augmentation with Guided Tissue Regeneration (Buccal and Cross-Sectional Views). **A, A′,** Incisions outlined. **B, B′, B″,** Views of ridge defect and/or implant exposure. **C, C′,** Decortification for bleeding. Small round holes are drilled into bone.

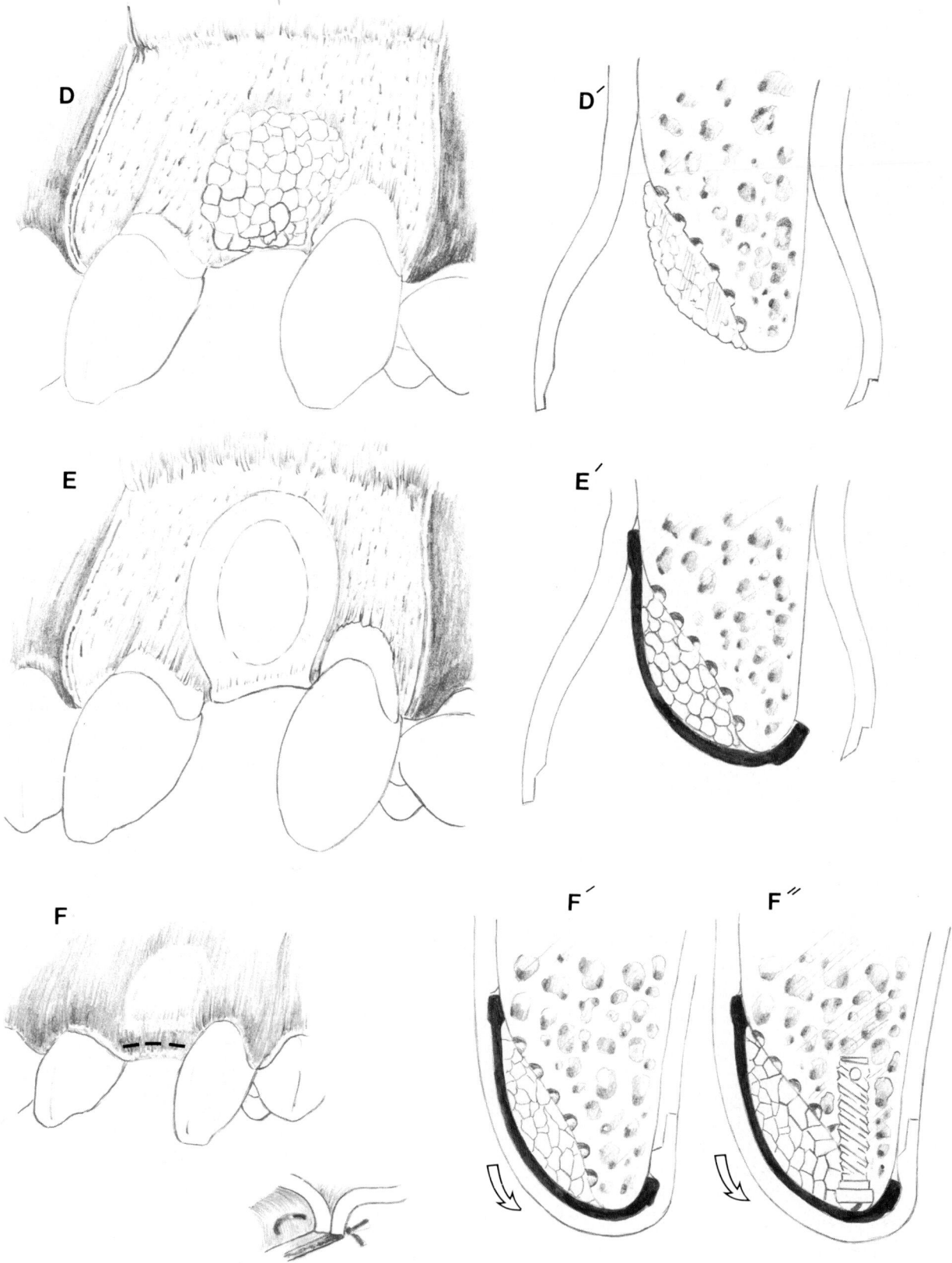

Fig. 13-18 (continued). **D, D′,** Graft material, usually DFDBA, placed in and over defects. **E, E′,** GTAM membrane placed over defect and material. Inner area must be wide enough for complete coverage. **F, F′, F″,** Final suturing. Primary coverage is desired.

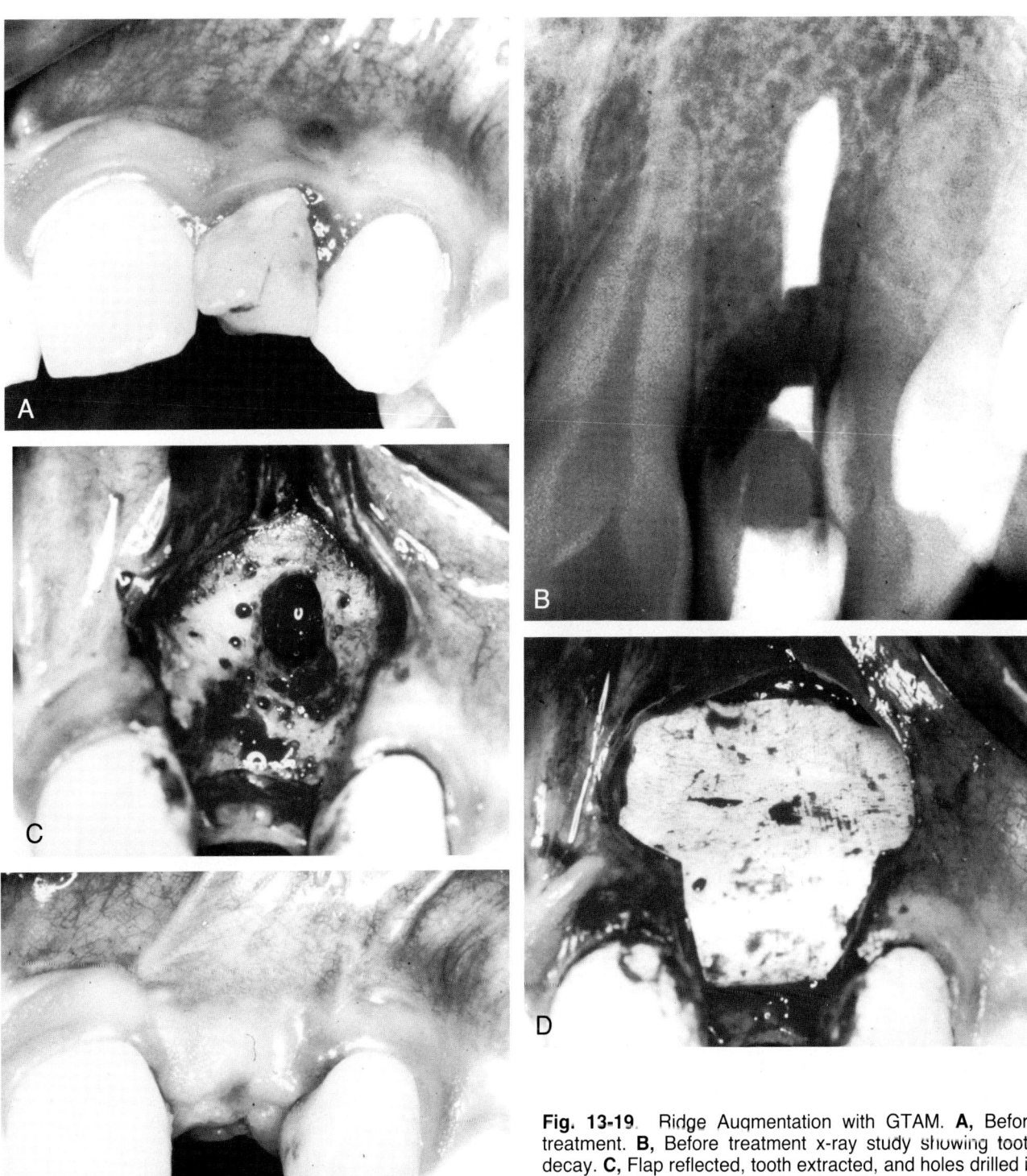

Fig. 13-19. Ridge Augmentation with GTAM. **A,** Before treatment. **B,** Before treatment x-ray study showing tooth decay. **C,** Flap reflected, tooth extracted, and holes drilled in cortical plate to promote bleeding. **D,** GTAM membrane positioned. **E,** Six-month view of healing.

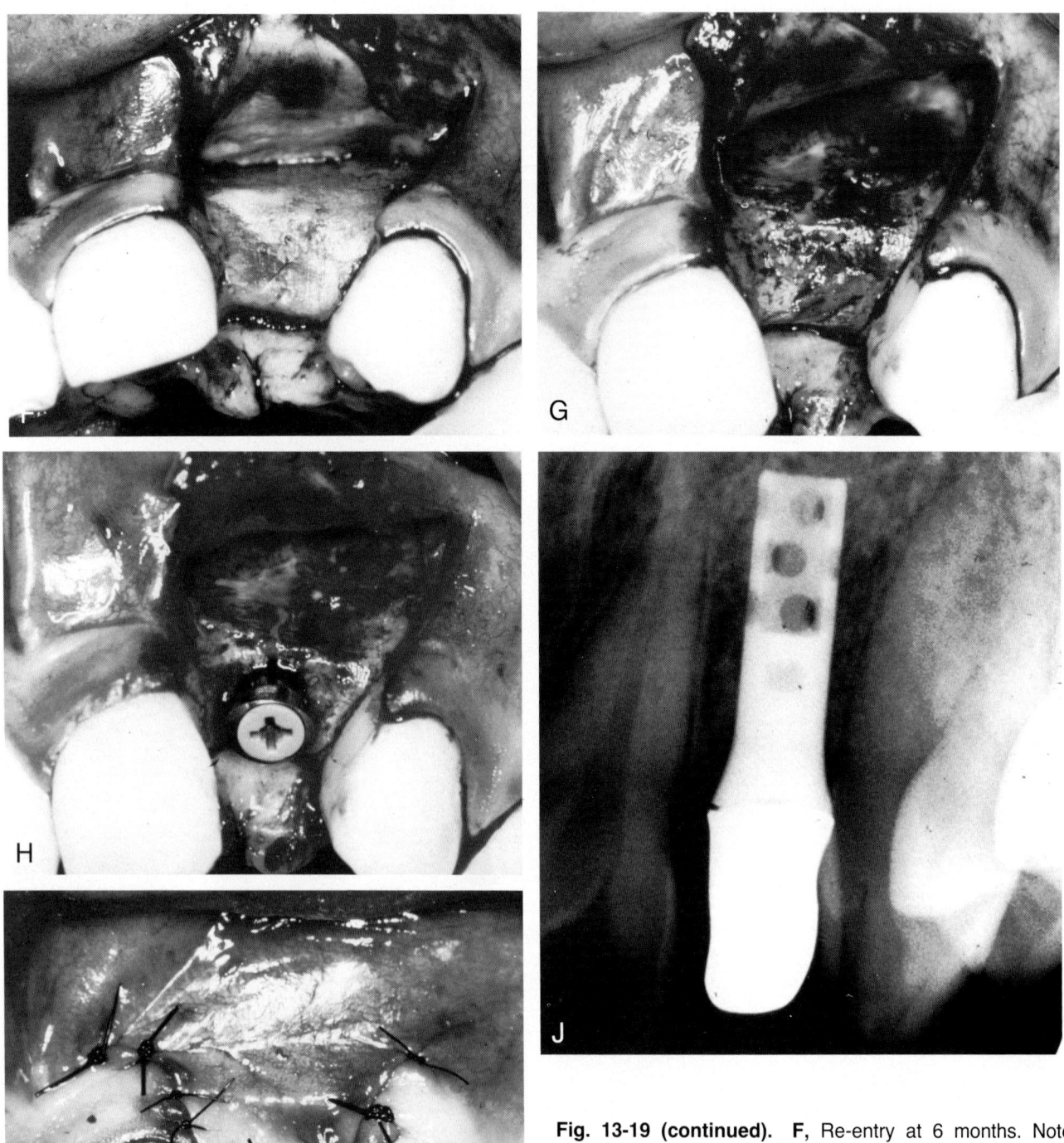

Fig. 13-19 (continued). F, Re-entry at 6 months. Note membrane position. **G,** GTAM removed. Note bone is in identical shape of GTAM material. **H,** Implant placed. **I,** Flaps reapproximated. **J,** Final X-ray study showing successful implant placement in enhanced ridge. (Courtesy of Dr. Daniel Buser, Bern, Switzerland.)

Guided Tissue Regeneration

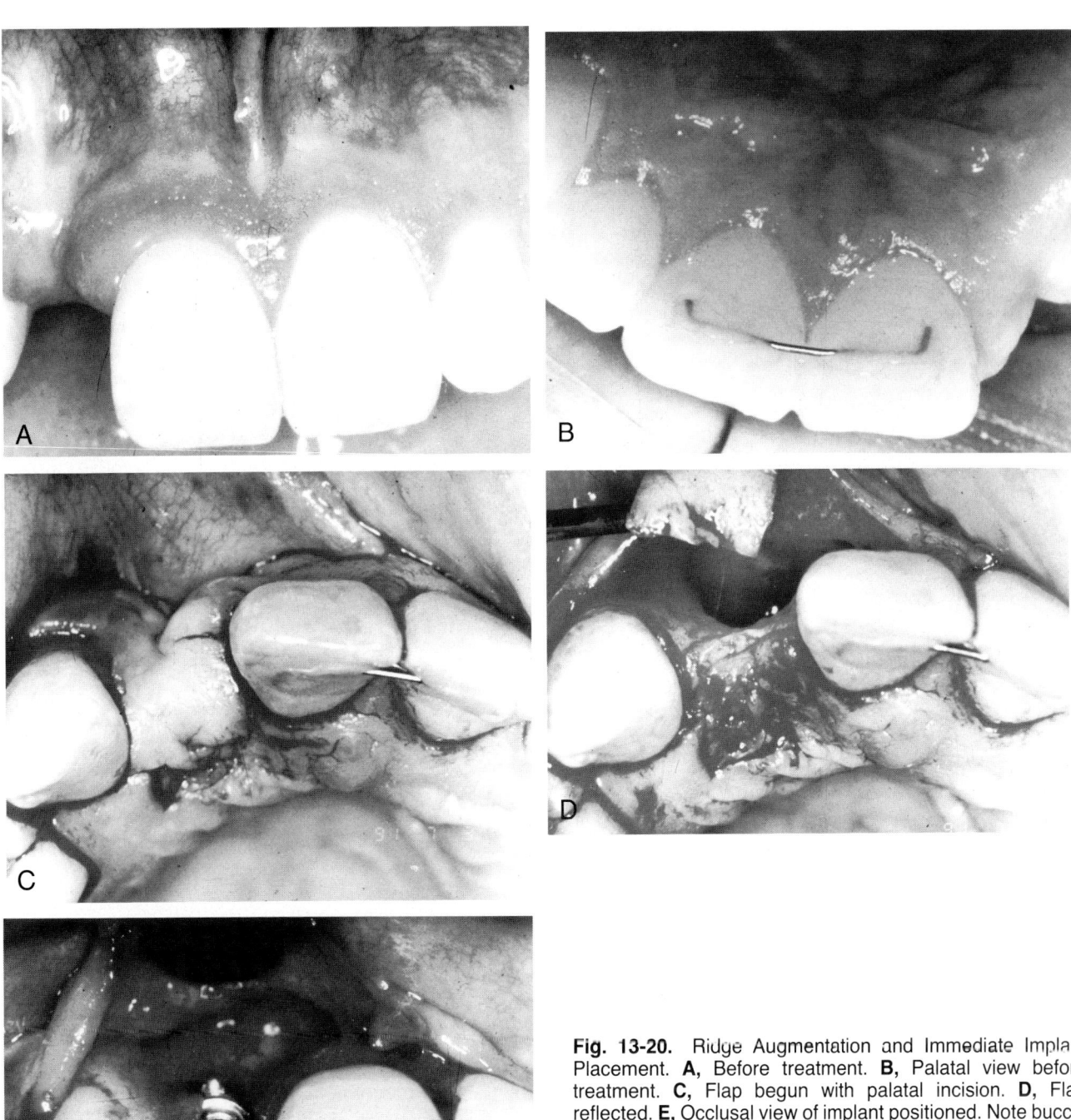

Fig. 13-20. Ridge Augmentation and Immediate Implant Placement. **A,** Before treatment. **B,** Palatal view before treatment. **C,** Flap begun with palatal incision. **D,** Flap reflected. **E,** Occlusal view of implant positioned. Note buccal dehiscence.

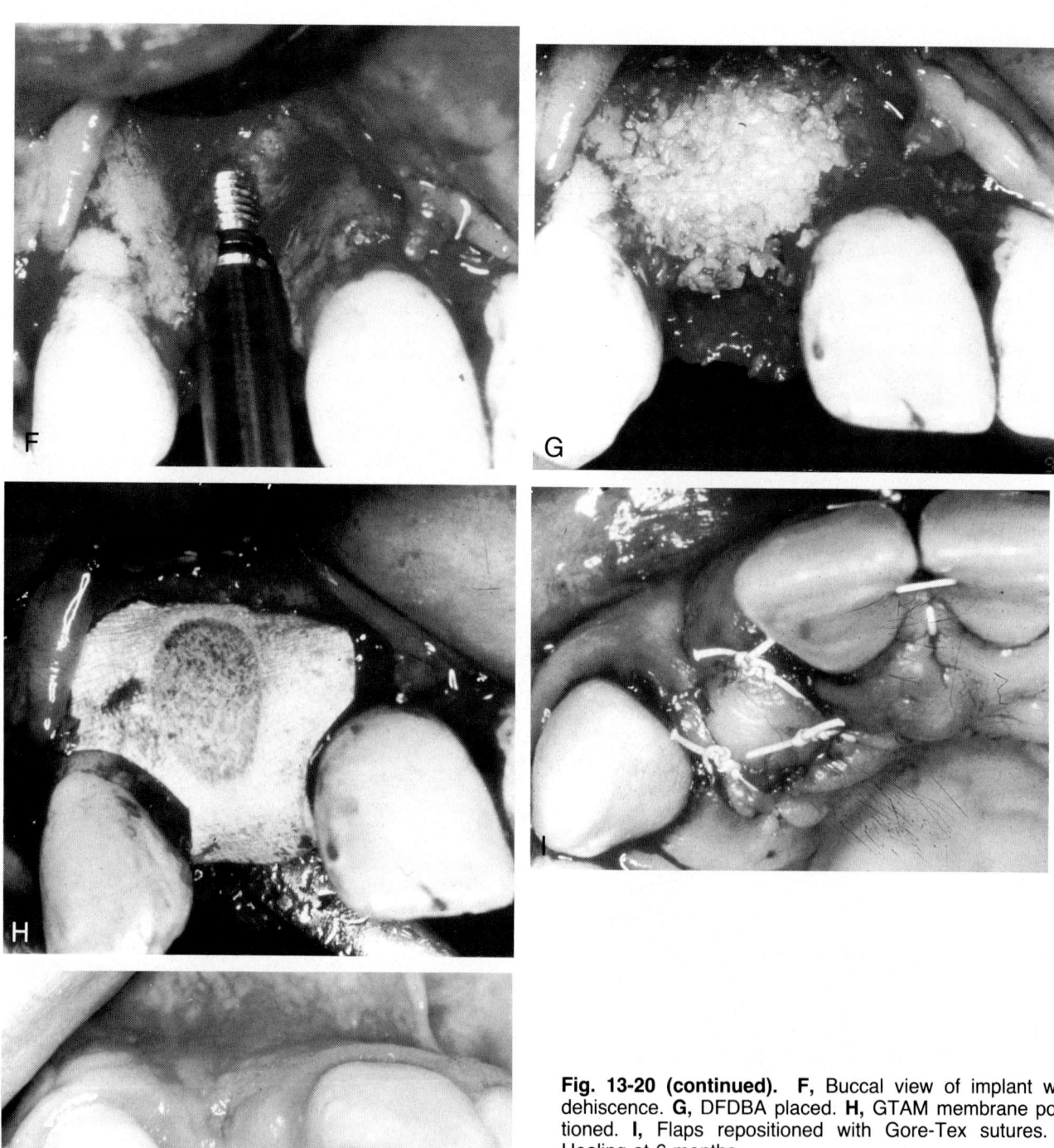

Fig. 13-20 (continued). F, Buccal view of implant with dehiscence. **G,** DFDBA placed. **H,** GTAM membrane positioned. **I,** Flaps repositioned with Gore-Tex sutures. **J,** Healing at 6 months.

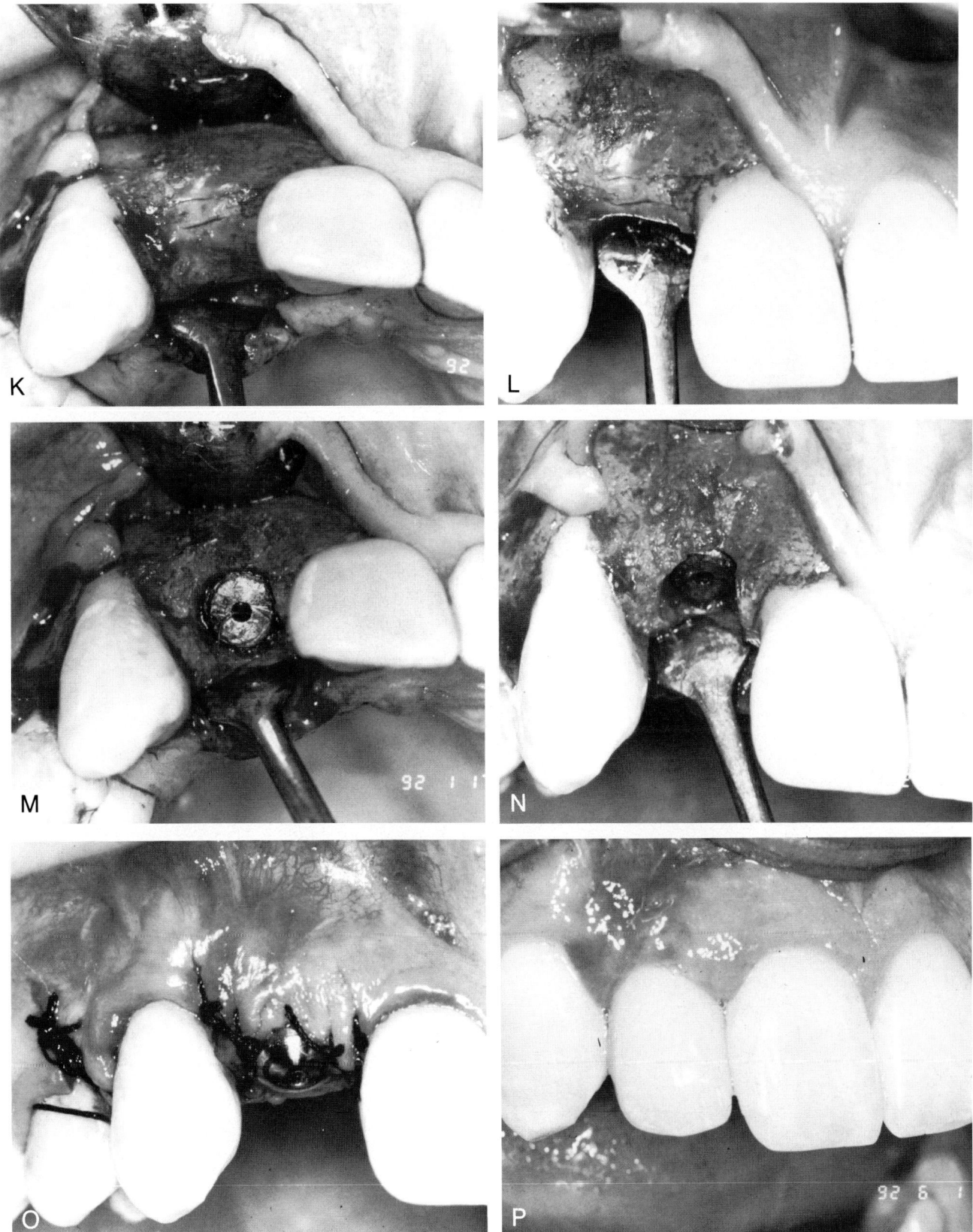

Fig. 13-20 (continued). K, L, Buccal and occlusal views of complete bone repair. **M, N,** Buccal and occlusal views showing implants exposed. Note in M the amount of bone that had to be removed overlaying the implant. **O,** Flap repositioned and sutured. **P,** Case completed. (Courtesy of Richard Shanaman, Reading, PA.)

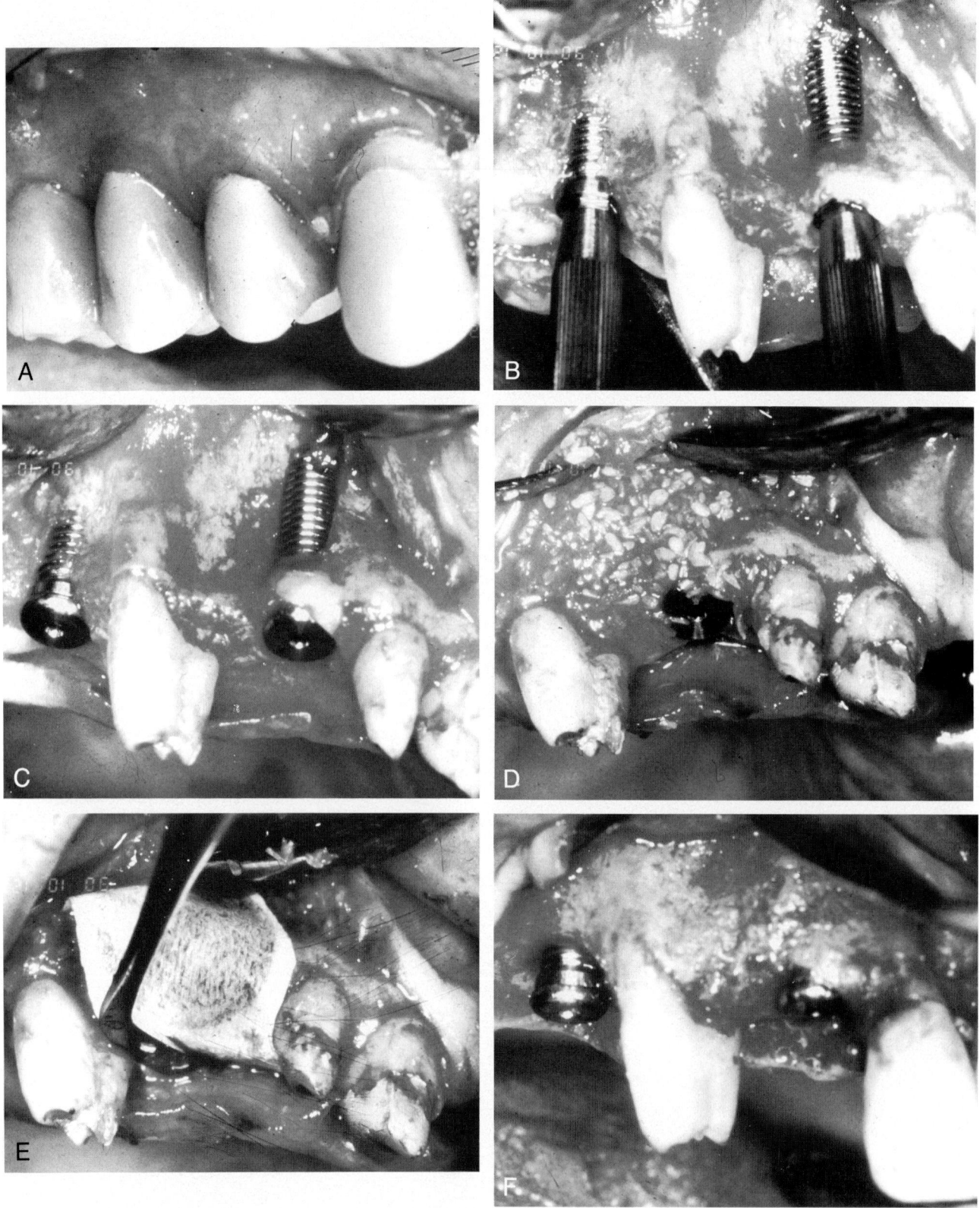

Fig. 13-21. Ridge Augmentation and Immediate Implant Placement. **A,** Before treatment. **B,** Implants placed with paralleling cones. Note almost complete buccal dehiscences. **C,** Implants with screw covers. **D,** DFDBA placed. **E,** GTAM positioned. **F,** Re-entry after 6 months. Note complete coverage of implant threads. (Contributed by Dr. Richard Shanaman, Reading, PA.)

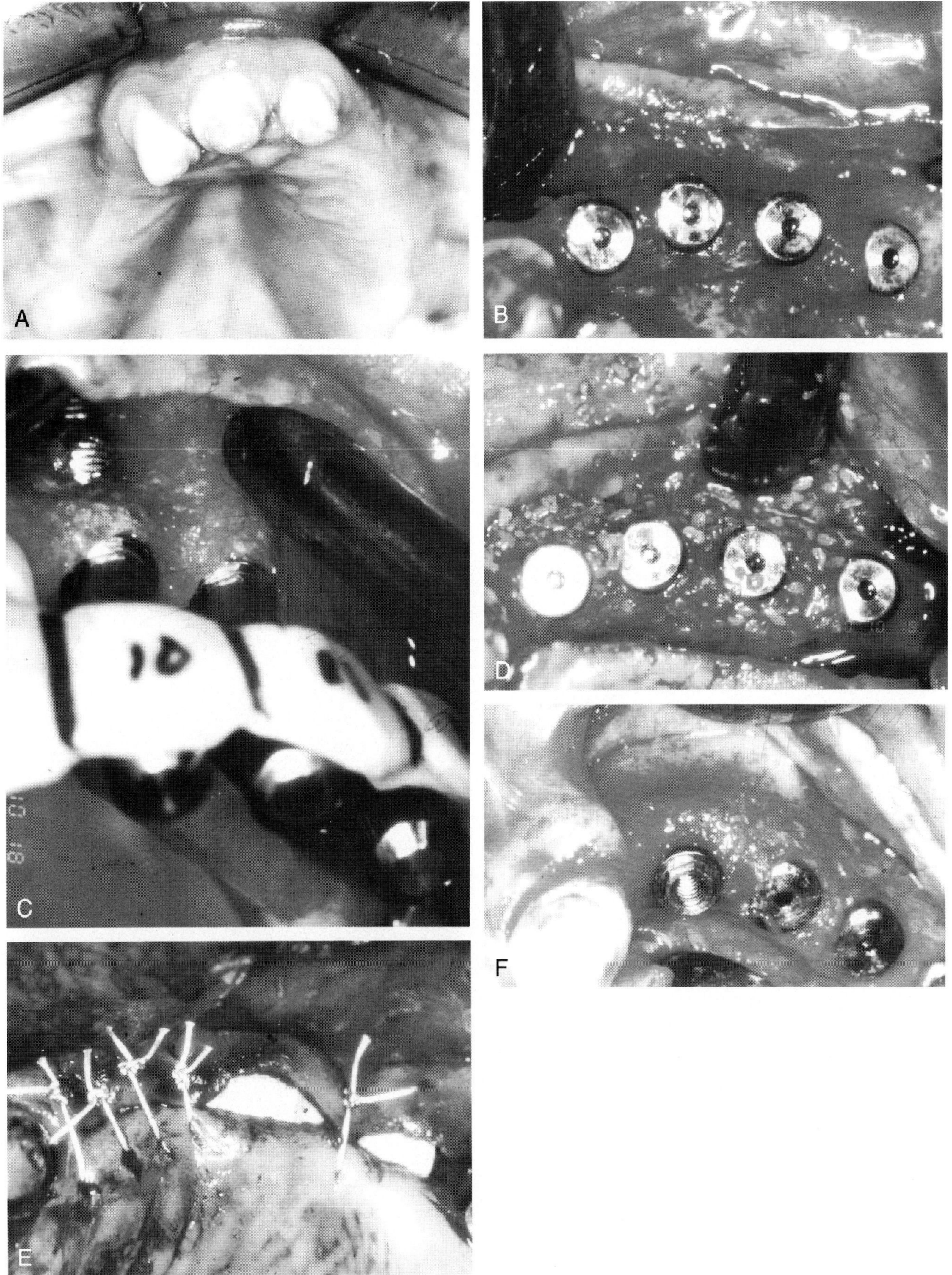

Fig. 13-22. Ridge Augmentation and Immediate Implant Placement. **A,** Before treatment. **B,** Implants positioned correctly over ridge. **C,** Note dehiscence over implant no. 10. **D,** DFDBA placed. **E,** GTAM positioned and sutured. **F,** Re-entry after 6 months. Note complete coverage of dehiscence. (Contributed by Dr. Richard Shanaman, Reading, PA.)

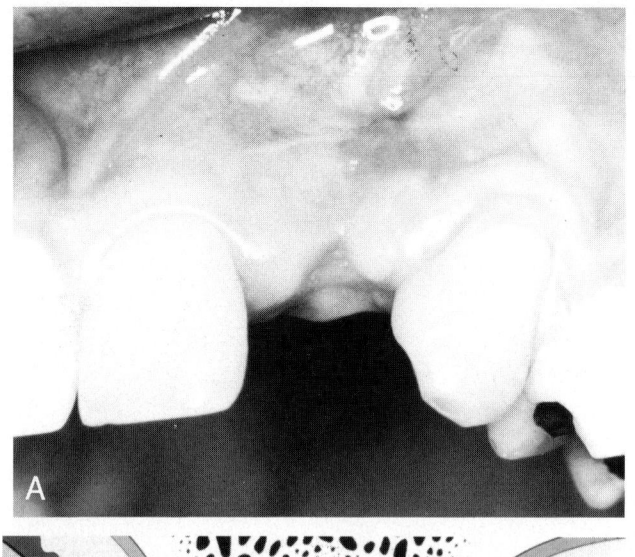

Fig. 13-23. Ridge Augmentation with GTAM and Stainless Steel Positioning Screws (ITI). **A,** Before treatment. **B, B′,** Diagrammatic and clinical views of palatal incision. **C, C′,** Flaps reflected.

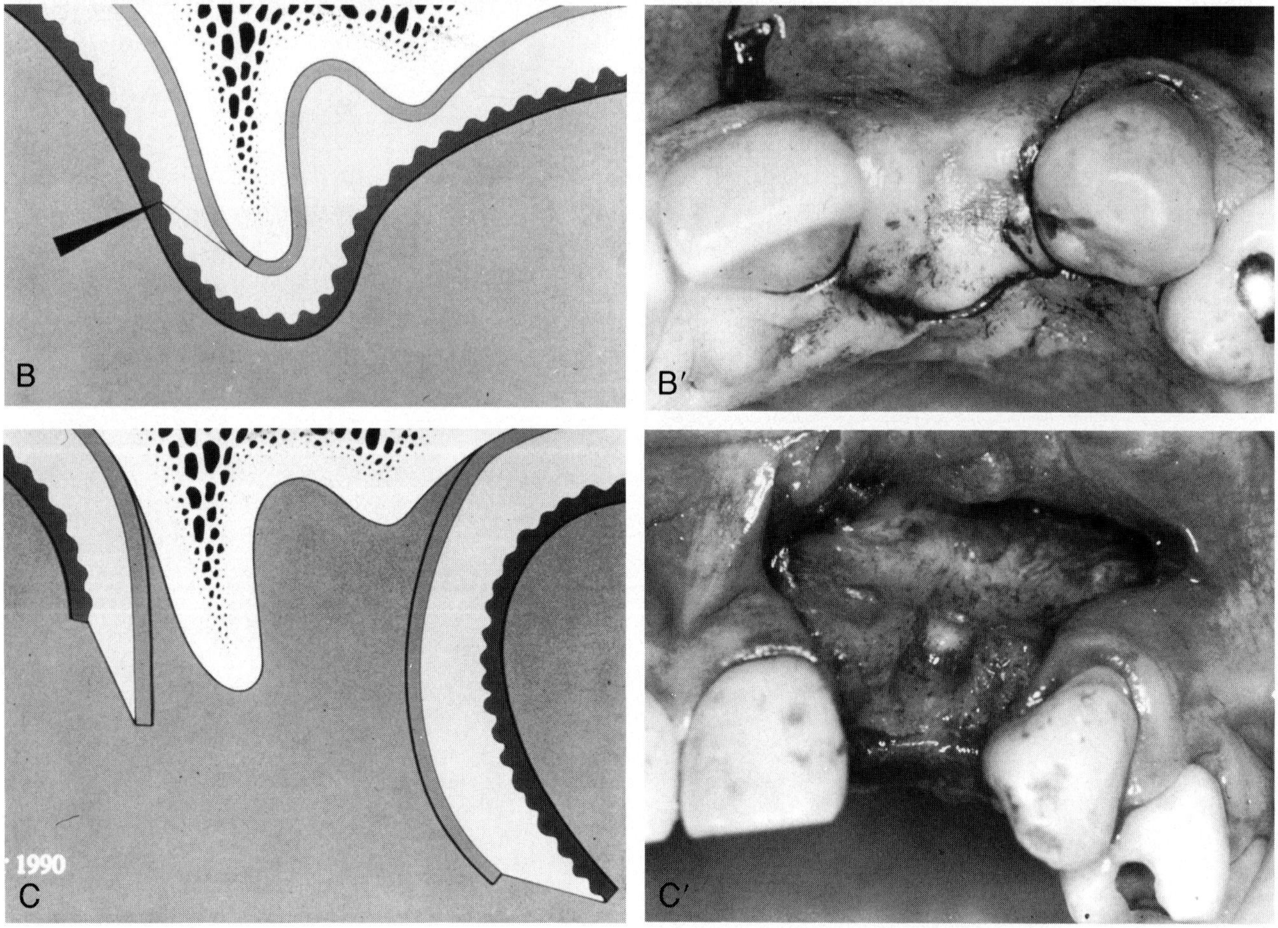

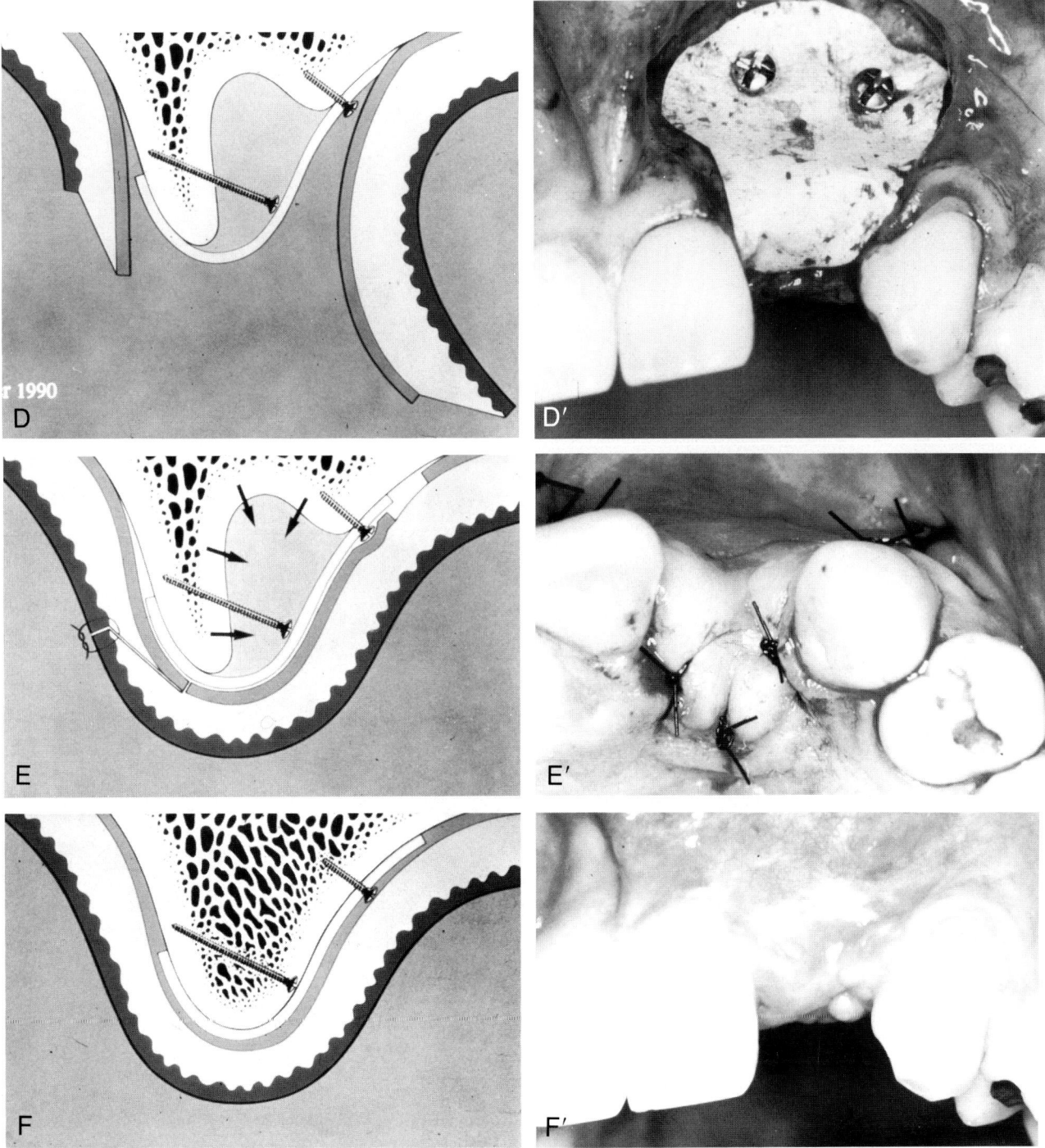

Fig. 13-23 (continued). **D, D'**, e-PTFE membrane positioned with stainless steel screws. **E, E'**, Flaps reapproximated and sutured. **F, F'**, Complete healing at 6 months.

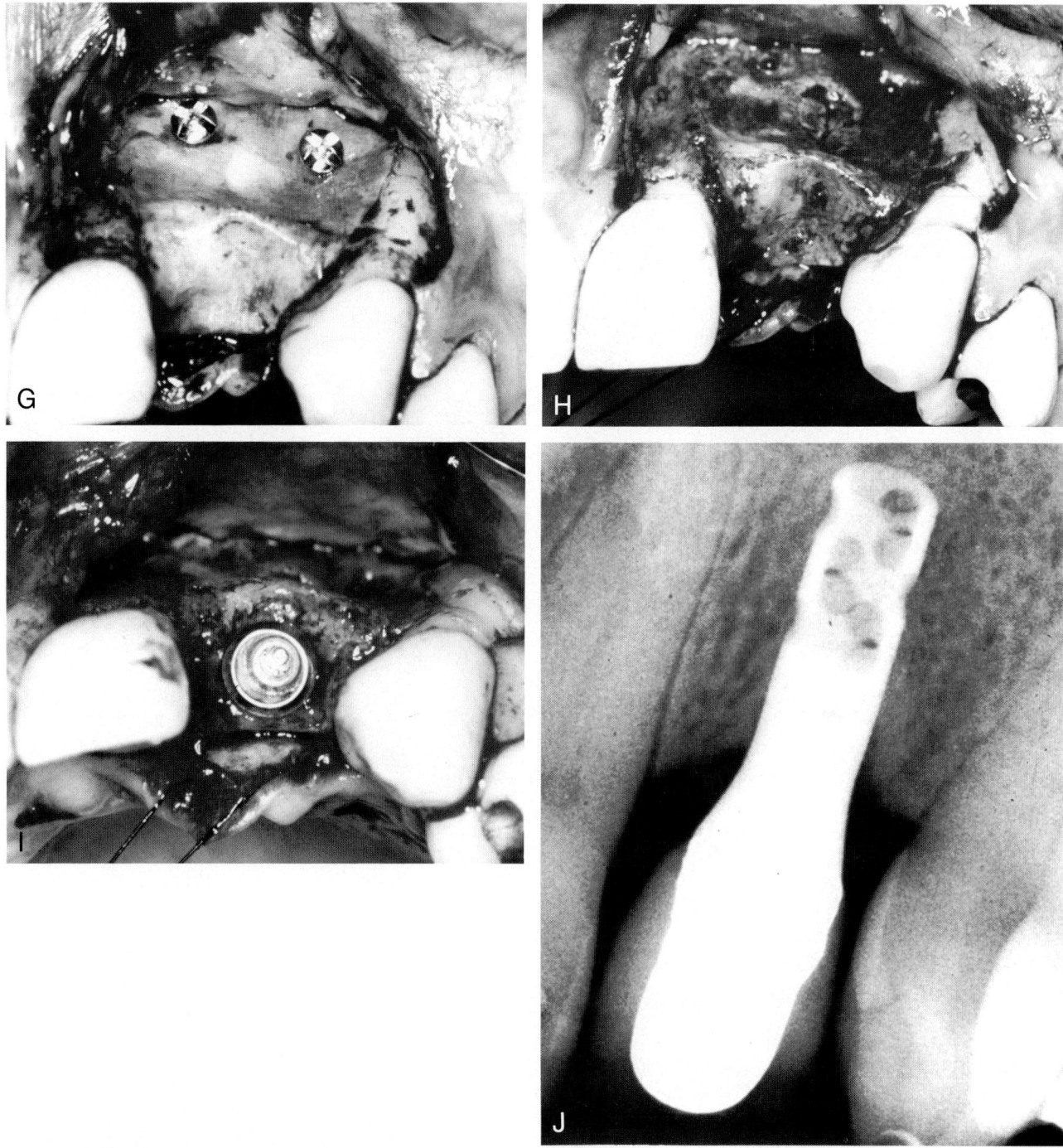

Fig. 13-23 (continued). **G,** Re-entry at 6 months showing membrane and screws. **H,** Membrane removed, exposing underlying bone. **I,** Implant properly positioned. **J,** X-ray study of case completed. (Contributed by Daniel Buser, Bern, Switzerland.)

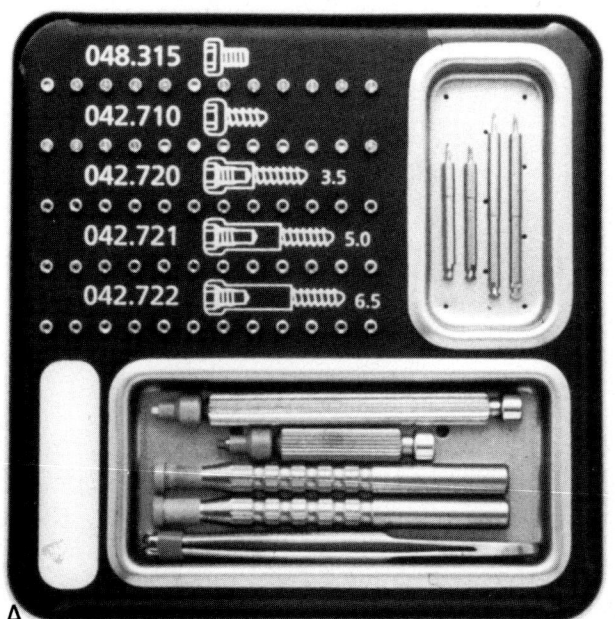
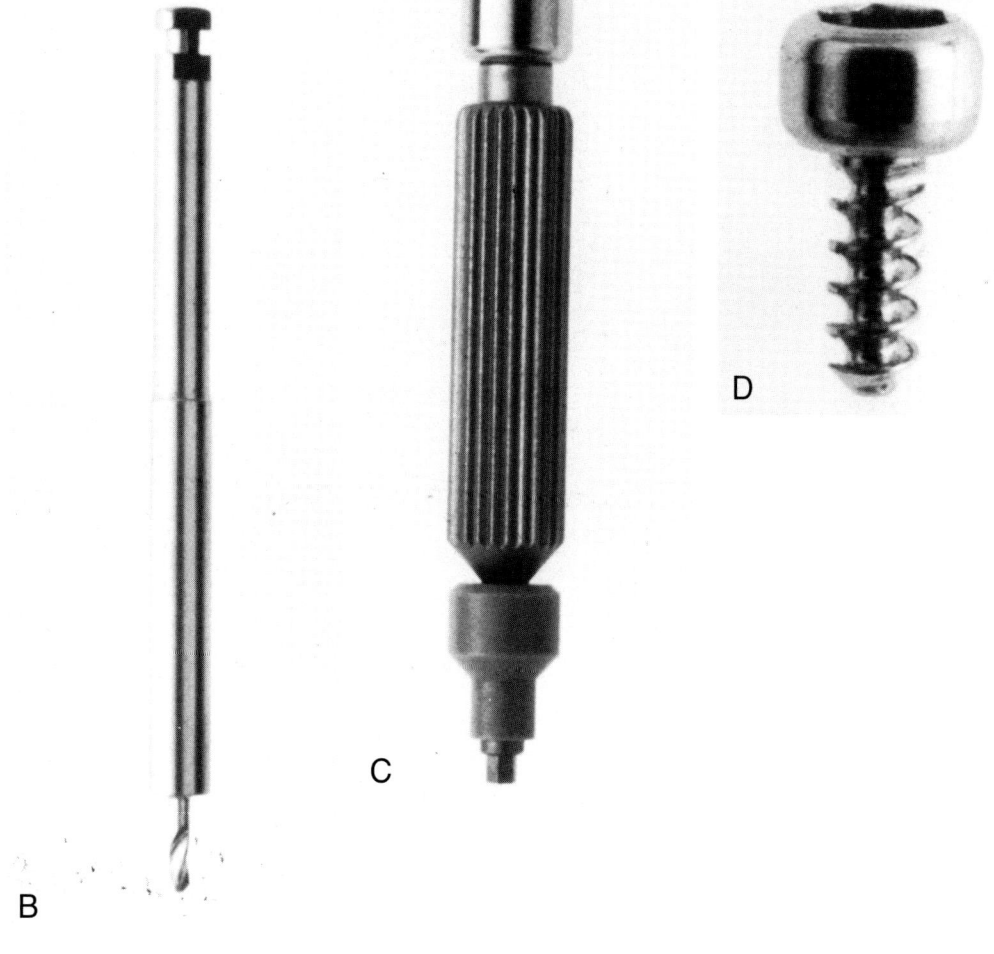

Fig. 13-24. Memfix-System Stainless Steel Bone Augmentation Kit. **A,** Complete kit. **B,** Drill. **C,** Screwdriver. **D,** Fixation screw.

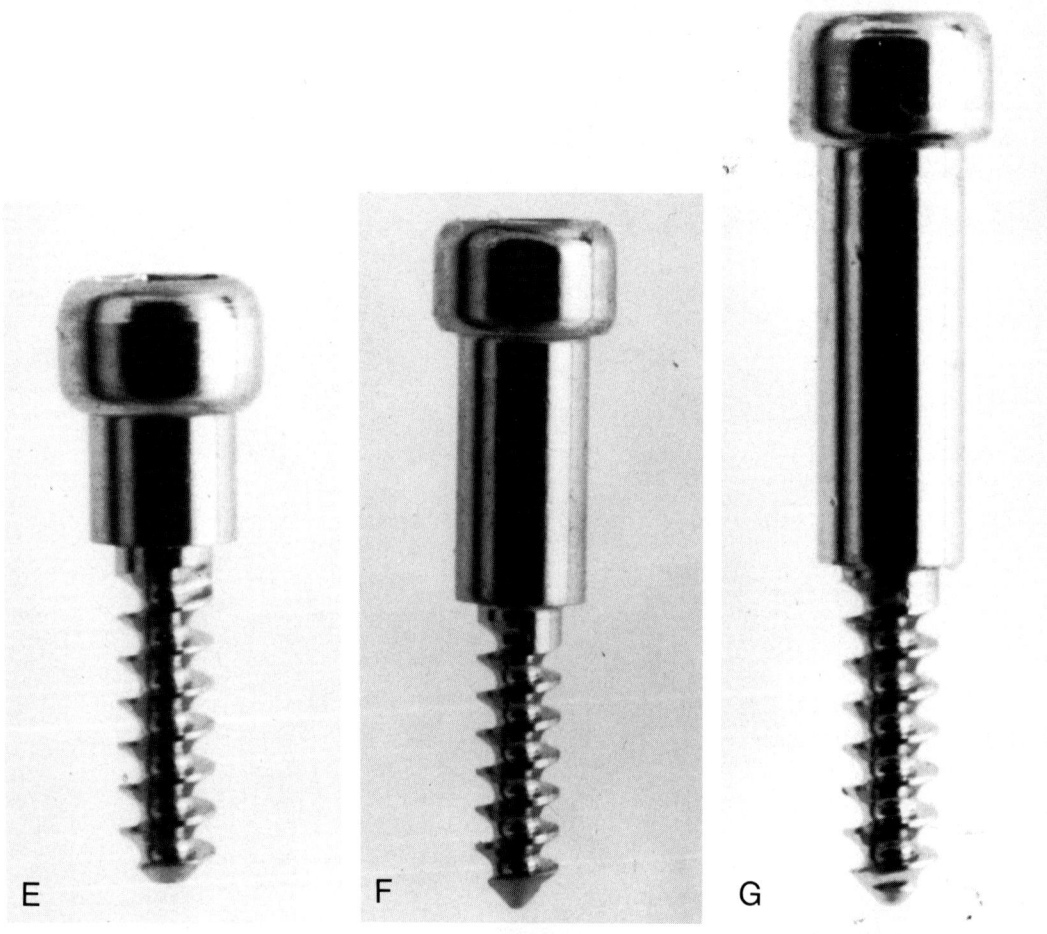

Fig. 13-24 (continued). **E, F, G,** Different sized spacing screws. (Contributed by ITT Straumann Company, Cambridge, MA.)

14

FURCATIONS

Multirooted teeth offer unique and challenging problems for the periodontist. The *furcation area,* because of the interrelationships between the size and shape of the teeth, the roots and their alveolar housing, and the varied nature and pattern of periodontal destruction, creates situations in which routine periodontal procedures are somewhat limited and special procedures are generally required. Waerhaug (1980) has shown that the best chance for success lies in early recognition and treatment.

DIAGNOSIS

Not counting the third molars, 24 potential furcations exist, and diagnosis is best made through use of radiography and clinical probing. Radiographs are not reliable when used by themselves. Most furcations can be detected clinically by probing with a No. 23 explorer or Nabers Nos. 1 and 2 curved probes (Fig. 14-1).

Diagnosis is made more difficult by certain anatomic factors. The trunk on the lingual aspect of the lower mandibular molars is longer than on the buccal aspect and greater on the second molar than on the first (Fig. 14-2A,B). The maxillary molars pose a special problem in that the mesial furcation, as opposed to the distal furcation, is located in the palatal third on the tooth (Fig. 14-2C). The mesial furcation can therefore be approached only from the palate. The distal furcation is higher than the mesial (Fig. 14-2D) and therefore more easily involved.

CLASSIFICATION

Newell (1981, 1984), in his reviews of the literature, notes that the classifications by Glickman (1958) Hamp, Nyman, and Lindhe (1975) and Lindhe (1983) are the most universally utilized. These classifications are based on horizontal loss of interradicular bone. To these, Newell adds one by Tarnow and Fletcher (1984), which is a subclassification, measuring vertical bone loss from the roof of the furcation.

1. Glickman (1958): Horizontal Classification
    Grade I   Incipient involvement into flute of furcation with suprabony pockets and no interradicular bone loss (Fig. 14-3A).
    Grade II   Any involvement of the interradicular bone without through-and-through probeability (Fig. 14-3A).
    Grade III Through-and-through loss of interradicular bone (Fig. 14-3B).
    Grade IV   Through-and-through loss of interradicular bone, with total exposure of furcation owing to gingival recession (Fig. 14-3C).
2. Lindhe (1983): Horizontal Classification
    Grade I   Loss of interradicular bone less than
    (initial) or equal to one-third (Fig. 14-4A).
    Grade II   Loss of interradicular bone greater
    (partial) than one-third but not through-and-through (Fig. 14-4B).
    Grade III Through-and-through loss of inter-
    (total)   radicular bone (Fig. 14-4C).
3. Tarnow and Fletcher (1984): Vertical Classification
    Grade A   Vertical loss of 1 to 3 mm
    Grade B   Vertical loss of 4 to 6 mm
    Grade C   Vertical loss of 7+ mm

For the purpose of clarity, the Lindhe classification (I, II, III) is used throughout the remainder of the text except where noted.

TREATMENT

Treatment is generally based on the nature and degree of furcation involvement. It is therefore important to understand which classification is being used in discussing treatment. The major classifications and the generally accepted modalities of treatment are outlined in Table 14-1. It is to be used only as a guide, because treatment selection varies according to the following considerations:

1. Size, shape, and divergence of roots
2. Size of crown
3. Length of root trunk (distance between cementoenamel junction and furcation area)
4. Crown–root ratio
5. Amount of remaining bone support

Scaling and Curettage, Gingivectomy, Odontoplasty

These procedures are used for incipient lesions where no interradicular bone involvement exists (Grade I, Glickman) and pockets are suprabony. Treatment is therefore limited to pocket reduction, gingivectomy, and possibly to reshaping of tooth structure, *odontoplasty* (Goldman, 1958), to widen the narrow furca entrance.

Furcation Plasty—Odontoplasty and Osteoplasty

Hamp, Nyman, and Lindhe (1975) described *furcation plasty* as raising a mucoperiosteal flap to provide access to the furcation area, and combining scaling and root planing, osteoplasty, and odontoplasty to remove local irritants and to open the furcation to allow the patient access to clean and maintain the area. The result should be a firm, well-contoured papilla to cover the interradicular space. This procedure is recommended for Grade I and early Grade II lesions (Figs. 14-5 and 14-6).

Odontoplasty should be used judiciously because it can result in hypersensitivity and possible pulpal involvement. Osteoplasty and ostectomy should also be performed cautiously to minimize the risk of further loss of attachment.

Grafting

The furcation area is characterized by defects, the walls of which are made primarily of tooth structure. Therefore, although the area is capable of holding a graft, it has little or no vascularity to support one. For this reason, the success of grafts is limited in furcations (Sepe et al., 1978; Saunders et al., 1983). Grafts may be indicated where the destruction of the furcation is only partial or where deep vertical lesions have still left some bone on the inner aspects of the roots.

Tunnel Preparation

Tunnel preparation is the surgical exposure of the furcation, which is indicated for advanced Grade II and Grade III lesions in which resection is not possible. It requires roots that are long and divergent and is generally indicated for the mandibular molars. It often fails because of decay in the furcation area (Lindhe, 1983).

Table 14-1. Classification and Treatment of Furcations

Glickman (1958)	I	II		III or IV
Lindhe (1983)	—	I	II	III
Tarnow (1984)	—	A, B, or C	A, B, or C	A, B, or C
Treatment	Scaling and root planing Gingivectomy Odontoplasty	Odontoplasty* Osteoplasty*† Root resection	Odontoplasty* Osteoplasty*† Root resection Tunnel preparation Grafting GTR‡ Flap and Ca Extraction	Root resection Tunnel preparation Grafting GTR‡ Extraction

*When done together, termed furcation plasty.
†Osteoplasty is used here to mean both osteoplasty and ostectomy.
‡Guided tissue regeneration.

Hellden et al. (1989) recently studied the long-termed prognosis of tunnel preparations on 149 teeth, with a range of 10 to 107 months (mean prognosis was 37.5 months). They showed that 75% were still caries free, 6.7% (10 teeth) were extracted, 4% (7 teeth) were hemisected, and 15.4% (23 teeth) showed initial or established caries. They concluded that teeth with tunnel preparations have a considerably better prognosis than that previously reported (Figs. 14-3C and 14-7).

Root Resection

This procedure involves removing one or more roots from a multirooted tooth. Proper tooth selection is important for success. The ideal tooth is one with well-developed long roots that have adequate divergence and a narrow root trunk. The furcation area should have a good deal of remaining bone, and the remaining roots should have adequate support and a favorable crown–root ratio (Fig. 14-8).

Indications

The following situations can be solved only by removal of one or more roots or extraction of the tooth. Extraction is not always desirable, especially if the tooth is a terminal abutment.
1. Grade II and Grade III lesions
2. Advanced decay
3. Severe gingival recession on a single root
4. Close root proximity with minimal interseptal bone (commonly seen between the maxillary first and second molars), preventing adequate embrasure space, as in the case of prosthetic restorations
5. Endodontic failure
6. Inability to perform endodontic therapy
7. Tooth fracture
8. Extensive root caries
9. Root resorption
10. Root perforation
11. Severe vertical bone loss about one or more roots

Contraindications

Success, as is failure, is based generally on tooth selection, and for this reason, preoperative evaluation is critical (Fig. 14-9).
1. Teeth with a poor crown–root ratio on remaining roots
2. Inadequate bone support on roots to be retained
3. Unfavorable roof anatomy of retained teeth
4. Long tooth trunks
5. Fused roots
6. Extensive webbing between roots
7. Bell-shaped crowns
8. Teeth in which endodontic treatment and restoration are not possible on the remaining roots
9. Poor surgical access
10. Inability to perform oral hygiene procedures
11. Poor form of remaining roots
12. Splinting is not possible
13. Severe vertical bone loss internally

Disadvantage

Need for additional complex restorative procedures.

Considerations

In considering which roots to remove, certain anatomic factors should be taken into consideration. The mesial buccal root of the maxillary first and second molars, although larger than the distal root, tends to have a deep concavity. This concavity makes prosthetic preparation and maintenance difficult. This is not true of the distal root, which is round or ovoid (Fig. 14-10).

When both the mesial and distal furcations are involved, a palatal root amputation should be considered if the buccal furcation is intact. This is because the palatal root has an unfavorable axial inclination as well as an unfavorable prosthetic relationship with the first bicuspid.

The mesial root of the mandibular molars, although larger, has two canals and a deep concavity, in contrast to the distal root, which has one canal and is ovoid. The distal root is easier to prepare prosthetically and involves a lesser chance of endodontic failure. Use of the distal root requires a bridge; this is not the case when using the mesial root (Fig. 14-11).

TERMINOLOGY

The two basic types of sectioning are *tooth sectioning,* which is defined as the division of the tooth into its individual roots, and *root resection* or *root amputation,* which is the removal of one or more roots from a tooth. Mandibular molars are usually treated by *hemisection* with or without root removal, whereas maxillary molars are generally treated by root amputation.

Both procedures may be carried out as *vital* or *nonvital* procedures. If vital sectioning is employed, provisions for final endodontic therapy should be made.

All tooth sectioning procedures require the use of buccal and lingual (palatal) flaps for access and visibility both for sectioning and osseous surgery. *Osseous surgery should always be performed at the time of sectioning.*

MANDIBULAR MOLAR FURCATIONS

Hemisection Procedure

With the patient under anesthesia, probing for the nature and extent of the furcation involvement and the outline of the surrounding osseous topography is completed prior to surgery. A mucoperiosteal flap is elevated buccolingually.

It is often convenient to draw a straight line in pencil on the tooth from both the buccal and lingual furcations to the occlusal surface where they are joined. The line is drawn with the same axial inclination as the tooth. This gives the clinician a perspective on sectioning the tooth, especially if the molar is tilted.

Using a friction-grip No. 701L enamel shaver or tapered No. 700 bur, the tooth is sectioned in a buccolingual direction. The initial cuts are made by starting at the furcation entrance and drawing the bur outward and upward along the pencil lines.

The sectioning is continued until the buccal and lingual grooves are joined together. A thin piece of the pulpal floor is still intact in the furcation area. *Note: High-speed burs should not be used on the thin pulpal floor for fear of damaging the remaining furcal bone.*

Using a dulled No. 4 rounded bur in a slow handpiece, the roof of the furcation is carefully perforated. A small chisel can then be placed in this area for final separation.

If one of the roots is to be removed, that is done, and the final tooth contouring in the furcation area is completed. Attention must be paid to removing any residual spurs of pulpal floor left attached to the root or undercuts and checking for and removing any *residual internal* furcations. *Without this final contouring, failure may result.*

Osseous surgery is completed by removing the residual internal osseous crater on the mesial or distal aspect of the remaining root. The broad residual ridge is now thinned buccolingually to facilitate pontic placement and plaque control. The distal root in general has a lower mesial bone level than the distal aspect of the approximating premolar or cuspid. This will often necessitate a leveling of the ridge. Some marginal bone may have to be removed for the final *positive* bony architecture.

The procedure is shown clinically in Figures 14-12, 14-13, and 14-14. If both roots are periodontally sound once hemisected, they can be separated orthodontally and used individually or splinted together (Fig. 14-15).

MAXILLARY FURCATIONS

Root Amputation Procedure

The maxillary molars and bicuspids are most often treated by root amputation and root resection, respectively. Tooth sectioning is generally used only in advanced periodontal and prosthetic cases.

Majzoub and Kon (1992) recently showed that in 86% of the distobuccal root resections in maxillary first molars, there was insufficient biologic width (<2.04 mm) remaining after tooth preparation.

In Figures 14-16A and 14-16A', the maxillary molar has severe bone loss about the the mesiobuccal root that requires root amputation. A mucoperiosteal flap is elevated buccally and palatally prior to starting.

The first step involves the use of a No. 4 or No. 6 round bur for removal of the bone overlying the affected root. This will facilitate the horizontal sectioning of the root below the fornix of the furcation, thus avoiding damage to the adjacent tooth structures (Figs. 14-16B and 14-16B').

In Figures 14-16C and 14-16C', a No. 7016 friction-grip enamel shaver or tapered diamond bur is used to section the root with a perpendicular or oblique cut, which is begun below the most coronal level of the furcation. The sectioning is completed in stages, each time a curved explorer is used to check for total separation. To prevent damage to adjacent roots, toothpicks or orthodontic wire are sometimes inserted into the open furcations to act as stops or guides.

An oblique cut is now made near the CEJ and angled into the initial cut (Figs. 14-16D and 14-16D'). This will facilitate the removal of the root tip and increase access to and visibility of the internal furcation.

The root is gently elevated with a small elevator (Figs. 14-16E and 14-16E'). Using the same bur, the remaining tooth structure in the furcation is smoothed to prevent any overhangs, and the coronal portion of the tooth is blended in (Figs. 14-16F and 14-16F').

Under direct visualization, the final osseous contouring is determined. Rosenberg (1988) recommends the following osseous management after a root amputation or trisection procedure:

1. Elimination of the residual bony ledge that extends into the exposed furcation to the facial plate at the root extraction site (Fig. 14-16F')

2. Removal of part of the facial plate in the extraction site so as to form a vertical groove (Figs. 14-16F and 14-16F')
3. Reduction of the facial lingual width of the interdental septum in the area of the extraction
4. Removal of any residual craters on the internal aspects of the remaining roots
5. Odontoplasty for elimination of internal furcations (Figs. 14-18F and 14-18G)
6. Osteoplasty and ostectomy for establishing final positive physiologic form with adjacent teeth

The final contour will allow a normal parabolic gingival form and will be open enough to permit adequate plaque control procedures (Figs. 14-16H and 14-16H'). The procedure is outlined clinically in Figures 14-17, 14-18, 14-19, 14-20, and 14-21.

Common Reasons for Failure

1. Root fracture because of
   a. Lack of conservative endodontic treatment—overinstrumentation
   b. Failure to restore teeth adequately with posts and crowns
   c. Inadequate provisional or final splinting for stabilization
2. Poor tooth selection
3. Incomplete sectioning
4. Failure to diagnose involvement of other furcations
5. Failure to correct osseous deformities, resulting in residual pockets
6. Failure to remove residual furcations
7. Inability to maintain an adequate level of oral physiotherapy about adjacent furcations

PERIODONTAL–ENDODONTAL PROBLEMS

Patients often have a large radiolucent furcation area, which to all appearances presents a periodontal problem. The tooth should be checked for possible endodontic involvement, and the rest of the mouth should also be examined to see if the finding is consistent with the patient's overall periodontal situation.

If this is a solitary lesion or the tooth has a large or recent restoration, an endodontic problem should be considered even if the tooth tests vital. Many accessory canals exist in the furcation area (some investigators report up to a 76% incidence), which are open to secondary pulpal involvement as periodontal inflammation moves apically. Generally, in cases of primary pulpal disease, endodontic therapy will resolve the problem (Figs. 14-22 and 14-23).

If periodontal therapy is attempted first, regeneration via endodontic therapy will be limited, if it occurs at all. Differential diagnosis is therefore very important.

The differential diagnosis of periodontal and pulpal disease is shown in Table 14-2.

Table 14-2. Differential Diagnosis of Periodontal and Pulpal Disease

Clinical	Pulpal	Periodontal
Age	Any	Older
Pain		
Presence	Yes	Sometimes
Quality	Sharp	Dull
Location	Localized	Diffuse
Pulp vitality	No	Yes
Tooth Mobility	No	Yes
Pocketing	No	Deep pockets about tooth
Fistula	Submarginal	Fistula leads to periodontal pocket
Probability		
Furcation	No	Yes
Radiolucency	No	Yes
Radiographic		
Interproximal bone loss	No	Yes
Furcation area	Yes	Yes
Apical radiolucency	Yes	No

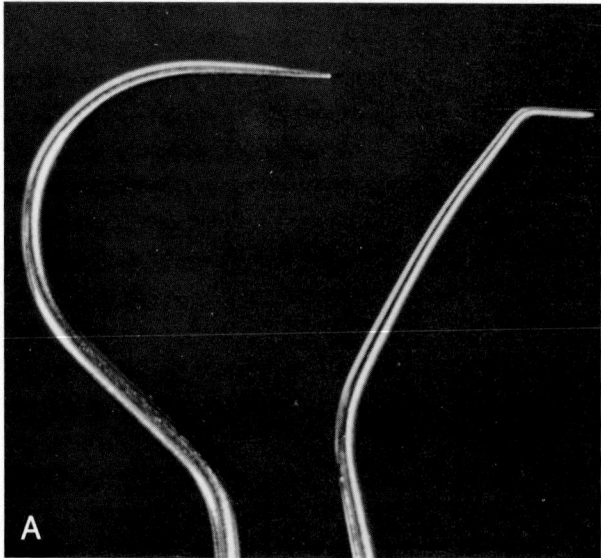
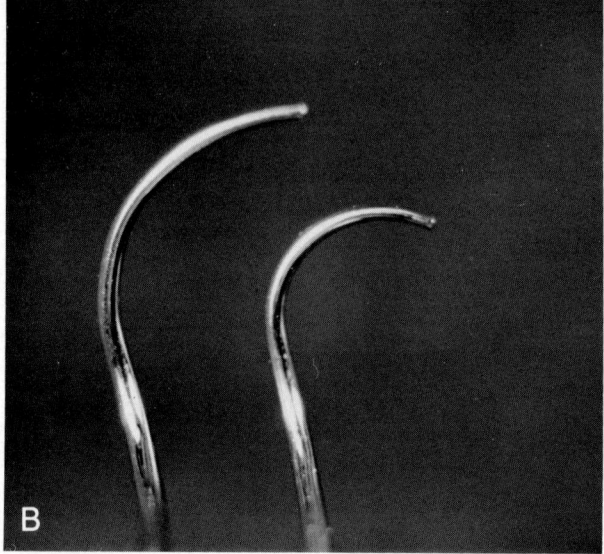

Fig. 14-1. Instruments Used for Furcation Deflection. **A,** No. 23 explorer. **B,** Nabers No. 1 and No. 2 curved probes.

Furcations

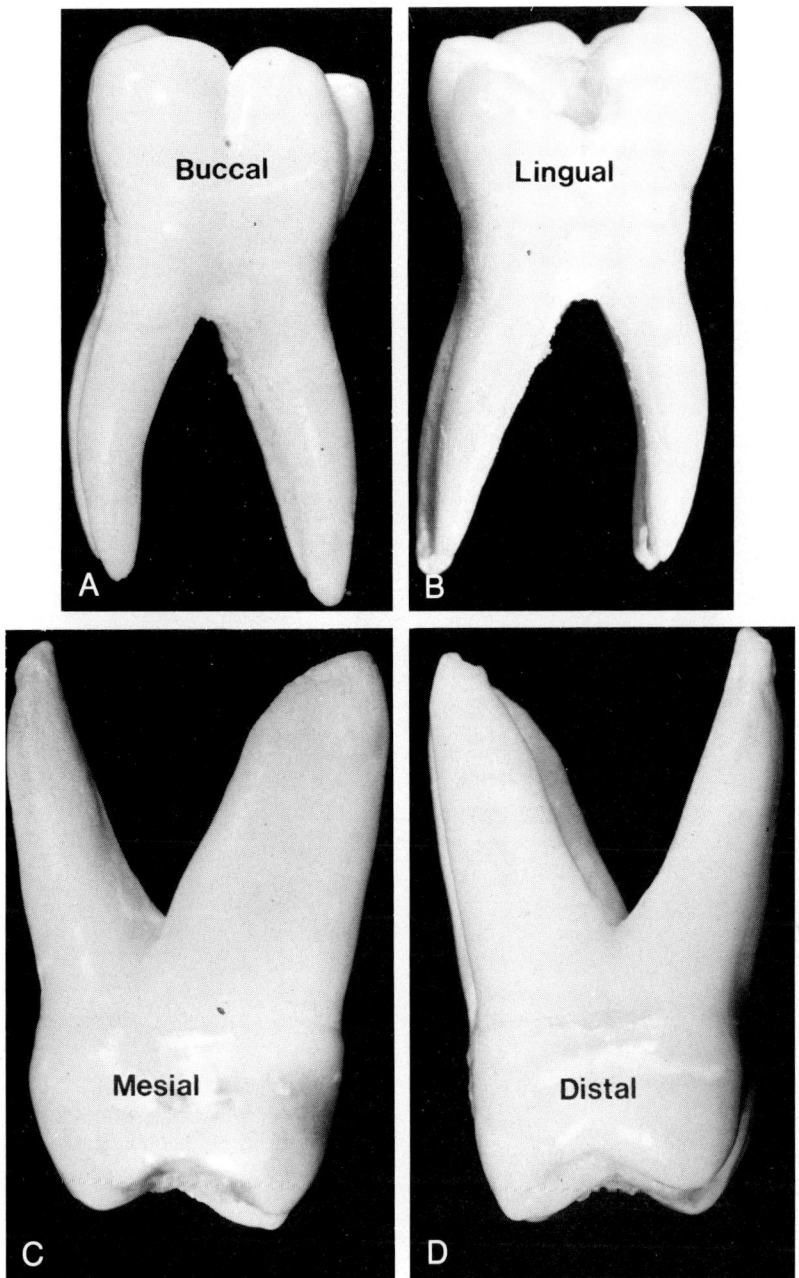

Fig. 14-2. Mandibular and Maxillary Molars. **A, B,** Buccal and lingual views of mandibular molar, showing that furcation is longer on the lingual than on the buccal aspect. **C, D,** Mesial and distal views of maxillary molar, showing mesial furcation to be palatal and the mesial root to be broader. Note that mesial and distal roots are as long as the palatal root.

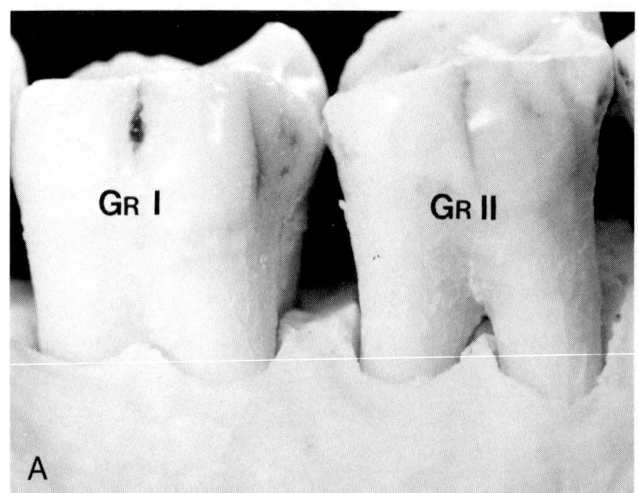
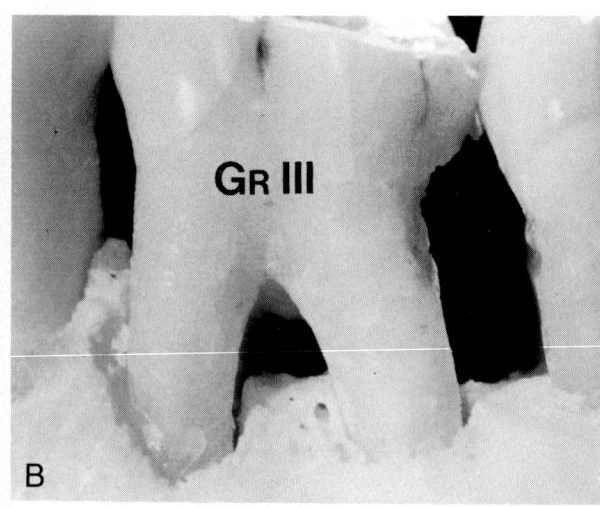
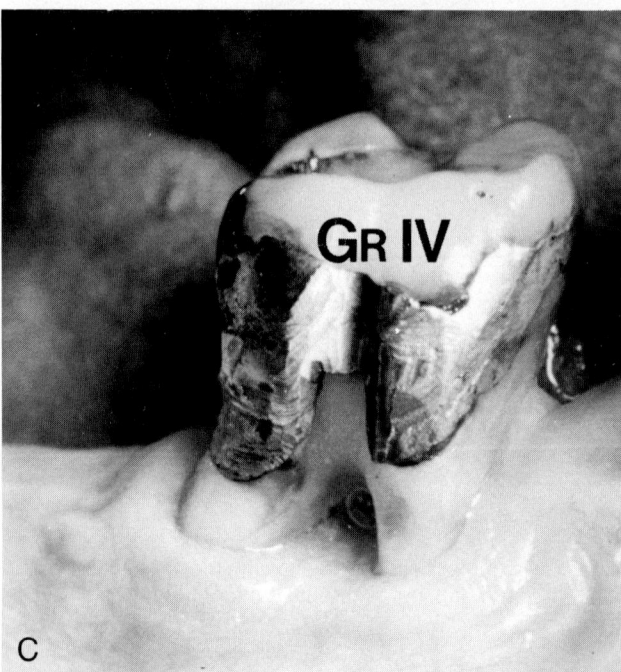

Fig. 14-3. Glickman Furcation Classification. **A,** Grade I and Grade II furcations. **B,** Grade III furcation. **C,** Grade IV furcation.

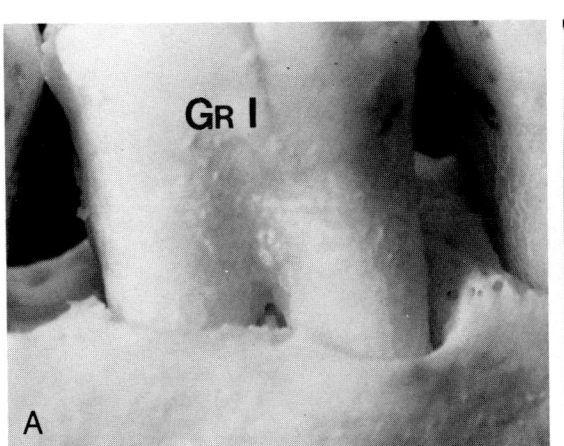
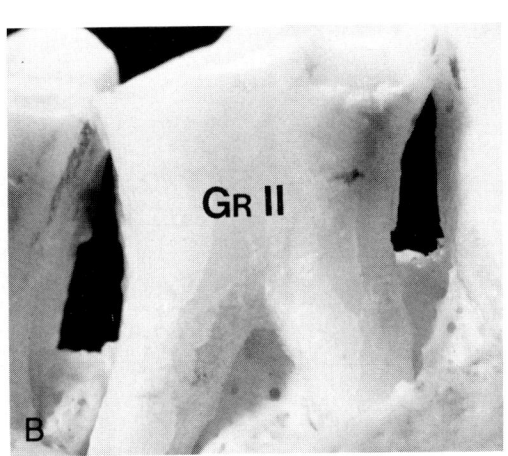
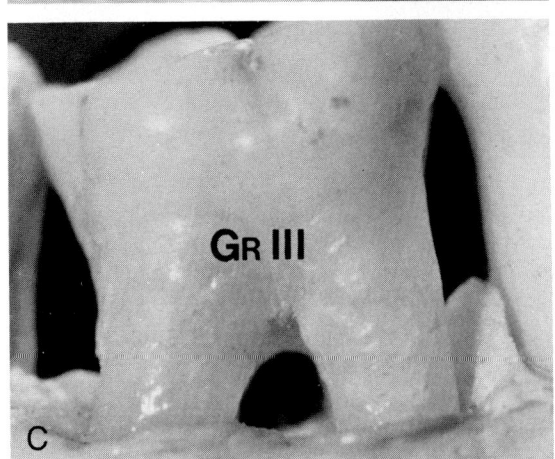

Fig. 14-4. Lindhe Furcation Classification. **A,** Grade I furcation. **B,** Grade II furcation. **C,** Grade III furcation.

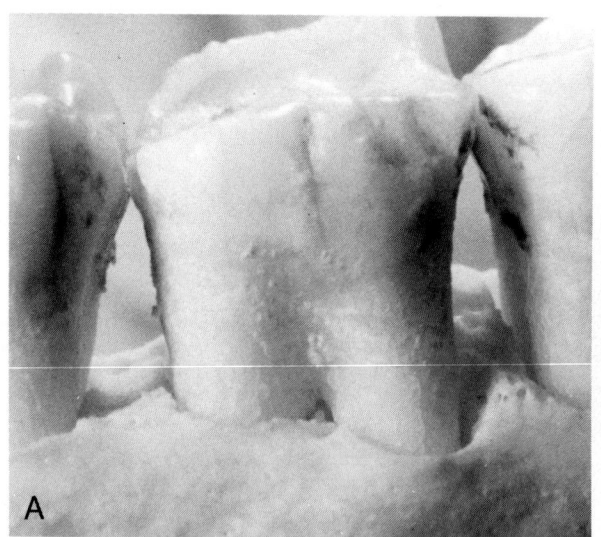
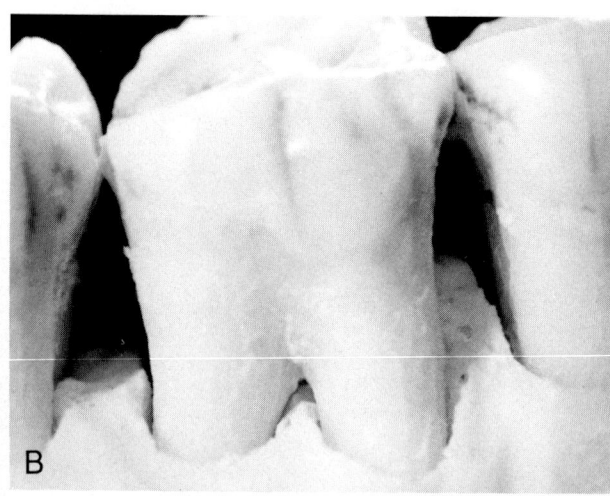
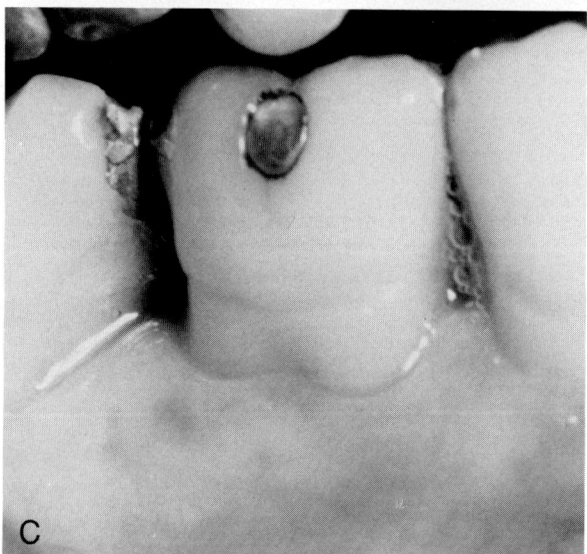

Fig. 14-5. Furcation Plasty of Grade I Furcation (Lindhe). **A,** Prior to treatment. **B,** Osteoplasty and ostectomy completed. **C,** Clinical representation of completed case. Note contour of tissue in furcation.

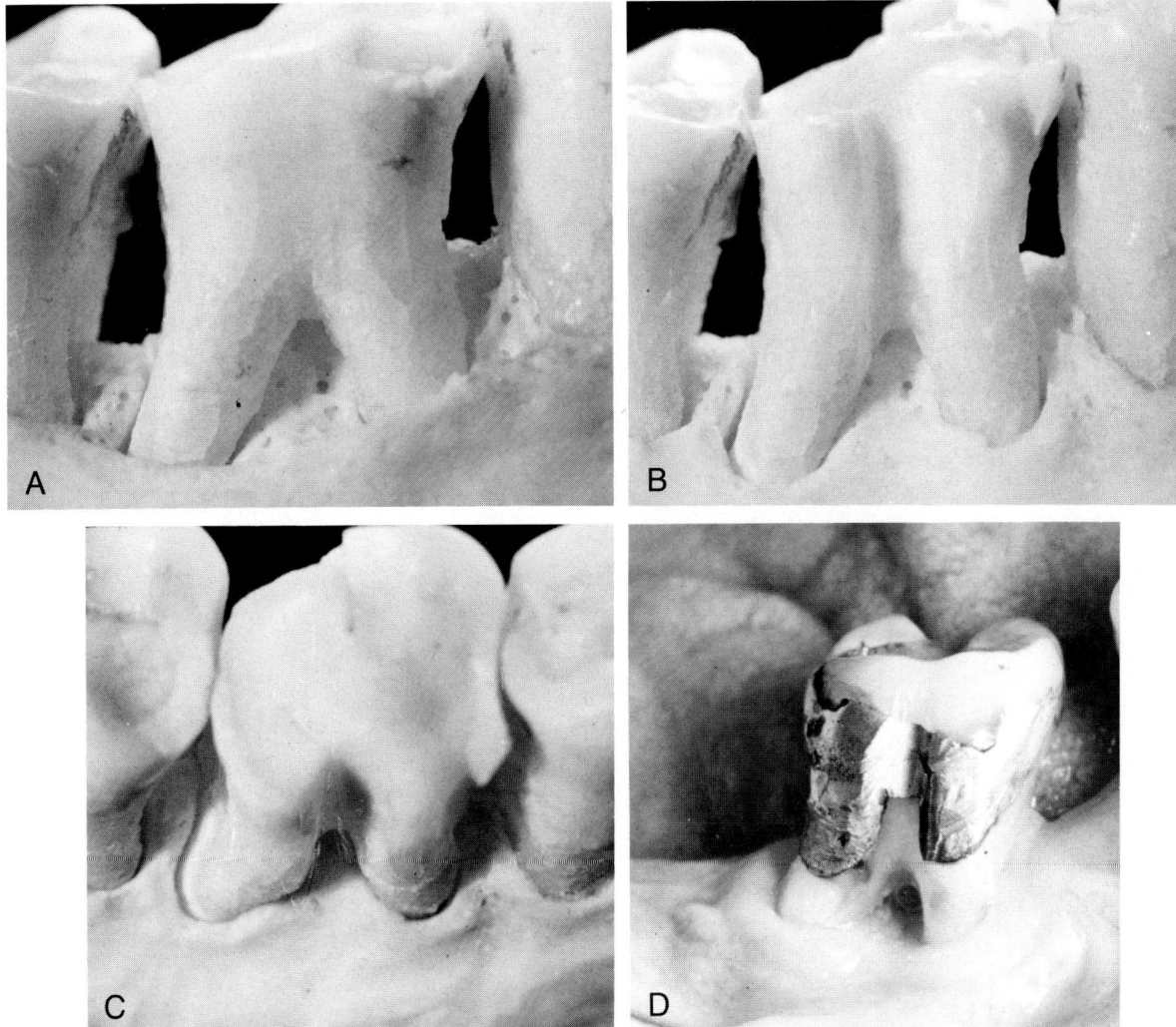

Fig. 14-6. Furcation Plasty of Grade II Furcation. **A,** Before treatment. **B,** Osteoplasty and odontoplasty completed. **C,** Occlusal view, showing extent of osteoplasty. **D,** Clinical representation of healed furcation plasty.

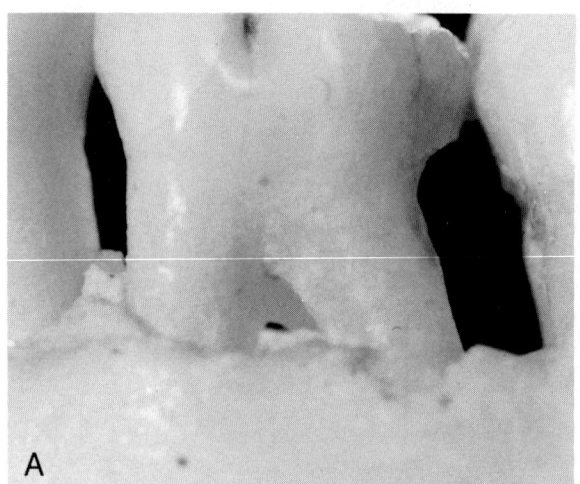
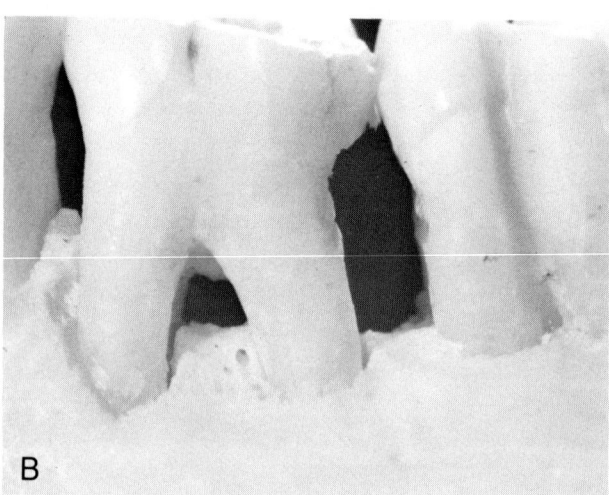
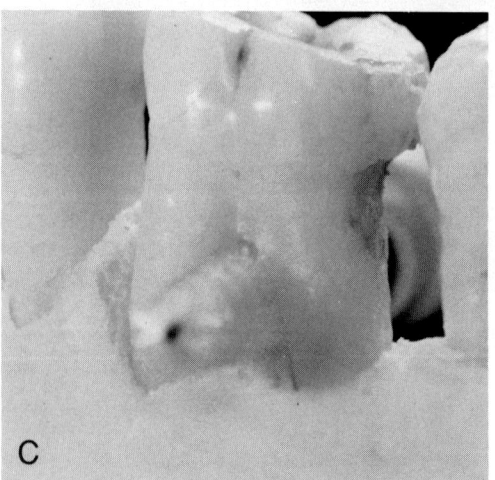

Fig. 14-7. Tunnel Preparation. **A,** Grade III furcation prior to correction. **B,** Tunnel preparation completed. **C,** Small interdental brush is inserted into and through the furcation to show that the inner portion of the furcation can be cleaned.

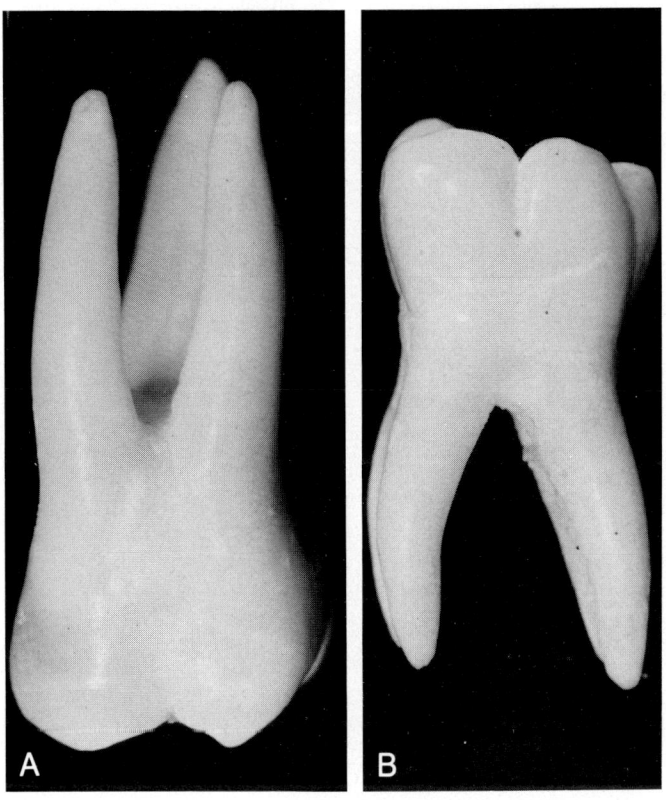

Fig. 14-8. Root Resection—Proper Tooth Selection. **A, B,** Maxillary and mandibular teeth showing adequate root length and divergence with narrow trunk and excellent crown–root ratio.

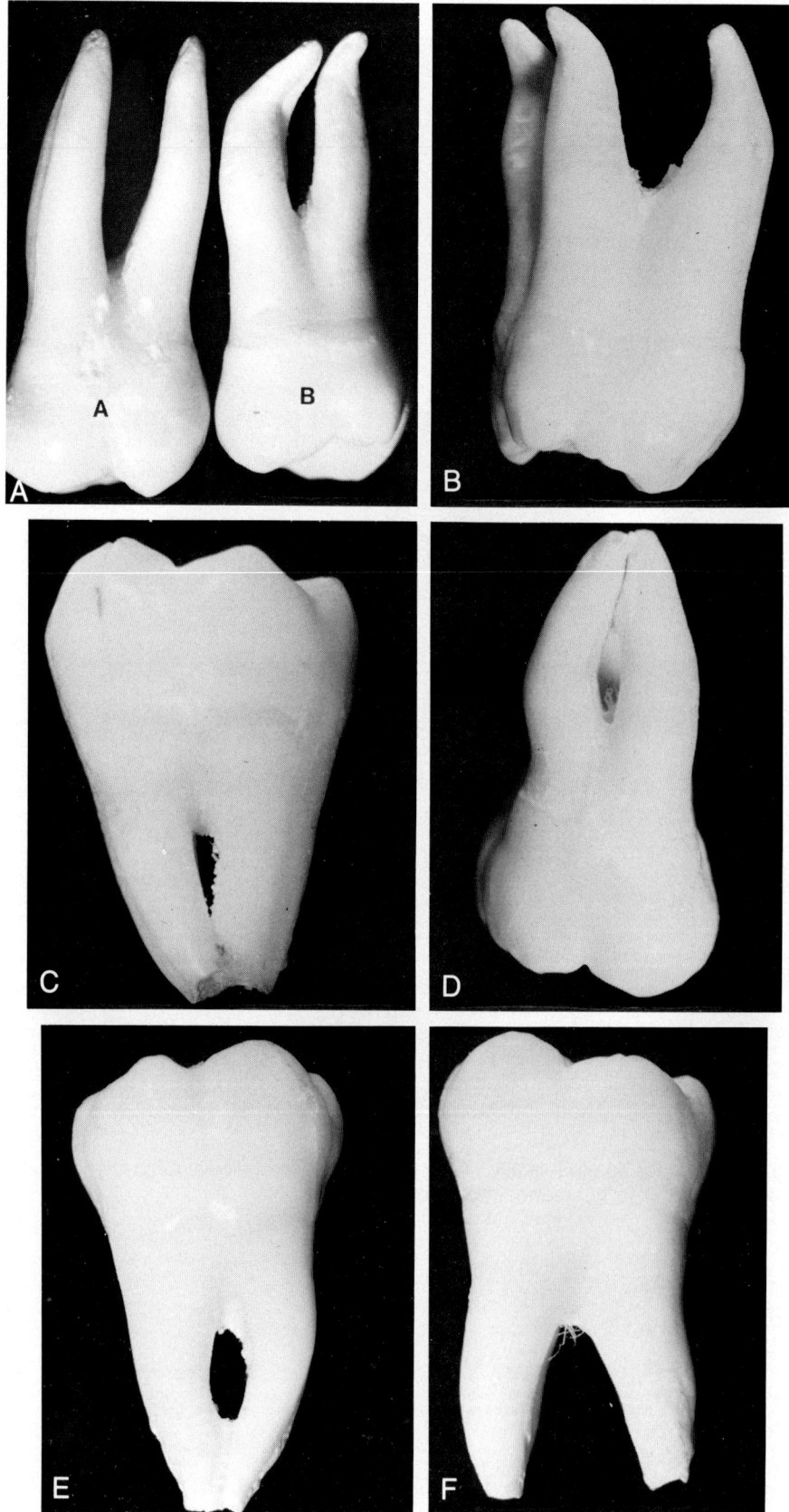

Fig. 14-9. Contraindications for Root Resection. **A,** Maxillary molar A with ideal crown–root relationship. Molar B has too long a root trunk and curved roots. **B,** Root trunk too long. **C,** Unfavorable crown–root ratio. Bell-shaped crown. **D,** Fused maxillary buccal roots. **E,** Fused mandibular roots. **F,** Roots too short.

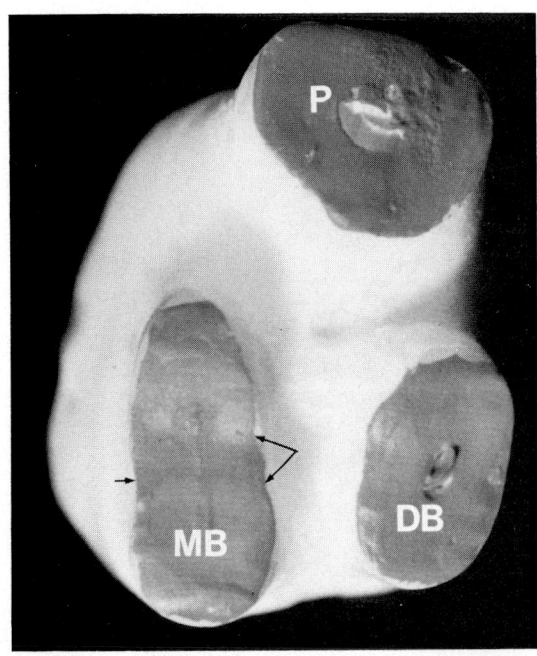

Fig. 14-10. Cross Section of Maxillary Molar. Arrows indicate concavities usually found on mesial root which make restoration more difficult.

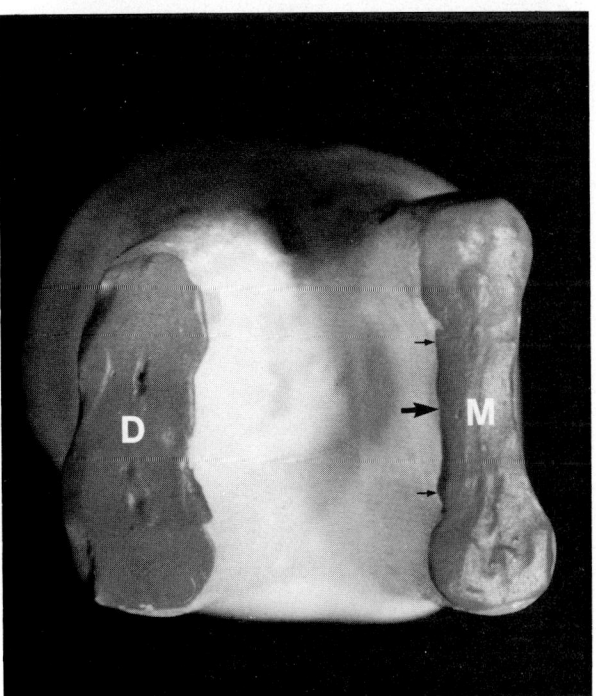

Fig. 14-11. Cross Section of Mandibular Molar. Arrows point to mesial concavity on mesial root which makes prosthetic treatment difficult.

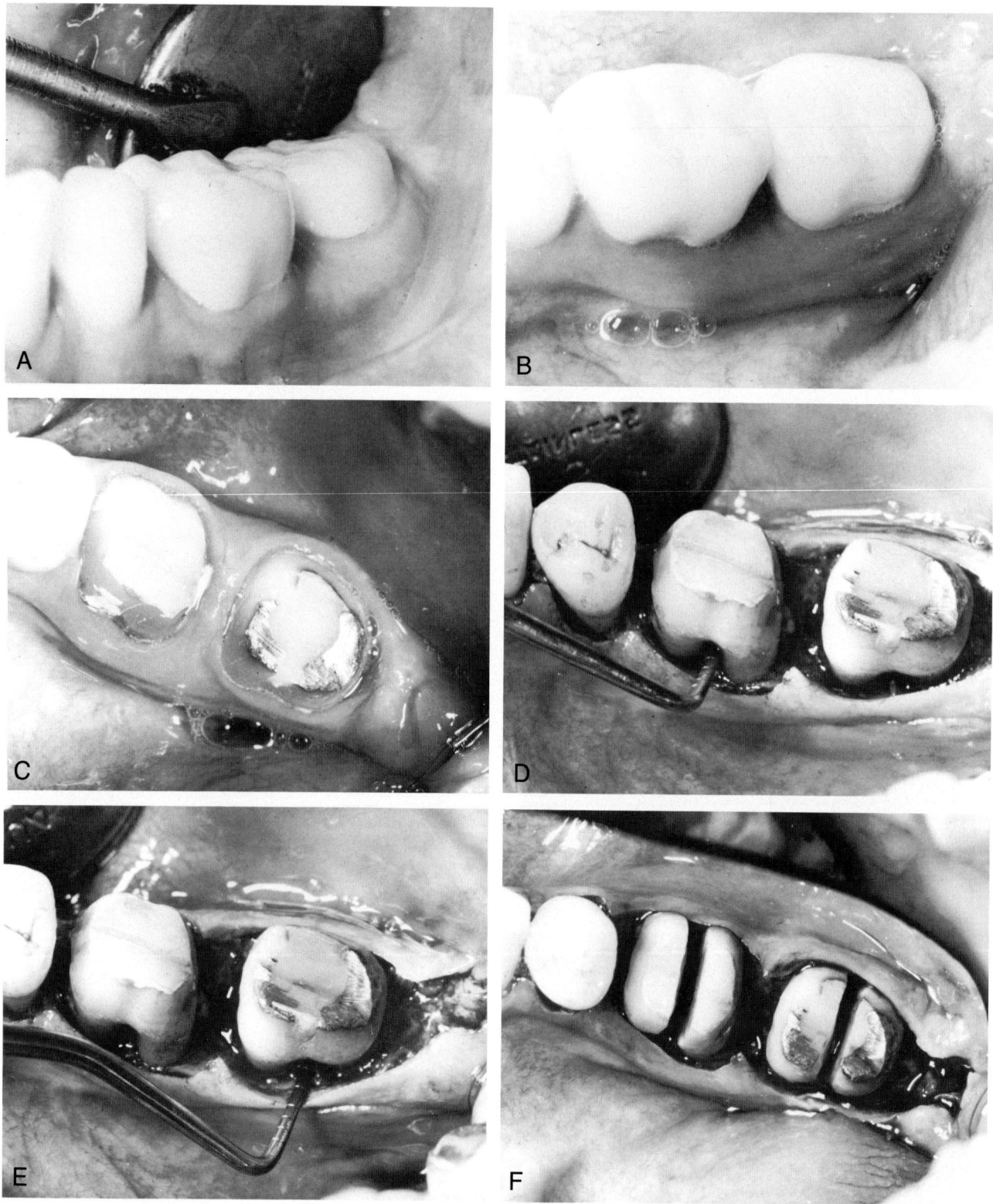

Fig. 14-12. Mandibular Hemisection. **A, B,** Buccal and lingual views prior to treatment. **C,** Temporary crowns removed. **D, E,** Periodontal probes positioned to show deep Grade II furcations. **F,** Occlusal view of teeth sectioned.

Furcations

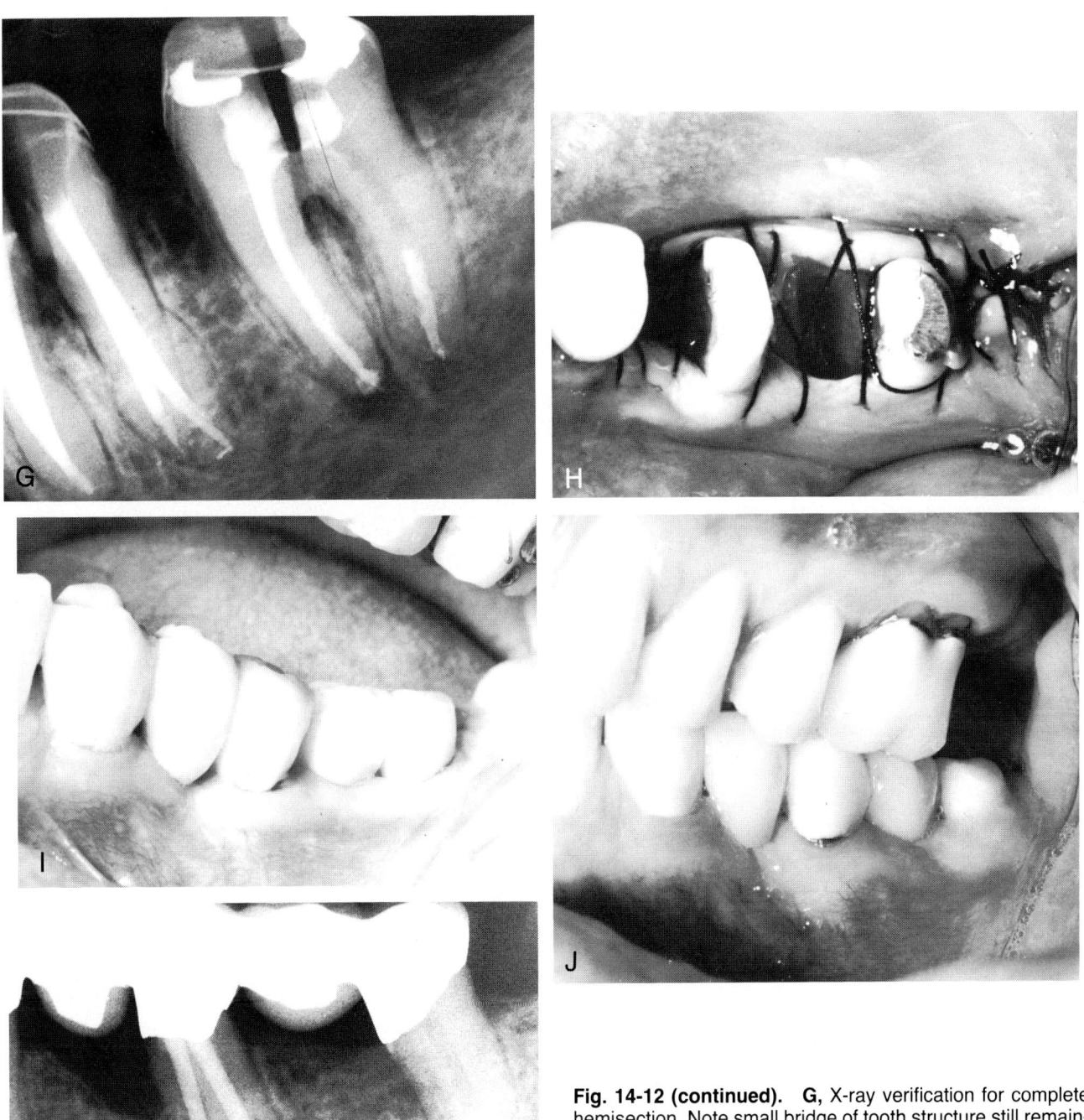

Fig. 14-12 (continued). **G,** X-ray verification for complete hemisection. Note small bridge of tooth structure still remaining on second molar. **H,** Mesial roots removed, teeth prepared, internal furcation contoured, osseous surgery completed, and flaps apically positioned. **I,** Temporization. **J,** Five years later; case complete. **K,** Final x-ray study 5 years later.

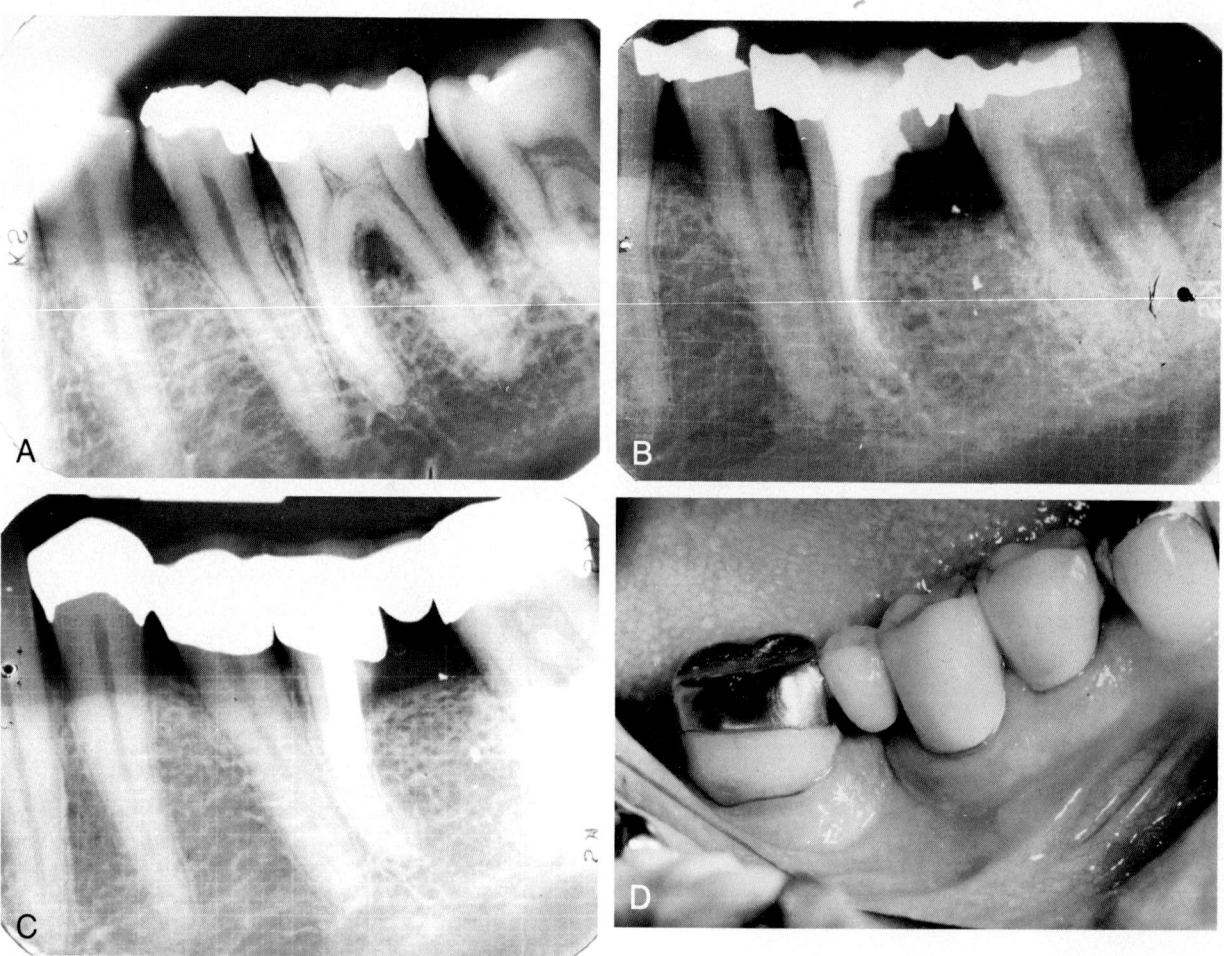

Fig. 14-13. Mandibular Hemisection. **A,** Pretreatment x-ray study showing severe involvement of distal root. **B,** Hemisection completed. **C, D,** Six years later, restoration is complete and bone has filled in about remaining root. (Prosthetics done by Dr. William Irving, Needham, MA.)

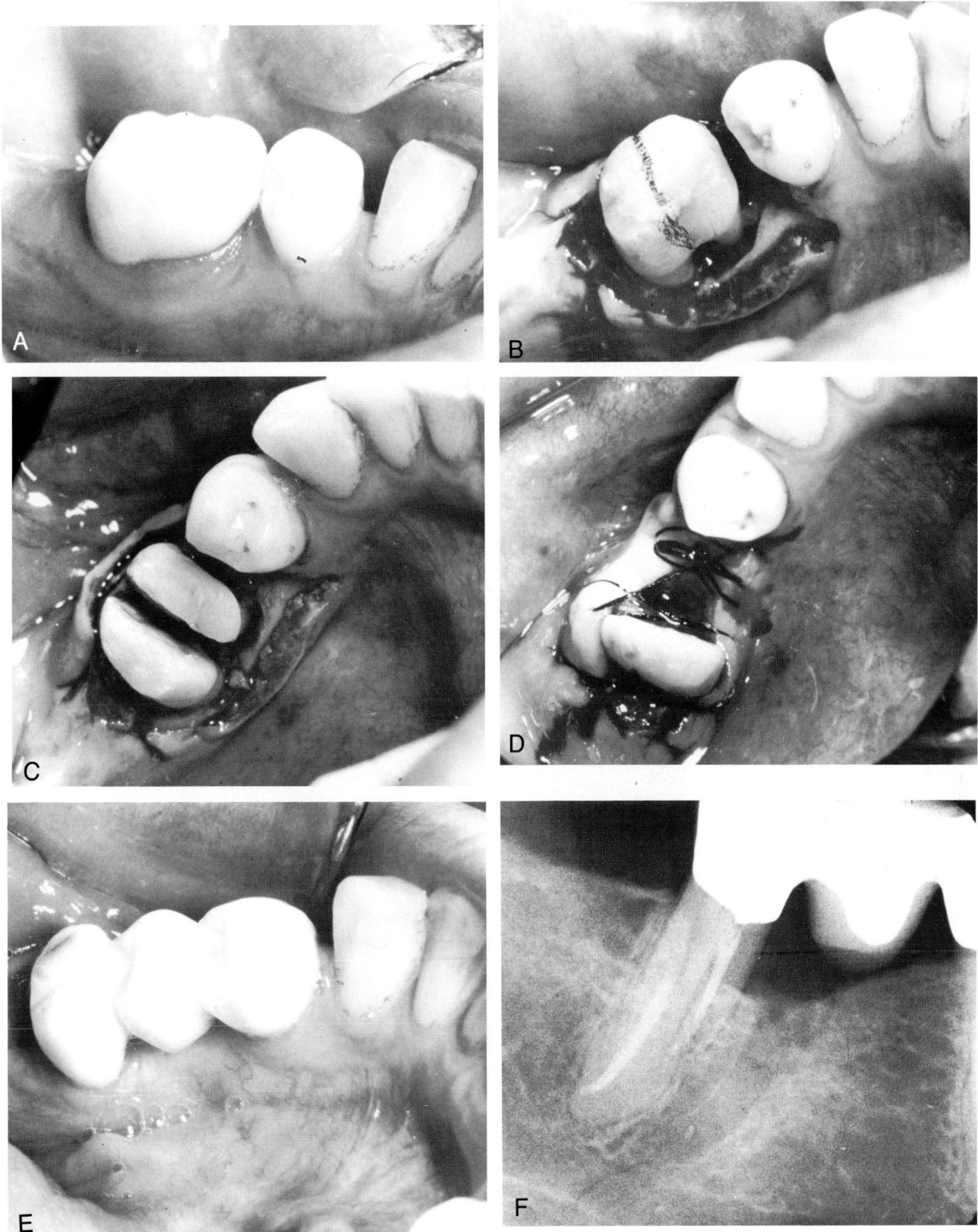

Fig. 14-14. Mandibular Hemisection. **A,** Before treatment. **B,** Flaps reflected exposing Grade II lingual furcation. Line drawn on tooth exposing Grade II lingual furcation. **C,** Sectioning completed. **D,** Mesial root extracted, internal furcation contour, osseous surgery completed, and flaps positioned apically. **E,** Temporization. **F,** X-ray study 5 years later.

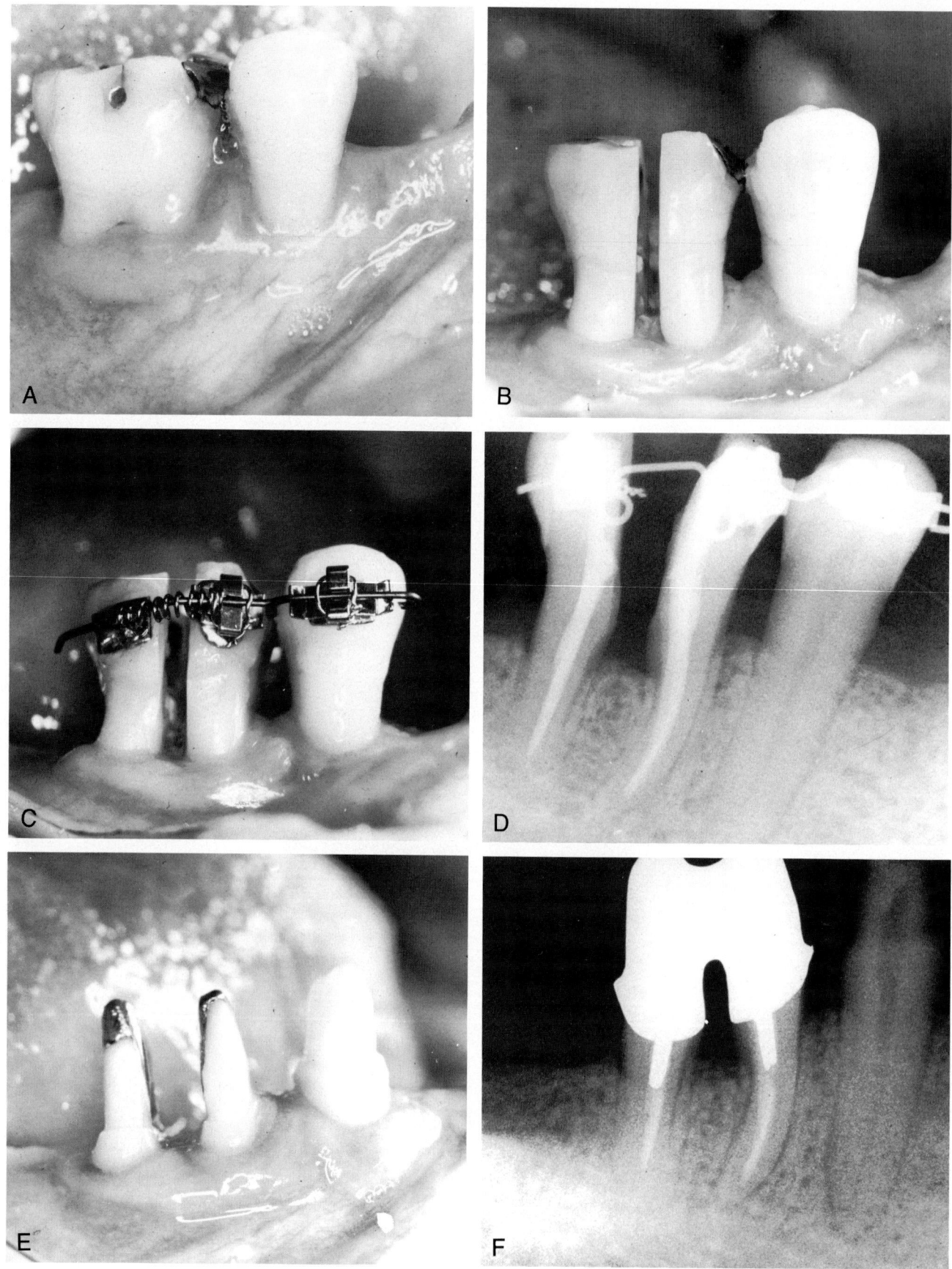

Fig. 14-15. Hemisection and Bicuspidization. **A,** Before treatment. **B,** Hemisection of roots. **C,** Orthodontic separation of roots for creation of adequate embrasure space. **D,** X-ray study showing final separation. **E,** Individual roots prepared for crowns. **F,** X-ray study showing final casting in place. (Contributed by Cary Golavic, Portsmouth, N.H.)

Furcations

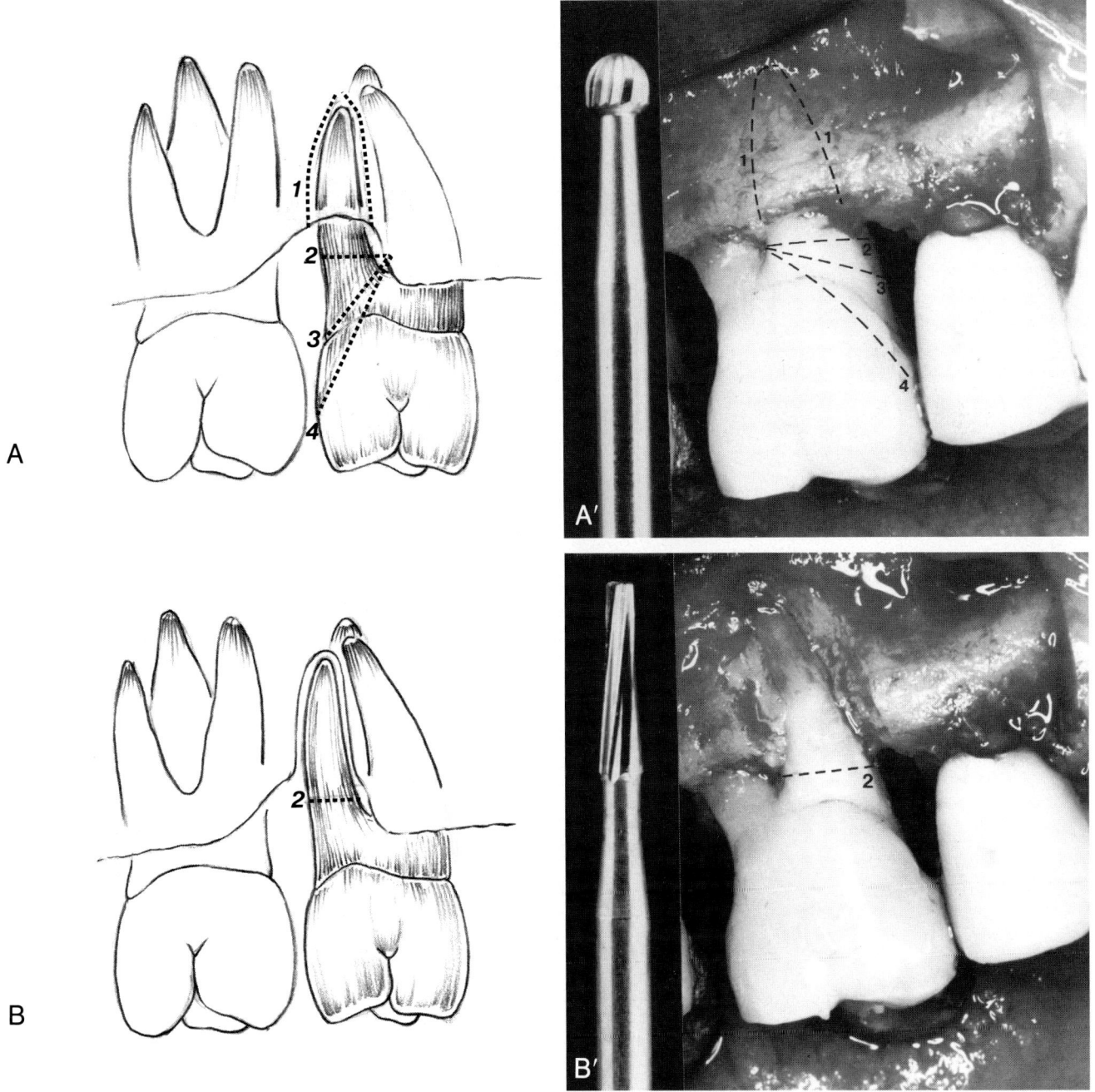

Fig. 14-16. Maxillary Root Amputation—Sequence of Treatment. **A, A′,** Before resection, with tooth cuts outlined. A round bur is used for bone removal over affected root. **B, B′,** 701L bur used for second cut.

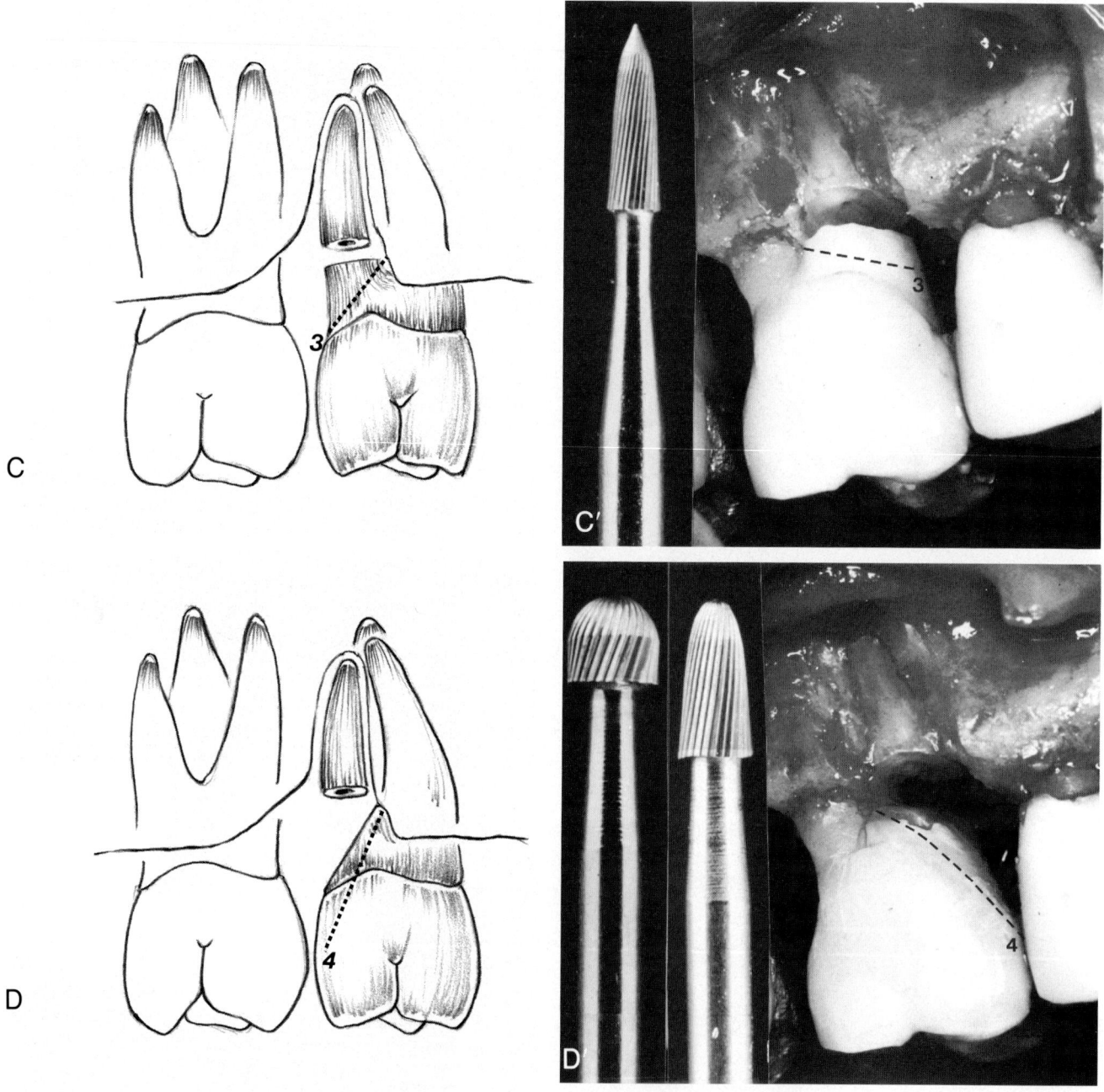

Fig. 14-16 (continued). **C, C′,** Flame-shaped enamel finishing bur used for oblique horizontal third cut. **D, D′,** Oblique cut completed and final internal contouring established with round and oval enamel finishing burs.

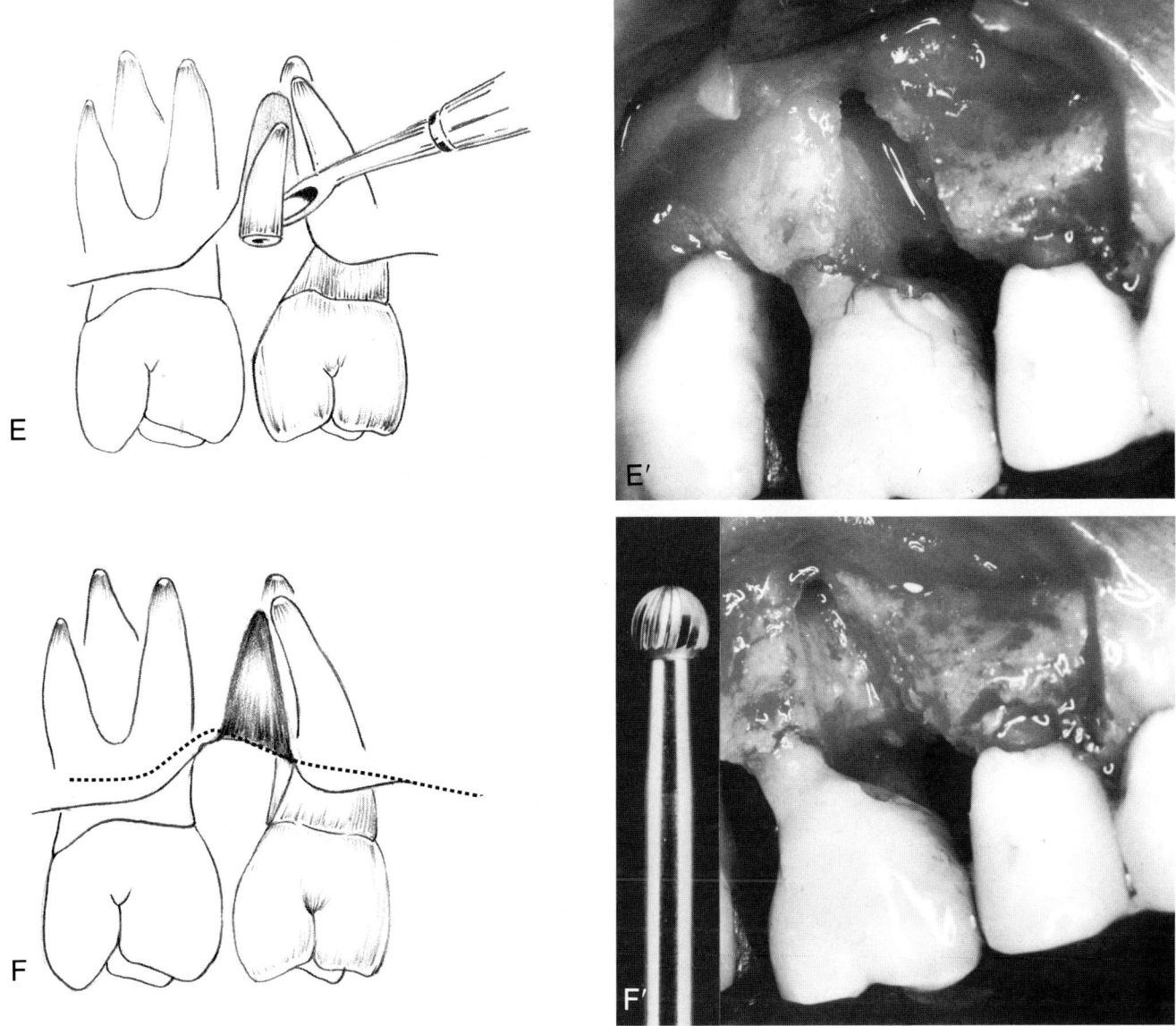

Fig. 14-16 (continued). **E, E′,** Root tip removed prior to osseous contouring. **F, F′,** Osseous contouring completed with No. 6 round bur, and final internal tooth contours established.

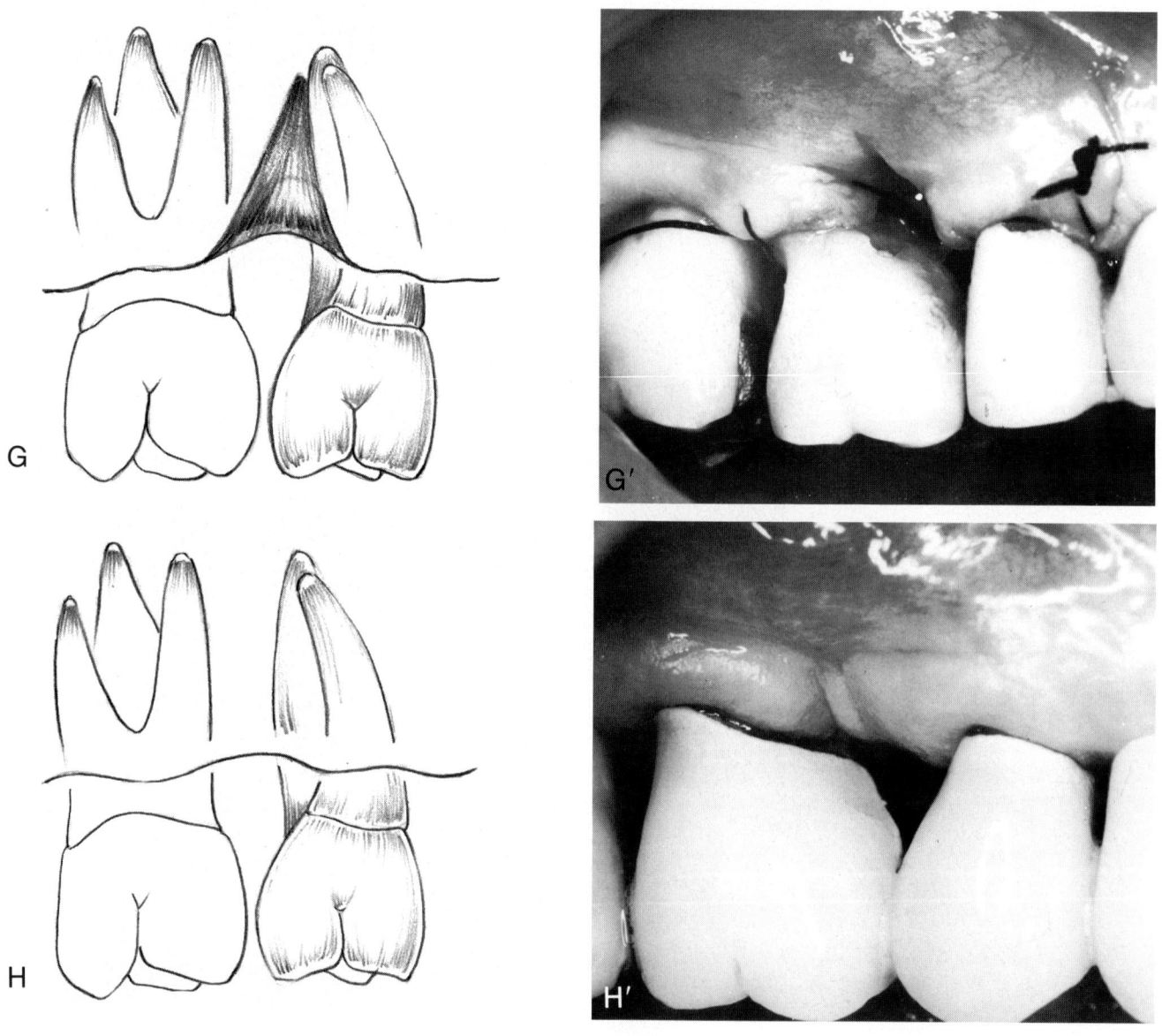

Fig. 14-16 (continued). **G, G′,** Final osseous contours established and flaps sutured. **H, H′,** Case completed.

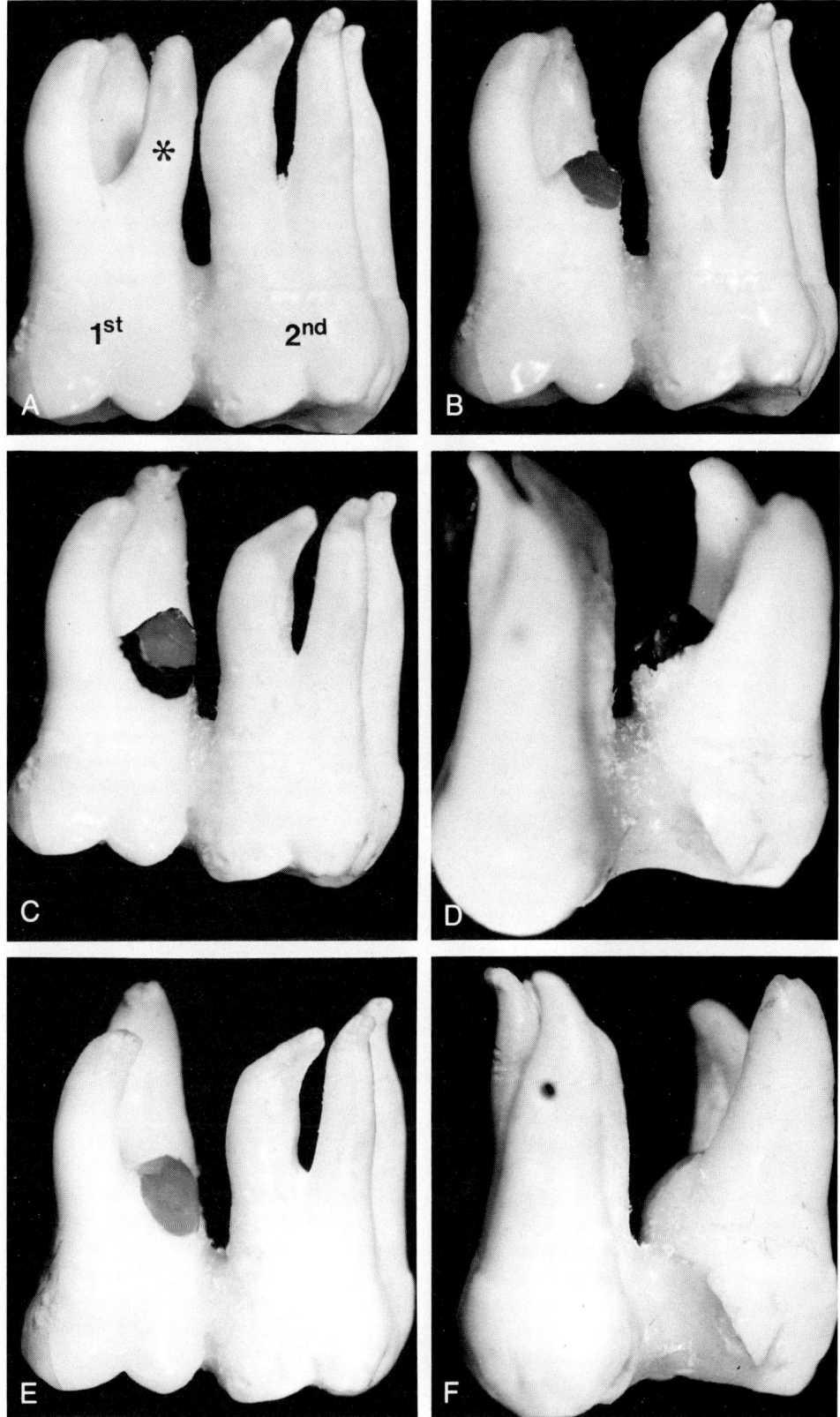

Fig. 14-17. Distobuccal Root Amputation Procedure. **A,** Before. Root to be removed is marked. **B,** Distobuccal root is removed. Cut root is shaded. **C,** Remaining portion of root to be removed is painted in black. **D,** Palatal view of root portion to be removed. **E,** Residual root portion reduced. **F,** Palatal view showing portion of root remaining.

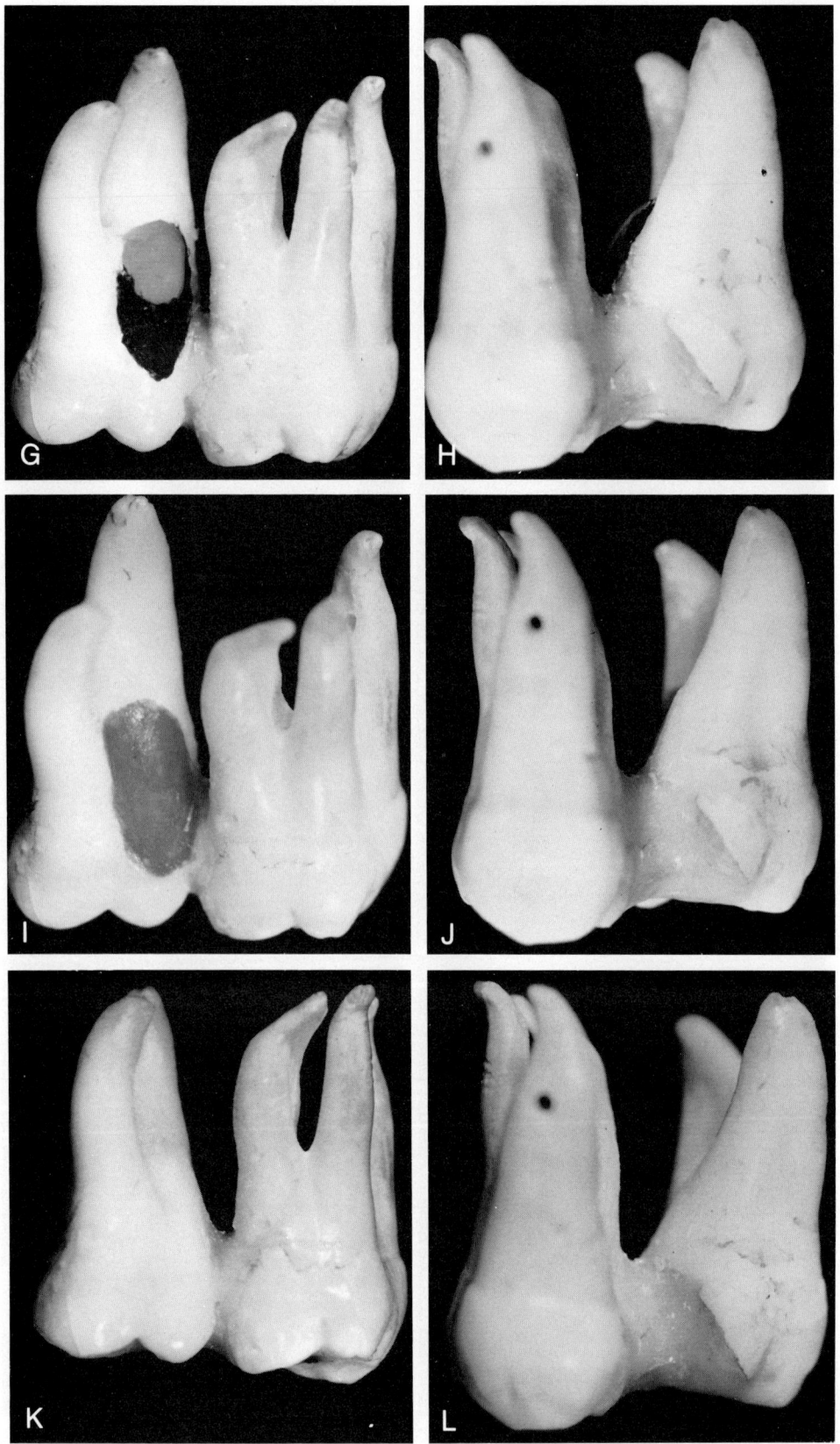

Fig. 14-17 (continued). **G,** Final areas to be contoured are painted black. **H,** Palatal view showing remaining root portion to be removed. **I,** Shaded area represents contoured portion of tooth. **J,** Palatal view, showing remaining root stump removed. **K, L,** Final buccal and palatal contour. Note how molar has been transformed into a bicuspid-like tooth. Compare with A.

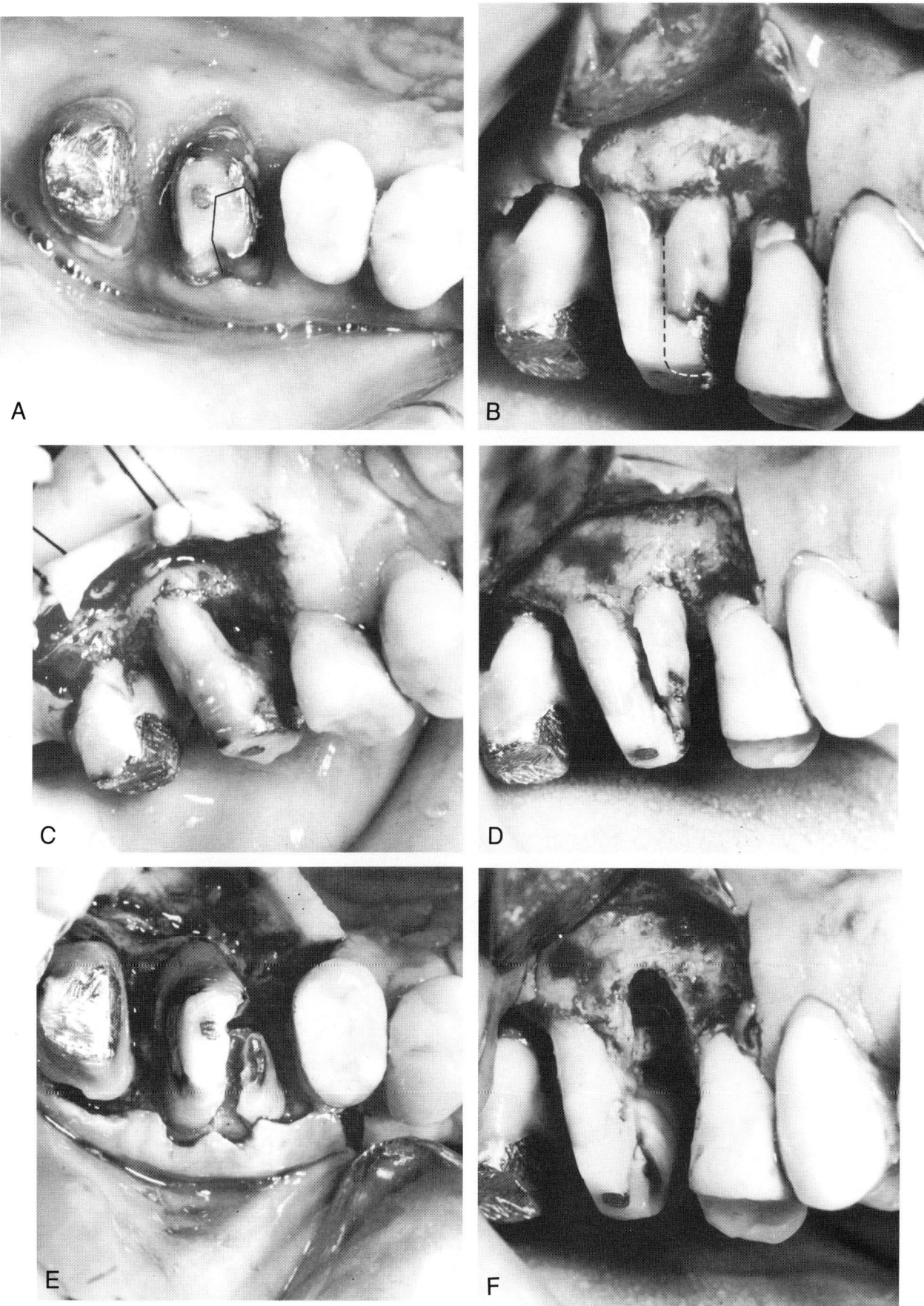

Fig. 14-18. Maxillary Root Amputation—Mesiobuccal Root. **A, B,** Occlusal and buccal views of crown preparation of maxillary first molar. **C,** Palatal view displaying deep Grade II mesial furcation. **D,** Buccal view of initial mesiobuccal root sectioning beginning at or near most coronal portion of furcation. **E,** Occlusal view shows the joining of the mesial and distal cuts. **F,** Mesiobuccal root removed and internal furcation prepared.

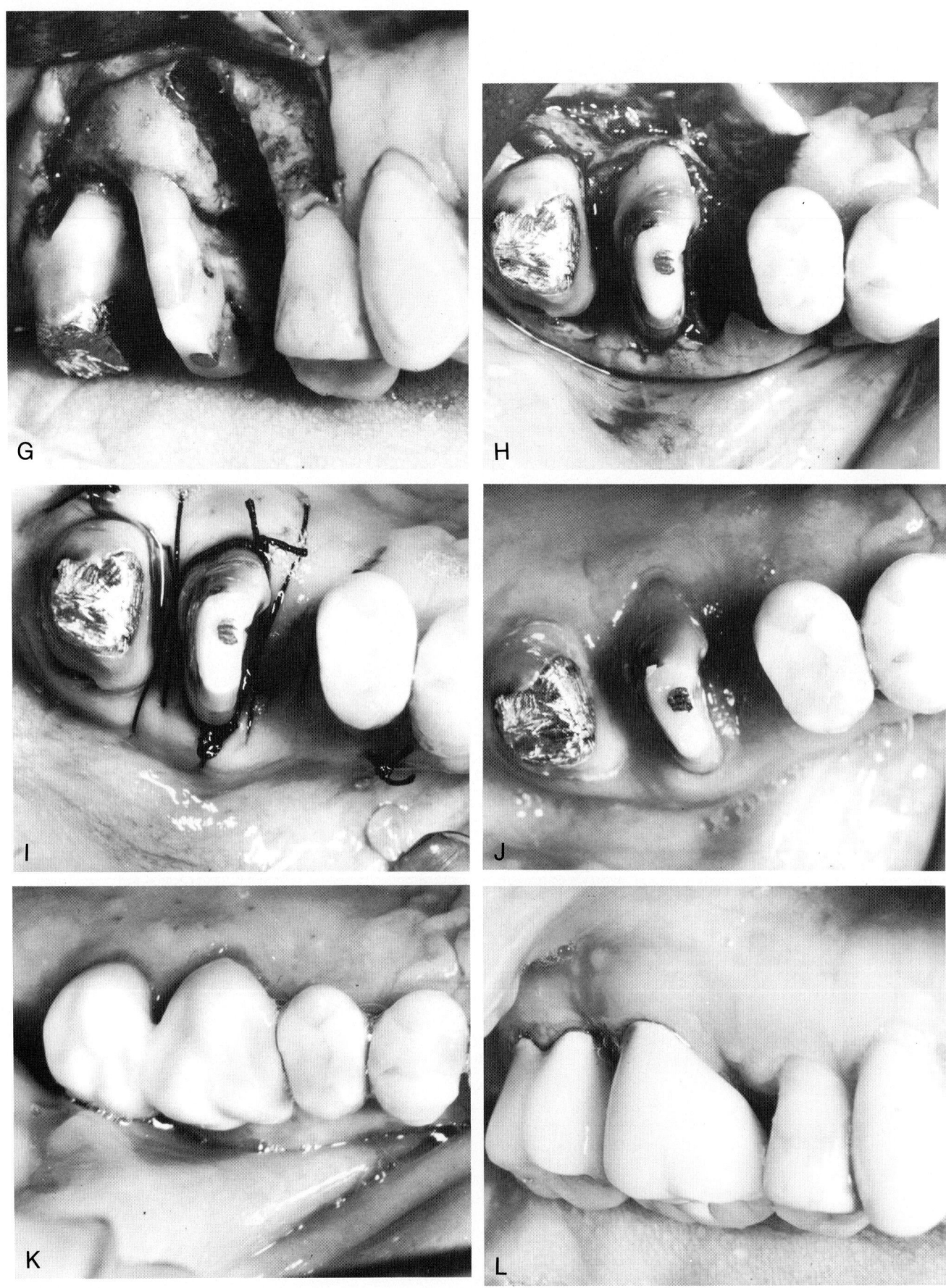

Fig. 14-18 (continued). **G,** Buccal plate removed over extracted root, final osseous contours established, and internal portion of furcation completely prepared. **H,** Occlusal view shows bicuspid contour established. **I,** Flaps apically positioned and sutured. **J,** Initial healing. **K,** Temporization. **L,** Case complete 1 year later. Note total opening of embrasure for patient access and that crown was not overcontoured. (Prosthetics by John Dolbec, Easton, MA.)

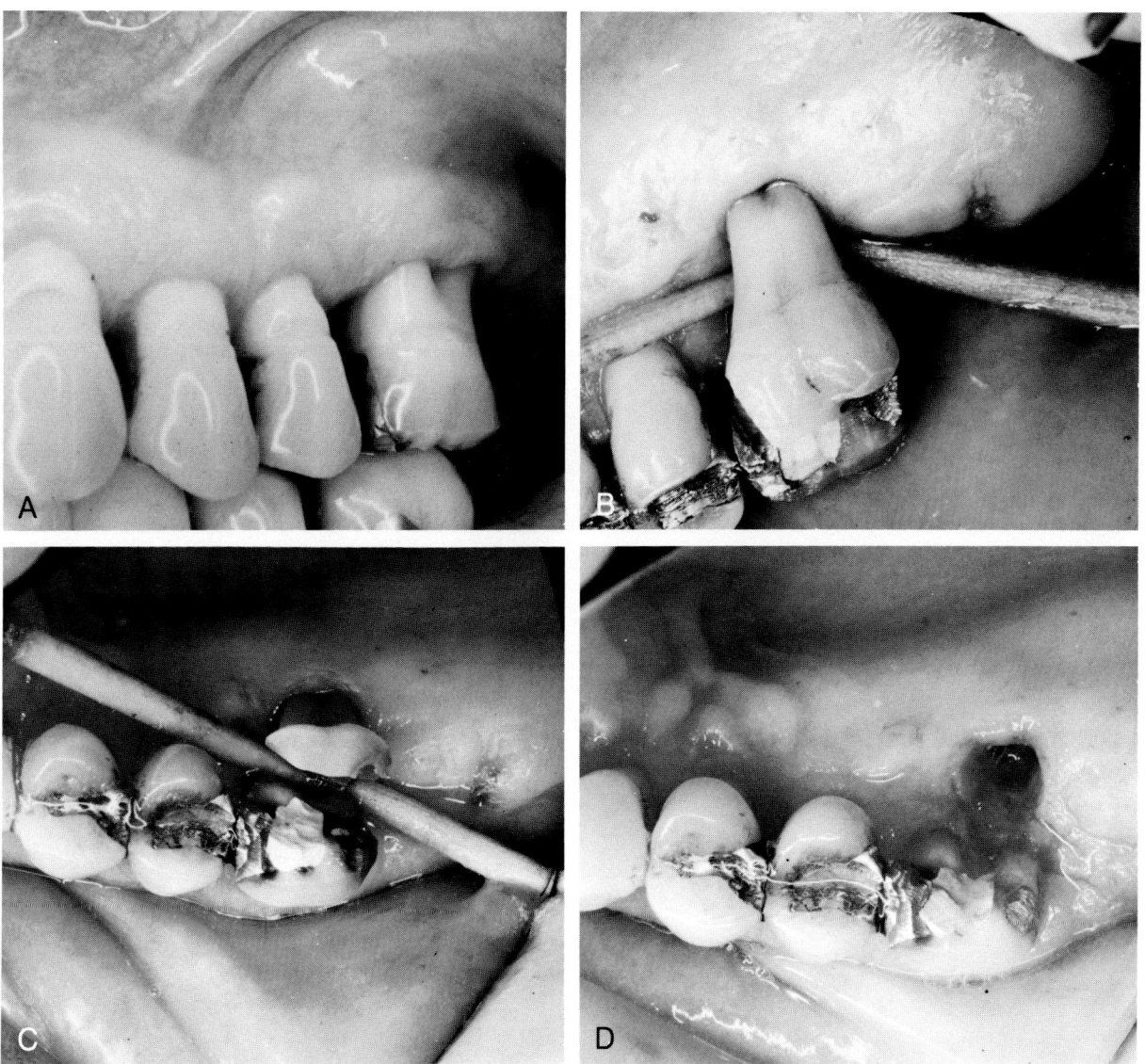

Fig. 14-19. Palatal Root Amputation. **A,** Before treatment. **B,** Toothpicks placed in mesial and distal furcations serve as reference points and protect surrounding tissue from damage. **C,** Tooth has been sectioned mesiodistally. The appearance of the toothpicks means that sectioning is complete. **D,** Palatal root has been removed.

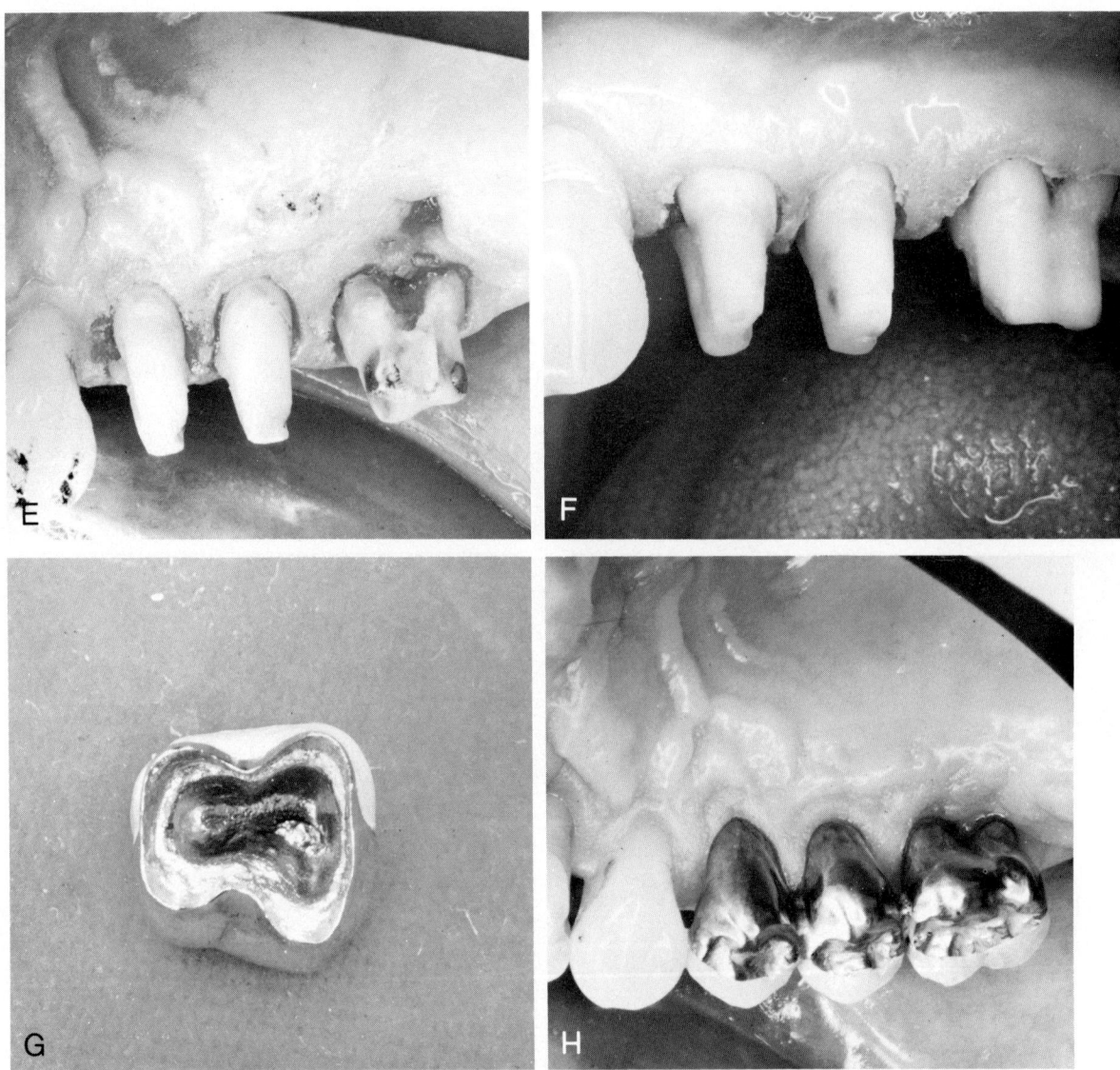

Fig. 14-19 (continued). **E, F,** Palatal and buccal views of teeth prepared for prosthetic treatment. Note resected molar is treated as a bicuspid. **G,** Occlusal view of crown with prominent contours that mirror tooth. **H,** Palatal view of final prosthetic restoration. (Prosthetics done by Dr. Bernard Croll, New York, NY.)

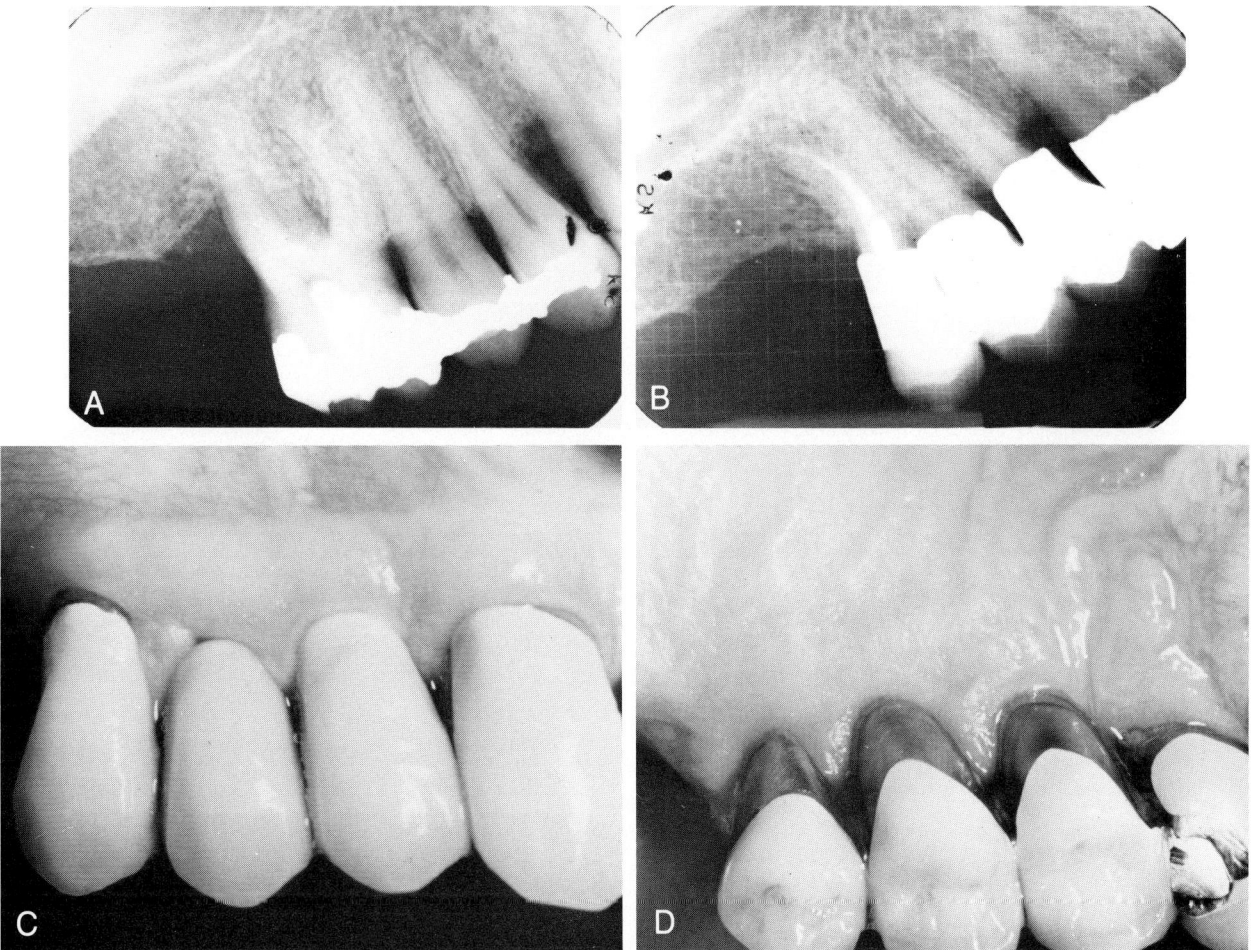

Fig. 14-20. Maxillary Distobuccal and Palatal Root Amputation. **A,** Pretreatment x-ray study, showing severe bone loss on distal and palatal roots. **B,** Five-year post-treatment x-ray study. Note total bone regeneration. **C, D,** Buccal and palatal views of completed restoration 5 years later. Note excellent contours and embrasures. (Prosthetics done by Dr. William Irving, Needham, MA.)

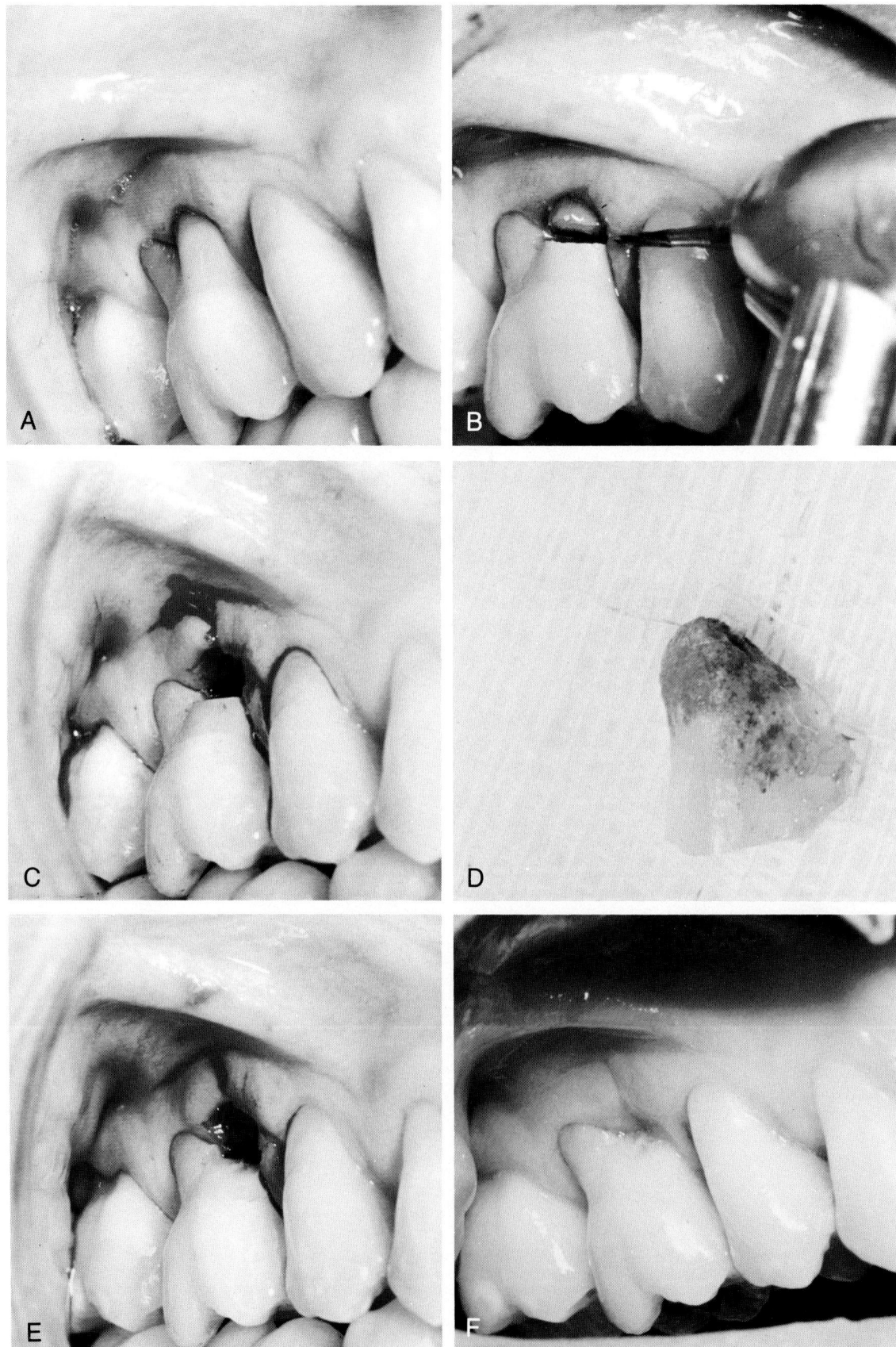

Fig. 14-21. Mesiobuccal Root Amputation. **A,** Before treatment. **B,** Root sectioned, using 701L bur. **C,** Root tip removed. **D,** Root tip with calculus. **E,** Tooth contoured. Mesial area beveled in. **F,** Four months later.

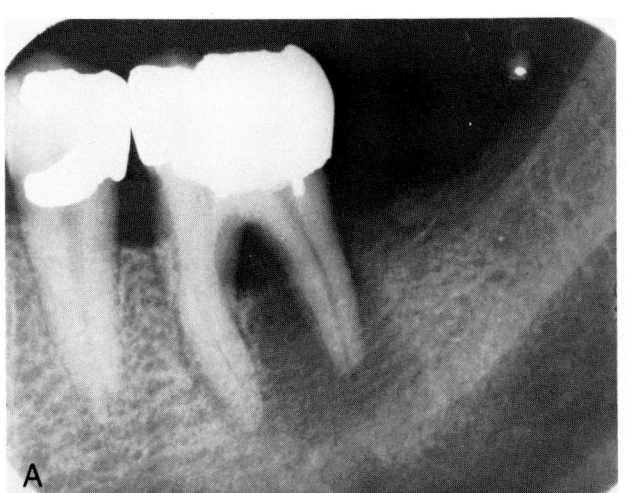
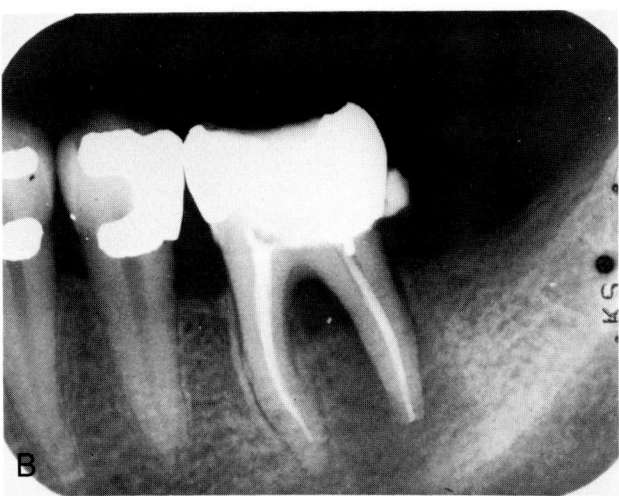
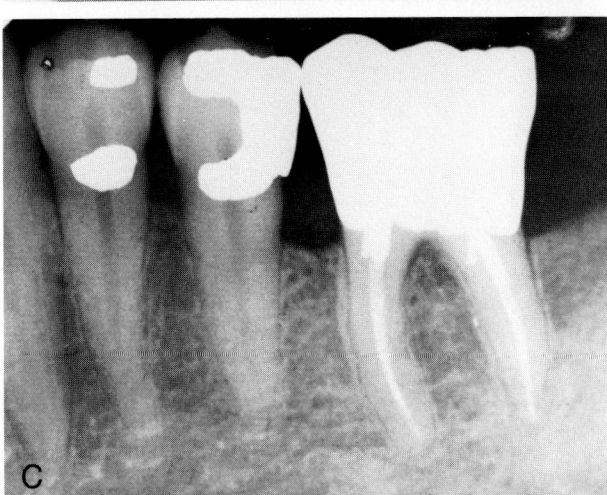

Fig. 14-22. Periodontal–Endodontal Interrelationships. **A,** Before treatment, showing total furcation bone loss and a large apical radiolucent area. **B,** Endodontic therapy completed. **C,** One year after treatment; total bone regeneration. (Contributed by Dr. Barry Jaye, Brockton, MA.)

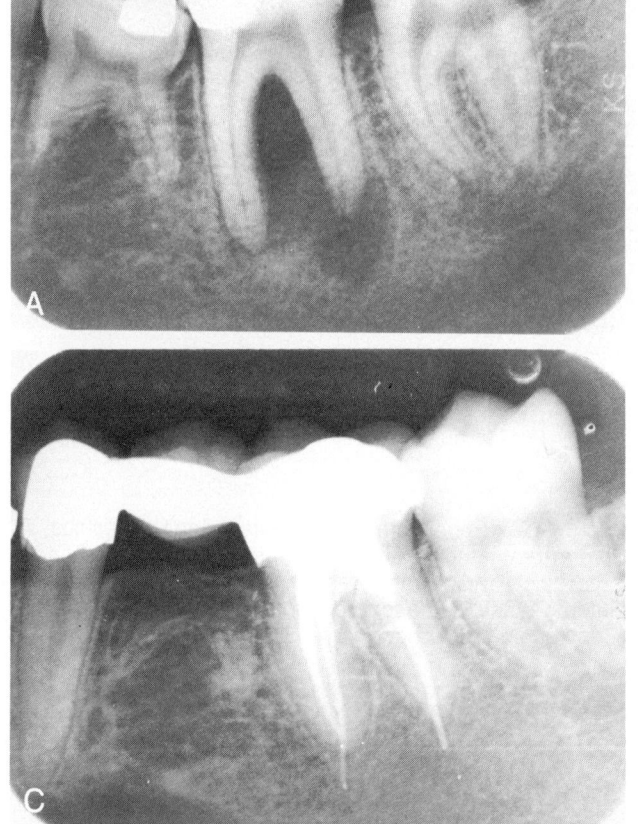
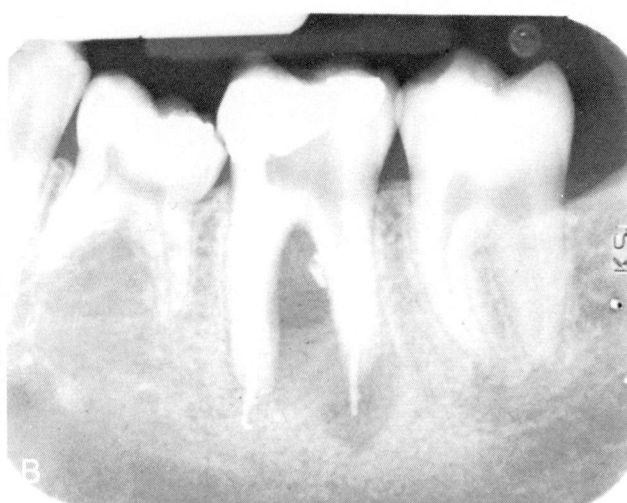

Fig. 14-23. Periodontal–Endodontal Interrelationships. **A,** Before treatment; total bone loss in furcation areas. **B,** Endodontic therapy completed, with lateral canal to furcation. **C,** One year later; total bone regeneration. (Contributed by Dr. Barry Jaye, Brockton, MA.)

BIBLIOGRAPHY

Abrams, L.: Augmentation of deformed residual edentulous ridge for fixed prosthesis. Compend. Contin. Ed. Gen. Dent., *1*:205, 1980.

Al-Ali, W., et al.: The effect of local doxycycline with and without tricalcium phosphate on regenerative healing potential of periodontal osseous defects in dogs. J. Periodontol., *60*:582, 1989.

Aleo, J.J., et al.: The presence and biologic activity of cementum-bound endotoxin. J. Periodontal., *45*:672, 1974.

Aleo, J.J., et al.: In vitro attachment of human gingival fibroblasts to root surfaces. J. Periodontol., *46*:639, 1975.

Aleo, J.J., DeRenzis, F.A., and Farber, P.A.: In vitro attachment of human gingival fibroblasts to root surfaces. J. Periodontol., *46*:639, 1975.

Aleo, J.J., and Vandersall D.C.: Cementum: Recent concepts related to periodontal disease therapy. Dent. Clin. North Am., *24*:627, 1980.

Alger, F.A., et al.: The histologic evaluation of new attachment in periodontally diseased human roots treated with tetracycline-hydrochloride and fibronectin. J. Periodontol., *61*:447, 1990.

Allen, E.P., and Miller, P.D.: Coronally positioning of existing gingiva. Short term results in the treatment of shallow marginal recession. J. Periodontol., *60*:316, 1989.

Allen, P.E., Gainza, A.C., Farthing, G.G., and Newbold, D.A.: Improved technique for localized ridge augmentation—A report of 21 cases. J. Periodontol., *56*:187, 1985.

Ammons, W., and Smith, D.: Flap curettage: Rationale, techniques and expectations. Dent. Clin. North Am., *20*:215, 1976.

Anderegg, C.R., et al.: Clinical evaluation of the use of decalcified freeze-dried bone allograft with guided tissue regeneration in the treatment of molar furcation invasions. J. Periodontol., *62(4)*:264, 1991.

Ariaudo, A.A., and Tyrell, H.: Repositioning and increasing the zone of attached gingiva. J. Periodontol., *28*:106, 1957.

Ariaudo, A.A., and Tyrell, H.: Elimination of pockets extending to or beyond the mucogingival junction. Dent. Clin. North Am., *4*:67, 1960.

Ariaudo, A.A.: Problems in treating denuded labial root surface of a lower incisor. J. Periodontol., *37*:274, 1966.

Aukhil, I., and Iglhaut, J.: Periodontal ligament cell kinetics following experimental regenerative procedures. J. Clin. Periodontol., *15(6)*:374, 1988.

Bahat, O., et al.: The influence of soft tissue on the interdental bone height after flap curettage. 1. Study involving six patients. Int. J. Periodont. Rest. Dent., *2*:9, 1984.

Bahat, O.: The transpositional flap in periodontal surgery. Int. J. Periodont. Rest. Dent., *10(6)*:473, 1990.

Baker, D.L., and Seymour, G.J.: The possible pathogenesis of gingival recession. A histological study of induced recession in the rat. J. Clin. Periodontol., *3*:208, 1976.

Baker, P.J., et al.: Minimal inhibitory concentration of various antimicrobial agents for human oral anaerobic bacteria. Antimicrob. Agents Chemother., *24*:420, 1983B.

Baker, P.J., et al.: Tetracycline and its derivatives strongly bind to and are released from the tooth surface in active form. J. Periodontol., *54*:580, 1983A.

Bang, H., et al.: Bone induction in excavation chambers in matrix of decalcified dentin. Arch. Surg., *94*:781, 1967.

Barnett, J.D., et al.: Comparison of freeze-dried bone allograft and porous hydroxylapatite in human periodontal defects. J. Periodontol., *60*:231, 1989.

Barsky, A.J., Kahn, S., and Simon, B.D.: Principles and Practice of Plastic Surgery. New York, McGraw-Hill, 1964.

Baum, B., and Wright, W.: Demonstration of fibronectin as a major extracellular protein of human gingival fibroblasts. J. Dent. Res., *59*:631, 1980.

Becker, B., and Becker, W.: Use of connective tissue autografts for treatment of mucogingival problems. Int. J. Periodont. Rest. Dent., *6(1)*:88, 1986.

Becker, W., and Becker, B.: Guided tissue regeneration for implants placed into extraction sockets and for implant dehiscences: Surgical techniques and case reports. Int. J. Periodont. Rest. Dent., *10(5)*:377, 1990.

Becker, W., et al.: Root isolation for new attachment procedures: A surgical and suturing method: Three case reports. J. Periodontol., *58(12)*:819, 1987.

Becker, W., et al.: New attachment after treatment with root isolation procedures: Report for treated Class III and Class II furcations and vertical osseous defects. Int. J. Periodont. Rest. Dent., *8(3)*:1988.

Becker, W., Becker, B.E., and Berg, L.: Repair of intrabony defects as a result of open debridement procedures. Report of 36 treated cases. Int. J. Periodontol. Rest. Dent., *8*:8, 1986.

Bell, H.W.: Resorptive characteristics of bone and bone substitutes. Oral Surg., *17*:650, 1964.

Bernimoulin, J.P., Luscher, B., and Muglemann, H.R.: Coronally repositioned periodontal flap. J. Clin. Periodontol., *2*:1, 1975.

Bertrand, P., and Dunlap, R.: Coverage of deep, wide gingival clefts with free gingival autografts: Root planing with and without citric acid demineralization. Int. J. Periodont. Rest. Dent., *8*:65, 1988.

Bjorn, H.: Free transplantation of gingiva propria. Sven. Tandlak Tidskr., *22*:684, 1963.

Bjorvatn, K.: In vitro study by fluorescence microscopy and microradiography of tetracycline-tooth interaction. Scand. J. Dent. Res., *91*:417, 1983.

Blumenthal, N.: The use of collagen membranes to guide regeneration of new connective tissue in dogs. J. Periodontol., *59*:830, 1988.

Blumenthal, N., and Steinberg, J.: The use of collagen membrane barriers in conjunction with combined demineralization bone–collagen gel implants in human infrabony defects. J. Periodontol., *61*:319, 1990.

Bogle, G., et al.: New attachment after surgical treatment and citric acid conditioning of roots in naturally occurring periodontal disease in dogs. J. Periodontol. Res., *16*:130, 1981.

Bogle, G., et al.: New connective tissue attachment in beagles with advanced natural periodontitis. J. Periodontol. Res., *18*:220, 1983.

Bohannan, H.M.: Studies in alteration of vestibular depth. II. Periosteum retention. J. Periodontol., *33*:354, 1962.

Bohannan, H.M.: Studies in alteration of vestibular depth. III. Vestibular incision. J. Periodontol., *34*:155, 1963A.

Bohannan, H.M.: The fixed, long, labial, mucosal flap in vestibular alteration. Periodontics, *1*:13, 1963B.

Borghetti, A., et al.: How much root planing is necessary to remove the cementum from the root surface. Int. J. Periodont. Rest. Dent., *7*:23, 1987.

Borghetti, A., and Gardella, J.P.: Thick gingival autograft for coverage of gingival recession: A clinical evaluation. Int. J. Periodont. Rest. Dent., *10(3)*:217, 1990.

Bowen, J.A., et al.: Comparison of decalcified freeze-dried bone allograft and porous particulate hydroxyapatite in human periodontal osseous defects. J. Periodontol., *60*:647, 1989.

Bowers, G.M., Schallhorn, R.G., and Mellonig, J.T.: Histologic evaluation of new attachment in human intrabony defects. J. Periodontol., *53*:509, 1982.

Bowers, G.M., et al.: Histologic evaluation of new attachment in humans—A preliminary report. J. Periodontol., *56*:381, 1985.

Bowers, G.M., et al.: Histologic evaluation of new attachment apparatus formation in humans. Part I. J. Periodontol., *60*:664, 1989A.

Bowers, G.M., et al.: Histologic evaluation of new attachment apparatus formation in humans. Part III. J. Periodontol., *60*:683, 1989B.

Boyko, G.A., et al.: Cell attachment to demineralized root surfaces in vitro. J. Periodont. Res., *15*:297, 1980.

Bragger, U., et al.: Surgical lengthening of the clinical crown. J. Clin. Periodontol., *19*:58, 1992.

Buchanan, S.A., and Robertson, P.B.: Calculus removal by scaling/root planing with and without surgical access. J. Periodontol., *58*:159, 1987.

Brustein, D.: Cosmetic periodontics. Coronally repositioned pedicle graft. Dent. Surv., *46*:22, 1970.

Burch, J.G., and Hulen, S.: A study of the presence of accessory foramina and the topography of molar furcations. Oral Surg., *38*:451, 1974.

Buser, D., et al.: Regeneration and enlargement of jaw bone using guided tissue regeneration. Clin. Oral Imp. Res., *1(1)*:22, 1990.

Buser, D., et al.: Titanium implants with a true periodontal ligament: An alternative to osseointegrated implants? Int. J. Oral Max. Imp., *5(2)*:113, 1990.

Buser, D., et al.: Formation of periodontal ligament around titanium implants. J. Periodontol., *61(9)*:598, 1990.

Buser, D., et al.: Localized ridge augmentation using guided bone regeneration. I. Surgical procedure in maxilla. Int. J. Periodont. Rest. Dent., *13(1)*:29, 1993.

Caffesse, R.G., et al.: The effect of citric acid and fibronectin application on healing following surgical treatment of naturally occurring periodontal disease in beagle dogs. J. Clin. Periodontol., *12*:578, 1985.

Caffesse, R.G., and Guinard, E.A.: Treatment of localized gingival recessions. Part II. Coronally repositioned flap with free gingival graft. J. Periodontol., *49*:357, 1978.

Caffesse, R.G., Sweeney, P.L., and Smith, B.A.: Scaling and root planing with and without periodontal flap surgery. J. Clin. Periodontol., *13*:205, 1986.

Caffesse, R.G., et al.: Cell proliferation after flap surgery, root conditioning and fibronectin application. J. Periodontol., *58*:661, 1978B.

Caffesse, R.G., et al.: Class II furcations treated by guided tissue regeneration in humans: Case reports. J. Periodontol., *61(8)*:510, 1990.

Caffesse, R., et al.: Periodontal healing following guided tissue regeneration with citric acid and fibronectin application. J. Periodontol., *62*:21, 1991.

Caffesse, S.B., et al.: Effects of citric acid and fibronectin and laminin application in treating periodontitis. J. Clin. Periodontol., *14*:396, 1987A.

Calura, G.: Ultrastructural observations on wound healing of free gingival connective tissue autografts with and without epithelium in humans. Int. J. Periodont. Rest. Dent., *11(4)*:283, 1991.

Carranza, F.A., Jr.: Glickman's Clinical Periodontology. 6th Ed., Philadelphia, W.B. Saunders, 1984.

Carvalho, J.C.M.: Clinical observations of suture techniques used for free gingival grafts. Rev. Fac. Odont. S. Paulo., *10(1):* 121, 1972.

Carvalho, J.C., Pustiglioni, F.E., and Kon, S.: Combination of a connective tissue pedicle flap with a free gingival graft to cover localized gingival recession. Int. J. Periodont. Rest. Dent., *4*:27, 1982.

Caton, J., et al.: Histometric evaluation of periodontal surgery II. Connective tissue attachment levels after four regenerative procedures. J. Clin. Periodontol., *7(3)*:224, 1980.

Chaiken, R.W.: Elements of surgical treatment in the delivery of periodontal therapy. Chicago, Quintessence, 1977.

Chamberlain, A.D.H., et al.: Healing after treatment of periodontal intraosseous defects. IV. Effect of a nonresective versus a partially resective approach. J. Clin. Periodontol., *12*:306, 1985.

Chung, K.M., et al.: Clinical evaluation of a biodegradable collagen membrane in guided tissue regeneration. J. Periodontol., *61*:732, 1990.

Clark, R.A., et al.: Fibronectin and fibrin provide a provisional matrix for epidermal cell migration during wound reepithelialization. J. Invest. Dermatol., *79*:264, 1982.

Coatoam, G.W., Behrents, R.G., and Bissada, N.F.: The width of keratinized gingiva during orthodontic treatment: Its significance and impact on periodontal status. J. Periodontol., *52*:307, 1981.

Cogen, H.S., et al.: Effect of various surface treatments on the viability and attachment of human gingival fibroblasts. J. Periodontics, *54*:277, 1983.

Cogen, R.B., et al.: Effect of various root surface treatments on the attachment and growth of human gingival fibroblasts: Histologic and scanning electron microscopic evaluation. J. Clin. Periodontol., *11*:531, 1984.

Cohen, D.W., and Ross, S.E.: The double papilla repositioned flap in periodontal therapy. J. Periodontol., *39*:65, 1968.

Cohen, H.V.: Localized ridge augmentation with hydroxylapatite: Report of case. J. Am. Dent. Assoc., *108*:54, 1984.

Cole, R.T., et al.: Connective tissue regeneration to periodontally diseased teeth. J. Periodont. Res., *15*:1, 1980.

Common, J., and McFall, W.T., Jr.: The effects of citric acid on attachment of laterally positioned flaps. J. Periodontol., *54*:9, 1983.

Corn, H.: Periosteal separation—Its clinical significance. J. Periodontol., *33*:140, 1962.

Corn, H.: Technique for repositioning the frenum in periodontal problems. J. Clin. North Am., *8*:79, 1964A.

Corn, H.: Edentulous area pedicle grafts in mucogingival surgery. Periodontics, *2*:229, 1964B.

Corsair, A.: A clinical evaluation of resorbable hydroxylapatite for the repair of human intra-osseous defects. J. Oral Implantol., *16*:125, 1990.

Cortellini, P., et al.: Guided tissue regeneration procedure in the treatment of a bone dehiscence associated with gingival recession: A case report. Int. J. Periodont. Rest. Dent., *11(6)*:461, 1991.

Cortellini, P., et al.: Periodontal regeneration of human infrabony defects. I. Clinical measures. J. Periodontol., *64*:254, 1993.

Cortellini, P., et al.: Periodontal regeneration of human infrabony defects. II. Re-entry procedures and bone measurements. J. Periodontol., *64*:261, 1993.

Coslet, J.G., Rosenberg, E.S., and Tisot, R.: The free autogenous gingival graft. Dent. Clin. North Am., *24*:651, 1980.

Cowan, A.: Sulcus deepening incorporating mucosal grafts. J. Periodontol., *36*:188, 1965.

Craig, M., et al.: Healing of periodontal connective tissues following surgical wounding and application of citric acid in dogs. J. Periodont. Res., *15*:314, 1980.

Crigger, M., et al.: The effect of topical citric acid application on the healing of experimental furcation defects in dogs. J. Periodont. Res., *13*:538, 1978.

Dahlberg, W.H.: Incisions and suturing: Some basic considerations about each in periodontal flap surgery. Dent. Clin. North Am., *13*:149, 1969.

Dahlin, C., et al.: Bone augmentation at fenestrated implants by an osteopromotive membrane technique. A controlled clinical study. Clin. Oral Imp. Res., *2(4)*:159, 1991.

Dahlin, C., et al.: Membrane-induced bone augmentation at titanium implants. Int. J. Periodont. Rest. Dent., *11(4)*:273, 1991.

Daly, C.G.: Anti-bacterial effect of citric acid treatment of periodontally diseased root surfaces. J. Clin. Periodontol., *9*:386, 1982.

Davis, J.S., and Davis, W.P.: Lewis' Practice of Surgery. Vol. 5. Hagerstown, Maryland: W.F. Prior Co., 1966.

Davis, J.S., and Kitlowski, E.A.: The immediate contraction of cutaneous grafts and its cause. Arch. Surg., *23*:954, 1931.

DeTrey, E., and Bernimoulin, J.P.: Influence of free gingival grafts on the health of marginal gingiva. J. Clin. Periodontol., *7*:381, 1980.

Diem, C.R., Bowers, G.M., and Moffitt, W.C.: Bone blending: a technique for osseous implants. J. Periodontol., *43*:295, 1972.

Dordick, B., Coslet, J.G., and Seibert, J.S.: Clinical evaluation of free autogenous gingival grafts placed on alveolar bone: 1. Clinical predictability: J. Periodontol., *45*:559, 1976.

Dorfman, H.S., Kennedy, J.E., and Bird, W.C.: Longitudinal evaluation of free autogenous gingival grafts. J. Clin. Periodontol., *7*:316, 1980.

Dorfman, H.S., Kennedy, J.E., and Bird, W.C.: Longitudinal evaluation of free autogenous gingival grafts. A four year report. J. Periodontol., *53*:349, 1982.

Dragoo, M.R., and Kaldahl, W.B.: Clinical and histological evaluation of alloplasts and allografts in regenerative periodontal surgery in humans. Int. J. Periodont. Rest. Dent., *2*:9, 1983.

Dragoo, M.R., and Sullivan, H.C.: A clinical and histological evaluation of autogenous iliac bone grafts in humans: Part I. Wound healing 2 to 8 months. J. Periodontol., *44*:599, 1973A.

Dragoo, M.R., and Sullivan, H.C.: A clinical and histological evaluation of autogenous iliac bone grafts in humans: Part II. External root resorption. J. Periodontol., *44*:614, 1973B.

Dubuc, F.I., and Urist, M.K.: The accessibility of the bone induction principle in surface-decalcified bone implants. Clin. Orthop., *55*:217, 1967.

Easley, J.: Methods of determining alveolar osseous form. J. Periodontol, *38*:112, 1967.

Edel, A.: Clinical evaluation of free connective tissue grafts used to increase the width of keratinized gingiva. J. Clin. Periodontol., *1*:185, 1974.

Egelberg, J.: Regeneration and repair of periodontal tissues. J. Periodont. Res., *22(3)*:233, 1987.

Egelberg, J.: Periodontics the Scientific Way. Synopsis of Human Clinical Studies. Copenhagen, Munksgaard, 1992.

Elden, A., and Mejchar, B.: Plastic surgery of the vestibulum in periodontal therapy. Int. Dent. J., *13*:593, 1963.

Ellegaard, B., et al.: Retardation of epithelial migration in new attachment attempts in intrabony defects in monkeys. J. Clin. Periodontol., *10*:399, 1983.

Ellegaard, B., and Loe, H.: New attachment of periodontal tissues after treatment of intrabony lesions. J. Periodontol., *42*:648, 1971.

Ellegaard, B., Karring, T., and Loe, H.: New periodontal attachment procedure based on retardation of epithelial migration. J. Clin. Periodontol., *1*:75, 1974.

Ellegaard, B., Karring, T., and Loe, H.: Retardation of epithelial migration in new attachment attempts in infrabony defects in monkeys. J. Clin. Periodontol., *3*:23, 1976.

Ellegaard, B., Karring, T., Listgarten, M., and Loe, H.: New attachment after treatment of interradicular lesions. J. Periodontol., *44*:209, 1973.

Ericsson, I., and Lindhe, J.: Recession in sites with inadequate width of keratinized gingiva. J. Clin. Periodontol., *11*:95, 1984.

Ethicon: Wound Closure Manual. Somerville, New Jersey, Ethicon, Inc., 1985, p. 9.

Everett, F.G., Waerhaug, J., and Widman, A.: Leonard Widman: Surgical treatment of pyorrhea alveolaris. J. Periodontol., *42*:571, 1971.

Evian, C.I., Corn, H., and Rosenberg, E.S.: Retained interdental papilla procedure for maintaining anterior esthetics. Compend. Contin. Ed. Gen. Dent., *6*:58, 1985.

Ewen, S.J.: Bone swaging. J. Periodontol., *36*:57, 1965.

Fardal, O., et al.: Initial attachment of fibroblast-like cell to periodontally diseased root surfaces in vitro. J. Clin. Periodontol., *13*:735, 1986.

Fernyhough, W., and Page, R.C.: Attachment, growth, and synthesis by human fibroblasts on demineralized or fibronectin-treated normal and diseased tooth roots. J. Periodontol., *54*:133, 1983.

Fine, D.H., et al.: Preliminary characterization of material eluted from the roots of periodontally diseased teeth. J. Periodont. Res., *15*:10, 1980.

Fine, D.H., and Oshrain, R.: Preliminary characterization of material eluded from the roots of teeth affected by juvenile periodontitis. J. Periodont. Res., *19*:146, 1984.

Fisher, M.R., Bowers, G.M., and Bergquist, J.J.: Effectiveness of the reverse bevel incision used in the modified Widman flap procedure in removing pocket epithelium in humans. Int. J. Periodont. Rest. Dent., *3*:33, 1982.

Frank, R.M., et al.: Cementogenesis and soft tissue attachment after citric acid treatment in a human. J. Periodontol., *54*:389, 1983.

Fredi, P.F., and Rosenfeld, W.J.: Excisional new attachment procedure. J. Missouri Dent., *57*:22, 1977.

Freeman, E., and Turnbull, R.S.: The value of osseous coagulum as a graft material. J. Periodontol. Res., *8*:229, 1973.

Friedman, N.: Periodontal osseous surgery: Osteoplasty and osteoectomy. J. Periodontol., *26*:257, 1955.

Friedman, N.: Mucogingival surgery. Texas Dent. J., *75*:358, 1957.

Friedman, N.: Mucogingival surgery: The apically repositioned flap. J. Periodontol., *33*:328, 1962.

Friedman, N., and Levine, H.L.: Mucogingival surgery: Current status. J. Periodontol., *35*:5, 1964A.

Friedman, N., and Levine, H.L.: Mucogingival surgery. Dent. Clin. North Am., *8*:70, 1964B.

Frisch, J., Jones, R.A., and Baskar, S.N.: Conservation of maxillary anterior esthetics: A modified surgical approach. J. Periodontol., *38*:11, 1967.

Froum, S.J.: Comparison of different autograft material for obtaining bone fill in human periodontal defects. J. Periodontol., *45*:240, 1974.

Froum, S.J., and Stahl, S.S.: Histologic evaluation of human intraosseous healing responses to the placement of tricalcium phosphate ceramic implants. J. Periodontol., *57*:211, 1986.

Froum, S., and Stahl, S.S.: Human intraosseous healing responses to placement of tricalcium phosphate ceramic implants. J. Periodontol., *58*:103, 1987.

Froum, S.J., Kushner, L., Scoop, I.W., and Stahl, S.S.: Human clinical and histologic responses to durapatite implants in intraosseous lesions. J. Periodontol., *53*:719, 1982.

Froum, S.J., Thaler, R., Scoop, I.W., and Stahl, S.S.: Osseous autografts. I. Clinical responses to bone blend or hip marrow grafts. J. Periodontol., *46*:515, 1975A.

Froum, S.J., Thaler, R., Scoop, I.W., and Stahl, S.S.: Osseous autografts. II. Histologic responses to osseous coagulum-bone blend grafts. J. Periodontol., *46*:656, 1975B.

Froum, S.J., et al.: Osseous autografts. III. Comparison of osseous coagulum-bone blend implants with open curettage. J. Periodontol., *47*:287, 1976.

Galgut, P.N.: Oxidized cellulose mesh used as a biodegradable barrier membrane in the technique of guided tissue regeneration. J. Periodontol., *61*:766, 1990.

Gantes, B., et al.: Treatment of periodontal furcation defects. (II) Bone regeneration in mandibular class II defects. J. Clin. Periodont., *15*:232, 1988.

Gantes, B.G., et al.: Treatment of periodontal furcation defects. Mandibular class III defects. *62*:361, 1991.

Garber, D.A., and Rosenberg, E.S.: The edentulous ridge in fixed prosthodontics. Compend. Cont. Ed. Gen. Dent., 2:212, 1981.

Gargiulo, A., and Arrocha, R.: Histochemical evaluation of free gingival grafts. Periodontics, 5:285, 1967.

Gargiulo, A.W., Wentz, F.M., and Orban, B.: Dimensions of the dentogingival junction in humans. J. Periodontol., 32:261, 1961.

Garrett, J.S., et al.: Effects of citric acid on diseased surface. J. Periodont. Res., 13:155, 1978.

Garrett, S., et al.: Treatment of periodontal furcation defects. (III) Coronally positioned flaps versus dura mater membranes in class II. J. Clin. Periodontol., 17:179, 1990.

Genon, P., and Bender, J.C.: Lambeau esthetique d'access en parodontie. L'Information Dent., 66:1047, 1984.

Glickman, I.: Clinical Periodontology. Philadelphia, W.B. Saunders, 1958.

Glickman, I.: Clinical Periodontology. 4th Ed., Philadelphia, W.B. Saunders, 1972.

Goldman, H.M.: A rationale for the treatment of the intrabony pocket; one method of treatment—subgingival curettage. J. Periodontol, 20:83, 1949.

Goldman, H.M.: The development of physiologic gingival contours by gingivoplasty. Oral Surg. Oral Med. Oral Pathol., 3:879, 1950.

Goldman, H.M.: Peridontia. 3rd Ed. St. Louis, C.V. Mosby, 1953.

Goldman, H.M.: Therapy of the incipient bifurcation involvement. J. Periodontol, 29:112, 1958.

Goldman, H.M., and Cohen, D.W.: The infrabony pocket: Classification and treatment. J. Periodontol., 29:272, 1958.

Goldman, H.M., and Cohen, D.W.: Periodontal Therapy. 6th Ed. St. Louis, C.V. Mosby, 1979.

Goldman, H.M., and Smukler, H.: Controlled surgical stimulation of periosteum. J. Periodontol., 49:146, 1978.

Goldman, H.M., et al.: Stimulated osteoperiosteal pedicle grafts in dogs. J. Periodontol., 54:36, 1983.

Goldman, H.M., Schluger, S., Fox, L., and Cohen, D.W.: Periodontal Therapy. 3rd Ed. St. Louis, C.V. Mosby, 1964.

Goldman, H.M., Shuman, A.M., and Isenberg, G.A.: Management of the partial furcation involvement. Periodontics, 6:197, 1968.

Goldman, H.M., Shuman, A., and Isenberg, G.: An Atlas of the Surgical Management of Periodontal Disease. Chicago, Quintessence, 1982.

Goldstein, R.E.: Esthetics in Dentistry. Philadelphia, J.B. Lippincott, 1976.

Golub, L.M., et al.: Tetracyclines inhibit tissue collagenase activity. A new mechanism in the treatment of periodontal disease. J. Periodontol. Res., 19:651, 1984.

Gordon, H.P., Sullivan, H.C., and Atkins, J.H.: Free autogenous gingival grafts. II. Supplemental findings—histology of the graft site. Periodontics, 6:130, 1968.

Gorman, W.J.: Prevalence and etiology of gingival recession. J. Periodontol., 38:316, 1967.

Gottlow, J., et al.: New attachment formation as the result of controlled tissue regeneration. J. Clin. Periodontol., 11(8):494, 1984.

Gottlow, J., et al.: New attachment formation in the human periodontium by guided tissue regeneration: Case reports. J. Clin. Periodontol., 12(6):604, 1986.

Gottlow, J., et al.: New attachment formation in monkey using Guidor, a bioabsorbable GTR-device. J. Dent. Res., 71(special issue):1535, 1992A.

Gottlow, J., et al.: Clinical result of GTR-therapy using a bioabsorbable device (Guidor). J. Dent. Res., 71(special issue):1537, 1992B.

Gottlow, J., et al.: Treatment of infrabony defects in monkeys with bioresorbable and non-resorbable GTR devices. J. Dent. Res., 72(special issue):823, 1993A.

Gottlow, J., et al.: Treatment of furcation degree II involvements in humans with bioabsorbable and nonresorbable GTR devices. J. Dent. Res., 72(special issue):825, 1993B.

Gottlow, J., and Karring, T.: Maintenance of new attachment gained through guided tissue regeneration. J. Clin. Periodontol., 19(5):315, 1992.

Gottsegen, R.: Frenum position and vestibular depth in relation to gingival health. Oral Surg. Oral Med. Oral Pathol., 7:1069, 1954.

Greenstein, G.: Repair of anterior gingival deformity with durapatite. J. Periodontol., 56:200, 1985.

Greenstein, G., Jaffin, R.A., Hilsen, K.L., and Berman, C.L.: Repair of anterior gingival deformity with durapatite: A case report. J. Periodontol., 56:200, 1985.

Grupe, H.E.: Horizontal sliding flap operation. Dent. Clin. North Am., 4:43, 1960.

Grupe, H.: Horizontal sliding flap operation. Dent. Clin. North Am., 8:43, 1964.

Grupe, H.: Modified technique for the sliding flap operation. J. Periodontol., 37:491, 1966.

Grupe, H.E., and Warren, R.F.: Repair of gingival defects by sliding flap operation. J. Periodontol., 27:92, 1956.

Haggerty, P.C.: The use of a free gingival graft to create a healthy environment for full crown preparation. Case history. Periodontics, 4:329, 1966.

Hall, W.B.: Present status of soft tissue grafting. J. Periodontol, 48:587, 1977.

Hall, W.B.: Pure Mucogingival Problems. Chicago, Quintessence, 1984.

Halliday, D.G.: The grafting of newly formed autogenous bone in the treatment of osseous defects. J. Periodontol., 40:511, 1969.

Hamp, S.-E., Nyman, S., and Lindhe, J.: Periodontal treatment of multirooted teeth. Results after 5 years. J. Clin. Periodontol., 2:126, 1975.

Handelsman, M., et al.: Guided tissue regeneration with and without citric acid treatment in vertical osseous defects. Int. J. Periodont. Rest. Dent., 11(5):351, 1991.

Hanes, P.J., et al.: Root and pulpal dentin after surface demineralization. Endo. Dent. Trauma., 2:190, 1986.

Hanes, P.J., and Polson, A.M.: Cell and fiber attachment to demineralized cementum from normal root surfaces. J. Periodontol., 60:188, 1989.

Hangorsky, U., and Bissada, N.F.: Clinical assessment of

free gingival grafts' effectiveness on the maintenance of periodontal health. J. Periodontol., *51*:274, 1980.

Harris, R.J.: The connective tissue and partial thickness double pedicle graft: A predictable method of obtaining root coverage. J. Periodontol., *63*:477, 1992.

Hars, E., and Massler, M.: Effects of fluorides, corticosteroids and tetracyclines on extraction wounds in rats. Acta Odontol. Scand., *30*:511, 1972.

Harvey, P.: Management of advanced periodontitis. Part I. Preliminary report of a method of surgical reconstruction. N.Z. Dent. J., *61*:180, 1965.

Hatfield, C.G., and Bauhammers, A.: Cytotoxic effects of periodontally involved surfaces of human teeth. Arch. Oral Biol., *16*:495, 1971.

Hattler, A.B.: Mucogingival surgery—utilization of interdental gingiva as attached gingiva by surgical displacement. Periodontics, *5*:126, 1967.

Hawley, C., and Staffilino, H.: Clinical evaluation of free gingival grafts in periodontal surgery. J. Periodontol., *41*:105, 1970.

Haynes, P.J., et al.: A morphological comparison of radicular dentin following root planing and treatment with citric acid and tetracycline HCL. J. Clin. Periodontol., *18*:660, 1991.

Heins, P.J.: Osseous surgery: An evaluation after twenty-five years. Dent. Clin. North Am., *13*:75, 1969.

Hellden, L.B., et al.: The prognosis of tunnel preparations in the treatment of Class III furcations, a follow-up study. J. Periodontol., *60*:182, 1989.

Herrmann, J.B.: Changes in tensile strength and knot security of suture materials. Am. Surg., *37*: 209, 1971.

Hiatt, W.H.: The repositioned alveolar ridge mucosal flap. Periodontics, *5*:132, 1967.

Hiatt, W.H., and Schallhorn, R.G.: Intraoral transplants of cancellous bone marrow in periodontal lesions. J. Periodontol., *44*:194, 1973.

Hileman, A.C.: Surgical repositioning of vestibule and frenums in periodontal disease. J. Am. Dent. Assoc., *55*:676, 1957.

Hileman, A.C.: Surgical repositioning of the vestibule and frenums in periodontal surgery. Dent. Clin. North Am., *4*:55, 1960.

Hirschfeld, L.: Subgingival curettage in periodontal treatment. J. Am. Dent. Assoc., *44*:454, 1952.

Holbrook, T., and Ochsenbein, C.: Complete coverage of the denuded root surface with a one-stage gingival graft. Int. J. Periodont. Rest. Dent., *3*:9, 1983.

Houston, F., et al.: Healing after root reimplantation in the monkey. J. Clin. Periodontol., *12*:716, 1985.

Ibbott, C.G., et al.: Effects of citric acid treatment on autogenous free graft coverage of localized recession. J. Periodontol., *56*:622, 1985.

Ingber, J.: Forced eruption. Part 1. A method of treating isolated one- and two-wall intrabony defects—rationale and case report. J. Periodontol., *45*:199, 1974.

Ingle, J.I.: Periodontal curettement in the premaxilla. J. Periodontol., *23*:143, 1952.

Isidor, F., et al.: New attachment-reattachment following reconstructive periodontal surgery. J. Clin. Periodontol., *12(9)*:728, 1985.

Isidor, F., et al.: The significance of coronal growth of periodontal ligament tissue for new attachment formation. J. Clin. Periodontol., *13(2)*:145, 1986.

Jahnke, P.V., et al.: Thick free gingival and connective tissue autografts for root coverage. J. Periodontol., *64*:315, 1993.

Jensen, O.T., and Greer, R.: Immediate placement of osseointegrating implants into the maxillary sinus augmented with mineralized cancellous allograft and Gore-tex: Second-stage surgical and histological findings. *In* Tissue Integration in Oral, Orthopedic, and Maxillofacial Reconstruction. (Laney, W.R., and Tolman, D.E., eds.) Carol Stream, Illinois, Quintessence, 1992.

Jones, A.W., and O'Leary, T.J.: The effectiveness of in vitro root planing in removing bacterial endotoxin from the roots of periodontally involved teeth. J. Periodontol., *49*:337, 1978.

Kaldahl, W.B., Tussing, G.J. Wentz, F.M., and Walker, J.A.: Achieving an esthetic appearance with a fixed prosthesis by submucosal grafts. J. Am. Dent. Assoc., *104*:449, 1982.

Karring, T., et al.: Conservation of tissue specificity after heterotropic transplantation of gingiva and alveolar mucosa. J. Periodont. Res., *6*:282, 1971.

Karring, T., et al.: Healing following implantation of periodontitis affected roots into bone tissue. J. Periodontol., *2*:96, 1980.

Karring, T., et al.: Healing following implantation of periodontitis affected roots into bone tissue. J. Clin. Periodontol., *7(2)*:96, 1980.

Karring, T.F., et al.: The significance of coronal growth of periodontal ligament tissue for new formation. J. Clin. Periodontol., *13*:145, 1986.

Karring, T., and Ellegaard, B.: New attachment attempts based on prevention of epithelial downgrowth in humans. J. Clin. Periodontol., *3*:44, 1976.

Karring, T., Lang, N.P., and Loe, H: Role of connective tissue in determining epithelial specificity. J. Dent. Res., *51*:1303, 1972.

Karring, T., Lang, N.P., and Loe, H.: The role of connective tissue in determining epithelial differentiation. J. Periodontol. Res., *10*:1, 1974.

Kazanjian, V.H.: Surgery as an aid to more efficient service with prosthetic dentures. J. Am. Dent. Assoc., *22*:566, 1935.

Kennedy, J.E., Bird, W.C., Palcanis, K.G., and Dorfman, H.S.: A longitudinal evaluation of various widths of attached gingiva. J. Clin. Periodontol., *12*:667, 1985.

Kenney, E.B., et al.: The use of porous hydroxylapatite implant in periodontal defects. I. Clinical results after six months. J. Periodontol., *56*:82, 1985.

Kenney, E.B., et al.: The use of a porous hydroxylapatite implant in periodontal defects. II. Treatment of class II furcation lesions in lower molars. J. Periodontol., *59*:67, 1988.

Kersten, B.G., et al.: Healing of the intrabony periodontal lesion following root conditioning with citric acid and wound closure including PTFE membrane. J. Periodontol., *63*:876, 1992.

King, K., and Pennel, B.M.: Evaluation of attempts to increase the width of attached gingiva. Presented at meeting of Philadelphia Society of Periodontology, April, 1964.

Kinoshita, S., and Wen, R.C.: Color Atlas of Periodontics. St. Louis, Mosby Year Book, 1985.

Kirch, J., Baderstein, A., and Egelberg, J.: Longitudinal observation of "unattached," mobile gingival areas. J. Clin. Periodontol., 13:131, 1986.

Kirkland, O.: The suppurative periodontal pus pocket; its treatment by the modified flap operation. J. Am. Dent. Assoc., 18:1462, 1931.

Kirkland, O.: Surgical flap and semiflap technique in periodontal surgery. Dent. Dig., 42:125, 1936.

Klebe, R.J.: Isolation of a collagen dependent cell attachment factor. Nature, 250:248, 1974.

Kleinman, H.K., et al.: Localization of the cell attachment region in types I and II collagens. Biochem. Biophys. Res. Comm., 72:426, 1976.

Kleinman, H.K., et al.: Role of collagen matrices in the adhesion and growth of cells. J. Cell Biol., 88:473, 1981.

Kleinman, H.: Interactions between connective tissue matrix macromolecules. Connect. Tiss. Res., 10:61, 1982.

Kohler, L., and Ranford, S.: Healing of gingival mucoperiosteal flaps. Oral Surg., 13:89, 1960.

Kozlovsky, A., et al.: Forced eruption combined with gingival fiberotomy. J. Clin. Periodontol., 15:534, 1988.

Kramer, G.M., and Schwartz, M.: A technique to obtain primary intention healing in pocket elimination adjacent to an edentulous area. Periodontics, 2:252, 1964.

Kramer, G.M., and Pollack, R.: Clinical application and histologic evaluation of microfibrillar collagen hemostat (Avitene) in periodontal surgery. Int. J. Periodont. Rest. Dent., 2:9, 1982.

Kronfeld, R.: Condition of alveolar bone underlying periodontal pockets. J. Periodontol., 6:22, 1935.

Kure, K., et al.: Influences of attached gingiva on plaque accumulation and gingival inflammation in monkeys. J. Dent. Res., 63:555, 1985.

Lai, H., et al.: The effect of different treatment modalities on connective tissue attachment. J. Periodontol., 57:604, 1986.

Lange, N.P., and Loe, H.: the relationship between the width of keratinized gingiva and gingival health. J. Periodontol., 43:623, 1972.

Langer, B., and Calagna, L.: The subepithelial connective tissue graft. J. Prosthet. Dent., 44:363, 1980.

Langer, B., and Calagna, L.: The subepithelial connective tissue graft. A new approach to the enhancement of anterior cosmetics. Int. J. Periodont. Rest. Dent., 2:23, 1982.

Langer, B., and Langer, L.: Subepithelial connective tissue graft technique for root coverage. J. Periodontol., 56:715, 1985.

Langer, B., and Langer, L.: The overlapped flap: A surgical modification for implant fixture installation, Int. J. Periodont. Rest. Dent., 10(3):209, 1990.

Langer, L., and Langer, B.: Mucogingival surgery: Esthetic treatment of gingival recession. In Advances in Periodontics. Singapore, Quintessence, 1992.

Laurell, L., et al.: Gingival response to Guidor. A bioabsorbable device In GTR-therapy. J. Dent. Res., 71(special issue):1536, 1992.

Laurell, L., et al.: Gingival response to GTR therapy in monkeys using two bioresorbable devices. J. Dent. Res., 72(special issue):824, 1993.

Lazzara, R.: Immediate implant placement into extraction sites: Surgical and restorative advantages. Int. J. Periodont. Rest. Dent., 9(5):333, 1989.

Leighton, J.: Collagen-coated cellulose sponge. In Tissue Culture, Methods and Applications. (Kruse, P.F., Jr., and Patterson, M.K., Jr., eds.) New York, Academic Press, 1982, pp. 367-371.

Lekovic, B., et al.: The use of autogenous periosteal grafts as barriers for the treatment of class II furcation involvements in lower molars. J. Periodontol., 61:775, 1991.

Lekovic, V., et al.: Evaluation of guided tissue regeneration in Class II furcation defects: A clinical re-entry study. J. Periodontol., 60(12):694, 1989.

Lekovic, V., et al.: Treatment of class II furcation defects using porous hydroxylapatite in conjunction with a polytetrafluoroethylene membrane. J. Periodontol., 61:575, 1990.

Lekovic, V., et al.: Treatment of Grade II furcation defects using porous HA in conjunction with a PTFE membrane. J. Periodontol., 62(9):575, 1990.

Levine, H.L., and Stahl, S.S.: Repair following periodontal flap surgery with retention of gingival fibers. J. Periodontol., 43:99, 1972.

Levine, H.L.: Periodontal flap surgery with gingival fiber retention. J. Periodontol., 43:91, 1972.

Levine, H.L.: Periodontal flap surgery. J. Periodontol., 43:91, 1972.

Libin, B.M., Ward, H.L., and Fishman, L.: Decalcified lyophilized bone allograft for use in human periodontal defects. J. Periodontol., 46:51, 1975.

Lie, T.: Periodontal surgery for the maxillary anterior area. Int. J. Periodont. Rest. Dent., 12(1):73, 1992.

Lindhe, J.: Textbook of Clinical Periodontology. Copenhagen, Munksgaard, 1983.

Lindhe, J., et al.: Connective tissue attachment as related to presence or absence of alveolar bone. J. Clin. Periodontol., 11:33, 1984.

Lindhe, J., and Nyman, S.: the effect of plaque control and surgical pocket elimination on the establishment and maintenance of periodontal health. A longitudinal study of periodontal therapy in cases of advanced disease. J. Clin. Periodontol., 2:67, 1975.

Lindhe, J., and Nyman, S.: Alteration of the position of the marginal soft tissue following periodontal therapy. J. Clin. Periodontol., 7:525, 1980.

Lindhe, J., Hamp, S.-E., and Loe, H.: Experimental periodontitis in the Beagle dog. J. Periodont. Res., 8:1, 1973.

Linghorne, W.: Studies in the regeneration and reattachment of supporting structures of the teeth. IV. Regeneration in epithelial pockets following organization of a blood clot. J. Dent. Res., 36:4, 1957.

Litch, J.M., O'Leary, T.J., and Kafrawy, A.H.: Pocket

epithelium removal via crestal and subcrestal scalloped internal bevel incisions. J. Periodontol., 55:142, 1984.

Livingston, H.: Total coverage of multiple and adjacent denuded root surfaces with a free gingival autograft. A case report. J. Periodontol., 46:209, 1975.

Loe, H., et al.: Experimental gingivitis in man. J. Periodontol., 36:177, 1965.

Lopez, N.J., et al.: Inflammatory effects of periodontally diseased cementum studied by autogenous dental root implants in humans. J. Periodontol., 51:583, 1980.

Louise, F., et al.: Histologic case reports of coralline hydroxyapatite grafts placed in human intraosseous lesions: Results 6 to 36 months postimplantation. Int. J. Periodont. Rest. Dent., 12(6):475, 1992.

Lowman, J.V., Burke, R.S., and Pellen, G.B.: Patent accessory canals; Incidence in molar furcation region. Oral Surg., 36:580, 1973.

Macht, S.D., and Krizek, T.J.: Sutures and suturing: Current concepts. J. Oral Surg., 36:710, 1978.

Madison, W.J.: A review of some surgical methods of treating pyorrhea. Am. J. Orthod. Oral Surg., 25:898, 1939.

Magnusson, I., et al.: Connective tissue repair in circumferential periodontal defects in dogs following use of a biodegradable membrane. J. Clin. Periodontol., 17:243, 1990.

Maitia, J.I., et al.: Efficiency of scaling of the molar furcation area with and without surgical access. Int. J. Periodont. Rest. Dent., 6:25, 1986.

Majzoub, Z., and Kon, S.: Tooth morphology following root resection procedures in maxillary first molar. J. Periodontol., 63:290, 1992.

Marggraf, E.: A direct technique with a double lateral bridging flap for coverage of denuded root surface and gingiva extension. Clinical evaluation after 2 years. J. Clin. Periodontol., 12:69, 1985.

Marks, S.C., Jr., and Mehta, N.R.: Lack of effect of citric acid treatment of root surfaces on the formation of new connective tissue attachment. J. Clin. Periodontol., 13:109, 1986.

Martin, M., et al.: Treatment of periodontal furcation defects. (I) Review of the literature and description of a regenerative surgical technique. J. Clin. Periodontol., 15:277, 1988.

Masileti, C., et al.: Healing after tooth replantation in monkeys. A radiographic study. Oral Surg., 39:361, 1975.

Matras, H.: Fibrin seal: The state of the art. J. Oral Maxillofac. Surg., 43:605, 1985.

Matter, J.: Creeping attachment of free gingival grafts—a five-year follow-up study. J. Periodontol., 51:681, 1981.

Matter, J., and Cimasoni, G.: Creeping attachment after free gingival grafts. J. Periodontol., 47:574, 1976.

Maynard, J.G., Jr.: Coronal positioning of a previously placed autogenous gingival graft. J. Periodontol., 48:151, 1977.

Maynard, J.G., Jr., and Ochsenbein, C.: Mucogingival problems: Prevalence and therapy in children. J. Periodontol., 46:543, 1975.

Maynard, J.G., Jr., and Wilson, R.D.: Physiologic dimensions of the periodontium significant to the restorative dentist. J. Periodontol., 50:170, 1979.

McFall, W.T., Jr., and Common, J.: The effect of citric acid on attachment of laterally positioned flaps. J. Periodontol., 54:9, 1983.

McClain, P.K., and Shallhorn, R.G.: Long-term assessment of combined osseous composite grafting, root conditioning, and guided tissue regeneration. Int. J. Periodont. Rest. Dent., 13:9, 1993.

McGuire, M.K.: Reconstruction of bone on facial surfaces: A series of case reports. Int. J. Periodont. Rest. Dent., 12(2):133, 1992.

McHugh, W.D.: The effect of exclusion from healing periodontal pockets. J. Periodontol., 59:750, 1988.

Meffert, R.M., Thomas, J.R., Hamilton, K.M., and Brownstein, C.N.: Hydroxylapatite as an alloplastic graft in the treatment of human periodontal osseous defects. J. Periodontol., 56:63, 1985.

Mehler, A.H.: On the repair potential of periodontal tissues. J. Periodontol., 47(5):256, 1976.

Melcher, A.H., and Dreyer, C.J.: Protection of the blood clot in healing circumscribed bone defects. J. Bone Joint Surg., 44B:424, 1962.

Mellonig, J.T.: Alveolar bone induction: Autografts and allografts. Dent. Clin. North Am., 24:719, 1980.

Mellonig, J.T.: Histologic evaluation of freeze-dried bone allografts in periodontal osseous defects (Programs and Abstracts). J. Dent. Res., 60:388, 1981.

Mellonig, J.T.: Decalcified freeze-dried bone allografts as an implant material in human periodontal defects. Int. J. Periodont. Rest. Dent., 6:41, 1984.

Mellonig, J.T., Bowers, G.M. Bright, R.W., and Lawrence, J.J.: Clinical evaluation of freeze-dried bone allografts in periodontal osseous defects. J. Periodontol., 47:125, 1976.

Mellonig, J.: Bone grafting (lecture). Boston, Yankee Dental Conference, 1992.

Mellonig, J.T., and Triplett, R.G.: Guided tissue regeneration and endosseous dental implants. Int. J. Periodont. Rest. Dent., 13(2):109, 1993.

Meltzer, J.A.: Edentulous area tissue graft correction of an esthetic defect: A case report. J. Periodontol., 50:320, 1979.

Mensing, H., et al.: A study of fibroblast chemotaxis using fibronectin and conditioned medium as chemoattractants. Eur. J. Cell Biol., 29:268, 1983.

Mergenhagen, S.E., et al.: Electron microscopic localization of endotoxin lipopolysaccharide in gram negative organisms. Ann. N.Y. Acad. Sci., 133:279, 1966.

Metzler, D.G., et al.: Clinical evaluation of guided tissue regeneration in the treatment of maxillary class II molar furcation invasions. J. Periodontol., 62:354, 1991.

Miki, Y., et al.: Mitogenic activity of cementum components to gingival fibroblasts. J. Periodont. Res., 66:1399, 1987.

Miller, P.D.: Root coverage using a free soft tissue autogenous graft following citric acid application. I. Technique. Int. J. Periodont. Rest. Dent., 2:65, 1982.

Miller, P.D., Jr.: Root coverage using a free soft tissue autograft following citric acid application. II. Treatment of the carious root. Int. J. Periodont. Rest. Dent., 3:38, 1983.

Miller, P.D.: A classification of marginal tissue recession. Int. J. Periodont. Rest. Dent., 2:9, 1985A.

Miller, P.D.: Root coverage using free soft tissue autografts following citric acid application. III. A successful and predictable procedure in areas of deep-wide recession. Int. J. Periodont. Rest. Dent., 2:15, 1985B.

Miller, P.D., Jr.: Root coverage with the free gingival graft. Factors associated with incomplete coverage. J. Periodontol., 58:674, 1987.

Miyasato, M., Crigger, M., and Egelberg, J.: Gingival condition in areas of minimal and appreciable width of attached gingiva. J. Clin Periodontol., 4:200, 1977.

Mlinek, A., et al.: The use of free gingival grafts for the coverage of denuded roots. J. Periodontol., 44:249, 1973.

Morris, M.L.: The unrepositioned mucoperiosteal flap. Periodontics, 3:141, 1965.

Morman, W., Meier, C., and Firestone, A.: Gingival blood circulation after experimental wounds in man. J. Clin. Periodontol., 6:417, 1979.

Nabers, C.L.: Repositioning the attached gingiva. J. Periodontol., 25:38, 1954.

Nabers, C.L.: When is gingival repositioning an indicated procedure? J. West Soc. Periodont. 5:93, 1957.

Nabers, C.L., and O'Leary, T.J.: Autogenous bone transplants in the treatment of osseous defects. J. Periodontol., 36:5, 1965.

Nabers, C.L., and O'Leary, T.: Autogenous bone graft: Case report. Periodontics, 5:251, 1967.

Nabers, J.M.: Extension of the vestibular fornix utilizing a gingival graft — case history. Periodontics, 4:77, 1966A.

Nabers, J.M.: Free gingival grafts. Periodontics, 4:243, 1966B.

Nelson, S.W.: The subpedicle connective tissue graft. J. Periodontol., 58:95, 1987.

Nery, E.B., Lynch, K.L. and Rooney, G.E.: Alveolar ridge augmentation with tricalcium phosphate ceramic. J. Prosthet. Dent., 40:668, 1978.

Nevins, M., and Mellonig, J.: Enhancement of the damaged edentulous ridge to receive dental implants: A combination of allograft and the Gore-tex membrane. Int. J. Periodont. Rest. Dent., 12(2):97, 1992.

Nevins, M., and Skurow, A.: The intracervicular restorative margin, the biologic width, and the maintenance of the gingival margin. Int. J. Periodont. Rest. Dent., 4(3):31, 1984.

Newell, D.H.: Current status of the management of teeth with furcation invasions. J. Periodontol., 52:559, 1981.

Newell, D.H.: The management of furcation invasions. Presented to the American Academy of Periodontology, New Orleans, (October) 1984.

Nilveus, R., and Egelberg, J.: The effect of topical citric acid application of the healing of experimental furcation defects in dogs. III. The relative importance of coagulum support, flap design, and systemic antibiotics. J. Periodont. Res., 15:551, 1980.

Nilveus, R., et al.: The effect of topical citric acid application of the healing of experimental furcations in dogs. II. Healing after repeated surgery. J. Periodont. Res., 15:544, 1980.

Nyman, S., Gottlow, J., Karring, T., and Lindhe, J.: The regenerative potential of the periodontal ligament. An experimental study in the monkey. J. Clin. Periodontol., 9:257, 1982A.

Nyman, S., Lindhe, J., Karring, T., and Rylander, H.: New attachment following surgical treatment of human periodontal disease. J. Clin. Periodontol., 9:290, 1982B.

Nyman, S., et al.: Healing following implantation of periodontitis-affected roots into gingival connective tissue. J. Clin. Periodontol., 7(5):394, 1980.

Nyman, S., et al.: New attachment following surgical treatment of human periodontal disease. J. Clin. Periodontol., 9(4):290, 1982.

Nyman, S., et al.: New attachment formation by guided tissue regeneration. J. Periodont. Res., 22(3):252, 1987.

Nyman, S., et al.: Bone regeneration adjacent to titanium dental implants using guided tissue regeneration: A report of two cases. Int. J. Oral Max. Imp., 5(1):9, 1990.

O'Leary, T.J., and Kafrawy, A.M.: Total cementum removal: A realistic objective. J. Periodontol., 54:221, 1983.

Obwegeser, H.: Operationstechnik der submukosen mundvorhofplastik in der Underkieferfront. Dtsch. Zahnarztl. Z., 11:1282, 1956.

Ochsenbein, C.: Osseous resection in periodontal therapy. J. Periodontol., 29:15, 1958.

Ochsenbein, C.: Newer concepts of mucogingival surgery. J. Periodontol., 31:173, 1960.

Ochsenbein, C.: Newer concepts of mucogingival surgery. J. Periodontol., 31:175, 1961.

Ochsenbein, C.: The double flap procedure. Periodontics, 1:1, 1963.

Ochsenbein, C.: Current status of osseous surgery. J. Periodontol., 45:577, 1977.

Ochsenbein, C.: A primer for osseous surgery. Int. J. Periodont. Rest. Dent., 6:8, 1986.

Ochsenbein, C., and Bohannan, H.M.: The palatal approach to osseous surgery. I. Rationale. J. Periodontol., 34:60, 1963.

Ochsenbein, C., and Bohannan, H.M.: The palatal approach to osseous surgery. II. Clinical application. J. Periodontol., 35:54, 1964.

Ochsenbein, C., and Ross, S.E.: A reevaluation of osseous surgery. Dent. Clin. North Am., 13:154, 1969.

Ochsenbein, C.: A primer for osseous surgery. Int. J. Periodont. Rest. Dent., 6(1):8, 1986.

Olsen, C.T., Ammons, W.F., and van Belle, G.: A longitudinal study comparing apically repositioned flaps, with and without osseous surgery. Int. J. Periodont. Rest. Dent., 4:11, 1985.

Orban, B.: Indications, technique, and postoperative management of gingivectomy in the treatment of periodontal pockets. J. Periodontol., 12:93, 1941.

Orban, B.: Oral History and Embryology. 6th Ed. St. Louis, C.V. Mosby, 1966.

Oreamuno, S., et al.: Comparative clinical study of porous hydroxyapatite and decalcified freeze-dried bone in

human periodontal defects. J. Periodontol., *61*:399, 1990.
Patur, B., and Blickman, I.: Gingival pedicle flaps for covering root surfaces denuded by chronic destructive periodontal disease—A clinical experiment. J. Periodontol., *29*:50, 1958.
Pennel, B.M., et al.: Oblique rotated flap. J. Periodontol., *36*:305, 1965.
Pennel, B.M., et al.: Free masticatory mucosa graft. J. Periodontol., *40*:162, 1969.
Pepelassi, E.M., et al.: Doxycycline-tricalcium phosphate composite graft facilitates osseous healing in advanced periodontal furcation defects. J. Periodontol., *62*:106, 1991.
Pitaru, S., et al.: The influence of the morphological and chemical nature of dental surfaces on the migration, attachment and orientation of human gingival fibroblasts in vitro. J. Periodont. Res., *19*:408, 1984.
Pitaru, S., et al.: The effect of partial demineralization and fibronectin on migration and growth of gingival epithelial cells on cementum in vitro. J. Periodont. Res., *23*:1386, 1988.
Pitaru, S., et al.: Partial regeneration of periodontal tissues using collagen barriers. J. Periodontol., *59*:380, 1988.
Polson, A.M., et al.: The production of a root surface smear layer by instrumentation and its removal by citric acid. J. Periodontol., *55*:443, 1984.
Polson, A.M.: The root surface and regeneration, present therapeutic limitations and future biologic potentials. J. Clin. Periodontol., *13*:995, 1986.
Polson, A.M., and Caton, J.: Factors influencing periodontal repair and regeneration. J. Periodontol., *53*:617, 1982.
Polson, A.M., and Proye, M.P.: Effect of root surface alterations of periodontal healing. II. Citric acid treatment of the denuded root. J. Clin. Periodontol., *9*:441, 1982.
Polson, A.M., and Proye, M.P.: Fibrin linkage: A precursor for new attachment. J. Periodontol., *54*:141, 1983.
Polson, A.M., Frederick, T.G., Ladenheim, S., and Hanes, P.J.: The production of a root smear layer by instrumentation and its removal by citric acid. J. Periodontol., *55*:443, 1984.
Pontoriero, R., et al.: Rapid extrusion with fiber resection: A combined orthodontic—periodontic treatment modality. Int. J. Periodont. Rest. Dent., *5*:31, 1987.
Pontoriero, R., et al.: Guided tissue regeneration in the treatment of furcation defects in man: Short communication. J. Clin. Periodontol., *14(10)*:619, 1987.
Pontoriero, R., et al.: Guided tissue regeneration in surgically produced furcation defects. An experimental study in the beagle dog. J. Clin. Periodontol., *19*:159, 1992.
Pontoriero, R., et al.: Guided tissue regeneration in the treatment of furcation defects in mandibular molars. A clinical study of degree III involvements. J. Clin. Periodontol., *16(3)*:170, 1989.
Postlethwait, R.W.: Wound Healing and Surgery. Somerville, New Jersey, Ethicon, Inc., 1971.
Prato, G.P., et al.: Human fibrin glue versus sutures in periodontal surgery. J. Periodontol., *58*:420, 1987.
Prato, G.P., et al.: Periodontal regeneration therapy with coverage of previously restored root surfaces: Case reports. Int. J. Periodont. Rest. Dent., *12*:451, 1992.
Price, P.B.: Stress, shear, and suture. Ann. Surg., *128*:408, 1948.
Prichard, J.F.: The infrabony technique as a predictable procedure. J. Periodontol., *28*:202, 1957.
Prichard, J.F.: Gingivoplasty, gingivectomy, and osseous surgery. J. Periodontol., *32*:275, 1961.
Prichard, J.F.: Advanced Periodontal Disease. 2nd Ed. Philadelphia, W.B. Saunders, 1965.
Prichard, J.F.: The etiology, diagnosis and treatment of the infrabony defect. J. Periodontol., *38*:455, 1967.
Prichard, J.F.: The diagnosis and management of vertical bony defects. J. Periodontol., *54*:29, 1983.
Proceedings of the World Workshop in Periodontics, 1989.
Proye, M.P., and Polson, A.M.: Effect of root surface alterations on periodontal healing. I. Surgical denudation. J. Clin. Periodontol., *9*:428, 1982.
Raetzke, P.B.: Covering localized areas of root exposure employing the "envelope" technique. J. Periodontol., *56*:397, 1985.
Ramfjord, S.P.: Experimental periodontal reattachment in Rhesus monkeys. J. Periodontol., *22*:67, 1971.
Ramfjord, S.P., and Nissle, R.R.: The modified Widman flap. J. Periodontol., *45*:601, 1974.
Ratertschak, K.H., Egli, U., and Fringeli, G.: Recession: A 4-year longitudinal study after free gingival grafts. J. Clin. Periodontol., *6*:158, 1979.
Ratcliff, P.A.: An analysis of repair systems in periodontal therapy. Periodont. Abstr., *14*:57, 1966.
Register, A.A.: Bone and cementum induction by dentin demineralized in situ. J. Periodontol., *44*:49, 1973.
Register, A.A., and Burdick, D.A.: Accelerated reattachment with cementogenesis to dentin, demineralization in situ. J. Periodontol., *46*:639, 1975.
Register, A.A., and Burdick, F.: Accelerated reattachment with cementogenesis to dentine demineralized in situ. J. Periodontol., *47*:497, 1976.
Renvert, S., and Egelberg, J.: Healing after treatment of periodontal intraosseous defects. II. Effect of citric acid conditioning of the root surface. J. Clin. Periodontol., *8*:459, 1981.
Renvert, S., Nilveus, R., and Egelberg, J.: Healing after treatment of periodontal intraosseous defects. V. Effect of root planing versus surgery. J. Clin. Periodontol., *12*:619, 1985A.
Renvert, S., et al.: Healing after treatment of periodontal intraosseous defects. III. Effect of osseous grafting and citric acid conditioning. J. Clin. Periodontol., *12*:441, 1985B.
Renvert, S., et al.: Healing after treatment of periodontal intraosseous defects. VI. Factors influencing the healing response. J. Clin. Periodontol., *12*:707, 1985C.
Ribault, A.F., Toto, P.D., Levy, S., and Gargiulo, A.W.: Autogenous bone grafts: Osseous coagulum and osseous retrograde procedures in primates. J. Periodontol., *42*:787, 1971.
Ripamonti, U., et al.: Regeneration of the connective tissue attachment on surgically exposed roots using a fibrin-fibronectin adhesive system. An experimental study

on the baboon (Papio urisnus). J. Periodont. Res., 22:320, 1986.

Ririe, C.M., et al.: Healing of periodontal connective tissues following surgical wounding and application of citric acid in dogs. J. Periodont. Res., 15:314, 1980.

Robinson, R.E.: Periosteal fenestration in mucogingival surgery. J. West. Soc. Periodont., 9:4, 1961.

Robinson, R.E.: The distal wedge operation. Presented to the Western Society of Periodontology, Palm Springs (November), 1963.

Robinson, R.E.: Utilizing an edentulous area as a donor site in the lateral repositioned flap. Periodontics, 2:79, 1964.

Robinson, R.E.: The distal wedge operation. Periodontics, 4:256, 1966.

Robinson, R.E.: Osseous coagulum for bone induction. J. Periodontol., 40:503, 1969.

Robinson, R.E., and Agnew, R.G.: Periosteal fenestration of the mucogingival line. J. Periodontol., 34:503, 1964.

Rosenberg, E.S., and Garber, D.A.: Tooth lengthening procedures. Compen. Contin. Ed. Gen. Dent., 1:161, 1980.

Rosenberg, M.M.: Repositioning the attached gingiva. J. Periodontol., 25:38, 1954.

Rosenberg, M.M.: Free osseous tissue autografts as a predictable procedure. J. Periodontol., 42:195, 1971.

Rosenberg, M.M., et al.: Tooth lengthening procedures. Comp. Cont. Dent., 1(3):243, 1980.

Rosenberg, M.M., et al.: Periodontal and Prosthetic Management for Advanced Cases. Chicago, Quintessence, 1988.

Rosenberg, S., Garber, D.A., and Rosenberg, E.S.: Treatment of gingival clefts—a modification of the laterally positioned partial-thickness flap, utilizing the multiple, interdental papillae and double papillae procedure. Compend. Contin. Ed. Gen. Dent., 5:106, 1984.

Rubin, M.P.: A biologic rationale for gingival reconstruction by grafting procedures. Quintessence, 11:47, 1979.

Ruoslahti, E., et al.: Current concepts of its structure and function. Coll. Rel. Res., 15:314, 1980.

Saadoun, A.P., Fox, D.J., Rosenberg, E.S., and Evian, C.I.: Surgical treatment of the short clinical crown in an area of inadequate keratinized gingiva. Compend. Contin. Ed., 4:71, 1983.

Saffar, J.L., et al.: Bone formation in tricalcium phosphate-filled periodontal intrabony lesions. Histological observations in humans. J. Periodontol., 61:209, 1990.

Salkin, M.L., et al.: A longitudinal study of untreated mucogingival defects. J. Periodontol., 58:164, 1987.

Sanchez-Corea, A.: History of surgical procedures in the control of periodontal lesions. Acad. Rev., 3:30, 1955.

Saroff, S.A., et al.: Free soft tissue autografts, hemostasis and protection of the palatal donor site with a microfibrillar collagen preparation. J. Periodontol., 53:425, 1980.

Sato, K., et al.: The effect of subgingival debridement on periodontal disease parameters and the subgingival microbiota. J. Clin. Periodont., 20:359, 1993.

Saunders, J.J., et al.: Clinical evaluation of freeze-dried bone allografts in periodontal osseous defects. Part III. Composite freeze-dried bone allografts with and without autogenous bone grafts. J. Periodontol., 54:1, 1983.

Schallhorn, R.G.: Eradication of bifurcation defects utilizing frozen autogenous hip marrow implants. Periodont. Abstr., 15:101, 1967.

Schallhorn, R.G.: The use of autogenous hip marrow biopsy implants for bony crater defects. J. Periodontol., 39:145, 1968.

Schallhorn, R.G.: Postoperative problems associated with iliac transplants. J. Periodontol., 43:3, 1972.

Schallhorn, R.G.: Osseous grafts in the treatment of periodontal osseous defects. In Periodontal Surgery. Edited by S.S. Stahl. Springfield, Illinois, Charles C Thomas, 1976.

Schallhorn, R., and McClaine, P.: Combined osseous composite grafting, root conditioning, and guided tissue regeneration. Int. J. Periodont. Rest. Dent., 8(4):8, 1988.

Schluger, S.: Osseous resection—a basic principle in periodontal surgery. Oral Surg., 2:316, 1949.

Schluger, S.: Surgical techniques in pocket elimination. Texas Dent. J., 70:246, 1952.

Schmid, M.O.: The subperiosteal vestibular extension: Literature review, rationale and technique. J. West. Soc. Periodontol., 24:89, 1976.

Seelich, T., and Redl, H.: DAS fibrinklebesystem biochemische grandlagen der klebemetode. Dtsch 2 Mund-Kiefes-Gesichts-Chir., 3:22, 1979.

Seibert, J.S.: Soft tissue grafts in periodontics. In Clinical Transplantation in Dental Specialties. Edited by P.J. Robinson and L.H. Guernsey. St. Louis, C.V. Mosby, 1980.

Seibert, J.S.: Reconstruction of deformed, partially edentulous ridges, using full-thickness onlay grafts. Part I. Technique and wound healing. Compend. Contin. Ed. Gen. Dent., 4:37, 1983A.

Seibert, J.S.: Reconstruction of deformed, partially edentulous ridges, using full-thickness onlay grafts. Part II. Prosthetic/periodontal interrelationships. Compend. Contin. Ed. Gen. Dent. 4:549, 1983B.

Selvig, K.A., et al.: Fine structure of new connective tissue attachment following acid treatment of experimental furcation pockets in dogs. J. Periodont. Res., 16:123, 1981.

Selvig, K.A., et al.: Scanning electron microscopic observations of cell population and bacterial contamination of membranes used for guided periodontal tissue regeneration in humans. J. Periodontol., 61:515, 1990.

Sepe, W.W., et al.: Clinical evaluation of freeze-dried bone allografts in periodontal osseous defects. Part II. J. Periodontol., 49:9, 1978.

Shahmiri, S., et al.: Clinical response to the use of the HTR polymer implant in intrabony lesions. Int. J. Periodont. Rest. Dent., 12(4):295, 1992.

Shanaman, R.H.: The use of guided tissue regeneration to facilitate ideal prosthetic placement of implants. Int. J. Periodont. Rest. Dent., 12(4):257, 1992.

Shiloah, J.: The clinical effects of citric acid and laterally positioned pedicle grafts in the treatment of denuded root surface. A pilot study. J. Periodontol., 51:652, 1980.

Simon, B., et al.: The role of endotoxin in periodontal disease. II. Correlation of the amount of endotoxin in human gingival exudate with the clinical degree of inflammation. J. Periodontol., *41*:81, 1970.

Simon, B., et al.: The role of endotoxin in periodontal disease. III. Correlation of the amount of endotoxin in human gingival exudate with the histologic degree of inflammation. J. Periodontol., *210*:1971.

Smith, B.A., et al.: Effect of citric acid and various concentrations of bironectin on healing following periodontal flap surgery in dogs. J. Periodontol., *58*:667, 1987.

Smith, D., Ammons, W., and Van Belle, G.: A longitudinal study of periodontal status comparing osseous recontouring and flap curettage. J. Periodontol., *51*:367, 1980.

Smukler, H., and Goldman, H.M.: Laterally repositioned "stimulated" osteoperiosteal pedicle grafts in the treatment of denuded roots. J. Periodontol., *50*:379, 1979.

Snyder, A.J., Levin, M.P., and Cutright, D.E.: Alloplastic implants of tricalcium phosphate ceramic in human periodontal osseous defects. J. Periodontol., *55*:273, 1984.

Soehren, E.E., Allen, A.L., Cutright, D.E., and Seibert, J.S.: Clinical and histologic studies of donor tissues for free grafts of masticatory mucosa. J. Periodontol., *44*:727, 1973.

Somerman, M.J., et al.: Effects of minocycline on fibroblast attachment spreading. J. Dent. Res., *23*:154, 1988.

Somerman, M.J., et al.: Enhancement by extracts of mineralized tissues of protein production by human gingival fibroblasts in vitro. Arch. Oral Biol., *32*:879, 1987.

Staffileno, H., Jr.: Management of gingival recession and root exposure problems associated with periodontal disease. Dent. Clin. North Am., *8*:113, 1964.

Staffileno, H., Jr.: Palatal flap surgery: Mucosal flap (split thickness) and its advantages over the mucoperiosteal flap. J. Periodontol., *40*:547, 1969A.

Staffileno, H., Jr.: Surgical management of furca invasion. Dent. Clin. North Am., *13*:103, 1969B.

Stahl, S.S.: Healing following stimulated fiber retention procedures in rats. J. Periodontol., *48*:67, 1977.

Stahl, S.S.: Repair potential of the soft tissue and root interface. J. Periodontol., *48*:545, 1977.

Stahl, S.S.: Speculations on periodontal attachment loss. J. Clin. Periodontol., *13*:1, 1986.

Stahl, S.S., and Froum, S.S.: Human clinical and histologic repair responses following the use of citric acid in periodontal therapy. J. Periodontol., *48*:261, 1977.

Stahl, S.S., and Froum, S.: Human intrabony lesion responses to debridement, porous hydroxyapatite implants and teflon barrier membranes. Histologic case reports. J. Clin. Periodontol., *18(8)*:605, 1991.

Stahl, S.S., and Froum, S.: Human suprabony healing following root demineralization and coronal flap anchorage. Histologic responses in 7 sites. J. Clin. Periodont., *18*:685, 1991.

Stahl, S.S., and Froum, S.J.: Healing of human suprabony lesion treated with guided tissue regeneration and coronally anchored flaps. J. Clin. Periodontol., *18*:149, 1991A.

Stahl, S.S., and Tarnow, D.: Root resorption leading to linkage of dentinal collagen and gingival fibers. A case report. J. Clin. Periodontol., *12*:399, 1985.

Stein, M.D., Salkin, L.M., Freedman, A.L., and Glushko, V.: Collagen sponge as a topical hemostatic agent in mucogingival surgery. J. Periodontol., *56*:35, 1985.

Steinberg, A.D., and Willey, R.: Scanning electron microscopy observations of initial clot formation on treated root surfaces. J. Periodontol., *59*:403, 1987.

Stern, I.B., Everett, F.G., and Robicsek, K.: S. Robicsek—A pioneer in the surgical treatment of periodontal disease. J. Periodontol., *36*:265, 1965.

Sterrett, J.D., et al.: Optimal citric acid concentration for dental demineralization. Quintessence Int., *22*:371, 1991.

Sterrett, J.D., et al.: Dentine demineralization. The effect of citric acid concentration and application time. J. Clin. Periodont., *20*:366, 1993.

Stewart, H.T.: Partial removal of cementum and decalcification of the tooth in the treatment of pyorrhea alveaolaris. Dent. Cosmos, *41*:617, 1899.

Stewart, J.M.: Reattachment of vestibular mucosa as an aid in periodontal therapy. J. Am. Dent. Assoc., *19*:283, 1954.

Sullivan, H.C., and Atkins, J.H.: Free autogenous gingival grafts. I. Principles of successful grafting. Periodontics, *6*:121, 1968A.

Sullivan, H.C., and Atkins, J.H: Free autogenous gingival grafts. III. Utilization of grafts in the treatment of gingival recession. Periodontics, *6*:152, 1968B.

Sullivan, H.C. and Atkins, J.H.: The role of free gingival grafts in periodontal therapy. Dent. Clin. North Am., *13*:133, 1969.

Synderman, R.: Role of endotoxin and complement in periodontal tissue destruction. J. Dent. Res., *51*:356, 1972.

Takei, H.H.: The interdontal space. Dent. Clin. North Am., *24*:169, 1980.

Takei, H.H., et al: Flap technique for periodontal bone implants: Papilla preservation technique. J. Periodontol., *56*:204, 1985.

Takei, H.H.: The use of a porous hydroxylapatite implant in periodontal defects. II Treatment of class II furcation lesions in lower molars. J. Periodontol., *59*:67, 1988.

Takei, H.H.: Surgical techniques for reconstructive periodontics. Dent. Clin. North Am., *35*:531, 1991.

Takei, H., et al.: Maxillary anterior esthetics. Preservation of the interdontal papilla. Dent. Clin. North Am., *33*:263, 1989.

Tarnow, D.P.: Semilunar coronally positioned flap. J. Clin. Periodontol., *13*:182, 1986.

Tarnow D., and Fletcher, P.: Classification of the vertical component of furcation involvement. J. Periodontol., *55*:283, 1984.

Tarnow, D., Chrisser, M., and Langer, B.: Management of the multirooted tooth. Presented at the American Academy of Periodontists Meeting, 1983.

Taylor, I.W.: Surgical knots. Ann. Surg., *107*:458, 1938.

Terranova, V.: A biochemical approach to periodontal regeneration. J. Periodontol., *58*:247, 1987.

Terranova, V., and Lundquist, G.: A possible role for

attachment proteins in periodontal reattachment. J. Dent. Res., 60(Abst.):320A, 1981.

Terranova, V.P., and Martin, G.F.: Molecular factors determining gingival tissue interaction with tooth structure. J. Periodontol. Res., 17:530, 1982.

Terranova, V.P., et al.: Role of laminin in the attachment of PAM 212 (epithelial) cells to basement membrane collagen. Edll., 22:719, 1980.

Terranova, V.P., et al.: A biochemical approach to periodontal regeneration: Tetracycline treatment of dentin promotes fibroblast adhesion and growth. J. Periodontol. Res., 21:330, 1986.

Thacker, J.G., et al.: Mechanical performance of surgical sutures. Am. J. Surg., 130:374, 1975.

Theilade, E., et al.: Experimental gingivitis in man. II. A longitudinal clinical and bacteriologic investigation. J. Periodont. Res., 1:1, 1966.

Tibbets, L., Ochsenbein, C., and Loughlin, D.M.: Lingual approach to mandibular osseous surgery. Dent. Clin. North Am., 20:61, 1976.

Tinti, C., et al.: Guided tissue regeneration in the treatment of human facial recession. A twelve-case report. J. Periodontol., 63:54, 1992.

Tolmie, P.N.: The predictability of root coverage by way of free gingival autografts and citric acid application: An evaluation by multiple clinicians. Int. J. Periodont. Rest. Dent., 11(4):261, 1991.

Tonetti, M.S., et al.: Periodontal regeneration of human infrabony defects. III. Diagnostic strategies to detect bone gain. J. Periodontol., 64:269, 1993.

Urist, M.R.: Bone formation by autoinduction. Science, 150:893, 1965.

Urist, M.R.: Surface-decalcified allogeneic bone (SDAB) implants. Clin. Orthop., 56:37, 1968.

Urist, M.R.: Bone histogenesis and morphogenesis in implants of demineralized enamel and dentin. Oral Surg., 29:88, 1971.

Urist, M.R., and Lietze, A.: A non-enzymatic method of preparation of soluble bone morphogenetic protein (BMP). J. Dent. Res., (Special Issue A): 415, 1980.

Urist, M.R., and McLean, F.: Osteogenic potency and new bone formation by induction in transplants to the anterior chamber of the eye. J. Bone and Joint Surg., 34:443, 1952.

Urist, M.R., and Strates, B.S.: Bone formation in implants of partially and wholly demineralized bone matrix. Clin. Orthop., 71:271, 1970

Urist, M.R., and Strates, B.S.: Bone morphogenetic protein. J. Dent. Res., 50:1392, 1971.

Urist, M.R., et al.: The bone inductive principle. Clin. Orthop., 53:243, 1967.

Urist, M.R., et al.: Inductive substrates for bone formation. Clin. Orthop., 59:59, 1968.

Urist, M.R., MacDonald, N.S., and Jowsey, J.: The function of the donor tissue in experimental operations with radioactive bone grafts. Ann. Surg., 147:129, 1958.

Varma, S., et al.: Comparison of seven suture materials in infected wound. An experimental study. J. Surg. Res., 17:165, 1974.

Viljanto, J., et al.: Fibronectin in early phases of wound healing. Acta. Chir. Scand., 147:7, 1981.

Wade, A.B.: Where gingivectomy fails. J. Periodontol., 25:289, 1954.

Wade, A.B.: Vestibular deepening by the technique of Edlan and Mejchar. J. Periodont. Res., 4:300, 1969.

Waerhaug, J.: Review of Cohen: Role of periodontal surgery, J. Dent. Res., 50:219, 1971.

Waerhaug, J.: Healing of the dentoepithelial junction following subgingival plaque control. II. As observed on extracted teeth. J. Periodontol., 49:119, 1978.

Waerhaug, J.: The furcation problem. Etiology, pathogenesis, diagnosis, therapy and prognosis. J. Clin. Periodontol., 7:73, 1980.

Wagenberg, B.D., et al.: Exposing adequate tooth structure for restorative dentistry. Int. J. Periodont. Rest. Dent., 9(5):323, 1989.

Walker, A., and Ash, M.M.: A study of root planing by scanning electron microscopy. Dent. Hygiene, 50:109, 1976.

Ward, V.J.: A clinical assessment of the use of the free gingival graft for correcting localized recession associated with frenal pull. J. Periodontol., 45:78, 1974.

Wennström, J.L.: Status of the art of mucogingival surgery. Acta Paradontologica, 95:343, 1985.

Wennström, J.L.: Lack of association between width of attached gingiva and development of soft tissue recession. J. Clin. Periodontol., 14:181, 1987.

Wennström, J.L. and Lindhe, J.: Plaque-induced gingival inflammation in the absence of attached gingiva in dogs. J. Clin. Periodontol., 10:266, 1983.

Wennström, J.L., Lindhe, J., and Nyman, S.: Role of keratinized gingiva for gingival health. J. Clin. Periodontol., 8:311, 1981.

Wennström, J.L., Lindhe, J., and Nyman, S.: The role of keratinized gingiva in plaque-associated gingivitis in dogs. J. Clin. Periodontol., 9:75, 1982.

Werbitt, M.J., and Goldberg, P.V.: The immediate implant: Bone preservation and bone regeneration. Int. J. Periodont. Rest. Dent., 12(3):207, 1992.

Widman, L.: The operative treatment of alveolar pyorrhea. Br. Dent. J., 37:105, 1917.

Wikesjo, U.M.E., et al.: A biochemical approach to periodontal regeneration: Tetracycline treatment conditions dentin surfaces. J. Periodont. Res., 21:322, 1986.

Wikesjo, U.M.E., et al.: Periodontal repair in dogs. Effect of heparin treatment in the root surface. J. Clin. Periodontol., 18:60, 1991.

Wilderman, M.N.: Exposure of bone in periodontal surgery. Dent. Clin. North Am., 8:23, 1964.

Wilderman, M.N., and Wentz, F.M.: Repair of dentogingival defect with a pedicle flap. J. Periodontol., 36:218, 1965.

Wilderman, M.N., Wentz, F.M., and Orban, B.J.: Histogenesis of repair after mucogingival surgery. J. Periodontol., 31:283, 1960.

Wilson, T.G., Jr.: Guided tissue regeneration around dental implants in immediate and recent extraction sites: Initial observations. Int. J. Periodont. Rest. Dent., 12(3):185, 1992.

Wirthlin, M.R.: The current status of new attachment therapy. J. Periodontol., 52:529, 1981.

Yeomans, J.D., and Urist, M.R.: Bone induction by decalcified dentine implanted into oral, osseous, and muscle tissues. Arch. Oral Biol., *12*:999, 1967.

Younger, W.J.: Some of the latest phases in implantation and other operation. Dent. Cosmos, *35*:102, 1893.

Younger, W.J.: Lactic acid in pyorrhea. Am. J. Dent. Sci., *31*:334, 1897.

Yukna, R.A.: Longitudinal evaluation of the excisional new attachment procedure in humans. J. Periodontol., *49*:142, 1978.

Yukna, R.A.: HTR polymer grafts in human periodontal osseous defects. I. 6-month clinical results. J. Periodontol., *61*:633, 1990.

Yukna, R.A., and Lawrence, J.L.: Gingival surgery for soft tissue new attachment. Dent. Clin. North Am., *24*:705, 1980.

Yukna, R.A., and Williams, J.E.: Five year evaluation of the excisional new attachment procedure. J. Periodontol., *51*:382, 1980.

Yukna, R.A., Bowers, G.M., Lawrence, J.J., and Fredi, P.F.: A clinical study of healing in humans following the excisional new attachment procedure. J. Periodontol., *47*:696, 1976.

Zemsky, J.: Surgical treatment of periodontal diseases with the author's open-view operation for advanced cases of dental periclasia. D. Cosmos, *68*:465, 1926.

Zentler, A.: Suppurative gingivitis with alveolar involvement. JAMA, *71*:1530, 1918.

INDEX

Page numbers in *italics* indicate figures; page numbers followed by t indicate tables.

A

Absorption, of suture material, 10t
Acids, biomechanical root preparation with, 177, *178-180*, 181-182, *181-184*, 185-186, *186-187*, 188
Acquired immune deficiency syndrome, protection against, 7
Allografts, in inductive osseous surgery, 308t, 308-309, *312-318*
Alloplasts, ceramic, in inductive osseous surgery, 297, *305-312*, 308
Apically positioned partial-thickness flap, 68-69, *79-83*
    advantages, 68-69
    disadvantages, 69
    indications, 68
    procedure, 69, *79-83*
Autogenous bone marrow graft, 296-297, *298-304*
    extraction site, 297, *303-304*
    extraoral site, 296, *298-299*
    intraoral site, 297, *300-302*

B

Bacteria, wicking of, and knot tying, 12
Bending, of needle, with incorrect handling, *16*
Biodegradable membrane, for guided tissue regeneration, 342-343, *344-350*
Biologic width, 263, *278-281*
Biomechanical root preparation
    citric acid, 177, 181, *181*, 182, *183-184*, 185, *186*
        animal studies, 182, *183-184*
        human clinical studies, 185, *186*
        collagen fibril, citric acid, 182, *184*
    epithelial proliferation, with healing, 177, *178-189*
    fibronectin, 186, *187*, 188
    hypermineralizing, of diseased root surface, 177, 181
    mat-like surface, 181, *181*
    periodontal regeneration, *187*, 188
    "smear layer", of residual debris, 181, *181*
    tetracycline hydrochloride, 185-186
Bioresorbable membrane, for guided tissue regeneration. *See* Guided tissue regeneration
Blunted interdental septa, with thick bone margin, osteoplasty for, 260-261, *266-267*
Body of surgical needle, 14
Bone
    infected/necrotic, removal of. *See* Resective osseous surgery
    nonsupporting, reshaping of. *See* Osteoplasty
    radicular/interradicular supporting, removal of. *See* Ostectomy
    supporting, removal of. *See* Ostectomy
Buccal approach, disadvantages of, compared to palatal flap approach, 137

C

Cementum, biomechanical root preparation for, 177, *178-180*, 181-182, *181-184*, 185-186, *186-187*, 188
Chemotherapeutic agents, topical, for biomechanical root preparation, 177, *178-180*, 181-182, *181-184*, 185-186, *186-187*, 188
Chromic gut, as suturing material, 10
Circumferential suture, with gingival augmentation, 190, *202*
Citric acid
    in biomechanical root preparation, 177, 181, *181*, 182, *183-184*, 185, *186*
    hypermineralizing, of diseased root surface, 177, 181
    mat-like root surface, biomechanical root preparation for, 181, *181*
Class I-II classification, gingival recession, 190-191, *197*, *199-202*
Class I-III classification, ridge defects, 233, *236*
Classification, furcations
    Glickman horizontal classification, 369, 370t, *376*
    Lindhe horizontal classification, 369, 370t, *377*
    Tarnow and Fletcher vertical classification, 369, 370t
Closed procedures, open procedures, compared, 5t
Coated Vicryl, as suturing material, 10
Collagen fibril, and biomechanical root preparation, citric acid, 182, *184*
Connective tissue pedicle graft, gingival augmentation, 223-224, *231-232*
Consent form, for surgery, 7
Continuous sutures, 19-20, *26-30*
    advantages, 19
    disadvantages, 19
    independent sling suture, 20, *26-29*
    locking suture, 20, *30*
    mattress suture, 20, *26-27*
    technique, 20
    types of, 19

Contour, parabolic, creation of. *See* Resective osseous surgery
Coronally positioned flap, for gingival augmentation, 191, *205-206*
Coronally positioned flap/citric acid, furcation treatment, 309-310, *319-321*
Cosmetic root coverage: gingival augmentation
　circumferential suture, 190, *202*
　connective tissue pedicle graft, 223-224, *231-232*
　with creeping attachment, 191, *203-204*
　dead space, from routine suturing, 191, *202*
　deep-narrow, deep wide gingival recession (Class II), Miller classification, 190, *192*
　gingival augmentation, contraindications, 207
　gingival recession, classification, 189-190, *192-193*
　grafting, for root coverage, overview, 189
　guided tissue regeneration, 224
　history of, 191, 207
　interdental concavity suture, 190, *202*
　interproximal bone loss with gingival recession (Classes III, IV), Miller classification, 190, *193*
　Miller classification, of gingival recession, 189-190, *192-193*
　procedural modifications, 190-191, *194-200*
　procedures, overview of, 189
　semilunar flap, 214, 223, *225-227*
　　disadvantages, 223
　　indications, 214
　　procedure, 223, *225-227*
　　requirements, 223
　shallow-narrow, shallow wide gingival recession, Miller classification, 189, *192*
　subepithelial connective tissue graft, 191, 207, *208-213*, 214
　　disadvantages, 207
　　donor site, 207, *209-213*
　　failure, 214, *215-218*
　　graft placement, *208*, 214
　　history of, 191, 207
　　indications, 207
　　procedure, 207
　　recipient site, 207, *208*
　subpedicle connective tissue graft, 214, *219-222*
　　advantages, 214
　　disadvantages, 214
　　procedure, 214, *219-222*
　suturing, modification of, for root coverage, 190-191, *197*, *199-200*
　transpositional flap, 223, *228-230*
　　advantages, 223
　　disadvantages, 223
　　procedure, 223, *228-230*
Craters, ostectomy for, 261-262, *268-272*
Creeping attachment, for gingival augmentation, 191, *203-204*
Curettage, 31-32, *35-39*
　contraindications, 32
　defined, 1, *4*, 31
　furcations, 370
　indications, 31-32
　procedure, 32, *36-39*
Curtain procedure, for maxillary anterior pocketing, 165-166, *167-171*
　advantages of, 165
　criteria for treatment, 165
　disadvantages of, 165
　procedure, 165-166, *167-171*
Cutting needles, surgical, 14, *15*

D

Dacron, as suturing material, 10
Dead space, from routine suturing, in gingival augmentation, 191, *202*
Debridement surgery, flap, 32
Deep-narrow, deep wide gingival recession (Class II), Miller classification, 190, *192*
Demineralized freeze-dried bone allografts, 308t, 308-309, *312-316*
Design, of surgical needle, 14, *14-15*
Dexon, as suturing material, 10
DFDBA, bone allograft, in inductive osseous surgery, 308t, 308-309, *312-316*
Diagnosis, furcations, periodontal disease, vs. pulpal disease, 373, 373t, *401-402*
Diagnostic probing, palatal flap, 137-138, *143-145*
Distal wedge, palatal flap, 140, *155-159*
Double papilla laterally positioned flaps, 121-122, *123-130*
　advantages, 121
　disadvantages, 121
　failure, 122, *129*
　horizontal lateral sliding papillary flap, 122, *130*
　indications, 121
　procedure, 121, *123-126*
　root coverage variation, 122, *127-128*
Duralon, as suturing material, 10

E

Ears of knot, 12, *13*
Edentulous area, gingivectomy, 52, *61*
Edentulous ridge
　modification, pedicle flap, laterally positioned, *100-113*, 100
　resective osseous surgery for, 263, *278*
Egyptians, use of suturing materials, 9
ENAP. *See* Excisional new attachment procedure
Endotoxin, biomechanical root preparation for, 177, *178-180*, 181-182, *181-184*, 185-186, *186-187*, 188
Epithelial proliferation, with healing, 177, *178-189*
Eruption, forced, resective osseous surgery, 264, *282-283*
Ethibond, as suturing material, 10
Ethilon, as suturing material, 10
Excisional new attachment procedure, 32-33, *40-43*
　advantages, 32
　contraindications, 32
　disadvantages, 32
　indications, 32
　modifications, of technique, 33, *43*
　procedure, 33, *40-43*
Eye, of surgical needle, 14

F

FDBA, bone allograft, in inductive osseous surgery, 309, *317-318*
Festooning, in osteoplasty, 260, *266*
Fibroblasts, biomechanical root preparation for, 177, *178-180*, 181-182, *181-184*, 185-186, *186-187*, 188
Fibronectin, biomechanical root preparation, 186, *187*, 188
Figure-eight interrupted suture, 17, 19, *21-22*
Flap
　apically positioned full-thickness, modified, 68, *75-78*
　apically positioned partial-thickness, 68-69, *79-83*
　coronally positioned, for gingival augmentation, 191, *205-206*
　curettage, 68
　debridement surgery, 32
　double papilla laterally positioned, 121-122, *123-130*
　full-thickness, 66-68
　　defined, 1, *4*
　　partial-thickness, compared, 5t
　modified full-thickness, defined, 1, *4*
　palatal, surgical procedures, 137-141, *142-163*
　palatal flap, 137-141, *142-163*
　partial-full-thickness. *See* Full-thickness flap

pedicle flap, laterally positioned, surgical management of, 99-101, *102-120*
procedures, gingivectomy, compared, 5t
semilunar, for gingival augmentation, 214, 223, *225-227*
surgical procedures, 3t, 66-69, *70-83*
suturing, Guidor matric barrier, for guided tissue regeneration, 343, *349*
tertiary. *See* Full-thickness flap
transpositional, gingival augmentation, 223, *228-230*
Widman, modified, 33-34, *44-50*
Forced eruption resective osseous surgery, 264, *282-283*
Free soft-tissue autograft, 84-87, *88-98*
 advantages, 84
 disadvantages, 84
 graft failure, 86-87, *96*
 historical background, 84
 preparation of donor tissue, 85-86, *90-95*
  graft thickness, 85, *92*
 preparation of recipient site, 84-85, *88-89*
 procedure, 84-86, *88-95*
 recipient modification, 87, *97-98*
  full-thickness recipient site, 87, *97*
  periosteal separation, 87, *98*
  vertical osseous clefts, 87, *98*
Free-soft tissue autograft, recipient modification of, 87, *97-98*
Freeze-dried bone allograft, in inductive osseous surgery, 309, *317-318*
Frenulectomy, 131, *132*
Frenulotomy, 131, *133-135*
Full-thickness flap
 advantages, 67
 contraindications, 67
 defined, 1, *4*
 disadvantages, 67
 incision placement, 67, *70*
 indications, 67
 partial-thickness flap, compared, 5t
 procedure, 67-68, *71-74*
Full-thickness soft-tissue grafts, for ridge augmentation, 233, *247-239*
Furcation plasty, 370, *378-379*
Furcations, 369-373, 370t, 373t, *374-402*
 classification, 369, 370t, *376-377*
  Glickman, horizontal classification, 369, 370t, *376*
  Lindhe, horizontal classification, 369, 370t, *377*
  Tarnow and Fletcher, vertical classification, 369, 370t
 considerations, 371, *383*

contraindications, 371, *382*
coronally positioned flap/citric acid, treatment with, 309-310, *319-321*
diagnosis, 369, *374-375*
disadvantage, 371
edentulous ridge, 263, *278*
grafting, 370
guided tissue regeneration, 327-328
hemisection, term usage, 371
hemisection procedure, in mandibular molar furcation, 372, *384-388*
indications, 371
mandibular molar, 262-263, *273-277*, 372, *384-388*
maxillary molar, 262
nonvital procedure, term usage, 371
odontoplasty, 370, *379*
osteoplasty, 370, *378-379*
periodontal disease, vs. pulpal disease, differential diagnosis, 373, 373t, *401-402*
periodontal-endodontal problems, 373, 373t, *401-402*
resective osseous surgery for, 262-263, *273-278*
root amputation, term usage, 371
root amputation procedure, in maxillary furcation, 372-373, *389-400*
root resection, 371, *381*
 term usage, 371
terminology, 371-372
tooth sectioning, term usage, 371
treatment, 370t, 370-372
 curettage, 370
 furcation plasty, 370, *378-379*
 gingivectomy, 370
 odontoplasty, 370
 scaling, 370
tunnel preparation, 370-371, *376, 380*
vital procedure, term usage, 371

G

Gingival augmentation
 connective tissue pedicle graft, 223-224, *231-232*
 contraindications, 207
 coronally positioned flap, 191, *205-206*
 creeping attachment, 191, *203-204*
 dead space, from routine suturing, 191, *202*
 deep-narrow, deep wide gingival recession (Class II), Miller classification, 190, *192*
 gingival recession, classification, 189-190, *192-193*
 "graft stretching" suture, 190, *202*
 grafting, for root coverage, overview, 189
 guided tissue regeneration, 224

 interdental concavity suture, 190, *202*
 interproximal bone loss with gingival recession (Classes III, IV), Miller classification, 190, *193*
 Miller classification, of gingival recession, 189-190, *192-193*
 procedural modifications, 190-191, *194-200*
 procedures, overview of, 189
 semilunar flap, 214, 223, *225-227*
  advantages, 214
  disadvantages, 223
  indications, 214
  procedure, 223, *225-227*
  requirements, 223
 shallow-narrow, shallow wide gingival recession, Miller classification, 189, *192*
 subepithelial connective tissue graft, 191, 207, *208-213*, 214
  disadvantages, 207
  donor site, 207, *209-213*
  failure, 214, *215-218*
  graft placement, *208*, 214
  history of, 191, 207
  indications, 207
  procedure, 207
  recipient site, 207, *208*
 subpedicle connective tissue graft, 214, *219-222*
  advantages, 214
  disadvantages, 214
  procedure, 214, *219-222*
 suturing, modification of, for root coverage, 190-191, *197, 199-202*
 transpositional flap, 223, *228-230*
  advantages, 223
  disadvantages, 223
  procedure, 223, *228-230*
Gingival recession, classification, 189-190, *192-193*
Gingival reconstruction, biomechanical root preparation in, 177, *178-180*, 181-182, *181-184*, 185-186, *186-187*, 188
Gingival surgical procedures, comparative analysis of, 6t
Gingivectomy
 advantages, 51
 contraindications, 51
 defined, 1, *4*, 51
 disadvantages, 51
 edentulous area, 52, *61*
 failure, reasons for, 52-53
 flap procedures, compared, 5t
 furcations, 370
 incisions, 52, *55-57*
 indications, 51
 partial-thickness palatal flap, 139, *150*
 pocket marking, 52, *54*
 presurgical phase, 51-52, *54*

Gingivectomy (cont.)
  retromolar area, 52, *62*
  tuberosity area, 52, *63*
Gingivoplasty, 52, *57-60*
  advantages, 51
  contraindications, 51
  defined, 51
  disadvantages, 51
  indications, 51
Glickman horizontal classification, furcations, 369, 370t, *376*
Gore-Tex
  Augmentation Material
    for guided tissue regeneration, 351-352, *353-368*
    ridge augmentation, 351-352, *353-368*
  barrier, guided tissue regeneration. *See* Guided tissue regeneration
  as suturing material, 10
Graft
  connective tissue pedicle graft, for gingival augmentation, 223-224, *231-232*
  failure
    in free soft-tissue allograft, 86, *96*
    free soft-tissue autograft, 86-87, *96*
  full-thickness soft-tissue graft, for ridge augmentation, 233, *237-239*
  furcations, 370
  "graft-stretching" suture, with gingival augmentation, 190, *202*
  material, inductive osseous surgery, 296-297, *298-304*
  material selection, inductive osseous surgery, 296-297, *298-304*
  for new attachment, in inductive osseous surgery, for intrabony defects, 287, 296-297, *298-304*
  for root coverage, in gingival augmentation, overview, 189
  subepithelial connective tissue graft, for gingival augmentation, 191, 207, *208-213*, 214
  subepithelial tissue graft, for ridge augmentation, 234, *246-254*
  subpedicle connective tissue graft, for gingival augmentation, 214, *219-222*
  thickness, free soft-tissue autograft, 85, *92*
  tissue
    obtaining, for free soft-tissue allograft, 85-86, *86*
    preparation, for free soft-tissue allograft, 85-86, *91, 93-95*
"Graft stretching" suture, with gingival augmentation, 190, *202*
Granny knot, 13
Grasping area of surgical needle, 14
Grooving, horizontal, in ostectomy, 261-262, *268*
Guided tissue regeneration, 310, 323, *324-326*, 327-330, *331-341*, 342-343, *344-349*, 351-352, *353-368*
  animal studies, 323, 327
  bioresorbable membrane, 342-343, *344-350*
  biodegradable membrane, 342-343, *344-350*
    Guidor matric barrier, 342-343, *344-350*
      adaptation, 343
      flap suturing, 343, *349*
      ligature tying, 343, *348*
      postoperative considerations, 343, *350*
      trimming, 342, *347*
  combination grafts, 328
  furcations, 327-328
  for gingival augmentation, 224
  human studies, *324-325*, 327-328
  intrabony defect, 327
  nonresorbable membranes, 328-330, *331-341*
    Gore-Tex barrier, 328-330, *331-341*
      contraindications, 329
      defect preparation, 329, *332*
      defect selection, 329
      indications, 329
      material removal, 330, *334*
      material selection, 329, *333*
      patient selection, 328
      postoperative considerations, 330, *335-341*
      surgical procedure, 329, *332*
      suture material, 329, *333*
      suturing technique, 329-330, *333*
  ridge augmentation, 351-352, *353-368*
    contraindications, 351
    defect selection, 351
    Gore-Tex Augmentation Material, 351-352, *353-368*
    material, 351, *354*
    osseous defects, 351
    peri-implant defects, 351
    postoperative considerations, 352
    predictability, 351, *359-362, 364-366*
    surgical procedure, 351-352, *355-368*
  type-specific cell repopulation theory of healing, 323, *326*
Guidor matric barrier, for guided tissue regeneration, 342-343, *344-350*
Gut
  chromic, as suturing material, 10
  plain, as suturing material, 10

H

Handling
  ease of, sutures, 11t
  suture needles, 14, *16*
Healing
  epithelial proliferation with, 177, *178-189*
  type-specific cell repopulation theory of, 323, *326*
Hemisection
  procedure, in mandibular molar furcation, 372, *384-388*
  term usage in furcations, 371
Hemiseptae, ostectomy for, 261-262, *268-272*
Hepatitis, protection against, 7
Historical review, of treatment, *2-3*
Holder, surgical needle, 14, *16*
Horizontal grooving, in ostectomy, 261-262, *268*
Horizontal mattress continuous suture, 20, *26-27*
Horizontal mattress interrupted suture, 17, 19, *21, 23*
Hypermineralizing, of diseased root surface, 177, *181*

I

Implant placement, palatal approach, 140-141, *161-163*
Incisions
  basic, 1, *2-4*, 5t-6t
  for gingivectomy, 52, *55-57*
Indecision, about incision type, consequences of, 7
Independent sling suture, continuous suture, 20, *26-29*
Inductive osseous surgery, 285-287, *288-295*, 296-297, *298-307*, 308-310, *311-321*
  allografts, 308t, *308-309, 312-318*
  alloplasts, ceramic, 297, *305-312*, 308
  autogenous bone marrow graft, 296-297, *298-304*
    extraction site, 297, *303-304*
    extraoral site, 296, *298-299*
    intraoral site, 297, *300-302*
  demineralized freeze-dried bone allografts, 308t, *308-309, 312-316*
  freeze-dried bone allograft, 309, *317-318*
  furcation, coronally positioned flap/citric acid, treatment with, 309-310, *319-321*
  graft, material, 296-297, *298-304*
    classification, 296
    selection, 296-297, *298-304*
  guided tissue regeneration, 310
  intrabony defects, 285-297, *288-295*, *298-304*
    bone regeneration failure, 287
    bone regeneration/new attachment, preparation for, 285-286, *289*

grafting for new attachment
advantages of, 287
rationale/selection, 287
success/failure of, factors affecting, 287
treatment procedure, 286-287, 289-295
bone, 286, 289-295
root surface, 286, 289-291
soft tissue, 286, 289-291
linkage, defined, 285
new attachment, defined, 285
reattachment, defined, 285
regeneration, defined, 285
repair, defined, 285
Infected bone, removal of. *See* Resective osseous surgery
Interdental concavity suture, with gingival augmentation, 190, 202
Interdental septa, blunted, with thick bone margin, osteoplasty for, 260-261, 266-267
Interproximal bone loss with gingival recession (Classes III, IV), Miller classification, 190, 193
Interradicular supporting bone, removal of. *See* Ostectomy
Interrupted sutures, 17, 21-25
Intrabony defects, 285-297, 288-295, 298-304
bone regeneration failure, 287
bone regeneration/new attachment, preparation for, 285-286, 289
grafting for new attachment
advantages of, 287
disadvantages of, 296
rationale/selection, 287
guided tissue regeneration, 327
success/failure of, factors affecting, 287
treatment procedure, 286-287, 289-295
bone, 286, 289-295
root surface, 286, 289-291
soft tissue, 286, 289-291
Intrapapillary placement, interrupted suture, 17, 19, 21

K

Knot/knot tying, 12, 13
bacteria, wicking of, 12
components of, 12, 13
ears of knot, 12, 13
granny knot, 13
loop of knot, 12, 13
square knot, 13
strength of, surgical suture, 11t
surgeon's knots, 13
"throws" of knot, 12, 13

L

Ligature tying, Guidor matric barrier,

for guided tissue regeneration, 343, 348
Lindhe horizontal classification, furcations, 369, 370t, 377
Lipopolysaccharides, biomechanical root preparation for, 177, 178-180, 181-182, 181-184, 185-186, 186-187, 188
Locking suture, continuous suture, 20, 30
Loop of knot, 12, 13

M

Mandibular molar
furcations, 372, 384-388
resective osseous surgery for, 262-263, 273-277
Mat-like root surface, biomechanical root preparation for, 181, 181
Material, suture, 9, 10t-11t
Mattress continuous suture, 20, 26-27
Mattress interrupted suture, 17, 19, 21, 23
Maxillary anterior pocketing, 165-166, 167-176
curtain procedure, 165-166, 167-171
advantages of, 165
criteria for treatment, 165
disadvantages of, 165
procedure, 165-166, 167-171
modified flap technique, 165
papillary preservation technique, 166, 172-176
semiflap technique, 165
Maxillary molar, resective osseous surgery for, 262
Medical history, presurgical, 7
Mersilene, as suturing material, 10
Miller classification, of gingival recession, 189-190, 192-193
Modified apically positioned full-thickness flap, mucogingival surgery, 68, 75-78
Modified flap technique, for maxillary anterior pocketing, 165
Modified full-thickness (mucoperiosteal) flap, defined, 1, 4
Modified new attachment procedure, 32-33, 43
Modified resective technique, for maxillary anterior pocketing. *See* Curtain procedure
Modified Widman flap, 33-34, 44-50
advantages of, 33
disadvantages of, 33
procedure, 33-34, 44-50
Molar
mandibular
furcations, 372, 384-388
resective osseous surgery for, 262-263, 273-277

maxillary, resective osseous surgery for, 262
Monocryl, as suturing material, 10
Mucogingival surgery, 65-69, 70-83, 84-87, 88-98, 99-101, 102-120, 121-122, 123-130, 131, 132-135
apically positioned partial-thickness flap, 68-69, 79-83
advantages, 68-69
disadvantages, 69
indications, 68
procedure, 69, 79-83
classification of procedures, 66
double papilla laterally positioned flaps, 121-122, 123-130
advantages, 121
disadvantages, 121
failure, 122, 129
horizontal lateral sliding papillary flap, 122, 130
indications, 121
procedure, 121, 123-126
root coverage variation, 122, 127-128
flap curettage, 68
free soft-tissue autograft, 84-87, 88-98
advantages, 84
disadvantages, 84
graft failure, 86-87, 96
historical background, 84
preparation of donor tissue, 85-86, 90-95
graft thickness, 85, 92
preparation of recipient site, 84-85, 88-89
procedure, 84-86, 88-95
recipient modification, 87, 97-98
full-thickness recipient site, 87, 97
periosteal separation, 87, 98
vertical osseous clefts, 87, 98
frenulectomy, 131, 132
frenulotomy, 131, 133-135
full-thickness flap, 66-68, 70-78
advantages, 67
contraindications, 67
disadvantages, 67
incision placement, 67, 70
indications, 67
procedure, 67-68, 71-74
modified apically positioned full-thickness flap, 68, 75-78
objective of, 66
partial-full-thickness flap. *See* Full-thickness flap
pedicle flap, laterally positioned, 99-101, 102-120
advantages, 99
contraindications, 99
disadvantages, 99
donor site preparation, 99, 103
edentulous ridge modification, 100-113, 100
failure, 100, 108
historical review, 99, 102

Mucogingival surgery (cont.)
　oblique rotated pedicle flap, 100-101, *114*
　partial-full-thickness pedicle flap, 101, *116-117*
　periosteally stimulated pedicle flap, 101, *115*
　preparation of pedicle flap, 99-100, *104-107*
　procedure, 99-100, *103-107*
　submarginal incisions, 101, *118-120*
　periodontal flaps, 3t, 66-69, *70-83*
　principles of, 66
　purpose of, 65
　tertiary flap. *See* Full-thickness flap
　tissue barrier concept, 65-66
　width, keratinized attached gingiva, 65
Mucoperiosteal flap. *See* Full-thickness flap

N

Necrotic bone, removal of. *See* Resective osseous surgery
Needle holder, 14, *16*
Needles, surgical, 14, *14-15*
　handling of, 14, *16*
　needle holder, 14, *16*
　placement in tissue, *16*, 17
Negative osseous architecture, ostectomy, 261-262, *268-271*
Nonresorbable membranes, guided tissue regeneration, 328-330, *331-341*
Nonsupporting bone, reshaping of. *See* Osteoplasty
Nylon, as suturing material, 10

O

Oblique rotated pedicle flap, pedicle flap, laterally positioned, 100-101, *114*
Odontoplasty, furcations, 370, *379*
Open procedures, closed procedures, compared, 5t
Osseous surgery
　inductive. *See* Inductive osseous surgery
　resective. *See* Resective osseous surgery
Ostectomy, 261-262, *268-272*
　advantages, 261
　contraindications, 261
　for craters, 261-262, *268-272*
　disadvantages, 261
　for hemiseptae, 261-262, *268-272*
　horizontal grooving
　　defined, 261
　　demonstrated, 261-262, *268*
　indications, 261
　parabolizing, defined, 261
　procedure, 261-262, *268-272*
　scribing, defined, 261
　spheroiding, defined, 261

Osteoplasty, 260-261, *265-267*
　for blunted interdental septa, with thick bone margin, 260-261, *266-267*
　festooning, 260, *266*
　furcations, 370, *378-379*
　vertical interradicular grooving, 260, *266*
Overview, surgical procedure classification, 5-7

P

Palatal flap
　advantages of approach, 137
　contraindications, 137
　diagnostic probing, 137-138, *143-145*
　disadvantages of buccal approach, 137
　distal wedge, 140, *155-159*
　historical review, 137, *142*
　implant placement, palatal approach, 140-141, *161-163*
　indications, 137
　partial-thickness palatal flap, 138-139, *146-149*
　　advantages, 138
　　common mistakes, 139, *154*
　　presurgical phase, 138, *146-147*
　　surgical phase, 138-139, *146-149*
　　　Stage I: gingivectomy, 139, *150*
　　　Stage II: partial-thickness flap, 139, *151-153*
Papillary flap, horizontal lateral sliding, in double papilla laterally positioned flaps, 122, *130*
Papillary preservation technique, for maxillary anterior pocketing, 166, *172-176*
Parabolic contour, physiologic, creation of. *See* Resective osseous surgery
Parabolizing, defined, 261
Partial-full-thickness flap. *See* Full-thickness flap
Partial-thickness flap, full-thickness flap, compared, 5t
Partial-thickness palatal flap, 138, *146-149*
　advantages, 138
　common mistakes, 139, *154*
　presurgical phase, 138, *146-147*
　surgical phase, 138-139, *146-149*
　　Stage II: partial-thickness flap, 139, *151-153*
PDS, as suturing material, 10
Pedicle flap, laterally positioned, 99-101, *102-120*
　advantages, 99
　contraindications, 99
　disadvantages, 99
　donor site preparation, 99, *103*
　edentulous ridge modification, *100-113*, 100
　failure, 100, *108*

historical review, 99, *102*
oblique rotated pedicle flap, 100-101, *114*
partial-full-thickness pedicle flap, 101, *116-117*
periosteally stimulated pedicle flap, 101, *115*
preparation of pedicle flap, 99-100, *104-107*
procedure, 99-100, *103-107*
submarginal incisions, 101, *118-120*
Periodontal-endodontal problems, furcations, 373, 373t, *401-402*
Periodontal flaps, 3t, 66-69, *70-83*
Periodontal probe, for pocket marking, in gingivectomy, 52, *54*
Periodontal regeneration, biomechanical approach, 187, *188*
Periosteal suturing, 17, *18*
Periosteally stimulated pedicle flap, pedicle flap, laterally positioned, 101, *115*
Physiologic parabolic contour, creation of. *See* Resective osseous surgery
Picket fence appearance, maxillary anterior pocketing, curtain procedure for, 165-166, *167-171*
Placement, in tissue, surgical needle, *16*, 17
Plaque, biomechanical root preparation for, 177, *178-180*, 181-182, *181-184*, 185-186, *186-187*, 188
Platelet activation
　biomechanical root preparation, citric acid, 182
　in root preparation, biomechanical, citric acid, 182
Pocket marking, gingivectomy, 52, *54*
Pocketing, maxillary anterior, cosmetic treatment of. *See* Maxillary anterior pocketing
Point of surgical needle, 14, *15*
Polydioxanone, as suturing material, 10
Polyester, as suturing material, 10
Polyglactin 910, as suturing material, 10
Polygycolic acid, as suturing material, 10
Polypropylene, as suturing material, 10
Pouch procedure, for ridge augmentation, 233, *240-242*
Presurgical considerations, 7
Prolene, as suturing material, 10
Pulpal disease, vs. periodontal disease, differential diagnosis, 373, 373t, *401-402*

Index

R

Radicular supporting bone, removal of. *See* Ostectomy
Raw materials, for suture material, 10t
Reaction to suture, by tissue, 11t
Recipient modification
    free soft-tissue autograft, 87, *97-98*
    of free-soft tissue autograft, 87, *97-98*
Removal of sutures, 12
Resective osseous surgery, 259-264, *264-283*
    biologic width, 263, *278-281*
    forced eruption, 264, *282-283*
    for furcation, 262-263, *273-278*
    furcations, edentulous ridge, 263, *278*
    historical review of, 259
    for mandibular molar, 262-263, *273-277*
    for maxillary molar, 262
    objectives of, 259, *264-265*
    ostectomy, 261-262, *268-272*
    osteoplasty, 260-261, *265-267*
    rules of, overview, 263
    terminology, 260
    tissue management, 259-260
Retromolar area, gingivectomy, 52, 62
Ridge augmentation, 233-235, *236-257*
    full-thickness soft-tissue grafts, 233, *237-239*
    guided tissue regeneration
        contraindications, 351
        defect selection, 351
        material, 351, *354*
        osseous defects, 351
        peri-implant defects, 351
        postoperative considerations, 352
        predictability, 351, *359-362, 364-366*
        surgical procedure, 351-352, *355-368*
    improved technique, 233-234, *243-245*
    pouch procedure, 233, *240-242*
    socket preservation, 234-235, *255-257*
    subepithelial tissue graft, 234, *246-254*
Ridge defects
    Class I classification, 233, *236*
    Class II classification, 233, *236*
    Class III classification, 233, *236*
    classification, ridge augmentation, 233, *236*
Root amputation
    procedure, in maxillary furcation, 372-373, *389-400*
    term usage in furcations, 371
Root coverage variation, in double papilla laterally positioned flaps, 122, *127-128*
Root demineralization, 177, *178-180,* 181-182, *181-184,* 185-186, *186-187,* 188
Root planing, defined, 31
Root preparation, biomechanical, 177, *178-180,* 181-182, *181-184,* 185-186, *186-187,* 188
    citric acid, 177, 181, *181,* 182, *183-184,* 185, *186*
        animal studies, 182, *183-184*
        human clinical studies, 185, *186*
    collagen fibril, citric acid, 182, *184*
    epithelial proliferation, with healing, 177, *178-189*
    fibronectin, 186, *187,* 188
    hypermineralizing, of diseased root surface, 177, 181
    mat-like surface, 181, *181*
    periodontal regeneration, *187,* 188
    "smear layer", of residual debris, 181, *181*
    tetracycline hydrochloride, 185-186
Root resection
    furcations, 371, *381*
    term usage in furcations, 371

S

Scaling, 35-39
    defined, 31
    furcations, 370
Scribing, in ostectomy, defined, 261
Security, of suture, 12, *13*
Semiflap technique, for maxillary anterior pocketing, 165
Semilunar flap, gingival augmentation, 214, 223, *225-227*
    advantages, 214
    disadvantages, 223
    indications, 214
    procedure, 223, *225-227*
    requirements, 223
Shallow-narrow
    shallow wide gingival recession, Miller classification, 189, *192*
    shallow wide gingival recession (Class I), Miller classification, 189, *192*
Silk, surgical
    disadvantages of, 12
    as suturing material, 10
Sling suture, 19, *24-30*
Slippage, of suture, 12, *13*
"Smear layer", of root debris, biomechanical root preparation against, 181, *181*
Socket preservation, ridge augmentation, 234-235, *255-257*
Sounding, palatal flap, 137-138, *143-145*
Spheroiding, defined, 261
Square knot, *13*
Strength
    knot, surgical suture, 11t
    of suture, 10t
Subepithelial connective tissue graft
    gingival augmentation, 191, 207, *208-213,* 214
        contraindications, 207
        disadvantages, 207
        donor site, 207, *209-213*
        failure, 214, *215-218*
        graft placement, *208,* 214
        history of, 191, 207
        indications, 207
        procedure, 207
        recipient site, 207, *208*
    history of, 191, 207
Subepithelial tissue graft, for ridge augmentation, 234, *246-254*
Submarginal incisions, pedicle flap, laterally positioned, 101, *118-120*
Subpedicle connective tissue graft
    for gingival augmentation, 214, *219-222*
    advantages, 214
    disadvantages, 214
    gingival augmentation, procedure, 214, *219-222*
Supporting bone, removal of. *See* Ostectomy
Surgeon's knots, *13*
Surgical procedures
    biomechanical root preparation, 177, *178-181,* 181-182, *183-184,* 185-186, *186-187,* 188
    classification, 5-7
    cosmetic root coverage, root augmentation, 189-191, *192-206,* 207, *208-213,* 214, *215-222,* 223-224, *225-232*
    curettage, 31-34, *35-50*
    furcations, 369-373, 370t, 373t, *374-402*
    gingivectomy, 51-53, *54-57, 61-63*
    gingivoplasty, 51-52, *57-60*
    guided tissue regeneration, 323, *324-326,* 327-330, *331-341,* 342-343, *344-350,* 351-352, *353-368*
    historical review, 2-3
    incisions
        basic, 1, *2-4,* 5t-6t
        indecision regarding, 7
    inductive osseous surgery, 285-287, *288-295,* 296-297, *298-307,* 308t, 308-310, *311-321*
    maxillary anterior pocketing, cosmetic treatment of, 165-166, *167-176*
    mucogingival surgery, 65-69, *70-83,* 84-87, *88-98,* 99-101, *102-120,* 121-122, *123-130,* 131, *132-136*
    palatal flaps, 137-141, *142-163*
    resective osseous surgery, 259-264, *265-283*
    ridge augmentation, 233-235, *236-257*

Surgical procedures *(cont.)*
  root planing, 31-34, *35-50*
  scaling, 31-34, *35-50*
  selection of, factors based on, 7
  sutures/suturing, 9-30, *10-11t, 13-16, 18, 21-30*
Surgical silk
  disadvantages of, 12
  as suturing material, 10
Surgilon, as suturing material, 10
Suture/suturing
  absorption, 10t
  circumferential, with gingival augmentation, 190, *202*
  circumferential interrupted suture, 17, 19, *21-22*
  continuous suture, 19-20
  continuous sutures, 19-20, *26-30*
  dead space, from routine suturing, in gingival augmentation, 191, *202*
  ease of handling, 11t
  Egyptian use of, 9
  figure-eight interrupted suture, 17, 19, *21-22*
  goals of, 9
  "graft stretching" suture, with gingival augmentation, 190, *202*
  horizontal mattress interrupted suture, 17, 19, *21, 23*
  interrupted sutures, 17, *21-25*
  intrapapillary placement, interrupted suture, 17, *19, 21*
  knot/knot tying, 12, *13*
  knot tensile strength, 11t
  material, qualities of ideal, 9
  mattress suture, 17, 19, *21, 23*
  modification of, for root coverage, in gingival augmentation, 190-191, *197, 199-202*
  needles, 14, *14-15*
  periosteal suturing, 17, *18*
  principles of, 12
  raw materials, for suture material, 10t
  removal of suture, 12
  sling suture, 19, *24-30*
  technique, 17, *18,* 19-20, *21-30*
  tensile strength of sutures, 10t
  tissue reaction, to suture, 11t
  types of, 11t
  uses of, 11t
  vertical mattress interrupted suture, 17, 19, *21, 23*

T

Tarnow and Fletcher vertical classification, furcations, 369, 370t
Tensile strength
  knot, surgical suture, 11t
  of suture, 10t
Tertiary flap. *See* Full-thickness flap
Tetracycline hydrochloride, as biomechanical root preparation, 185-186
"Throws" of knot, 12, *13*
Tissue barrier concept, 65-66
Tissue reaction, to suture, 11t
Tissue regeneration, guided. *See* Guided tissue regeneration
Transpositional flap, gingival augmentation, 223, *228-230*
  advantages, 223
  disadvantages, 223
  procedure, 223, *228-230*
Treatment. *See also* Surgical procedures
  historical review of, *2-3*
Trimming, Guidor matric barrier, for guided tissue regeneration, 342, *347*
Tuberosity area, gingivectomy, 52, *63*
Tunnel preparation, furcations, 370-371, *376, 380*
Type-specific cell repopulation theory of healing, 323, *326*
Types of sutures, 11t

V

Vertical interradicular grooving/festooning, in osteoplasty, 260, *266*
Vertical mattress continuous suture, 20, *26-27*
Vertical mattress interrupted suture, 17, 19, *21, 23*
Vicryl, coated, as suturing material, 10

W

Widman flap, modified. *See* Modified Widman flap